In praise of Alan Tillotson

"Dr. Alan Tillotson is a trailblazer at integrating the key tenets of the great traditional systems with current scientific understanding. Working side by side with Alan over the years, I can tell you that he is uncompromisingly committed to and consistently successful in finding high quality clinical outcomes for individuals with severe, chronic and degenerative diseases. His thinking goes far beyond recipes and simplified protocols."

Salvatore D'Angio, M.D.
Former Medical Director and Chief of Staff
Cherokee Medical Center, Cherokee, North Carolina
Co-Founder, Asheville Wellness Center, Asheville, North Carolina

"An important resource for researchers and physicians, while at the same time accessible to the general reader. An outstanding and unique treatise on herbalism and the complicated subject of chronic disease. Thorough, enjoyable, enlightening."

Cynthia Husted, Ph.D.
Director, Center for the Study of Neurodegenerative Disorders
University of California, Santa Barbara

"Alan has independently developed safe natural medicine treatment strategies for hypoglycemia, multiple sclerosis, and uveitis, and demonstrated their usefulness with patients. He has brought important treatments for retinal bleeding, hepatitis C, allergic rhinitis, and glaucoma to America for the first time. Alan is a skilled thinker, writer, and worker in his chosen field, and enjoys the respect of world leaders in the field of herbal medicine."

Albert Schatz, Ph.D.
Discoverer of Streptomycin
Professor Emeritus
Temple University
Philadelphia, Pennsylvania

"Get beyond those other diluted and plagiaristic herbals. Wow! Get this book."

Robyn Klein, A.H.G.
Editor, *Robyn's Recommended Reading,* Bozeman, Montana

"Alan's book is one of the rare gems of new herbals that speaks to the needs of the educated patient and the neophyte herbalist, as well as the seasoned clinical practitioner and researcher. Indeed, his insights are rich, his perspectives broad, his research comprehensive, and his personal style so accessible that we all might wish he were a practitioner and teacher in our own neighborhoods."

Aviva Jill Romm, A.H.G.
Author, *The Natural Pregnancy Book* and *ADHD Alternatives*

THE ONE EARTH HERBAL SOURCEBOOK

Everything You Need to Know About Chinese, Western, and Ayurvedic Herbal Treatments

ALAN KEITH TILLOTSON, Ph.D., A.H.G., D.Ay.
with **Nai-shing Hu Tillotson**, O.M.D., L.Ac.
and **Robert Abel Jr.**, M.D.

TWIN STREAMS
Kensington Publishing Corp.
http://www.kensingtonbooks.com

KENSINGTON BOOKS are published by

Kensington Publishing Corp.
850 Third Avenue
New York, NY 10022

All Kensington titles, imprints and distributed lines are available at special quantity discounts for bulk purchases for sales promotion, premiums, fund raising, educational or institutional use.

Special book excerpts or customized printings can also be created to fit specific needs. For details, write or phone the office of the Kensington Special Sales Manager: Kensington Publishing Corp., 850 Third Avenue, New York, NY 10022. Attn. Special Sales Department. Phone: 1-800-221-2647.

Kensington and the K logo Reg. U.S. Pat. & TM Off.
Twin Streams and the TS logo are trademarks of the Kensington Publishing Corp.

ISBN 1-57566-617-0

First Printing: July, 2001
10   9   8   7   6   5   4   3   2   1

Printed in the United States of America

Dedicated to my beloved Dr. Mana (Vaidya Mana Bajra Bajracharya),
whose soul entered eternity in January 2001.

CONTENTS

CONTENTS

SECTION THREE
HERBS TO TREAT THE WHOLE BODY

FOREWORD

by Robert Abel Jr., M.D.

The One Earth Herbal Sourcebook reveals the truth behind centuries of herbal medicine from around the world. The World Health Organization estimates that nature's botanicals are used by 80% of the people of the earth and are being incorporated into the fabric of Western medicine. In fact, our earliest chemicals and cures came from the rain forest, savannas, and plains and are well recognized today to provide relief from the symptoms of contemporary diseases.

Comfortable consumerism has come at the cost of both our environment and our health. We have epidemics of viral, cardiac, neurological, and cancerous diseases which have spawned an enormous pharmaceutical industry. But, to tell the truth, in order to truly deal with these 21st-century plagues, we must step out of our current medical mind-set and return to the resources of nature. *The One Earth Herbal Sourcebook* helps us to understand herbs and how to use them.

Alan Tillotson has created a primer of nature's botanical answers which have served people through two centuries. He has assembled the best of Chinese, Ayurvedic, and Western herbs and described the principles behind their use in one volume in an easy-to-read, informative style. His case histories demonstrate the depth of his ability to work with Western physicians to determine the best therapeutic options for their patients. Many times these options are less expensive and less toxic, and can be discontinued within weeks, instead of years.

Alan Tillotson's humor, insights, case histories, and research reporting enhance every page, from his description of the body's amazingly varied systems to his fascinating descriptions of the best herbs for common diseases. The result is a book offering inspiration and insight to every reader, from those who have had limited knowledge of herbal medicine to those who are experts in the field. Few authors command such a level of knowledge about this multicultural field, which connects our botanical past, current prescribing patterns, and future therapies.

Although I have worked closely with Alan Tillotson over the past ten years, I have learned much by participating in this wonderful reference book on herbs. *The One Earth Herbal Sourcebook* should be on every physician's shelf, taught to every medical and pharmaceutical student, and serve as a guide to all of us who have ever been or will be patients. Unlike those in modern medical textbooks, the principles and facts in *The One Earth Herbal Sourcebook* will remain relevant throughout this—and future—millennia.

ROBERT ABEL JR., M.D.

ACKNOWLEDGMENTS

No one person can produce this kind of book. I have been fortunate in having close relationships with masters in each of three fields. First, I must single out for the utmost praise Robert Abel Jr., M.D., for his—and I do not say this lightly—remarkable and almost daily support at every level, and especially for his genius at innovative medical thinking. His friendship has been a constant blessing to me.

I have learned so much from my dear, dear teacher Dr. Mana (Vaidya Mana Bajra Bajracharya), the great Ayurvedic sage of Kathmandu, heir to perhaps the world's oldest living father-to-son lineage. I do not have words to describe his loving support. Little did he know when he saved my life in 1976 that I would dedicate *my* life to his herbal medicine, and be singing his praises in the year 2001. I only hope I can be one-tenth the herbalist that he is. This book is one step in my goal of saving his precious tradition and plants, which are today under threat of extinction.

I have been further blessed to have a wife who taught Chinese medicine at China's third-largest medical complex at Chengdu City in Sichuan Province. Working with Nai-shing on a daily basis at our clinic for over a decade has allowed me to learn Chinese medicine in the most practical of ways, dealing with real patients and real diseases.

The magnificent Dr. James Duke has, for reasons I cannot comprehend, decided to help me at every turn, providing volumes of detail and insight, sometimes within minutes of a simple e-mail request. Incredible.

I'd also like to thank Lee Heiman of Kensington Books for having faith in me and convincing me to do this book when I was reluctant to take on such a massive job. My editor, Claire Gerus, has remained lovingly supportive throughout, putting up with my plodding single-minded focus on details, and giving me key support at critical times. Marjorie Gabriel did a yeoman's job putting my words and work into usable form.

What can I say about my medical mentors, from family physicians such as Dr. Sal D'Angio, who taught me Western medicine as we worked together for five years, to Dr. David Jezyk, who put up with me for another two years after that. Without them, how would I know the difference between penicillin and penicillamine? Fixing my errors in chemical thinking with the speed of light were biochemistry professor Jon Narita, Ph.D., and his wife, molecular biologist Thianda Manzara, Ph.D.

Throughout the book you will also see the influence of some of today's great clinical herbalists. Many of them I know and am proud to call friends and teachers, such as David Winston, Michael and Lesley Tierra, Terry Willard, K. P. Singh, Robyn Klein, Ed Smith, and Aviva Romm. David Winston provided key information in many areas, especially with regard to Eclectic and Cherokee herbs, and patiently answered many difficult questions for me at several critical junctures (thanks, David). Robyn helped write a key section in Chapter 3 and part of the Resource Guide (thanks, Robyn). Phytochemist Steve Dentali helped with an important part of Chapter 6 (thanks, Steve). Chiropractor Douglas Briggs and rolfer Ellen Freed helped straighten out Chapter 15 (thanks, Doug; thanks, Ellen).

Other herbalists have helped me with their books, tapes, and lectures, little suspecting that I was their secret devotee, spending countless hours poring over their writings. These include both contemporary experts and timeless herbal masters like Rudolph Weiss, Michael Murray, Sun Si Miao, Donald Yance, Joseph Pizzorno, Li Bo Ning, Harvey Felter, William Mitchell, Dan Bensky, Bhagawan Punarvasu Atreya, Kerry Bone, Cascade Anderson-Geller, Virender Sodhi, Amanda McQuade Crawford, Zhang Zhong Jing, Jill Stansbury, Patrick Quillin, Paul Bergner, John Christopher, John Heinerman, Vriddha Susruta, Subhuti Dharmananda, Roy Upton, David Frawley, Mark Blumenthal, Finley Ellingwood, Richard Noble, and John Uri Lloyd. Equally important were the contributions of spiritual thinkers with impeccable scientific credentials whose ideas and thoughts guide me every day. These include professors Albert Schatz, Jeffery Bland, Idries Shah, and Wolfgang Schad, and T'ai Chi master Ray Hayward.

My heartfelt thanks to all of them across space and time. [Alan closes his eyes and says a prayer.]

Introduction

As a medical herbalist with a busy private practice, I encounter on a daily basis patients who are confused by the bewildering and rapidly growing modern herbal marketplace. Patients ask me the same basic questions about herbal medicine time and again. They typically come to my office with a list of medical complaints and a bag containing 10 or more remedies that they think will solve their health problems. Seldom do they have a good combination of herbs, in proper dosage, at good cost, and in harmony with their individual needs. If they did, they probably wouldn't be coming to me.

Most of these patients sincerely want to believe in the power of natural herbal medicines but require clarification about the proper applications and uses of these products. They often remind me of well-intentioned but ill-equipped jungle explorers who wish they had known in advance to bring along mosquito nets and maps.

I think it is crucial to get properly oriented before you jump into herbal treatment. You need context as well as information to avoid the many pitfalls that await consumers. This book contains lots of information that can be used as a self-treatment guide for simple problems. However, my deeper purpose is to provide you with the global perspective you need to understand how highly trained doctors of herbal medicine from all parts of the world work with their patients. Many serious health conditions considered incurable here in North America have known solutions in other parts of the world. For example, it is little known in this part of the world that Chinese doctors have promising medicines to treat or control leukemia, Ayurvedic doctors have effective, time-tested medicines to cure chronic hepatitis, and Nigerian doctors have medicines routinely used to dramatically reduce sickle cell anemia symptoms. I want you to know how to locate and work with the right physician(s), so you can get the best medicines for your condition.

My partners in this process are three people who offer diverse medical perspectives, representing the three largest medical systems on our planet. The first is my wife, Nai-shing Tillotson, L.Ac., O.M.D., who will help us understand the Chinese perspective on herbal medicine. The second is Robert Abel Jr., M.D., a holistic Western-trained doctor who has maintained a firm grip on science. The third is Dr. Mana Bajra Bajracharya (Dr. Mana), a Nepalese master of Ayurvedic medicine.

My Background and Qualifications

I bring to this project a richly diverse cross-cultural background. I have studied Traditional Ayurvedic Medicine (TAM) with Dr. Bajracharya of Kathmandu, Nepal, since 1976, and in the early 1980s I trained in Western herbal medicine with Drs. Michael and Lesley Tierra. My wife (and teacher) is a doctor of Traditional Chinese Medicine (TCM) trained in Sichuan Province. I still see 40 to 50 patients each week at my clinic.

Over a decade ago I opened and directed Delaware's first multispecialty holistic health center, bringing together acupuncturists, nutritionists, M.D.'s, and various other specialists. In recent years I have spoken at numerous herbal medicine and hospital conferences, have worked as a formulator of herbal medicines, and have acted as consultant to the herbal medicine industry. I have also spent countless hours sharing information via the Internet with many prominent herbalists from all parts of the world. In addition, I have spent almost a decade working directly with M.D.'s to develop herbal programs for serious and challenging diseases.

I am also an herbal medicine patient, as well as a clinician. I developed juvenile diabetes at the age of 11, almost 40 years ago, and was on a downhill slide when I met my first teacher, Ayurvedic master Dr. Mana. Back then, I began to use herbal medicine and adopted a sensible lifestyle to help myself, and I am proud to say that today I have escaped all the normal problems associated with this disease. I have no problems with my eyes, my heart, my skin, my nerves, or my energy.

Science and Nature: Our Health Depends on Both

You will often hear me repeat a key point, my long-held belief that coexistence between science and nature is the surest road to health. Virtually all systems of herbal medicine hold that one must respect the healing power of nature and the teachings of our herbalist ancestors. At the same time, science and technology prize and use knowledge obtained from modern scientific research. While I believe that good herbal medicine should be based on philosophy and tradition, it should also strive to maintain harmony with scientific insights.

But this is not as simple as it sounds. The blinding nature of technology and "progress" is creating a world where we often never see the sky or breathe clean air. All good herbalists choose to look at the subject of herbal medicine as an entity integrated with nature. We cannot ignore that as herbal medicine science advances, the plants and traditional healers of the world are dying. Science leads us to question and change our beliefs as new evidence comes into the picture.

Those who share a love of nature need also to become acutely aware of issues such as pollution and global warming, which threaten our natural world. These issues should tie into our choices about which industries we patronize. Moreover, I see the greatest health challenge of the next century to be the global changes to our environment. We need our *planet* to be healthy if we are to be healthy.

How This Book Is Organized

This book is divided into three sections:

Section One: An Orientation Guide to Herbal Medicine

This section will provide you with the basic information you will need to understand the different types of herb doctors and herbal systems, manufacturing methods, advertising and marketing, and environmental issues. I will also describe safety issues of herbal usage in great detail.

Section Two: Getting to Know Your Herbs

Here I will introduce you to the herbal medicines, their components, and how to use them. I'll review 96 herbs commonly used in my practice, emphasizing the safest and most effective herbs from around the globe.

Section Three: Herbs to Treat the Whole Body

Sections One and Two will prepare your mind for Section Three. Here, I will discuss herbal protocols for treating some common diseases, introduce you to a variety of strategies for healing from different traditions, and give you deeper insights into how an herbalist thinks and works. When you know how to "put herbs together," you'll have far more freedom and diversity of choice than if you were simply buying over-the-counter herbal remedies. You will be empowered to handle your own health care.

Resource Guide

At the end of the book, I will share with you some of the best herbal resources available, including herbal organizations, herbal manufacturers and distributors, herbal books and magazines, herbal doctors, and herbal Internet sites.

SECTION

ONE

AN ORIENTATION GUIDE TO HERBAL MEDICINE

CHAPTER 1

Principles and Traditions of Herbal Medicine

Demonstrate the unknown in terms of what is called "known"
by the audience.

— Ibrahim Khawwas

What is an herb?

*W*ebster's *New World Dictionary* defines an herb as "any seed plant whose stem withers away to the ground after each season's growth." It further defines an herb as "any such plant used in medicine." However, the use of the word *herb* in natural healing has broadened to mean any substance from the plant kingdom that is used as medicine. Many of the world's herbal traditions also use a limited number of mineral and animal substances under the heading "herbal medicines."

What is herbal medicine?

The pioneering European phytotherapist Rudolph Weiss, M.D., tells us that "herbal medicine, or phytotherapy, is the science of using herbal remedies to treat the sick." I would add that it is also the art and tradition of using herbal medicines to protect and augment health, and to prolong healthy life.

How long have people been using herbs?

A long, long time. There is educated speculation that prehistoric humans used herbs for illness by following the example of animals. German medical scholar Paul Unschuld tells us that in the Shang Empire, about 16 centuries before the birth of Christ, we find the first written evidence of the Chinese use of herbs for healing. Two of the most important diseases were "curse of an ancestor" and "blow of a demon." Although we do not know what these ailments were, we do know that to protect against them the ancient Chinese burned incense, used simple aromatic herbs, and made a ritual offering of roast pig. All the above were intended to appease their ancestors, who had become "hungry ghosts."

What is an herbalist?

An herbalist is a practitioner of and contributor to the field of herbal medicine. Hailing from all parts of the world, herbalists include native healers, shamans, scientists, naturopaths, holistic medical doctors, nutritionists, pharmacists, growers, collectors, writers, and many others.

What are the world's herbal traditions?

Every society, in all parts of the world, has its own herbal tradition which has evolved over time. Among these are Traditional Chinese Medicine (TCM), Traditional Ayurvedic Medicine (TAM), European phytotherapy, naturopathy, Eclectic medicine, Native American medicine, Arabic medicine, and African Traditional Medicine, as well as many others. All the well-known major systems became legitimate learned professions at some point in time, producing doctors, theories, medicines, standards of practice, and results.

What is traditional Chinese medicine?

Traditional Chinese Medicine (TCM) is the traditional medicine system of China, developed from its ancient beginnings in shamanistic medicine. It is the second-largest medical system in the world after Western medicine. Today, TCM doctors go through extensive training—4 to 9 years—in theory and practice, including thousands of classroom hours, in large universities in each of the Chinese provinces, learning herbal therapy and acupuncture. In recent times, schools of TCM and/or acupuncture have been training professionals in the United States. Many states now license acupuncturists, giving them the professional title L.Ac. Some acupuncture schools do not teach herbal medicine. TCM doctors trained in China or those who have completed higher levels of training in herbal medicine in the United States often use the additional title O.M.D. or D.O.M. (doctor of Oriental medicine).

What is traditional Ayurvedic medicine?

Traditional Ayurvedic Medicine (TAM), or Ayurveda, is the traditional medical system of India and Nepal. It is the third-largest medical system in the world today. Ayurveda was founded when a group of sages gathered in the Himalayan Mountains before the birth of Christ and broke up into eight committees led by an expert practitioner. Over a 3-year period, each committee wrote a voluminous medical textbook. These books were used as the foundation for a group of teaching ashrams (schools). Today, doctors of TAM treat more than 80% of the people on the Indian subcontinent. The rich history of Ayurveda has still not been brought intelligibly to the West, though a few of the best Ayurvedic herbs are now available here. Ayurvedic doctors are given the title Vaidya, which is derived from the Sanskrit word for "wisdom." Properly trained TAM doctors go through extensive training that can last as long as 12 years.

What is Eclectic medicine?

Few are aware that America had an extensive herbal tradition, known as Eclectic medicine. This was an extension of early American herbal medicine traditions, such as Thompsonian medicine in the early 1800s, and Native American medicine. In 1827, a doctor named Wooster Beach founded an alternative medical society and later opened the first Eclectic school. The Eclectics were doctors with a philosophy of "alignment with nature," learning from and using concepts from other schools, and opposing the practices of bleeding and purging common among the other doctors of that time. The Eclectic doctors eventually numbered in the thousands, published numerous books and journals, and treated millions of patients over many decades, primarily with herbal medicines. Their popularity ended in the early 1900s with the overwhelmingly rapid growth of the strength of allopathic medicine, fueled by the funneling of millions of dollars into their schools by institutions such as the Carnegie and Rockefeller foundations. The knowledge they developed is still practiced in Europe by professional herbalists and more recently has been embraced by naturopaths and medical herbalists in America.

What is naturopathic medicine?

Naturopathic medicine shares historical roots with Eclectic medicine, and today integrates traditional natural therapeutics with modern scientific medical diagnoses and standards of care. Naturopaths complete premedical university training, then attend naturopathic college for 4 years. They are awarded the title N.D, or doctor of naturopathic medicine and are currently licensed in an increasing number of states. The natural therapies used by naturopaths include botanical medicine, clinical nutrition, homeopathy, acupuncture, traditional oriental medicine, hydrotherapy, and naturopathic manipulative therapy. Today, naturopaths, along with European and American medical herbalists, are among the leaders in carrying forward the traditions of Eclectic medicine.

What is a holistic M.D.?

A holistic M.D. is a licensed physician who has completed standard Western medical training and then gone on to additional education in the philosophies and methods of natural healing. The natural therapeutics holistic M.D.'s study are similar to those of naturopathic medicine, but N.D.'s are educated at workshops or through self-study instead of through university attendance. Some of the more advanced holistic doctors have completed fellowships or have gone on to get additional education or degrees in oriental medicine, chiropractic, or clinical nutrition.

What is a medical herbalist?

Medical herbalists are present in the United States and in most of the nations in the European Union (where they are also called phytotherapists). Training for practice is offered today by university programs throughout European countries, as well as in several new schools in the U.S.A. Medical herbalists generally must study both the traditional uses of herbs and basic medical sciences of biochemistry, nutrition, anatomy, and so on, as well as diagnosis and prescription. In America, those who have successfully passed the accreditation process of the American Herbalists Guild are given professional status and the right to use the title AHG.

Here is a list of the most common titles given to medical herbalists around the world:

AHG: Professional Member, American Herbalists Guild
MCPP: Member, College of Practitioners of Phytotherapy
FNIMH: Fellow, National Institute of Medical Herbalists
MNIMH: Member, National Institute of Medical Herbalists
FNHAA: Fellow, National Herbalists Association of Australia

Finding a Qualified Medical Herbalist

Currently, there is a shortage of properly trained medical herbalists in the United States. The best herbalist holds a license or has had valid training, as described above. Most have learned from a foreign or domestic school or by apprenticeship. However, there are also a select few self-taught geniuses.

The American Herbalists Guild is now working on linking and listing herbalists from different traditions to help the public identify qualified practitioners. According to their web site, "The American Herbalists Guild (AHG) was founded in 1989 as a nonprofit, educational organization to represent the goals and voices of herbalists. It is the only peer-review organization for professional herbalists specializing in the medicinal use of plants."

Herbalists from any tradition with sufficient education and at least 4 years of treating patients, and who pass the AHG credentialing process, receive professional status and the title Herbalist, AHG. I have included specific information on how to find qualified herbalists in the Resource Guide at the end of the book.

In my opinion, a qualified herbalist is more than someone who is knowledgeable about plants and diagnostics, as important as these are. He or she must also be able to move beyond barriers of culture, language, and emotion to achieve deep emotional, physical, and spiritual connections and understanding.

To do this, there must be an underlying philosophy and spirituality, a connection to and reverence for nature. This is the common link shared by herbalists from around the world which allows them to identify each other.

Although this idea is often mentioned in the field of holistic health, it is difficult to put this concept down in writing. It is a feeling that is intensely personal. Start by spending time in nature as often as you can. Most of the herbalists I know got started this way. This is one of the experiences that will help lead to your choice of philosophies, and it is your philosophy that will help you find a healer you can trust. This understanding is not limited to herbalists. You can have it too.

An Herbalist's Philosophy

Although it takes about 15,000 hours of training to become a TCM or a TAM doctor, I am going to try to give you a simplified essence of the key points from Chinese, Ayurvedic, and Western herbal philosophies in less than 200 words.

The human being is a small hologram, or model, of the larger universe in which he or she lives. Outside are the energies of sunshine, day and night, the moon and stars, and the forces of nature, all existing within the external ebb and flow of life. Inside, we have our internal organs, our structural organs and our minds. These also flow and change in response to the outside world and to each other. Outside, there are no diseases; there is no pneumonia, and no cancer. The weather is simply too hot, too cold, too damp, too dry, or too windy. In the same way, our lungs can be hot and windy (a fever with cough) or hot and damp (fever with mucus). These characteristics can be applied to any other organ or system.

Herbs act to heat, cool, moisten, dry, nourish, and calm our organs. Therefore, we want to use our herbs to heat, cool, moisten, dry, nourish, and calm our organ systems back into balance.

This sort of language is the basis of herbalism. Chapter 6 will provide you with a brief overview and a glossary of herbal terms to help you understand the language of herbal medicine. These are terms you will encounter throughout this book and the rest of your journey through the world of herbal medicine. To me, it is a human language, not a scientific one. It does not require double-blind studies for people to grasp its basic meanings.

Centuries of observations have led to general agreement that herbs nourish, warm, cool, reduce pain, detoxify, stimulate, sedate, and so forth. The language of herbalism is constantly in a stage of evolution from its humble roots. Rather than discarding the teachings of the past and replacing them with modern science, herbalists are continuously balancing and reconstructing the wisdom of their elders through their own experiences. These observations take on new power when science looks at them and adds its perspectives to the echoes from the past. Those who ignore the teachings of the past do so at the peril of their own health.

Science versus Herbal Philosophy

Are you saying that the naturalistic and spiritual philosophies of traditional herbal medicine systems are superior to science?

No, and we need not think the two are in competition. Herbal medicine without a rational or practical basis is no better than science without a philosophical basis. I believe we should root ourselves in a philosophy that respects the healing power of nature, yet strives always to be in harmony with scientific findings.

One of the scientific findings that drives this point home is that religious and spiritual people who attempt to love others are healthier than nonreligious people. They actually experience lower incidences of cancer and heart attacks, and they live longer.

I don't have much experience with herbs. How concerned should I be about their safety?

Knowledge is the best road to safety. Until recently, it was quite difficult for anyone to get accurate information about safety. In 1998 and 1999, a very important book was published that made this information available to consumers and doctors. It is entitled the *Botanical Safety Handbook* and is sponsored by the American Herbal Products Association (AHPA). The book provides safety data for over 600 commonly used and prescribed herbs, with complete up-to-date information regarding international regulatory status, standard dosage, and certain common toxicity concerns. The AHPA web site accurately states: "The editors of this book are among the most respected leaders in the herbal products industry. Their experience includes years of clinical practice, manufacturing and industry governance, and significant writing and lecturing about herbs."

Also useful for safety data are the following books: *PDR for Herbal Medicines;* the *Time-Life Drug and Natural Medicine Advisor;* the *German Commission E Monographs;* and *Herb Contraindications and Drug Interactions.* On the Internet you can consult the web site of the Dietary Supplement Quality Initiative (http://www.dsqi.org/home/home.htm). Health World Online's Vitamins and Dietary Supplement Center lists information about many botanicals and also includes information on dosage, safety, and toxicity (http://www.healthy.net/index.html). An interactive CD on herb/drug interactions was recently published by IBIS software; contact them at (503) 641-6419.

I strongly suggest that you make sure the health food store you use or the health practitioners with whom you work have, at the very least, a copy of the *Botanical Safety Handbook* on their shelves. I have found in my clinical practice that documented safety information is very effective at reassuring patients that they are not in danger when they use herbs appropriately. In addition, I often provide them with information to show their doctors, if they have concerns. We'll be talking a lot more about safety in Chapters 4 and 5.

How can I know if a particular herb will work for me?

It's best to have a good understanding of your diagnosis or health needs before you start choosing herbs. Once you have determined your particular needs, refer to Section Two for a description of the herb you are interested in using. You will find a brief statement titled "WHAT IT DOES." This will tell you what you can expect the herb to do if your body responds to it. The more you know, the better you will be able to answer this question for yourself.

If you are fortunate, you will be one of the millions of people who have found solutions to health problems with over-the-counter herbal products. But don't be too disappointed if a particular herb doesn't work for you. There are no guarantees in herbal medicine. Rest assured that there is most likely another herb out there that will help you if you do not abandon your search prematurely. The more complex the problem, the more complex the solution. In Section Three, we will discuss how to combine and use herbs to treat more serious health conditions. This will give you insights about your options and make it clear where you can find the help you need.

CHAPTER 2

Growth, Manufacture, Storage, and Quality Control

Without an integrated understanding of life, our individual and collective problems will only deepen and extend.
—Jiddu Krishnamurti

In this chapter, I will answer common questions consumers ask me about how to buy herbs safely and economically. To my knowledge, few, if any, other herbal books have tackled this aspect of herbs in the marketplace.

How can I know I am getting good-quality herbs?

A good rule of thumb is that a good-quality product gives you results within a reasonable period of time based on its expected action(s). You should understand, however, that there are infinite good ways to prepare and manufacture herbs, infinite bad ways, and infinite ways in between. Read labels, and ask your store manager or health care practitioner about the company. Check the Resource Guide to find a list of companies who make high-quality products.

How many herbal medicine companies are there?

In its 1999 *Source Book, Whole Foods* magazine listed more than 2,000 companies and organizations—a virtual explosion in recent years, with sales into the billions of dollars.

How do we know these companies are doing a good job of manufacturing their products?

The FDA is responsible for regulation of the herbal medicine industry. There is currently controversy about the quality of the job the FDA is doing. Some critics say the FDA is not strict enough, while others say the government is too oppressive. In an ideal world, we would know that if a company follows government GMPs (good manufacturing practices) and other regulations, we could be reasonably certain the product was safe in terms of correct plant material content, potency, and purity. In the real world, government regulation is sparse, and it is difficult for an individual to know, without a private investigation, whether or not a particular company is following good manufacturing practices. Recent changes in the herbal medicine and supplement industry have led to the creation of independent third-party certifications. We will discuss the system, started by the National Nutritional Foods Association (the industry's largest trade association), in more detail when we talk about safety.

What has the government done about regulation so far?

In 1994 Congress passed the Dietary Supplement Health and Education Act (DSHEA), regulating labeling and sales of herbs and other supplements. This was a great relief to those who fought hard for its passage because it broke a long-standing FDA policy of either restricting natural medicines as if they were drugs or treating them as simple foods.

If the government does a good job of regulating herbal manufacturing, which may involve changing the laws, it will winnow out the good company practices from the bad. Fortunately, herbal medicines have rarely caused serious harm. We all want that to continue. However, it is true that while most herbs heal, there are still herbs that can kill. Positive changes are taking place rapidly, but this process is far from complete, so your best bet right now is to educate yourself as much as you can.

How is a quality product made?

The first and most essential step in making good-quality end products is the growing and harvesting of good-quality herbs. What exactly does the phrase "good-quality" mean? Let's look at another natural product—grapes for wine—as an example. Bardolino is a light red, slightly sweet wine produced in the Veneto region of Northern Italy and is best drunk when young. On the other hand, Barolo, a premium Italian red wine, is made from Nebbiolo grapes grown in the Piedmont. The wine is dark and full-bodied, and it improves over decades of aging. With this analogy we can see at once that not all wine is the same, nor are all grapes the same. This holds true for herbs as well.

There are many, many variations of herb quality which depend on numerous factors. The Chinese have a saying that illustrates one part of this puzzle. "Ginseng root grown in Sichuan is a laxative." This means that the energizing tonic herb ginseng (*Panax ginseng*), which usually grows in the cold North, loses its energy-increasing properties when grown in different soil and a warmer climate and becomes a laxative, which may be undesirable. If you wanted a laxative, you'd choose rhubarb, which is far less expensive.

Herbs grown from seeds with good genetics under the correct climatic conditions, in healthy soil, with clean air, and nurtured by a skilled grower who knows when and how to harvest the plants at their peak, will be the best possible quality and provide the best medicine. I hope that in the future good herb growers become as identified and well-known as the French vintners.

How are herbs processed and stored?

Like the different kinds of grapes and methods of preparing and bottling we find in winemaking, there are many different methods to process herbs, all with subtle differences too complex and numerous to mention here. Naturally, each manufacturer will claim its processes and products are the best.

There are at least three rich sources of historical knowledge of herb storage and preparation. The first is the writings of the Eclectic physicians. The second and third are the medicine-making traditions of Ayurvedic and Chinese medicine. The knowledge of Ayurvedic medicine making, barely arrived in this part of the world, is usually handed down by apprenticeship to only the most trusted students. In China, medicine making is a four-year university course.

In all traditions, once harvested, the herbs are extracted and prepared, which includes drying, separating, isolating, and many other processes. Herbs that have been collected in the wild (a discipline called "wildcrafting"), or grown and then only dried, are called "crude herbs." Crude herbs have not been shredded, ground, crushed, mixed, or extracted. Each company has its own methods and proprietary processes for preparing their herbal products.

Traditional herbal doctors have their own methods of processing and storage, and have done just fine without modern intervention. Researchers in Nara, Japan, actually process stored samples of ginseng root *(Panax ginseng)*, licorice root *(Glycyrrhiza glabra)*, and rhubarb root *(Rheum emodi)* that have retained their active properties for over 1,200 years! Similarly, in India there are samples of stored ghee (clarified butter) over 100 years old which physicians report to be medicinally effective. On the other hand, herbs such as red clover blossoms *(Trifolium pratense)* or echinacea *(Echinacea species)* can have vital components damaged or lost within minutes of harvesting if extreme care is not used.

This takes us back to one of my earlier points, the importance of possessing a reverence for nature as well as a respect for science. In the last century, the first scientific food processors gave us the gift of a new purified chemical: white sugar. We took the bait and ran with it, adding sugar to thousands of food products. Further down the road, we were told that adding pesticides to our soil would control the growth and proliferation of insects but would not harm us. Then, we were informed that chemical preservatives added to foods would make them last forever on the shelf and would do us no harm. What have we learned since?

What does "quality control" mean?

Quality control is the process of ensuring that herbal products actually have the characteristics the manufacturers claim. All herbal manufacturers must have some form of quality control. This will vary depending on the size of the company and the type of product it is manufacturing. While there is no simple formula for quality, there are some basics you should be aware of:

First, you have to distinguish "suppliers" from "distributors" and "manufacturers." Suppliers of raw materials are the farmers or collectors in the wild who sell their products to manufacturers. Manufacturers may sell directly to the public or to stores or may sell to co-packers or distributors, who then forward the product to the public or to stores. *Responsibility for quality control starts with growers, moves to manufacturers, and ends up in the hands of distributors and retailers.*

Once the product ends up in your home, you yourself become responsible for quality control. For example, you must discard products that have expired and make sure products are properly stored and refrigerated.

What happens in the lab?

To stay in business today, companies must align with government-regulated GMPs, or good manufacturing practices. This requires access to a lab. The job of the lab is to ensure two things: purity and potency.

The laboratories in which herbal products are manufactured are quite large and sophisticated. They usually range from 1,000 to 2,000 square feet in size, have two or more well-trained employees on site, and house several major pieces of equipment with names like HPLC (high-performance liquid chromatography), GC (gas chromatography), UV/VIS (ultraviolet/visible spectrophotometer), and AA (atomic absorption spectroscopy). They also need hardness testers, analytical balances, rotoevaporators, disintegration/dissolution apparatus, chemicals and solvents, and so on.

The cost of all this space and equipment runs into the hundreds of thousands of dollars. The larger companies that can afford this expense do all the analysis in house using their own equipment, while the others use outside testing labs. As a matter of fact, even the companies with labs on the premises utilize outside third-party analysis to ensure objectivity.

The company, once it has access to a lab, must then set up standard operating procedures unique to its own needs. Safety equipment might include hoods to exhaust particles and fumes, and explosion-proof areas for gas chromatography and other volatile tests. Documentation standards are also part of this process, to ensure that there are traceable lot numbers and paper trails that identify the movement of each herb, bottle, chemical, or other material.

How does quality control work?

1. The first essential step in quality control is correct identification of raw material. This requires that every manufacturer have someone on staff who is trained to check each batch of product when it arrives to ensure that it is what it's supposed to be. This practice is standard everywhere. When I lived in Nepal at my teacher's herbal

medicine clinic, one of the family members (an herbalist) was assigned to make sure that arriving material was of good quality and was the correct plant substance.

2. The second step in quality control is microbiological testing to see if the levels of bacteria are within normal limits. In traditional cultures, the products are cooked down and concentrated to make them hygienic. The modern lab can perform chemical tests to check for undesirable components such as insecticides, pesticides, heavy metals, and solvents.

3. Then comes disintegration/dissolution testing. Here in the United States, various pills and capsules are tested to see if your body can absorb them. It is the same for Nepal, where the size, softness, and ingredients of pills are established with good absorption in mind.

4. "Assays" (chemical tests) are performed to ensure potency. This means both that there is enough of a particular substance at the time of manufacture and that there is some allowance for degradation. The type, the form, and the method of packaging each product must be researched to determine the expiration date, which is then stamped on the bottle.

5. At the end of each test, the company records results and creates a certificate of analysis (C of A) for each batch.

What does "standardization" mean?

Standardization is the hottest issue in the world of herbal manufacturing. Companies have invested a lot of money in convincing consumers to believe in "standardization," a term used to describe the process of testing for certain chemical markers to make sure herbs are potent enough.

There are high-quality and low-quality herbs. You want to be sure that the herb you buy is of high quality, ensuring that you get enough of it to do its job. Therefore, scientific testing is done to ensure quality control. The concept of standardization is relatively simple. If a product contains specified chemical components, then it will work. If the essential constituents are absent, or are present in insufficient amounts, it will not work.

Although standardization has a place in herbal medicine, herbs are not simply containers for chemicals. They are living things. Therefore, there will be natural differences in chemical composition depending on soil conditions, genetics, rainfall, age, and the time of day or season of collection.

When I was young, I wanted to make sure I got a delicious watermelon. My dad, who grew up on a farm, taught me that if the watermelon was picked at the right time, was properly sized, had a nice color, and made a good thumping sound when I tapped it, it would taste good. In the same way, good starting material, good soil, good farming, absence of poisonous chemicals, and good harvesting make for a healthy plant, and if the plant is healthy, it will most likely have the right amounts of the essential constituents.

And, to throw a fascinating fact into the mix, we now know that in the presence of certain stressors such as low water levels and poor soil conditions, plants will actually increase the production of certain phytochemicals that are beneficial to humans, as a defensive reaction.

Are there problems with standardization?

Although many effective methods of making herbal medicines have worked fine in the past, the important test of identifying an individual marker must be performed for quality assurance. Knowing how to determine which constituents to look for as markers is a hotly debated issue, and methods vary from company to company.

One obvious drawback is the existing practice of "spiking"—adding some of the marker substance before testing to create the illusion of a healthy batch of plants or medicines. As each new chemical becomes more popular with the public, there is a rush to believe that this component is the "right" one, the only one that can ensure results.

One of the little-known problems with standardization can be illustrated with St. John's wort, which is standardized to 0.3% of a chemical called "hypericin," long believed to be the key antidepressant chemical in the herb. If you see this marker on the label, you will know that you have a consistent batch of herb that should produce the intended (but unlisted) result, a reduction in depression. The other 99.7% of the product is comprised of various other substances.

However, a problem developed when it turned out that hypericin is an antiviral compound and has nothing to do with depression. So it must be assumed that the presence of hypericin ensures the presence of whatever antidepressant compound or group of compounds makes St. John's wort effective. It may even be that the antidepressive effect comes from a detoxification effect on the liver. Only time will tell.

There are no set rules in the industry on how to standardize for each herb. Because each plant is unique, it will take an estimated 5 years to "standardize" standardization for the most popular herbs, and decades to do the rest. Each plant is unique. As I write this book, even though standards are placed on bottles, each company is using its own methods, and there are large variations from batch to batch, from bottle to bottle, and even in the same bottle over time. However, nearly everyone agrees that standardization is inevitable. Done well, it can be valuable, but it is not the final answer to quality.

Is "standardizing" standardization important?

The great American herbalist David Winston warns us that standardization has not been "standardized" yet. Different companies use different markers, or different levels of the same markers, or different methods of testing for marker compounds. He also points out that whenever different compounds are chosen as "active ingredients" for different herbs, there is a chance that suppliers will get a substandard batch (low on the chemical markers) and mix it with a batch higher in the desired marker to compensate for the difference. Some bulk suppliers have told me that they have detected chemicals in plant batches that were added to fool the testing labs into accepting low-quality materials from dubious sources. Standardized herbs from "organic" sources (assuming the word remains meaningful) would be preferred.

I distrust commercial herbal crops grown with pesticides, purchased from underpaid third-world workers, then cooked up and concentrated until certain chemical markers reach standardization levels. The end result may have the right amount of XYZ acid, but who is fooling whom? If you don't believe me, take an organic carrot and a supermarket one of similar size and place them on the counter of your kitchen. Find out which one tastes sweeter, and which one rots first. In other words, trust your senses.

How do you make good medicine?

One of the time-honored traditions of making a good medicine is to simply tincture (extract with alcohol) healthy plants. This extracts some of the plants' numerous ingredients to make the medicine. If the plants are of good quality, and the method of production is consistent, the results will be equally consistent. The assumption here is that using the whole plant is the best way to go. I mention this because I am afraid that we may lose sight of the fact that there is much more to making good herbal medicines than standardization. Standardizing herbs will not replace the importance of the soil, the genetics, and the aging process.

Shelf Lives of Herbal Products

The shelf life of a product should be stamped on the container. If it is not, these general guidelines can be used:

- **Crude herbs** stored in tightly closed containers made of plastic or dark glass will retain their properties for at least 6 months if they are placed in a cool, dark, dry location.
- **Alcohol-based liquid tinctures** are usually good for up to 3 years. They may still be good for several more years, but different chemicals in the tincture may cause subtle changes over time, as wine bottlers well know. For this reason I keep tinctures for a maximum of 3 years.
- **Glycerin-based herb tinctures** are good for 6 months to 1 year.
- **Capsules and tablets** should be used within 3 to 6 months of opening, and within 1 year of manufacture.
- **Salves and oils** are good for 6 months to 1 year and should be stored in the refrigerator after you get them home.

Why is feedback so important?

Nature is variable, and it is not natural or even possible to take exactly the same amount of a particular natural chemical into your system each time. Even if you standardize the herbs, you can't standardize the patient. Dr. Mana, my Ayurvedic teacher, told me many years ago that some patients are large, some small, some weak, some strong, some nervous, some sluggish, some irritable, some old, and some young. All patients have a different digestive capacity, which determines how they assimilate the herbs. Even in the same patient, this will change from morning to night, and from day to day. The herbs themselves vary depending on the genetics, the method of preparation, and the length of time elapsed from production to market.

The traditional herbalist handles this by figuring out the digestive capacity and individual needs of the patient, and prescribing a starting dose of herbs. In 3 days or a few weeks the patient comes back, and the dosage is adjusted according to the results. This is a "feedback system." In this way, the medicines are adjusted until each individual patient gets exactly what his or her system needs. This system takes our individuality into account.

What makes a good company?

Companies that have good philosophies to guide them and good scientists to figure out the details are likely using science appropriately and making good products. Those who think only of the bottom line are likely to repeat the mistakes of the early food processors. That said, there are many enlightened consumers and companies demanding high-quality herbs from trusted natural sources. Many of them now depend on their own network of growers working under contract to ensure the integrity of the plant materials. The raw material suppliers must provide certificates of analysis with their deliveries to manufacturers.

Other companies have gone beyond this and have found innovative ways to make good products. Natrol, an example of a good company with strong philosophical roots, has developed a testing system using multiple markers to ensure quality, while still paying strict attention to other quality issues.

Wolfgang Aulenbucher, vice president of sales and marketing for the well-respected raw materials company East Earth Herbs, offers a very interesting outlook in an article entitled, "Quality Is Key with Herbal Extracts." In it, he describes how his company actually sends horticulturists into the field on a daily basis to determine when to pick the herbs.

What's the bottom line on herbal healing?

In spite of all this, I go back to my basic experience of having my health restored by drinking plain old dried or fresh herbs brewed into a tea. I agree with Jim Duke, Ph.D., renowned phytochemist and former director of the USDA's botanical division, who says that eventually science will find a health benefit and value for virtually every component we find in herbs. Until then, I think our priority should be finding healthy organic herbs, using the wisdom of science and tradition to make them palatable, and consuming them with love.

Please refer to the Resource Guide for a list of companies that have been identified as following safe manufacturing practices.

CHAPTER 3

How to Evaluate Information on Herbs

The truth is more important than the facts.
—Frank Lloyd Wright

Information on herbs is now voluminous. Some days I get 10 e-mails trying to sell me herbal products, a phone call or two from salespersons, and a few pounds of catalogs. Unless you are cross-trained in science, traditional medicine, and advertising psychology, it is very difficult to clearly judge every piece of information you come across. Information comes to us from diverse sources: magazine articles, books, friends, TV advertising, Internet advertising, physicians, health care practitioners, and health food store employees. Current herbal information available to consumers ranges from the most precise and accurate articles to outright falsehoods and deceptions. I am going to share my understanding of the ins and outs of this information with the hope that it will afford you some protection against misconceptions and common errors. We will look at:

- Advertising
- Evidence-based medicine
- Dishonesty in media
- Pricing issues
- Labeling
- Dosing
- Combination products
- Naming and substitution issues

Before we explore all these issues, I want to again mention the "good guys." These are the many herbal companies and health food stores that distribute promotional information that accurately describes the nature, quality, and expected actions of their products. They employ well-trained sales representatives who can answer questions clearly and responsibly. There are many books and Internet sites that distribute reliable information. In the Resource Guide, I have listed many that I have personally evaluated.

At home, I like to shop at Harvest Market, a local health food store in Delaware, run by two wonderful guys named Art and Bob. When I go to their store, the first thing I notice is that they get almost all of their products from well-known, high-quality suppliers. Bob keeps a copy of the *Botanical Safety Handbook* on the shelf and a good variety of magazines and articles on hand. Most impressive to me was an incident that occurred one day when I saw several copies of a best-selling herbal cancer treatment book I strongly believed was misleading to the general public. When I voiced my concerns to Bob, he promptly took the books off his shelf. His action reflected his genuine concern and care for his clients. There are a lot of good guys in the natural foods and herbal medicine world. "Good" doesn't just mean good-hearted. To me, it means good-hearted, well-read, and endowed with critical thinking skills.

Don't Be Duped

A few years ago I took a defensive driving course. I liked to think I was a pretty good driver and therefore had little to fear on the road, so I was taking the course merely to save money on my car insurance premiums. In the first class my instructor said, "When you turn on your engine, imagine you will be driving through a pit of snakes . . . and if you are not afraid of snakes, you should be." I would recommend heeding this same advice any time you initially encounter anyone or anything, human or electronic, that sells herbs and vitamins.

While there are many honest and skilled salespeople in the herbal marketplace, dishonest or overzealous retailers are in great supply. Ever since Madison Avenue realized, "Thar's gold in them thar holistic hills," there has been a deluge of herbal marketing messages from TV, radio, magazines, catalogs, Internet sites, books, billboards, audiotapes, and videos. If you are suffering from illness, the natural desire to get better places you at increased risk for believing some of the magical accounts of the healing powers of herbs.

Do not underestimate the persuasive powers of a determined salesperson. I remember a particular patient to whom I had explained for over an hour how to heal her skin condition. I provided extensive documentation and clear explanations for my entire course of recommended action, which involved over $75 worth of rare and uniquely useful herbs. I was confident my suggestions would help her, though I expected it to take several months.

She never returned for her second visit, and when I called her she confessed tearfully that a multilevel marketing salesperson had convinced her I was a thief who was only trying to "get my hands on her money and string her along." He claimed that his single product would absolutely solve her problem within a few weeks. I may have been a better herbalist, but he was obviously a better salesman. She returned 6 months later, no better, of course, and I was able to improve her skin condition in a few months.

In order to protect your health and your wallet from predatory salespeople, you must have a nose for fantastic claims, as well as the ability to recognize appeals to your desire to avoid pain. Many of these fantastic pitches claim to be backed up by scientific research.

Take a look at the adjoining box to read an ad I created based on real ads I have in my files. Sadly enough, if I ran this "ad," I'd probably sell a lot of juice.

By the way, if you think I am exaggerating, one of the real ads I am parodying claims that by diluting their special juice with different amounts of water, it will cure different parts of your body. The water dilution supposedly changes its cosmic vibrations. If you dilute it 2:1 it will cure your skin, if you dilute it 3:1 it will cure your bowels, and so on . . . Amazing!

The Incredible Super Purple, Green, Yellow Magnetic Anti-Carcinoma Volcanic Colloidal Desert Juice

I would like to share with you a remarkable new discovery I made last week that shows how YOU can slow the onset of all your health problems and live exactly 29.7% longer.

Wandering in the deserts of Nevada, I by chance discovered a rare desert plant so powerful it was the only plant or animal that did not wither or die from the United States nuclear testing programs of the 1940s! Natives originally used the juice derived from this plant to dye their hair purple and cure diarrhea. After months of research, we have proven that this product works miraculously for everyone suffering from the following ailments: cancer, arthritis, heart disease, pain, sexual problems, fatigue, high blood pressure, diabetes, age spots, wrinkles, high cholesterol, depression, digestive or gas problems, anemia, angina, heart disease, athletic injuries, back pain, bronchitis, diabetic retinopathy, emphysema, diarrhea, eczema, epilepsy, fibromyalgia, fungal infections, glaucoma, cataracts, herpes, headaches/migraines, immune disorders, menstrual disorders, prostate problems, sciatica, skin disorders, and flatus. This product has sent shock waves through leading scientists at major medical universities around the world.

Months of research have revealed how this product works. Super Purple, Green, Yellow Magnetic Anti-Carcinoma Volcanic Colloidal Desert Juice enters the colon, and the suspended particles attach magnetically to the colon membrane. There, the unique purple, green, and yellow structure causes them to absorb all sorts of foods, juices, vitamins, minerals, trace elements, fats, carbohydrates, proteins, anthraquinones, glycosides, and cosmic vibrations and transforms them into pure energy. The juice also transmutes all negative energy, including industrial filth, air pollution, and even sugar, into a subatomic state, where it is hydrolyzed and hydrogenated into amino acid carbon chains which re-form into energized spring water particles which your cells can absorb without producing waste products.

Evidence-Based Medicine

It is very common to extrapolate minor achievements in animal or test tube experiments into the wildest of advertising claims. Without undergoing the proper scientific training and then going back to check the literature yourself, it is difficult for you, the consumer, to know what to make of scientific evidence. This is why I generally (but not always) prefer time-tested herbs over newer discoveries. If an herb has a history of effective use in humans, then scientific evidence can add to our understanding. Remember that pharmaceutical companies often spend hundreds of millions of dollars on research with products that initially look promising, then turn out to be duds. If the information presented in an ad sounds too good to be true, it probably is.

In an article appearing in the *Journal of the American Medical Association* entitled "Technology Follies: The Uncritical Acceptance of Medical Innovation," the authors argue that many physicians are untrained in the need for critical reading of the scientific literature and lack necessary skills to practice evidence-based medicine. If physicians have problems in this area, what does this imply about our own shortcomings?

Here are a few simple guidelines that can help you to sort out the scientific information you will encounter in the marketplace.

1. Don't believe everything you read in books. When you encounter a piece of medical information concerning an issue relevant to you, such as an herb you might want to try, you need to evaluate the information critically. If, for instance, a friend tells you about an herb for "arthritis," you might ask to read the original article from which he or she got the information. If the article quotes a scientific study, you might want to go to the original study and evaluate its validity and relevance for yourself. Some studies are poorly done. For example, one study on the safety of Prozac in nursing mothers "measured" results by *asking the mothers* if their babies' behavior had changed.

2. If you have Internet access, look up studies about different herbs or illnesses using the wonderful and massive PubMed databases provided by the United States government. Go to: *http://www.ncbi.nlm.nih.gov/entrez/query.fcgi.* This source provides easy-to-access information of high quality.

3. Anecdotal accounts have great appeal, but they are not scientific proof. Do not expect scientists to be swayed by this type of evidence. Yes, these accounts are valuable, and I will give many from my personal experience, but at best, they point to the need to pursue futher study. Anecdotes, especially expert clinical observation are of great value as the first step to discovering new truths.

4. Medical studies are ranked by certain criteria. Randomized, placebo-controlled, double-blind clinical studies are the gold standard and should therefore rank high in your estimation. These studies eliminate many sources of error. Best, however, is *meta-analysis,* a statistical process that takes a large number of studies and combines their results to assess the validity of the theory being tested. Ten studies on echinacea, for example, might be collected and then ranked according to their quality. A few are thrown out for not meeting quality-control restrictions, and the results for the rest are tabulated.

5. Remember that studies done on living human beings are far superior to studies done on animals. *In vivo* means the study was performed on living creatures, while *in*

vitro means it was performed in an artificial environment, like a test tube. Although they provide valuable information, studies done in test tubes are the least clinically relevant and most likely to mislead. For example, it is much easier to shrink a tumor in a test tube than in a human being. Human studies, on the other hand, are limited by the fact that certain variables, such as diet or external environment, are much harder to assess and control.

6. If a study is well done, accept and use its findings only if they are clinically relevant to you. Ask yourself, "Does this study have a direct bearing on my health problem?" For example, a study that shows that a particular herb "strengthens the immune system" is not nearly as useful as one that shows that a particular herb has helped real people with your condition in a clinical setting.

7. Scientific studies are not the only evidence used in herbal thinking. Traditional teachings, which have persisted over several generations of dedicated herbalists, are considered reliable information.

The next section shows what happens when new media and sometimes even journal sources do not follow these simple rules.

Dishonesty in the Media

In the late 1980s a media trend appeared that was generally very favorable to and supportive of herbal medicine. Since then, the general public has been solidly and steadily moving toward accepting natural products as a very important part of health care.

In recent years, however, there has been a trend of "warning" articles about herbal medicines. While we all want to hear valid warnings, these can be very confusing if the media do not use good judgment.

Perhaps the funniest "warning" was the one published in the March 1999 edition of the journal *Fertility and Sterility*. News reports said that **St. John's wort** *(Hypericum perforatum),* **echinacea** *(Echinacea* species), and **ginkgo leaf** *(Ginkgo biloba)* might have a negative impact on human fertility. Researchers from the Loma Linda University School of Medicine in California reported that directly dosing human sperm with large amounts of these herbs in a test tube caused these sperm to lose their ability to penetrate *hamster* eggs! The lead author of the study, Richard R. Ondrizek, M.D., was upset and "flabbergasted" that the media were using his research to claim that these herbs could cause infertility in humans.

Herbalist Robyn Klein, AHG, instructor at the Sweetgrass School of Herbalism, has been vigilant in exposing the strategies used by dishonest critics, and she sent me the following synopsis of her investigations. By the way, Robyn publishes *Robyn's Recommended Reading,* which is a great way to keep up on the best literature in the field of herbal medicine. See the Resource Guide for a comprehensive list of Robyn's suggestions.

Following are some examples of the less-than-truthful tactics that have been used by critics of herbal medicine.

- Convince the public that an adverse effect of an herb was discovered through credible research. The study mentioned above, published in *Fertility and Sterility,* suggested that **echinacea** and **St. John's wort** cause sterility and mutation of cells. This test tube study certainly cannot support this conclusion because it does not resemble real-life conditions.

- Base claims of toxicity on single parts of the herbs, while ignoring the whole herb. Carotoxin, found in tiny amounts in garden carrots, is toxic to lab rats. However, this does not prove that garden carrots are dangerous. People don't eat the purified active constituents, although they do ingest teas, tablets, and liquid extracts made from whole plants.

- Focus on an unusual use of the poisonous part of an herb instead of the gentler, more commonly used part of the herb. Many critics ignore the gentle parts of an herb completely and instead focus on the uncommon use of the more potentially poisonous parts of the herb. This is like saying that rhubarb stem is dangerous because the leaves are toxic.

- Use a rare herb not usually found in herbal products to prove that herbs in general pose a danger to the public. In fact, many critics talk about poisonous plants that are not even found in herbal products. For example, they warn against using **uzara root,** which contains cardiac glycosides. This product is rarely used in herbal medicine today.

- Use examples of overdose or misuse of an herb instead of appropriate properly prescribed dosage. **Ephedra** has been used for centuries in China to safely treat asthma. But companies here in the United States began to add the extracted alkaloids in high doses to weight-loss products, causing serious problems.

- Present flawed or incomplete scientific research as if it is conclusive evidence. One study showed that **echinacea** wasn't effective for treating or shortening colds. What the report didn't reveal was that the researchers studied ridiculously low doses.

- Ignore any literature that does not come out of Western scientific research, even though there might be an overwhelming amount of evidence from traditional and ethnobotanical literature. This happens all the time.

- Use one case of an adverse reaction to imply that such reactions are commonplace. Critics constantly warn that **chamomile flower** can cause anaphylactic shock, though this occurs only in one out of millions of doses.

- Demand that herbal medicine meet standards that have never been applied to Western medicine. Critics of herbal products claim that they have not been proven efficacious or safe using the objective, scientific methods of placebo-controlled double-blind studies and rigorous testing. Yet such critics conveniently ignore the fact that some 85% of everyday medical treatments have never been scientifically validated! For example, each year 700,000 children have tubes inserted into their ears to treat inner ear infections. However, several research groups have raised doubts as to the usefulness of this procedure.

- Use hypothetical interactions of an herb with a drug to alarm clinicians when no such interactions have been reported. For example, skeptics warn against using **ginseng root** with estrogen or corticosteroids. They also purport that dangerous **licorice root**–digoxin interactions exist. However, there are no reports of any kind to support these warnings.

- Blame an innocent herb by association with a blemished herb. One case of toxicity caused by a product containing **echinacea** and **skullcap** led to an incorrect deduction that **echinacea** caused the toxicity. However, at that time **skullcap** *(Scutellaria lateriflora)* was commonly adulterated with **germander** *(Teucrium chamaedrys),* an herb known to be toxic to the liver.

- Use products that are *not* herbs as examples of toxicity. An animal product called Kyushin is a Chinese medicine rarely seen in the West. It contains dried toad venom and has been shown to be toxic. Kyushin is not an herb, so its dangers have no revelance to herbal medicines.

- Overstate hypothetical adverse reactions for an herb used to treat a condition for which dangerous Western drugs are typically prescribed. **Hawthorn** used alone has shown absolutely no dangerous effects on the heart or vascular tissue. Nor are there any clinical reports of **hawthorn** interacting with any cardiac medicine.

- Blame an herb for adverse effects commonly associated with medicine taken at the same time. **Evening primrose** and **borage oils** have been blamed for epileptic episodes in patients undergoing treatment with phenothiazines. While there is no evidence to support the claim that these oils are responsible, there *is* scientific research showing that *phenothiazines* can cause epileptic episodes!

Robyn found evidence of these tactics while reading articles in such respected and prestigious publications as the *New England Journal of Medicine*, the *Journal of the American Medical Association*, the *New York Times*, and *Archives of Internal Medicine*.

The problem of misleading reporting can be solved if we insist that only accurate science and scientific reporting be used to evaluate herbal medicines. On August 4, 1999, the Associated Press reported that Congress had reinforced this idea when it announced that the FDA had used sloppy science to justify some of its proposed rules for the use of ephedrine.

As I mentioned earlier, most journalists attempt to write honest evaluations of their understanding of herbal safety issues, while some do not. However, I have seen magazine articles appearing in early 2000 which defy all sense of propriety. When you mix moderate amounts of accurate information with large amounts of innuendo, speculation, and discredited information, you remove the public's ability to judge that information and replace it with fear.

In late 1999, a writer took every available negative fact known about herbal medicine and mixed them all together with the worst possible slant. It sounded as if anyone who dared to take an herb was in danger of being immediately poisoned or blinded. Fortunately, I knew the truth behind each of the 30 or so negative points brought up in this article, and now so do you, since we will have discussed each and every one in this book.

How Pricing is Determined

We are now in a revolution where low-cost Internet and catalog shopping are taking significant market share from the health food stores. Because of mass buying and lower infrastructure costs, they can offer things at lower cost, and often with great convenience.

However, there are several pitfalls. There is wide disparity in the costs of different herbs, so it is worth your while to carry a calculator.

Here is an example of milk thistle capsules offered by two companies. Which is the better-priced product?

Imagine you are buying a car, but you cannot see it because it is covered by a huge capsule. You must depend on the information on the outer label. This puts you

Milk Thistle Prices

Product 1 contains 120 capsules of milk thistle extract, 150 mg (80% flavonoids), and costs $13.50.

Product 2 contains 90 capsules of milk thistle extract, 200 mg (80% flavonoids), and costs $12.50.

We need to calculate how much each product costs per gram.

Product 1: 120 capsules x 150 mg = 18,000 mg for $13.50

If we divide by 1,000, we see that this product costs $13.50 for 18 grams, or 75¢ per gram.

Product 2: 90 capsules x 200 mg = 18,000 mg for $12.50

If we divide by 1,000, we see that this product costs $12.50 for 18 grams, or 69.5¢ per gram.

This is the basic calculation method for determining the true cost of an herbal product. However, in Product 1, the 150 mg of milk thistle extract was packaged in a capsule containing 350 mg of an inexpensive filler herb. In other words, there may have been 500 mg of total herb in each capsule as stated on the label, but only 150 mg of it was milk thistle. **You must read the labels carefully to make accurate calculations.**

at a huge disadvantage over the retailer, who knows what went into the capsule before it was sealed. A $25,000 car capsule containing a new Mercedes would be a bargain, while a $6,000 car capsule containing a used bicycle would be a rip-off. Similarly, you can buy the Mercedes of herbs, or you can buy an expensive rip-off.

For example, I'm looking at a catalog right now. Let's assume the catalog offers only good-quality products. Two common herbs, ginkgo leaf and echinacea, are being offered at very good prices. However, the prices for other herbs in this particular catalog are much higher. Ginkgo and echinacea are known as "loss leaders," offered at a low cost in the hopes of gaining your trust, so you will assume that everything else is fairly priced.

To identify good prices, you must do a little comparison shopping. Read the labels carefully to make sure the products contain the same herbs in the same form. Then use a calculator to compare. For a detailed example, go back to the milk thistle example in the box above.

Labeling

Labeling is supposed to be controlled by the government. Ideally, it means that the herbs listed on the label match what the laboratory has determined to be inside. If the label says 200 mg of dandelion root per capsule, then each capsule contains 200 mg of dandelion root. Right? Maybe so, but labels can be literally true and still misleading. Just because the product contains a *total weight* of an herb, it doesn't tell you anything about the source, form, and level of concentration.

Therefore, starting in Spring 2000, the FDA required all labels to list the full contents of a product, its common and scientific (Latin) names, the parts used, the form used, and the potency. This important step will help end a lot of confusion. You will still have to read labels carefully, paying special attention to the statements that warn you when not to use a particular product. It is also important to check the expiration date—a common oversight.

Beware Labeling Trickery

In spite of the positive changes mentioned above, product labeling is currently a hot issue in the herbal medicine industry. Even with the new labeling laws, manufacturers have found many ways to fool consumers into buying their products.

Some typical tricks include:

- **"Three tablets contain."** I love this one. The "three tablets contain" is listed in small print so that people who are not used to reading 8-point type do not even notice the notation and end up believing each capsule or tablet contains a larger quantity of the active ingredient than it really does. This is allowed because 3 tablets is a serving.

- **Formulating a product with a much lower concentration of the active ingredient than recommended.** One patient complained to me that her $8 bottle of ginkgo leaf was not working, and implied that I had cheated her because I had tried to sell her "the same thing" for $18. However, her $8 preparation contained a 5:1 "gingko leaf dry concentrate," while mine had the stronger recommended 50:1 concentrate. Essentially, her $8 bottle really cost $80. The label on the product was telling the truth, but the manufacturer probably knew that many consumers would not know the difference between that minimal 5:1 (if they even noticed it) and the standard 50:1. In these cases, the manufacturer is concerned only with selling the product, without regard to whether it will actually benefit consumers. Unfortunately, many will never try this product again, when it could be of great benefit.

- **A product is promoted for its ability to increase energy when it actually contains herbal forms of caffeine.** Improved energy levels may result from taking herbs like **black tea** *(Camellia sinensis)* or **guarana** *(Paullinia cupana),* but people should be told that the herbs contain caffeine. Other herbs like this include **yerba mate** *(Ilex paraguariensis),* **oolong tea**, **green tea**, and **cola** *(Cola nitida, C. acuminata).*

- **A low-quality component is combined with a better one in the same product.** Sometimes manufacturers will mix a small amount of a standardized ingredient with crude herb. The label might read "milk thistle, 500 mg, standardized to contain 80% flavonoids." The small print on the label reveals that the product is actually a mixture of 80 mg of standardized herb and 420 mg of herb that is not standardized, possibly making the product weaker and less effective.

Beware of "Synergistic," "Balanced," "Natural," and "Best"

Labels often contain lots of words that are full of sound and fury, yet signify next to nothing. If something is "synergistic," it means that the combined effect of all the parts working together is stronger than that of the individual elements. For example, adding an herb that aids digestion to one that is hard to digest would increase the medical activity of the second. Unfortunately, words like "synergistic" are generally used without discrimination or definition.

The uses of "balanced" and "best" also have no consistent meaning. "Natural" sometimes describes a product derived from natural sources as opposed to synthetic, but I have seen it used to describe white sugar. Nonetheless, consumers are attracted to herbs that are "the highest-quality, best-selling, most synergistically balanced and completely natural formula you can buy today."

Problems with Dosing

Each herb requires proper dosing, which is listed on the label. There would be few problems if companies would just put the standard effective adult dose on the label of a product and provide enough pills in the package to last for 2 weeks to a month. However, consumers like low prices, and manufacturers like high returns. It is a well-known fact in the mass market that when product prices go beyond about $9 per bottle, items become more difficult to sell. So even if manufacturers indicate on the label that each pill contains a low (read: ineffective) dose, people will still buy the seemingly low-cost product. If consumers were aware of the dose required for the proper effect, they might find themselves finishing off a bottle every 3 or 4 days. The manufacturers are justified in one sense, in that they could argue (and in court must argue) that they are selling nutritional supplements, not medicines, and so are not required to put effective dose levels for treating diseases on their labels.

Therefore, the doses listed on many herbal product labels are far below what is needed to obtain a therapeutic effect, especially in acute cases. I found general agreement in China, India, and Nepal with regard to dosage levels. In China, you would usually leave the herb doctor's office with about 4–8 ounces of dried plants—a 3-day supply. You would then go home and brew them into tea, using one-third of the batch to make 2 or 3 cups of dark, intense tea. Whew! Then, you would have to drink it. In Nepal, the routine was similar, but they used concentrated powders, and you would take 1–2 teaspoons of powder (about 3–6 grams) straight, or make a tea with it.

Often the effective dose for an herb is 10–20 grams per day, which equals taking 20–40 capsules. The same is true for tinctures. Echinacea tincture seems quite inexpensive at $9 per 1-oz. bottle, until you start taking 1 teaspoon every 2 hours, required when you have a cold. This will use up a bottle in a day and a half. Standardized herbs like ginkgo leaf and saw palmetto berries don't require large numbers of pills due to concentration, though I often need double the label dosages to get results.

Combination Products

Another aspect of herbal medicine that is challenging to the novice concerns combination products, otherwise known as **formulas**. Unless you're a professional, it is next to impossible to determine whether a group of herbs in a formula designed to support the prostate or the kidneys will be good for you. Some of these formulations are well thought out, while others simply mix everything "good for the pancreas," no matter how far this stretches credulity. Good companies hire well-paid experts to formulate their products.

Often these are marketed using names like "Livr-Pure" or "Hepato-Magic." I suggest that potential buyers look up the individual ingredients one by one, or try to find literature explaining the history and scientific or traditional basis behind the formulation. Beware of formulas that use the word "secret," or that were handed down from an ancient Indian formula revealed in a trance to the company president's dead uncle.

Polypharmacy or Good Formula Writing?

The random mixing together of herbs was dubbed **polypharmacy** by the Eclectic physicians of the last century, who looked down on it as an ill-conceived practice.

Well-constructed herbal formulas are put together to match the needs of the individual patient, and should be based upon a solid system of diagnosis or scientific reasoning. Each herb in the formula should have a stated and specific purpose.

For example, putting six diuretics into a formula for the kidneys is not the correct way to treat a kidney infection. Some of the diuretics may be mild, while others, such as **uva ursi** leaf *(Arctostaphylos uva-ursi),* may be irritating and therefore not recommended. A better formula might contain two nonirritating diuretics, along with one or two herbs that reduce inflammation, one that soothes the ureters, and one that stimulates the immune system.

To make a formula for a general purpose or particular organ instead of a specific condition is certainly allowable and can work well, as long as you are aware of the drawbacks. Formulas that are designed for the liver, for example, must take into account that hepatitis is a different liver problem than elevated cholesterol or cirrhosis, distinctions that may escape the layperson. Herbs that are beneficial for one liver condition might be harmful or ineffective for another. This does not mean, however, that there aren't a few very safe liver herbs that can be used without much worry.

Good medicine making and new formula construction still exist. Well-trained herbalists, physicians, nutritionists, and biochemists are creating new combination products all the time. As new information comes to light, new formulas are constructed.

When Nai-shing first came to this country, she examined a group of TCM formulas I had been using. By reading the ingredients, she immediately knew what the formula was and what it treated. It seems the company I was working with had copied a core group of traditional formulas known by every well-trained TCM doctor. Upon examination, Nai-shing said that the company had also done a good job with the literature provided along with the formulas, which I found reassuring.

Today, we have three basic groups of formulas: those formulated at random with little thought, those handed down through an herbal tradition, and those formulated by a knowledgeable herbalist or physician in modern times. Unfortunately, consumers without the specialized knowledge of an expert like Nai-shing or myself cannot distinguish among these groups. Therefore, it would be most helpful if the name of the formulator or the text in which the formula first appeared is on the label. If such information does appear on the label, there is a good chance that you are getting a superior product.

Today, we have a new form of polypharmacy. It occurs when people wander from pharmacy to pharmacy picking up every new wonder herb until their countertop is full of herbs. This is actually more of a disease than a mere habit. In the advanced stages, you run out of counter space and lose all memory of what the herbs you bought 3 months ago are supposed to do.

What's in a Name?

There are many ambiguities in herbal naming systems. A single international body of botanists is responsible for establishing the Latin names of herbs in the world, which are always *italicized* and are the best way to identify herbs. Common names vary from place to place, and a Latin-named herb may have a variety of common names. A single well-known name may refer to several related or even unrelated plants. Each country has its own common names in its own language. This leaves plenty of room for mistakes and even trickery. Some examples:

- **Substituting one plant for another.** After the Chinese herb **ephedra** *(ma huang)* got a bad reputation after people died from diet products containing ephedrine, many diet pills became suspect. Ephedrine is a stimulant that can be dangerous for some people. When it was discovered that the Ayurvedic plant **bala** *(Sida cordifolia)* also contains ephedrine (though less), manufacturers substituted it for the **ephedra.** Now consumers who for medical reasons should avoid taking ephedrine might be fooled into taking an ingredient that can endanger their health. The label may be "accurate," but the result could be disastrous.

- **Hiding ingredients by using little-known common names.** Perhaps I want to make a laxative formula using **aloe leaf** *(Aloe vera)*. I don't want anyone to know, because they might copy my formula, so I use a little-known common name, like "socotrine aloes," or even a foreign name like "kumari." The average consumer would never figure out what plant it really is. This creates lots of confusion for both patients and doctors if a problem develops. I'm looking at one I still can't figure out—"rain deity bark." Contact me if you know what it is.

- **Associating your product with a more popular one.** For a time, **wild red desert "ginseng"** was sold before people realized it was not **ginseng root** at all. It came from a different plant family and had no relationship whatsoever to **ginseng**. The same trick was used to promote **Siberian ginseng root bark**, although this plant does share some tonic actions with real Chinese or American **ginseng root.**

- **Using made-up names.** In an attempt to get around legal restrictions against claiming disease benefits for particular herbs, sometimes manufacturers will make up new names. I saw a French product that contained an herb I could not identify by common name. The Latin name given was something like *Turina anticarcinoma*. In another case, in an attempt to promote the supposed sexual-potency-enhancing properties of the Ayurvedic herb **gokshura fruit** *(Tribulus terrestris)*, some manufacturers changed the Latin name to *Tribulus erectus*. In fact, there is an herb called *Trillium erectum*. Unfortunately it is used to treat female problems and to induce vomiting. Its common name is **"stinking benjamin."**

More on Substitution

When performed by growers in the wild, substitution can cause major problems with safety (more on this in Chapters 4 and 5). Most often, however, the problem is not one of safety but one of effectiveness. In ancient times, herbalists studying and working in one part of a country sometimes could not find a particular plant when they moved to another region. They may have gotten around this problem by substituting another plant with similar qualities or of similar appearance. This is not a major problem if both herbs are effective and the herbalists in each region know how to use them.

Some substitutions, however, can mean big problems for consumers. For example, **dang gui root** *(Angelica sinensis)* is sold all over America as a "women's" herb. Although this herb is used for many female problems, its traditional Chinese use as a warming, blood-nourishing herb for both men and women has been put in the background in favor of the modern and less correct use as a treatment for menopausal hot flashes.

This problem is compounded by the fact that in 1957, a large amount of European **dang gui root** *(Levisticum officinale)* was planted in China to meet demand. This process began in the area around Beijing and then spread to the rest of the country, in large measure supplanting the local **dang gui.** The reasons were financial. The European variety was larger, yielding more plant per acre. In 1983 the Chinese government stopped this process. It is still assumed that the European **dang gui** may enter the market at times. To make matters even more complicated, the Chinese name **dang gui** is also spelled "tang kuai" and "dong quai" on many bottles.

CHAPTER 4

Safety and Regulation:
Who's Watching the Herbal Store?

*Observe that the things which are considered to be right today
are those which were considered impossible yesterday. The
things which are thought wrong today are those which will be
esteemed right tomorrow.*

—Hudhaifa

Does anyone regulate the safety of the herbal industry?

Reports in the media have spread the untruth that the herbal medicine industry is not well regulated. In fact, the Food and Drug Administration (FDA) regulates it very closely. The FDA reviews an herbal product's labels, manufacturing standards, and contents. It also collects reports of adverse effects, issues warnings, and pulls products off the shelves if problems are reported.

In addition, the National Nutritional Foods Association (the industry's largest trade association), has developed a program to examine the herbal products and factory conditions of its member companies and give them the right to display GMP (good manufacturing practices) seals of approval on their products. This program resembles the certification process used to accredit hospitals and will be in operation by July 2002.

While regulation of the herbal medicine industry could be more extensive, herbs generally do have an excellent safety record. As with everything else in life, there is no such thing as "total safety" with herbs, but you can certainly raise your odds of success when you know what to look for.

You do not need to be a professional herbalist to be safe. A combination of background knowledge and common sense will be your most important safeguard. Read labels carefully, and check with your doctor before tampering with your prescriptions or changing over to herbal alternatives.

Once you have the facts, you can make sound judgments about whom and what to trust in this "marketplace of occult medicine sellers."

The Guiding Light

In 1993, the World Health Organization published its "Research Guidelines for Evaluating the Safety and Efficacy of Herbal Medicines." They stated that the long-term use of an herbal substance is valid proof of its safety unless there is scientific evidence of danger: "A guiding principle should be that if the product has been traditionally used without demonstrated harm, no specific regulatory action should be undertaken unless new evidence demands a revised risk-benefit assessment."

Natural Poisons Found in Plants

Many plants are poisonous, despite the safety statistics on commercial herbal preparations. In fact, about 5% of all poisonings, or over 10,000 incidents per year, are caused by the ingestion of plants. Most of these poisonings occur when children ingest household or outdoor plants. Parents should learn how to recognize toxic household plants, and children should be trained never to eat a plant unless an adult first teaches them how to identify and use it. Everyone should know how to contact regional poison control centers. For information on finding your local poison control center, refer to the Resource Guide.

> According to the Cherokee Indians, all plants belong to one of three classifications:
>
> **Foods:** to be eaten freely
> **Medicines:** to be used in times of ill health
> **Poisons:** to be avoided at all times
>
> By teaching this to our children, thousands of annual poisonings could be avoided.

Under conditions of drought, livestock may also consume poisonous plants for their moisture content. As a result, they will sometimes end up dying. Of course, such obviously poisonous plants are not put into capsules and sold to unsuspecting consumers at the health food store, but there are some important lessons to learn here. In a 1989 report, the Data Collection System of the American Association of Poison Control Centers identified the 15 most frequently ingested plants, with numbers of ingestion episodes and information about toxicity. Most of them either are sold for household use or are extremely common in the wild. If you have any of these plants in or near your home, make sure your kids know that they are dangerous. For a complete list of the plants and their effects, refer to the Appendix.

Contaminants and Adulteration

A "contaminant" is an impurity, an extraneous material associated with an herb that can cause problems. Contaminants exert their effects by interacting with your cells, where they distort the manner in which the cells function. Some common contaminants are pesticides, fumigants, irradiation, sterilizing gases, viruses, heavy metals, Western drugs, insects, hairs, additives, bacteria, and fungal toxins. Obtaining foods and herbs from organic manufacturers should lessen your exposure to these toxins, especially pesticides and heavy metals.

Contaminants can inflame, irritate, or burn cell membranes, causing redness, pain, swelling, or itching. These effects can be delayed or remote, meaning that the contaminant enters your body through the gastrointestinal tract, the lungs, or the skin and then goes through several metabolic steps before making you sick when it arrives at a target organ such as the liver or kidneys. Some contaminants can also harm unborn children.

The most important determinant of the true toxicity of a substance is dosage. Everything that exists has the potential to be toxic. In toxicology, this is called the **dose-response relationship**. Scientists determine how toxic a substance will be by performing tests on animals to identify the **LD50**, or lethal dose (the amount necessary to kill 50% of the animals). The only way to avoid contaminants in herbs is to depend on top-quality manufacturing.

An "adulterant" is an intentionally introduced additive that dilutes or alters the desired character of an herbal product. Adulteration is usually accomplished by adding a less pure form of a given herb into a batch, or even substituting another species (usually a cheaper one). For instance, **ginseng root** *(Panax ginseng)* is expensive, so **ginseng leaves** are often added to the brew. David Lytle, lab director of Peak Botanical Laboratories, reports: "**Guarana** *(Paullinia cupana)* is the seed of a creeping shrub native to the Amazon region and a popular botanical stimulant. A significant number of **guarana extracts** on the market today are adulterated." Adulteration is not necessarily a health concern, as the adulterants themselves may not be toxic. However, if a toxic species is substituted, such as the **germander/skullcap** or **stephania/aristolochia** mix-ups mentioned, sometimes poisoning can occur.

In fact, in an editorial in the fall of 1998 pharmacist and TCM physician Dennis Awang stated, "The overwhelming majority of adverse events recorded from herbal treatments has involved adulteration with, or substitution of, toxic plant material from relatively innocuous components. . . . Careful characterization of botanical material, whether being assessed for activity or implicated in adverse health effects, is an absolute prerequisite to authoritative judgement."

Remember, however, that the overall safety record of herbal medicines is generally good, especially when companies meet the GMP standards we mentioned in our discussion of manufacturing. These problems are what quality control standards are designed to prevent.

Heavy Metals

How do heavy metals and pesticides contaminate foods and herbs?

Most heavy metals and all pesticides come from industrial sources. These substances can enter the food chain and contaminate soil, air, foods, and herbs. Each year, for example, thousands of tons of lead are dumped into the atmosphere. Cadmium and lead can be found in cigarette smoke. Mercury can come from contaminated fish. Aluminum can come from antacids and kitchen utensils.

According to a recent review, "Epidemiologic studies on pesticides have found associations with long-term effects on health mainly in three fields: cancer (especially hematological cancer), neurotoxic effects (polyneuropathy, neurobehavioral hazards, Parkinson's disease), and reproductive disorders (infertility, birth defects, adverse pregnancy outcomes, perinatal mortality)."

Therefore, we recommend that you purchase foods and herbs from organic sources. Also, it is important to know that some people react to minute amounts of these metals that are harmless for most of us, due to genetic susceptibility or impaired detoxification capacity.

What can you say about reports stating that "significant amounts of heavy metals" have been found in Chinese herbs?

Virtually all animal products and herbs contain small amounts of various naturally occurring heavy metals, including **lead, mercury, cadmium, arsenic, nickel,** and **aluminum**. These do not pose a health concern unless they exceed safe levels (remember, dosage is everything). While not all Chinese and Ayurvedic herbs contain excessive amounts of heavy metals, some batches have shown concentrations of heavy metals that exceed safe levels, sometimes to an alarming degree.

Most reports of seriously high levels of heavy metals in Chinese herbs, when investigated, are based upon the fact that certain patented Chinese medicine formulas have purified heavy metals added intentionally for medicinal purposes, just as we do here with, for example, calcium and zinc. Chinese and Ayurvedic doctors purify these heavy metals with methods developed in ancient times. The supposedly "toxic" herbs are prescribed and consumed in China without apparent side effects. These methods have not, to my knowledge, been verified by Western science.

It is possible to be exposed to heavy metals if you take herbs that are processed by companies that do not meet United States GMP (good manufacturing practice) standards. Therefore, **I would avoid all patent medicines made outside the United States unless manufactured by companies that follow GMP standards.** This warning does not apply to individual herbs imported and used to make formulas inside the United States. **The best way to do this is to consult with a professional herbalist who is able to assess the companies from which they purchase their products.**

Pharmaceutical Contamination

There have been reports that some imported Chinese herbs contain pharmaceuticals. This problem is limited to imported patent medicines. In China, pharmaceuticals are often added to patent medicines to make them stronger, a practice considered acceptable there. For example, a formula for colds may have Chinese herbs combined with aspirin or perhaps an antibiotic. Like medicines containing heavy metals, such medicines are illegal to import into the United States. However, they sometimes make it into the United States when the pharmaceuticals are not listed on the labels or are removed from the list to avoid detection, or kept in the Chinese language so you cannot understand them.

Fortunately, the FDA is aware of this problem, and the number of poisonings has been very small. I consider the practice of changing labels or removing ingredient information to be a criminal offense.

This is a real concern. Physicians at King's College Hospital in London found that several TCM skin creams for eczema contained a synthetic steroid called dexamethasone. The patients who were using these products had no idea that the steroid had been added to their herbs. The concentrations of the steroid were above levels considered safe for use in children. Steroid creams applied to the face can lead to thinning of the skin. I would therefore again advise against purchasing over-the-counter Chinese patent medicines without consulting with a trained TCM doctor. The larger importing firms that cater to acupuncturists and physicians (such as Mayway Co., Nuherbs, Sun Ten, Spring Wind, and Min Tong) strictly follow GMP standards and are subject to FDA inspections.

The American Association of Oriental Medicine (AAOM) has, for several years, called for a boycott of patent medicines contaminated with heavy metals and pharmaceuticals.

CHAPTER 5

Actions, Interactions, and Reactions: Guidelines for the Safe Use of Herbs

Only two things are infinite, the universe and human stupidity,
and I'm not sure about the former.

—Albert Einstein

I have read warnings in well-respected publications that herbal medicines can pose serious dangers. How concerned should I be?

This question was answered very clearly by Jim Duke, Ph.D., former head of the USDA's botanical division and author of numerous best-selling books on herbal medicine. On one of his many web sites, he published the list in the accompanying box, comparing the use of herbs with other possible causes of death.

Dr. Duke's Herbal Death List

Herbs: 1 in 1,000,000
Supplements: 1 in 1,000,000
Mushrooms: 1 in 100,000
Food poisoning: 1 in 25,000
NSAID: 1 in 10,000
Murder: 1 in 10,000
Hospital surgery: 1 in 10,000
Car accident: 1 in 5,000

Improper use of medication: 1 in 2,000
Angiogram: 1 in 1,000
Alcohol: 1 in 500
Cigarettes: 1 in 500
Western medicines: 1 in 333
Medical mishap: 1 in 250
Iatrogenic hospital infection: 1 in 80
Bypass surgery: 1 in 20

Every year about 100,000 people die from prescription drug reactions. As you can see, by comparison, the chance of being killed by herbs is small.

I'm still not convinced.

Good, because there are two more things that need to be made clear. First, herbs contain chemicals and, though generally safe, can cause severe allergic reactions and even death, just like foods. Most but not all of these reactions are preventable if you educate yourself, as you are now doing.

Rules to Follow When Using Herbs

- Consult with someone who is properly trained before using herbs to treat a medical condition.
- Consult with your doctor or herbalist if you are also taking Western prescription medications.
- Always read labels carefully.
- Read about an herb in at least two different sources before taking it.
- Don't believe claims about miraculous cures.
- Follow dosage recommendations. More is not always better. Start with moderate doses and increase over time if necessary.
- Heed contraindications, which are there for your safety. Note that contraindications are often understated in clinical settings and on written instructions, so you may have to do some of your own research.
- Monitor yourself for reactions, and discontinue herbs if you notice any adverse effects.
- If you have a serious reaction to an herb, call 911.

Second, you must take responsibility for your own health. This means you must take the time to learn to listen to your own body, find good sources of information, and check with your physician before you change or stop any prescription medicines you are taking. Make sure that all your caregivers know exactly what you are doing. I am always very impressed when new patients show up with clearly written lists describing all the medications, prescription or natural, that they are taking. Dr. Duke tells me that his HMO doesn't even want to hear about the herbs he takes—which is all he took in 1998 except for seven Aleve tablets—so you must be sure to inform your doctors about any herbs you are taking.

Allergic and Hypersensitivity Reactions to Herbs

Theoretically, it is possible to have an allergic or hypersensitive response to any substance. In practice, certain herbs are more likely than others to cause allergic reactions. I estimate that in my practice one patient in a thousand experiences an unexpected allergic reaction. So far, all except one have recovered within 24 hours simply by stopping the herbs. (The remaining case required steroids to relieve the itching caused by a reaction to the herbs.)

It is impossible to predict such reactions in advance, but the mild level of the reactions compared to, say, a bee sting is probably because the concentration of allergens is relatively low in most herbs consumed orally. It is equally probable that an allergic response might occur as a result of exposure to an unexpected contaminant in the preparation, rather than the herb itself. If you suspect you are having an allergic reaction to an herb or herbal preparation, stop taking it immediately and call your health care practitioner.

In the adjoining box you will see a short list of medicinal plants related to ragweed, from the aster plant family, which might evoke allergic responses in some people. Unfortunately the aster herbs and shrubs are the largest family of flowering plants, comprising about 1,100 genera and 20,000 species. Interestingly, some of the plants from this family are used to *treat* allergies. Dr. Duke's database also lists individual phytochemicals that have been reported to be allergenic (see Resource Guide).

Hypersensitivity is a more common problem, affecting perhaps 1% of people who take herbal medicines. These are unexpected reactions of various sorts that other people do not have. Symptoms may develop such as elevated liver enzymes, nervousness, changes in blood pressure, or fatigue. If such responses occur, they are unpredictable, and patients should always discontinue the herbs and consult with their doctors.

Allergic and other negative reactions to herbs sometimes indicate imbalances in the intestinal flora. People suffering from intestinal dysbiosis or chronic intestinal infections will often find themselves becoming increasingly allergic to more and more things, including the herbs that are supposed to help them. Chronic intestinal inflammation leads to an increased challenge to the immune system. I discuss this in Chapter 11.

Drug Interactions

Can I take herbs along with the other medicines given to me by my doctor?

This is perhaps the most common question people ask me. Historically, herbs and pharmaceutical drugs have been developed independently, and only in the past 40 years has there been widespread concurrent use of these two forms of medicines. It is now very common for patients to consult more than one allopathic doctor, and for patients to turn to herbalists for information and take supplements purchased at health and nutrition stores. Many people are taking multiple drugs, herbs, and vitamins at the same time. It is very difficult to predict in advance any side effects that may occur as a result of such combinations, yet it is unreasonable to ask people to just give up potential solutions to their health problems. Skilled observers are now saying that it is important to learn and report as much as we can about drug-herb combinations.

In our clinic, we often prescribe herbs side by side with Western medications, and we see few problems. When problems do occur, they are invariably quickly resolved. Nonetheless, we should pay close attention to certain areas where interactions are likely, such as with cardiac medications.

Plants That May Cause Allergic Reactions

Arnica flowers (*Arnica montana*)
Artichoke leaves (*Cynara scolymus*)
Boneset (*Eupatorium perfoliatum*)
Burdock (*Arctium lappa*)
Chamomile, German (*Matricaria chamomilla*)
Chicory (*Cichorium* species)
Dandelion root/leaves (*Taraxacum officinale*)
Echinacea (*Echinacea* species)
Feverfew (*Tanacetum parthenium*)
Goldenrod flowers (*Solidago* species)
Wormwood (*Artemisia absinthium*)
Yarrow leaves/flowers (*Achillea millefolium*)
Zi wan root (*Aster tataricus*)

Believing that herbs are categorically safe or unsafe is insufficient. While it is true that herbs may harm only one person in a thousand, and kill only one in a million, it is my job to make sure you are not that one.

In the rest of this chapter we will review every major concern with regard to herbal medicine toxicity of which I am currently aware. By the end you will know more than enough to protect yourself.

I will provide lists of herbs for which there may be some concerns in each section. However, these lists are not exhaustive. For more exhaustive coverage, I suggest you get a copy of the *Botanical Safety Handbook*, the *PDR for Herbal Medicines,* or *Herb Contraindications and Drug Interactions*.

Herbs and Their Effect on Medication

Herbs can increase or decrease your absorption of nutrients and Western medications. Being aware of this possibility will help you to spot such a problem if it occurs. This can be critically important if you are taking medicines that have a high danger potential, such as cardiac glycosides (heart medications) and blood-thinning agents.

Some herbs contain large amounts of mucilage and other types of fiber, and therefore may inhibit absorption of certain medications. Bulk-forming laxatives are the most common category of herbs to do this.

Herbs that strengthen digestion and absorption may increase absorption of medications. This alone may be the reason so many persons have reported being able to reduce their medications after taking herbs. Both **cayenne** and **black pepper** have shown to speed up absorption of various chemicals including phytochemicals.

It is also known that many herbs can change the way the body processes and eliminates drugs in the liver. Many herbs and common foods have effects on liver enzyme systems and can change blood levels of drugs. **St. John's wort** was implicated in January 2000 in lowering the blood levels of AIDS drugs and cyclosporine, a drug used to prevent organ rejection. In both of these cases, the results could be deadly.

Grapefruit juice contains a compound called "bergamottin," which inactivates cytochrome P450-3A4, a digestive enzyme that metabolizes up to 60% of all drugs, including antihistamines and various high blood pressure medicines. This may explain why grapefruit juice increases the effects of many prescription drugs. **When certain drugs are ingested with grapefruit juice, the blood levels of those drugs can reach five times their normal levels, which is especially dangerous with cardiac glycosides.**

These concerns are limited to people taking drugs where lowering below therapeutic levels is dangerous. If you are not taking such medicines you certainly can drink grapefruit juice.

Blood Thinners

Many herbs contain mild to moderate blood-thinning or -thickening properties. For example, foods and herbs containing vitamin K (which allows the body to produce proteins that clot blood) are widely distributed in nature. Because the actions by themselves are not strong, and because there are many steps in the pathway of coagulation, they almost never pose a danger. Nonetheless, strong blood-thinning and catalyzing herbs should be avoided if you are undergoing surgery, along with supplements like vitamin E. If you are taking a blood thinner such as Coumadin (warfarin), you must exercise caution both when taking herbs that may further thin your blood and when consuming foods that contain vitamin K. If your blood-clotting time changes too much, you could be in danger of hemorrhage or increased risk of stroke. I have provided a list of herb and food sources and their content of vitamin K, which may potentially counteract blood-thinning medications if used in excess (see the adjoining box).

Even if you are taking the herbs under professional guidance, the best way to deal with this situation is to have your doctor conduct clotting-time studies (prothrombin or PT time), which determine how fast your blood clots. This should be done about once a week for the first month you are taking the herbs. If the clotting time does not change significantly within the first few weeks, then it is safe for you to continue taking the herb. However, if the clotting time changes by more than a few seconds, you must discontinue the herb or ask your doctor to adjust the dosage of your blood-thinning medication. Be sure to talk to your doctor about this when you discontinue or restart any herb with significant blood-thinning actions. The use of herbs that strengthen blood vessels, such as **berries** (blueberries, raspberries, boysenberries and strawberries) and **tien chi root,** can help prevent problems. For a complete list of herbs that affect blood coagulation, see the Appendix.

> **Herbs and Foods High in Vitamin K**
>
> - Kale: 6.18 parts per million (ppm)
> - Parsley: 5.48 ppm
> - Spinach: 3.80 ppm
> - Cabbage (green): 3.39 ppm
> - Watercress: 3.15 ppm
> - Broccoli: 1.79 ppm
> - Soybean oil: 1.73 ppm
> - Brussels sprouts: 1.47 ppm
> - Rapeseed oil: 1.29 ppm
> - Mustard greens: 0.88 ppm

Blood Pressure Medications

Some herbs may lower or raise blood pressure. The effects of most nonprescription blood-pressure-changing herbs commonly available are minor. Clinically, I have seen several cases where patients taking herbs were able to reduce their Western prescriptions to avoid side effects by using lifestyle changes and mild herbs. If you are taking blood pressure medications along with herbs, check with your physician to see if your medication dosage needs to be modified. The only herbs I have seen actually raise patients' blood pressure to any significant degree (and this rarely occurs) are **astragalus root, yohimbe** *(Corynanthe yohimbe),* **ephedra,** and **ginseng root**. Commonly known herbs that lower blood pressure include **linden flower, mistletoe, rauwolfia root,** and **garlic**. For a complete list of herbs that affect blood pressure, refer to the Appendix.

Cardiac Glycosides

Cardiac glycosides are chemical medicines used by physicians, which are also found in plants. These chemicals affect the pumping action and rhythm of the heart muscle. **Foxglove** is the best known of these herbs and is the botanical source for pharmaceutical cardiac medications.

These herbs are dangerous because the amount needed to create a medicinal effect is very close to the amount that can cause immediate and sometimes deadly toxic reactions, including intoxication, hallucination, nausea, headache, vomiting, seizures, ventricular tachycardia, ventricular fibrillation, heart blockage, and death. **You should avoid herbal medicines containing cardiac glycosides or herbs that stimulate the heart unless prescribed by a doctor. If you are taking cardiac glycoside medicines you must avoid these herbal medicines.**

There are also some reports that the commonly used herb **hawthorn berry** (*Crataegus* species) may increase the action of digitalis, but I have not seen any adverse reports at this time. Dr. Weiss reports in his textbook *Herbal Medicine* that "a heart no longer giving an adequate response to digitalis or strophanthin becomes reactive again after intercurrent *Crataegus* therapy." A physician trained in the use of both herbs and heart medications may therefore be able to improve results of digitalis therapy without raising the dosage into a more dangerous range.

Herbs that increase digestion and absorption may intensify your cardiac medicine's effects (see the Appendix). **The following herbs may interact with cardiac glycosides**: **Aloe** (*Aloe* species*)*, **buckthorn bark** (*Rhamnus cathartica*), **cascara** (*R. purshiana*), and **senna** (*Senna* species*)*. All of these are laxatives that might reduce the absorption times of your medicines. From a traditional point of view, herbs that are very hot or toxic, such as **purified aconite,** may overstimulate the heart. **Ma huang root** (*Ephedra* species) can do the same.

Tranquilizers and Antidepressants

Patients are always coming to me with questions about the use of herbs like **St. John's wort** and **kava root** with their prescription antidepressants or tranquilizers. This is to be expected, as drugs like Prozac are associated with significant side effects. About 20% of patients experience nausea or headaches and about 15% anxiety, nervousness, or insomnia, while 17% of patients are forced to discontinue use due to side effects. Most of our mood-oriented herbs like **St. John's wort, kava root, milky oat seed, skullcap, Siberian ginseng root bark,** and **ashwagandha root** are safe to try as milder alternatives prior to taking psychiatric drugs.

Once you are taking one of the stronger drugs, it is important to check with your physician about monitoring and managing your dosages to see if you can benefit from combined or replacement therapy. In my experience, mild to moderate depression and anxiety can be controlled with herbs, but more severe problems cannot. In Section Three, we will examine the possibility of adopting a comprehensive holistic program to get some people off these drugs.

If you are considering combining herbal therapy with prescription medicines, recognize that additive effects (potentiation) or other problems are possible. Do this only with professional supervision. Don't tell yourself, "My doctor won't understand, so I'll do this without telling him." Try to find a physician trained in the use of herbal medicines.

Overuse or Improper Use of Laxatives

There are two areas to be concerned about from a biochemical perspective:

Selective serotonin reuptake inhibitors (SSRIs) are drugs like Paxil, Prozac, Zoloft, and Celexa. Herbs such as **St. John's wort** may interact with these medications and increase their action. On the other hand, if you are trying to come off these medications **St. John's wort** may be a gentle, helpful alternative during the transition period.

Monoamine oxidase inhibitors (MAOIs) are a class of enzymes used as antidepressant drugs, including Nardil, Parnate, Eldepryl, and Marplan. These drugs can potentially cause serious problems. It is a well-known fact that if you are taking one of these medications and you eat foods high in tyramine concentration, such as fermented cheeses, yeast-containing products, alcohol of any type, and pickled herring, you can experience a dramatic change in blood pressure (orthostatic hypotension) as well as headaches and irregular heartbeat.

Laxatives have two main actions. "Bulk-forming laxatives" are herbs or other substances that promote bowel movement by increasing the bulk of the stool. Overuse of these herbs can cause bowel obstruction, especially if they are not taken with enough fluids. They may also decrease absorption of your medications.

"Stimulant laxatives" contain chemicals called "anthraquinones," which act on the smooth muscles of the lower bowel. These chemicals gently stimulate peristalsis 8–12 hours after ingestion. Their effects on the gut are largely topical, and they flush out of the body without being absorbed. Long-term use can sometimes lead to dependence. They may also cause potassium loss, which could be dangerous if you are on heart medications.

Overuse or improper use of laxative herbs may cause loss of appetite, nausea, cramping, uterine contractions, diarrhea, and vomiting. It can also cause an electrolyte imbalance (loss of chemicals such as potassium) known by German doctors as "laxative colon." This condition can cause exhaustion and heart palpitations and may produce symptoms resembling paralysis. These problems increase parallel to the dosage, strength, and length of time the patient uses the herbs. If you are using laxatives and notice any symptoms remotely like those listed above, consult your doctor or herbalist.

Overuse or Misuse of Diuretic Herbs

If overused, strongly diuretic herbs may dehydrate the body or cause loss of potassium or other essential electrolytes. Dehydration itself can be a cause of inflammation, so I advise you to exercise caution if using these herbs long term. These herbs can also cause or worsen constipation by removing fluids from the intestines. TAM doctors warn that overuse of diuretics can weaken the kidneys. You must be especially careful if using these herbs along with commonly prescribed diuretic drugs (known as thiazide diuretics).

Digestive Problems Caused by Herbs

Some herbs can cause nausea, abdominal discomfort or burning, and diarrhea. This is especially true if they are taken in medicinal doses. Why does this happen? For the digestive system to function properly, the digestive fires should be regular in both amount and activity. Ayurvedic doctors tell us that anyone who digests food properly enjoys good health and plentiful energy. These people have a good appetite in the morning and evening when the stomach is empty; they experience regularity in peristaltic motion and defecation; there is a balance between the stomach and the intestine in which the acid and alkaline reactions act in harmony. A physician can diagnose problems in the digestive system simply through observation of these basic functions.

To maintain a strong digestive system, it is very important to follow a regular schedule for breakfast, lunch, and dinner, eating the appropriate amounts and varieties of healthy foods. The body naturally maintains its digestive strength when meals are regular. For example, if we always eat lunch at noon, the body will increase the secretion of digestive enzymes at that time.

**Common Food Sources
That Cause Goiter**

- Members of the cabbage family (*Brassica* species) including cabbage, turnip, rutabaga, and kale
- Cassava root (*Manihot* species), millet, peanuts, pine nuts, and raw soybeans
- Milk from cows that have eaten goitrogens
- Dietary excess of calcium or fluorine
- High levels of indigestible crude fiber, which may bind the thyroxine secreted in the bile and prevent its reabsorption

---

This phenomenon is easy to identify in people who have developed the unhealthy habit of eating a meal right before bed. If they force themselves not to eat at that time for a few weeks, they will find that their bedtime hunger disappears. Overeating or not eating at all when the stomach is empty will also damage the digestive power. In addition, large quantities of meats, sweets, greasy foods, and milk products tend to weaken digestion, especially if eaten when the stomach is already full.

Diarrhea can sometimes be caused by poor or incomplete digestion. When the body detects a foreign substance beyond its digestive capacity, such as bitter herbs that have been ingested suddenly, it simply lets go of the substance as a defensive reaction. Medicinal herbs, by definition, contain large quantities of various strong-tasting components. These preparations are highly concentrated vegetables. If the digestive system is overly sensitive or weak, the strong tastes are likely to upset the stomach, causing nausea or diarrhea. The simplest way to overcome this problem is to reduce the dosage until it matches your digestive capacity. Alternatively, drink some **ginger tea,** a reliable antinausea agent, or add some digestion-strengthening herbs.

If digestive problems continue, you need to identify the cause of the problem and correct it. We will examine digestion in more detail in Chapter 11.

Herbs That Modify Thyroid Function

"Goitrogens" are substances that may block the use of thyroid hormone and induce goiter formation. They include a wide variety of substances found in food and water, including industrial waste. Persons who have a history of goiter or diminished thyroid function, or are taking thyroid medications, may need to be careful with some of these herbs and foods. The cooking process is thought to inactivate many of the vegetable goitrogens, such as cabbage family plants, so only raw forms of these foods need to be avoided. Some herbs affect thyroid function in a variety of ways, and they can be used to treat thyroid disorders when prescribed by a qualified practitioner. These plants may raise, lower, or regulate thyroid function.

Herbs That May Alter Thyroid Function

Betel leaf *(Areca catechu):* dual role, inhibits or stimulates thyroid function depending on dosage

Bugleweed leaf *(Lycopus* species): inhibits thyroid function

Coleus root *(Coleus forskohlii):* may stimulate thyroid function

Guggul gum *(Commiphora mukul / Balsamodendron mukul):* may stimulate thryoid function

Holy basil leaf *(Ocimum sanctum):* may inhibit thyroid function

Lemon balm leaf *(Melissa officinalis):* may inhibit thyroid function

Lithospermum root *(Lithospermum* species): inhibits thyroid function, may reduce thyroid swelling

Mother of thyme plant *(Thymus serpyllum):* inhibits thyroid function

Stoneseed plant *(Lithospermum* species*):* inhibits thyroid function, may reduce thyroid swelling

Xing ren seed *(Prunus armeniaca):* inhibits thyroid function, may reduce thyroid swelling

Zi cao root *(Lithospermum* species): inhibits thyroid function, may reduce thyroid swelling

---

Herbs That Affect Blood Sugar

Many herbs have blood-sugar-lowering effects. Some of the herbs listed in the Appendix are based upon traditional usage for diabetes, some upon animal experiments documenting blood-sugar-lowering effects, and some upon experiments done with humans. The list is not complete, and there are likely hundreds of other plants that can lower blood sugar. Although these effects are often mild, they may cause problems for some hypoglycemics or diabetics. I have rarely seen this occur, but it is difficult for many people to identify the signs of low blood sugar. These include weakness, shakiness, dizziness, a drop in blood pressure, and sometimes ravenous hunger. The only three substances I have seen strongly affect blood sugars unexpectedly in our clinic are chromium picolinate, **ginseng root,** and **gymnema leaves** *(Gymnema sylvestre)*. I suggest you monitor your blood sugar carefully if you are taking any of these herbs. You can find a complete list in the Appendix.

Herbs that raise blood sugar when used in a therapeutic dosage are much rarer, though any sugar- or carbohydrate-containing fruit or plant will raise blood sugar if enough is consumed.

Essential/Volatile Oils

"Essential" or "volatile" oils are complex concentrated chemicals distilled from plants. There is an entire field of herbal medicine, called "aromatherapy," that describes the use of these oils. One drop of essential oil often requires 1 ounce of plant to produce it. In fact, it takes more than 60,000 **rose petals** to produce 1 ounce of **rose oil!**

Due to their range of strong scents, these oils have been studied extensively by perfume manufacturers. Chemically, they tend to be mixtures of oxygenated hydrocarbons, their polymers, and alcohols. A volatile oil from a specific plant will be a blend of a whole range of chemical components. In addition to producing strong odors, such oils are highly antiseptic and antifungal and can even be used as insect repellents. **These oils can really burn your skin if you are not careful. Never apply them or even touch them undiluted.**

If you decide to use them externally, handle the oils carefully. Wash your hands after each use and avoid eye contact. I do not recommend using the oils internally unless they are prescribed by a competent herbalist. If you take too much or use a preparation that is too concentrated, it can cause intestinal inflammation, kidney inflammation, and even kidney infection.

I got a call from a woman who had developed severely itchy hives and wanted to know if she could avoid steroids and use herbs to control the problem. I questioned her about her habits and found out that a multilevel marketer had convinced her that taking 25 drops of pure **eucalyptus oil** in water every day would cure her chronic toenail infections. She did this for 2 weeks before her skin developed the color and texture of lobster claws.

Using Herbs While Pregnant or Breast-Feeding

Using herbs when pregnant or breast-feeding is a serious subject. In the early stages of pregnancy, the fetus is highly susceptible to even minute amounts of chemicals. The cells of the newly formed miracle are changing rapidly and are thus open to many influences including enzymes, oxidative chemicals, and the like. Anything that influences cell division or fetal circulation can be problematic. Careless use of foreign substances such as coffee, alcohol, pills, or herbs is just plain irresponsible. Exercise extreme caution and consult professionals in these instances.

I do not recommend using herbs while pregnant, unless under the direction of a trained professional. The nutrition that comes from using a good prenatal multivitamin is usually sufficient supplementation. TCM doctors, naturopaths, and other herbal professionals are trained to prescribe some simple herbs during pregnancy for problems like morning sickness.

Personally I like the TAM philosophy concerning pregnancy. Ayurveda prefers that women and men prepare themselves for pregnancy prior to conception by using herbs and meditation practices to purify the system. Prayer and fasting are part of these practices in India and Nepal, but the basic idea could be modified according to your own beliefs. If this is done, hopefully there will be less need for medicine during pregnancy. I discuss this more in Chapter 19.

Breast-feeding is another concern. Strong herbs may pass through the breast milk. This can be good when using the safest herbs. TAM doctors, for example, say that small amounts of common bitter herbs such as **turmeric root** are good for purifying the breast milk. Other sources suggest avoiding herbs containing strong alkaloids. I have compiled a list of herbs, gathered from several authoritative sources, to avoid during pregnancy or breast-feeding. Many of these, such as **turmeric**, are not necessarily dangerous to use, but I see absolutely no reason to take any chances, so I have listed them all. Again, these lists cannot be totally exhaustive. Many of the herbs are listed based upon theoretical concerns. For example, **rosemary** contains volatile oils but probably would only be problematic if taken in high doses. Herbs that contain phytoestrogens are included, but theoretical concerns have not been proven. Some of the teratogenic research is done on animals, and at high doses. Remember, dosage is everything in toxicology. As time goes by, safety testing will no doubt show that some of the herbs on this list are indeed safe to use.

I do not want to put pregnant women with health problems in the unfortunate position of having to choose between herbal medicines, which have not undergone safety studies, and Western prescription medicines, which have undergone such studies, but which may potentially be more difficult for the body to handle. Therefore, again, **pregnancy is a time when it is very important to consult with a skilled professional herbalist, holistic physician, or naturopath trained in the use of herbs.** I fully expect that as knowledge in this field improves, we will rediscover ancient methods and also find new ways to use herbal medicines to benefit unborn children. See the Resource Guide to find a qualified herbalist. Also, refer to the Appendix for a comprehensive list of herbs to avoid during pregnancy and breast-feeding.

Herbs That Can Kill

Certain herbs used commonly in the past are now known to be poisonous and are no longer available except to professionals. **Belladonn**a *(Atropa belladonna),* for example, was once used in Europe and North Africa to dilate the pupils because people thought this would increase beauty. Excess use causes a blocking of the autonomic nervous system, dry eyes, rapid heartbeat, and even stupor and coma. Of course you can't find capsules of **belladonna** or **deathcap toadstool** in your health food store.

Some herbs should be avoided because they can be toxic to the liver, especially those with a high alkaloid content (for a complete listing of these herbs, refer to the Appendix). **Comfrey root** *(Symphytum officinalis)* and **coltsfoot flower** *(Tussilago farfara)* contain substances called "pyrrolizidine alkaloids" (PAs) that can cause obstructive liver damage. They have been shown to cause veno-occlusive disease, endothelial cell glutathione depletion, central vein necrosis, thrombosis, and fibrosis, all very serious conditions. It is probably safe to consider these herbs for short-term internal use under expert medical guidance in certain cases, but long-term use should be avoided.

There is currently controversy over whether the use of the PA-containing herbs for short periods of time is safe, considering the track records of use of many of these herbs in the past versus the fact that negative effects can accumulate over time. The jury is still out. Fortunately, some companies, such as Herb Pharm, now make pyrrolizidine-free comfrey. This can be used safely and confidently for longer periods of time. The herb extracts (which contain PAs) are run through an ion exchange bed that removes the PAs. The finished extract contains less than 1 ppm of PAs.

Germander *(Teucrium chamaedrys)* contains furanoditerpenoids, chemicals that have been shown to cause hepatitis, hepatocyte glutathione depletion, and apoptosis. In other words, it can severely damage your liver. This herb is not sold to the public, of course, but has been known in the past to be substituted for the commonly used herb **skullcap** *(Scutellaria laterifolia).* They look almost identical in the field.

Aristolochic acid is a chemical found primarily in plants from the genus *Aristolochia.* This chemical has been shown to cause rapid kidney failure. The Chinese herb *Aristolochia fangqi* has, in the past, commonly been substituted for **stephania root** *(Stephania tetranda)* and **magnolia bark** *(Magnolia officinalis).* There have been cases of serious poisoning in Europe resulting in death, and a ban of this herb was instituted in the European Union in 1999. Importation into the United States is now prohibited.

Yohimbe *(Corynanthe yohimbe)* is an African herb that has been used as an aphrodisiac and a weight-loss aid. Overdose can lead to numerous side effects, including paralysis. I would avoid this herb, especially as it is available as a prescription item, and there are other herbs that perform better for the same intended uses.

Some herbs are very toxic in their natural state and must be purified (neutralized) before use:

You might be surprised to learn that **ginkgo leaf** is mildly toxic until ginkgolic acids are removed. **Aconitum** species plants contain deadly poisonous alkaloids, and are used medicinally only in purified form.

One alkaloid called **aconitine** is extraordinarily poisonous. Ayurvedic doctors neutralize poisons in **aconite** by steaming in cow's or goat's milk for 3 hours and restricting dosage to $\frac{1}{40}$ gram (fatal dosage is only 1–2 grams). Chinese doctors neutralize the poisons by various means, such as soaking the herb in salt, then boiling it with **licorice root** and **black soybeans.**

These alkaloids initially stimulate your system, then cause paralysis in the motor and sensory nerve endings, as well as the central nervous system. Intestinal absorption of the alkaloids is rapid, so gastric lavage is recommended in overdose. Keep the patient warm and go immediately to the emergency room.

SECTION

TWO

GETTING TO KNOW
YOUR HERBS

CHAPTER 6

The Language of Herbs:
Essential Concepts and Vocabulary

Under the most rigorously controlled conditions of pressure, temperature, humidity, and other variables, the organism will do as it damn well pleases.

—Anonymous

We spent most of our time in Section One reviewing issues concerning the herbal marketplace, including how to obtain good-quality, safe herbal medicines. In this section we are going to learn more about what herbs actually do, and how to understand the way herbalists in America and other parts of the world think about them. To do this you need to have a basic herbal vocabulary. This will give you a definite advantage as you explore the literature and products in today's marketplace.

Each of the major traditions uses key concepts and words to describe how herbs work on the body. I am going to introduce some of these terms in this chapter. I would like to point out that certain concepts drawn from the Eastern herbal traditions may seem unfamiliar and perhaps even primitive to Western ears. Also, pharmacological words like *proanthocyanin,* though sometimes easier to accept as valid (because we all trust scientific terminology), often are more difficult to recall due to their complexity. Just sound out the words and don't worry too much about pronunciation.

Unfortunately, the language of our modern Western medical culture seems to have lost some of these descriptive terms illustrating ideas that plant-based societies have embraced over time. Think of this chapter as a map of a foreign country. All the words on the map seem unfamiliar at first, but you need to know some of them to get around. Once learned, they make the world of herbal medicine much easier to understand. My purpose in teaching these ideas is to provide you, as a consumer, access to the traditions of Eastern and Western herbal medicine through familiarity with basic ideas. This will allow you to choose and learn about herbs more effectively.

By introducing concepts from different traditions in the same chapter, I am not giving you license to mix them indiscriminately. This can prove unworkable, as illustrated quite well in the old tale about a young boy's experience in the jungle. He examines all the wild animals and identifies in each the one characteristic he believes is exceptional. The boy then travels throughout the jungle, taking the "best" feature of each animal. When all is said and done, he has transformed himself into a fantastic creature with the tail of a monkey, the trunk of an elephant, the claws of a lion, and the horn of a rhinoceros. Unfortunately, due to the bizarre nature of his new physical form, the boy is unable to walk and all the animals in the jungle are afraid of him.

Why Integrate Knowledge from Different Cultures?

I once saw a cartoon in which a beaker was filled with round billiard balls labeled "money" and square blocks labeled "politics." The caption underneath read, "Money and politics do not mix." In the same way, it is difficult to know how to successfully combine the principles of the different herbal traditions. How do you determine which Western herbs you should use to treat a patient whose health problem is best described by the Chinese as "deficiency of kidney Yin," or results from "reversed Vata," as determined by Ayurvedic diagnosis?

It is clear to those of us who have taken the time to study natural medicine systems from around the world that there is vast clinical benefit in these teachings. Much of what is called "scientific herbalism" is simply the result of scientists personally checking out certain traditional therapeutic claims and deeming them valid or invalid. The same principles will work for you; in time, your choices of herbs will become much more accurate and your results more consistently satisfying.

How to Learn from Other Cultural Systems of Herbology

I once challenged a Western-trained herbalist to take the 500 best-known herbs of TCM and, using the tools of pharmacology and Western scientific analysis, compound a formula that could stabilize chronic nephritis. He declined, knowing how daunting a task this would be. However, Chinese and Japanese scientists were easily able to identify a few formulas and herbs that could do exactly that, simply by asking trained TCM doctors to choose classic formulas based upon the theories of TCM.

Contrary to common belief, the human mind does not necessarily learn or store information in a purely sequential, logical form. Rather, we learn through a succession of experiences that ripen our understanding at each stage and consequently displace or enhance our knowledge with each progression. The human learns, albeit on a smaller scale, in a manner similar to that in which an entire culture acquires and integrates knowledge.

Humans have an innate desire to conserve energy, a characteristic that can inhibit intellectual growth and development. The manner in which we acquire, internalize, and apply new information requires us to tap into the body's precious energy stores. Therefore, we have a natural anthropological tendency to reject unfamiliar information or avoid opportunities to learn new things in the interest of conserving energy.

This not only is a detriment to the individual learning process, but also acts as a barrier to the growth and expansion of entire cultures. Oriental teachers thus always stress to their reluctant students the necessity of learning basic concepts in depth to build a solid educational foundation.

Upon examining various herbal medicine teachings from around the world, we discover a universal common thread—the focus of attention on the health of the human body. The advantage of this shared focus is simple. It is easier to accept and integrate concepts from different cultures once you reconcile the notion that, although you think your method is best, there is more than one way to skin a cat. Integrating concepts from other cultures

> According to Sufi teachings, we can use a simple question to illustrate the complexity of concept integration and acceptance. Is an orange a round, soft, sweet-smelling object, is it something to eat, or is it a container for genetic material useful for the growing of orange trees? It is, of course, all three (not to mention a good source of useful vitamin C and citrus bioflavonoids).

affords us the same variation of perspective as would seeing the world through a new pair of eyeglass lenses every day, each of a different color. Seeing the world through the green of Ayurveda provides a different slant from the yellow of modern science or the red of Chinese medicine.

By applying various principles from each system of thought we can find countless ways to approach the same problems. For instance, a Western-trained doctor might not accept the idea of "dampness" in the muscles or stomach as easily as a Chinese or Ayurvedic practitioner. Consequently, it would be difficult for this Western doctor to establish the correct remedy or even entertain the notion of using certain herbs to treat this problem, especially when the caregiver is not famil-

> I remember talking to Dr. Mana many years ago as he described the diagnostic breakdown of a particular disease into four groups, although further division into six groups was possible. When I asked why this was done, he told me, "These classifications are based upon the examinations of thousands and thousands of patients, through which doctors discovered that this disease usually fell into one of these four diagnostic categories, and rarely the other two."

iar with the nature of the complaint. However, if you introduce visible physical swelling into the equation, the same Western doctor will have a much easier time diagnosing and treating the problem. To be truly effective, a practitioner must come to understand the coexistence of different physical health principles. This type of acceptance can be reached only through a willingness to incorporate and apply the teachings of different healing traditions. In fact, we may already be doing this, but it is better if we make it a conscious effort.

The set of ideas through which we ascribe herbal actions and physical symptoms to particular conditions is known collectively as **herbal energetics.** Herbalists Michael and Lesley Tierra, developers of the "East-West Home Herbal Medicine" study course, were among the first herbal practitioners to identify the need for an eventual integration of the large world medical systems with the publication of their book *Planetary Herbology.* In the book, Michael writes about how he told his teachers in China that he believed there was a need for classification of our native North American herbs into the energetic system of Chinese medicine. They said that what he proposed could not be done, because it had taken the efforts of countless herbalists over many centuries to evolve such a complete system. Tierra tells us that after many years of pondering this problem, he agrees that a single individual cannot accomplish this process. "All I may hope to achieve is a modest beginning." But how do we even begin this process? Part of Dr. Tierra's effort entailed preliminary classification of many herbs from around the world according to energetic principles. Thanks to his efforts, *Planetary Herbology* still stands as an excellent model for integration.

A Note on Semantics

It is important when discussing herbs to know and trust the source of your information. In an editorial in *Modern Phyto-Therapist,* herbalists Kerry Bone and Nicholas Burgess point out the very important distinction between knowledge based upon anecdotal information and coincidence and traditional, proven knowledge. They tell us that "valid traditional use is the refined knowledge of many generations, carefully evaluated and re-evaluated by many of the practitioners of the craft. It is not just the anecdotal accounts of a few practitioners. When traditional use is part of a great system and culture, the information therein should be rated highly because it has evolved over many years and been tried on large numbers of people." This point can be applied not only to information on specific herbs, but also to the use of herbal concepts like Yin and Yang to differentiate different disease processes.

How Herbs Are Named

To navigate the herbal world successfully, it is very important to understand how herbs are named. The hundreds of thousands of plants and herbs in our world have an unbelievably wide variety of names. The name given to a plant in its local geographic region is known as the common name, and there are no rules for assigning these names. For example, the word **echinacea,** now a familiar term to many people venturing into the world of herbs, may describe any one of several species of coneflower plants. Fortunately, a plant usually has only one or two Latin names. However, one can easily become confused by common names, which can number into the dozens for a single plant.

To solve the problem of naming plants, the Swedish biologist Linnaeus developed our modern method of taxonomy in the 1700s, using the **Latin binomial** method. In this model, plants are divided into many different families. Within families, each plant is given at least two Latin names, which are always italicized. The first Latin name represents the genus—the main subdivision of a plant family—which is comprised of many different species.

The particular species of each plant is then reflected in the second Latin name. For example, the Latin name for the herb **kava root** is *Piper methysticum. Piper* is the name for the pepper genus, and *methysticum* is the particular species. *Piper nigrum*, on the other hand, refers to **black pepper.**

The Latin word ascribed to the species name describes some unique characteristic of the plant, such as its color. For example, *Paeonia rubra* is **red peony,** and *Echinacea purpurea* is **purple coneflower.** Due to its oval *(ovata)* shape, the **plantain leaf** is called *Plantago ovata.* Sometimes the geographical location is used to determine the species name, as in **poke root** *(Phytolacca americana),* a plant found in America. The Latin word *officinalis* or *officinale,* as in *Calendula officinalis* (**calendula flower**), is drawn from the historical knowledge that these plants were collected and categorized by European monks who kept them in small storerooms called officinae.

It is possible for a plant to have *two* different Latin names. This occurs because every few years, taxonomists revise the "International Code of Botanical Nomenclature," sometimes even adding new rules for naming plants. There is a transition period following these changes, during which both names are used. For example, **guggul gum** refers to the gum of the plant named guggul in Sanskrit, but guggul has two Latin names, *Commiphora mukul* and *Balsamodendron mukul.*

Rules for Pronunciation

- When pronouncing Chinese herb names, the two most important things to remember are (1) that the letter *x* sounds like "sh," and (2) that the letter *q* sounds like "ch." For example, the Chinese herb **huo xiang** *(Agastache rugosa)* is pronounced "who-oh she-ang," and the herb **huang qin** *(Scutellaria baicalensis* / Chinese skullcap) is pronounced "who-ang chin."
- Sanskrit words pretty much sound as they are written, with slight melodic tones.
- Latin is a dead language, so your pronunciation doesn't have to be perfect. (Just act as though you know what you're doing.)

To make it as easy as possible for you to follow along in this book, I will strive always to refer to herbs by their **common names,** printed in **bold letters** to make them easier to spot. You will most likely find the common names easiest to pronounce and understand. The Latin name will follow the common name when appropriate for the sake of proper identification. I will also identify the part of each plant that is actually used, whether it is the root, the leaf, the flower, or some other portion. If no part is specified, you can assume that we use either multiple parts or the entire plant, as in the case of **black cohosh** *(Cimicifuga racemosa).* Chinese and Sanskrit names will probably be the most difficult to grasp, so it will help if you apply your knowledge of common name, plant part, and Latin nomenclature to identify herbs. You will then be able to deduce that **carthamus flower** refers to the flower of *Carthamus tinctorius,* also known in Chinese as hong hua.

Understanding Herbs by Their Dispensing Forms

Herbs come in many different forms. The most common are crude herbs, powders, dried decoctions, tinctures, capsules, gelcaps, salves, oils, and teas.

Crude herbs are simply collected and dried, then cut and sifted. This is the original way herbs have been prepared since the dawn of time. Crude herbs are commonly found in traditional herb shops around the world, and in ethnic neighborhoods in major cities in the United States. The advantage of this form is that you can actually see, taste, and smell the herbs. Crude herbs are usually taken home and cooked into teas.

Powders are simply ground crude herbs. You can use powders to make herbal tea or simply ingest them in their natural form. I like powders because they allow you to experience the taste and smell of the herbs you are using. Another benefit of this form is that you can often take larger doses of the herbs. However, powdered herbs do not last as long in storage as the other forms.

Teas are aqueous extractions of crude herbs or herbal powders. Most herbs today come in pills or tinctures, so to make sure we do not forget our herbal roots, I always keep some loose herb teas in the house. There are several methods of preparation for herbal tea. **Infusion,** better for delicate leaves and flowers, entails bringing water to a light boil, turning off the heat, and letting the herbs steep in the water. Leaving the crude herbs out in the sun for a couple of hours in a tightly sealed container makes **sun tea.** Simmering the herbs for anywhere from 10 minutes up to an hour (longer is better for the much heavier barks and roots) makes a **decoction.**

Tinctures are extracts made by soaking herbs in solutions designed to draw out their virtues. Alcohol is the most common soaking solution for tinctures. Tincture manufacturers must have recipe books to guide them, as the exact method will differ for each herb. Tinctures are valuable because they are easy to digest and absorb. Some herbs can be used only in this form. The strength of a tincture should be listed on the bottle in the form of a ratio, such as 1:5 or 1:2. The first number tells you how much of the herb is present, and the second number tells you how much menstruum (the liquid used to dissolve the herb) is in the preparation. Therefore, a 1:5 tincture is weaker than a 1:2 tincture, because a larger volume of liquid is used.

Dried decoctions, also called **concentrated granules,** are used primarily by Chinese (TCM) herbalists. This method of preparing herbs was devised several decades ago in

Taiwan by a group of chemists and traditional doctors. Basically, the herbs are cooked as teas in large vats and the solid residues are removed, after which the remaining liquids are dried out until only powders remain. Sometimes certain important components (such as volatile oils) are collected separately by specialized equipment and then added back to the final product. **These powders are usually about four times as potent as the crude herbs.** The label may list a **ratio** of 4:1, but concentration can be as low as 2:1 or even as high as 10:1. Dried decoctions still retain the herbs' basic tastes and smells, and the concentrations of chemicals discourage bacterial growth so they tend to store well. I use these granules frequently in my practice.

Concentrated herbal extracts are now made using various methods. These extracts, in liquid or solid form, can be anywhere from 2 to 100 times as concentrated in certain components as crude herbs.

Capsules are simply powdered herbs, dried decoctions, or concentrated herbal extracts that have been put into gelatin capsules.

Tablets are simply powdered herbs, dried decoctions, or concentrated herbal extracts with a binding substance added. They are then pressed into tablets by a machine.

Gelcaps are sealed gelatin capsules that hold either tinctures or concentrated liquid herbal extracts.

Understanding Herbs by Their Chemical Actions

Each individual herbal medicine is a unique package of nutrients capable of acting on the human body in a variety of ways. Following is a list of some common chemical actions of herbal medicines.

- Herbs can promote the action (reduction) of antioxidants, capturing and eliminating the destructive energy of free radicals (unpaired electrons).

- Nutrients in many herbs can nourish specific tissues even to the point of helping repair damaged DNA strands.

- Chemicals found in certain herbs and foods can up- and down-regulate various biological activities, including cell division and genetic expression.

- Herbs can reduce and modulate various inflammatory processes.

- Herbs can alter the activity of the digestive flora, affecting the chemical balance of the digestive system.

- Nutrients found in certain herbs can enhance the action of adenosine triphosphate (ATP), the basic process necessary for the body to produce energy.

- Herbs can affect the chemical reactions taking place in the liver, necessary for neutralization of toxins.

- Herbs can stimulate all components of the body's immunity, including every aspect of immune function and every immune cell.

- Herbs can affect intracellular, intercellular, and extracellular communication.

- Herbs can stimulate or suppress specific bodily actions, such as urination, defecation, digestion, wake and sleep, night vision, breathing, and muscle tension.

Understanding Some Important Herbal Actions

The word **action** refers to the influence an herb exerts on the body. There are literally hundreds of terms used to describe herbal actions, but those listed below are the most common and are necessary for you to understand the process of healing. These words are derived chiefly from Western herbal traditions, and many of the terms are used in modern allopathic medicine.

Adaptogens are strengthening herbs that bring balance back to the body no matter what the direction of imbalance. They combine both tonic and balancing properties. Examples include **Siberian ginseng root bark** *(Eleutherococcus senticosus)* and **jiao gulan leaves/stem** *(Gynostemma pentaphyllum).*

Alteratives are herbs that increase elimination of metabolic waste via the liver, large intestine, lungs, lymphatic system, skin, and kidneys. Examples include **burdock root** *(Arctium lappa),* **dandelion root** *(Taraxacum officinale),* **red clover blossom** *(Trifolium pratense),* and **Tu fu ling rhizome** *(Smilax glabra).*

Amphoterics, from the Greek *amphoteros* or "both," are herbs that normalize hyper- or hypofunction of different organs or regulatory systems. Examples include **licorice root** *(Glycyrrhiza glabra),* **cordyceps mushroom** *(Cordyceps sinensis* / dong chong xia cao), and **Siberian ginseng** *(Eleutherococcus senticosus).*

Antimicrobials are herbs that reduce or diminish the activity of bacteria, fungi, and viruses. Examples include **isatis root** *(Isatis tinctoria),* **oregano** *(Origanum* species), and **horseradish** *(Armoracia rusticana).*

Antiseptic herbs are those that can be applied to the body externally to inhibit bacterial growth. Examples include **tea tree oil** and **oregano oil.**

Aphrodisiac herbs are those that stimulate sexual desire and potency. Examples include

potency bark *(Ptychopetalum olacoides* / Muira puama) and **ashwagandha root** *(Convolvulus* species / *Withania somnifera).*

Demulcents are soothing mucilaginous or oily substances that can be taken internally to soothe and protect damaged or inflamed tissue. One common example is **slippery elm bark** *(Ulmus rubra).*

Diuretics are herbs that stimulate the flow of urine and help remove fluids from the body. Common examples are **dandelion leaf** *(Taraxacum officinale)* and **coffee** *(Coffea arabica).*

Emollient herbs are those that are applied externally to soften and soothe the skin. One common example is **olive oil** *(Olea europaea).*

Emmenagogues are herbs that stimulate and promote menstruation. **Turmeric root** and **chaste tree berry** are emmenagogues.

Expectorants are herbs that assist the body in expelling mucus from the upper respiratory tract. One common example is **licorice root** *(Glycyrrhiza glabra).*

Hemostatic herbs are those that stop bleeding. One common example is **tien chi root** *(Panax pseudoginseng).*

Laxative herbs are those that stimulate or promote bowel movements. There are two classes of laxative herbs. **Bulk-forming laxatives** increase the water and bulk of the stool. One common example is **flaxseed** *(Linum usitatissimum).* **Stimulant laxatives** invigorate the muscles of the lower bowel. One common example is **rhubarb root** *(Rheum emodi).*

Nervines are herbs that calm and soothe the nervous system and emotions. Examples include **milky oat seed** *(Avena sativa)* and **skullcap** *(Scutellaria laterifolia).*

Stimulants are herbs that increase metabolism and mental activity. Examples include **ephedra** *(Ephedra sinica* / ma huang), **coffee bean** *(Coffea arabica),* and **ginseng root** *(Panax ginseng* / ren shen).

Tonics are herbs that strengthen or tone general energy, specific organs, or organ systems. They act to strengthen the immune system and can even help slow the aging process. Examples include **ginseng root, Siberian ginseng, astragalus root** *(Astragalus membranaceus* / huang qi), **shilajatu**, and **shou wu root** *(Polygonum multiflorum).*

Understanding Yin, Yang, and Qi

The triad of **Yin**, **Yang**, and **Qi** (pronounced "chee") serves as the basis for the medical theory of TCM. Entire textbooks have been written about this subject in China, and one could argue that similar mechanisms are found everywhere in the universe, even at the molecular level. For our purposes we are going to simplify this philosophy as much as possible, while describing the terms as understood by TCM doctors.

The essential thing to know is that TCM doctors use these broad general medical terms to orient their medical thinking, diagnose disease, and choose herbs. The purpose is to bring these three into balance. In Chinese theory this process is conceived as bringing Yin and Yang into balance with each other, which results in the production of Qi.

Yin represents the nutritive processes and substances of the body. When the Yin is strong, the body is strong, moist, well nourished, and fertile. When the Yin is in excess, the body, or the individual organ, becomes sluggish and damp. When the Yin is weak, the body is weak, dry, deficient, and can flare up with heat. There can be sensitivity to heat, weight loss, insomnia, hot flashes, dryness, and sometimes dizziness and heart palpitations.

This presentation of symptoms is known as **Yin deficiency**, a very important TCM medical concept. To treat Yin deficiency, TCM herbalists use **Yin tonic herbs**. These herbs generally nourish and moisten the tissues and increase nutritive forces.

Some of the most commonly used Yin tonics are **raw rehmannia root** (sheng di huang / *Rehmannia glutinosa*), **glehnia root** (sha shen / *Adenophora tetraphylla*), **scrophularia root** (xuan shen / *Scrophularia ningpoensis*), **ligustrum berry** (nu shen zi / *Ligustrum lucidum*), **American ginseng root** (xi yang shen /*Panax quinquifolius*), **ophiopogon root** (mai men dong /*Ophiopogon japonicus*), and **wild asparagus root** (tian men dong / *Asparagus lucidis*).

Notice that many of the Yin tonics are roots, used by plants to absorb nutrients from the soil. Interestingly, the Chinese use seeds, such as **sesame seeds,** as Yin tonics. At our clinic I often use nutritive oils like **flaxseed oil** *(Linum usitatissimum)* or **evening primrose oil** *(Oenothera biennis)* along with the above herbs to moisturize and reduce inflammation.

Yang represents the heat and metabolic processes of the body. When the Yang is strong the body is energetic, warm, and powerful. When the Yang is in excess, the body becomes inflamed. When the Yang is weak the body is fatigued, cold, and weak, often to the point of exhaustion. There can be symptoms of low back pain, impotence, diarrhea, and weakness in the four extremities. These symptoms are known as **Yang deficiency**. TCM doctors use **Yang tonic herbs** to treat Yang deficiency. These herbs are generally warming and drying. Chinese research has shown that many of these herbs benefit the endocrine system.

Some of the most commonly used Yang tonic herbs are **prepared aconite** (fu zi / *Aconitum palmatum*), **dried ginger root** (gan jiang / *Zingiber officinalis*), **cinnamon bark** (rou gui / *Cinnamomum zeylanicum*), **deer antler** (lu rong / *Cervus nipon*), and **morinda root** (ba ji tian / *Morinda officinalis*).

Qi (sometimes spelled as "Chi") represents the vital energy of the body flowing along invisible energy channels. The balance of Qi is dependent upon the functional relationship between Yin and Yang. When the Qi is strong, the digestion is strong, the organs are well regulated, and nourishment and energy flow through and vitalize the organs. When the Qi is weak or blocked, the digestion weakens, dampness accumulates, and the corresponding organs exhibit pain, spasm, or irregular functioning. There can be extreme fatigue, poor digestion, diarrhea, muscle atrophy, compromised immunity, or weakness in the lungs. This is called **Qi deficiency.** When Qi is weak, TCM doctors use herbs that supply Qi, known as **Qi tonics.** The most common Qi tonic herbs are **ginseng root, astragalus root, codonopsis root** (dang shen / *Codonopsis pilosula),* **licorice root,** and **white atractylodes rhizome**.

The easiest way to understand how these herbs work is to substitute the word *nutrient* when you see the word *Yin, metabolism or heat* when you see the word *Yang,* and *vital force* when you see the word *Qi.*

It may help you remember the triad by using the following analogy found in ancient Chinese medical texts. Think of the stomach as a pot of soup. The **Yin** represents the nutrients in the soup, and the **Yang** is the fire under the soup. The **Qi** is the nutrient-filled steam that rises up from the pot when Yin and Yang work together. This nutrient steam travels through tiny pathways in the body (meridians), carrying its warmth and nutrients to the organs. If the pathways are blocked, the restricted area becomes painful, and the organs beyond it wither from lack of energy and nutrition. If the blockage occurs in the larger channels flowing up and down between the trunk of the body and the brain, the person becomes depressed, constricted, and less creative. Because "the mind directs the Qi," one major goal of meditation is to strengthen the Qi energy and use the mind to feel and direct its flow throughout the body.

Understanding Ayurveda's Vata, Pitta, and Kapha

Vata, Pitta, and **Kapha** (called the Tridoshas) are terms central to the study of health in Traditional Ayurvedic Medicine (TAM). They correspond very closely with the TCM terms *Qi, Yang,* and *Yin,* respectively. Kapha and Pitta are the respective creative and destructive forces of the universe. Vata, the third principle, is an animating force that regulates the eternal interplay of the first two. From this basic philosophical idea Ayurvedic doctors proceed to an understanding of how the body works in a very specific and useful way. They understand these philosophical terms to represent both metaphysical and physical realities. Vata, Pitta, and Kapha operate at several levels simultaneously, from the universal to the specific, traversing several categories of Western thought.

The *Susruta Samhita,* written over 2,000 years ago, states, "Vata, Pitta and Kapha are the primary essential principles animating the human organism. . . . The human body is supported by the three fundamental principles in the same way a house is supported by its foundation."

How does this relate to our bodies? Vata, which regulates movement, can be equated with nervous system functioning. Kapha, which regulates creative processes, can be equated with (or seen in action within) the arterial supply of nutrients. Pitta, which regulates destructive processes, can be equated with venous and hepatic drainage of metabolic wastes. These direct physical associations make this system of understanding practical.

Specific treatments for specific diseases are recorded in all the major Ayurvedic treatment texts. Every disease is categorized in terms of its relationship to Vata, Pitta, and Kapha. When the patient visits the TAM doctor, a comprehensive diagnostic process is done to determine the location, degree of severity, and nature of any imbalances among these three.

Depending on the training and experience of the Ayurvedic physician, the examination might include various tests, tongue and pulse diagnosis, physical exams, review of symptoms, and extensive questioning. These would help identify physical, mental, emotional, and accidental causes or factors contributing to the problem.

Once the diagnostic profile was completed, the patient would usually be given medicines or treatments for the specific problem, along with treatments to balance the system as a whole, including counseling on diet and lifestyle.

Vata is linked to the nervous system. When Vata is out of balance, the result is Vata dosha, which is recognized by the general symptoms of dryness, sharp pain, shooting pulse, coldness, excess movement, and so on. Herbs that are used to correct Vata imbalances are generally nourishing (sweet), strengthening to the digestion, calming, and moisturizing. Important Ayurvedic herbs used to treat Vata imbalances include **ashwagandha root, bala, and gokshura fruit** *(Tribulus terrestris).*

Pitta is linked to inflammation and removal of metabolic wastes from the body. Pitta is recognizable by symptoms such as excess heat, movement, burning pain, strong odors, and racing pulse. Herbs that reduce Pitta are generally nourishing, cooling, detoxifying, and astringent. Important Ayurvedic herbs that correct Pitta imbalances include **licorice root** (madhukam /*Glycyrrhiza glabra),* **vasaca leaves** *(Adhatoda vasica),* **boswellia bark/gum** (shallaki / *Boswellia serrata),* **neem leaves** (nimba / *Azadirachta indica),* **guduchi stem** *(Tinospora cordifolia),* **turmeric root** (haridra / *Curcuma longa),* **red sandalwood** (rakta chandanam / *Pterocarpus santalinus),* and **white sandalwood** (chandanam /*Santalum album).*

Kapha is linked to the arterial supply of nutrients via the blood serum. Kapha disorders invariably involve disordered arterial supply of nutrients to the tissues and excess production of mucus. Herbs that reduce excess Kapha are generally purifying, warming, mucus-reducing, and astringent. Important Ayurvedic herbs that correct Kapha imbalances include **guggul gum** *(Commiphora mukul / Balsamodendron mukul),* **turmeric root** (haridra / *Curcuma longa),* **black pepper** (maricham /*Piper nigrum),* **long pepper** (pipali / *Piper longum),* and **vidanga seeds** *(Embelia ribes).*

Understanding Herbs by Their Tastes

Both TAM and TCM doctors describe herbs from the point of view of their tastes, believing that the flavor of the herb provides information about how it will act in the body. To me, any herbalist who doesn't know the taste of an herb but attempts to use it can be compared to a painter who doesn't know the colors of the rainbow, or a musician who doesn't know the scales. These terms are generalizations and must be used together with other markers to determine and define the actions of herbs. The following is a simplified version of how TAM doctors describe the basic tastes:

Sweet herbs and foods tend to nourish, cool, moisten, and heal the tissues and strengthen physical energy. They should be used more when the body is weak and emaciated, and less when the body is heavy and sluggish. Grape juice is sweet.

Sour herbs and foods tend to warm the body and strengthen digestion. They should be used more when the body is weak and dry, and less when the body is hot and damp. Lemons are sour.

Salty herbs tend to increase appetite, promote digestion, moisten tissues, and soften and dissolve blockages. They should be used more when the body is dry, and less when the body is hot and damp. Obviously, salt is salty. Most meat is sweet and salty.

Bitter herbs tend to stimulate appetite and digestion, reduce mucous membrane secretions and perspiration, reduce inflammation, and counteract toxins. They should be used more when the body is inflamed and damp, and less when the body is nervous and dry. Coffee and radishes are bitter.

Pungent (hot, acrid, spicy) herbs tend to warm the body, strongly stimulate the appetite and digestion, disperse blockages, and stimulate the senses. They should be used more when the body is heavy and sluggish, and less when the body is nervous and inflamed. **Ginger root** and **cayenne pepper** *(Capsicum frutescens)* are pungent.

Astringent herbs and foods tend to heal and strengthen tissues, slow digestion, slow fluid leakage, bowel movements, and urination, reduce exudation, and constrict capillaries (enough to stop bleeding in some cases). They should be used more when the body is inflamed and damp, and less when the body is nervous and dry. The astringent taste tends to accompany sweet and sour foods. **Pomegranate seeds** are sour and astringent. **Betel nuts** *(Areca catechu),* **guavas,** and unripe **bananas** are sweet and astringent.

Understanding the Heating and Cooling Properties of Herbs

All the major traditional systems of herbal medicine recognize that some herbs warm or heat the body, while others cool. Any herb can be classified in this way. Herbs that are warming tend to dilate the capillaries and bring vitality into tissues, while herbs that are cooling tend to constrict the capillaries and/or reduce heat and inflammation. The medical term *inflammation* is similar to the herbal medicine term *heat,* though there are differences in the way it is used in different traditions. For example, in TCM these terms are sometimes further divided according to the strength of the sign in the following sequence: cold, cool, neutral, warm, and hot. Neutral herbs can be used to treat either hot or cold diseases.

TCM doctors point out that there is more importance to this than meets the eye. They believe the human body developed as part of the natural cycle of day and night, living always in the heat of day alternating with the relative cool of night. However, when the body cannot properly regulate its temperatures, problems occur. Therefore, traditional herbal doctors might alter their view of specific symptoms and treat patients with different herbs depending on the seasons. Knowing whether an herb is warming or cooling is important when making treatment choices. During a spell of summer heat, for example, more cooling herbs may be indicated for use in a formula than are usually used during other seasons.

As simple as this seems, it can sometimes be confusing in application. In asthma, for example, it is necessary to dilate (warm) and relax the muscles surrounding the lungs. For menstrual cramping, it is necessary to relax the muscles of the uterus. For hepatitis, it is important to constrict (cool) the dilated vessels in the liver.

Following are some basic guidelines regarding the heating and cooling actions of herbs.

- "Heating herbs" tend to strongly affect the liver, heart, and brain. It is important to make sure that heating herbs do not worsen inflammation.

- "Cooling herbs" strongly affect the stomach and gastrointestinal (GI) tract, the kidneys, and the bladder. It is very important to make sure that cooling herbs do not harm digestion. Long-term use of very cold herbs can definitely weaken digestion.

- "Heating herbs" are generally used to treat cold diseases, while cooling herbs are applied with hot diseases.

- Heating and cooling effects are somewhat subjective, so formulas are adjusted after initial use to reflect changes in heat and cold as they occur in the body.

- If you use other herbs in the formula to balance the temperature characteristics, it is possible to use a cold herb in a cold condition, or a hot herb in a hot condition.

- Sweet, bitter, and astringent herbs tend to be cooling. Sour, salty, and pungent herbs tend to be heating.

Postdigestive Effects of Herbs

Ayurvedic doctors place great importance upon how herbs affect Vata (nerve function), Pitta (metabolic function), and Kapha (nutritive function) following digestion. Herbs often exhibit delayed or long-term effects, called **vipaka** in Sanskrit. This phenomenon is most clearly demonstrated with **cayenne pepper** and **ginger root**.

Both herbs are obviously pungent (hot) in taste when you eat them. But after the cooking process, which affects the physical properties of the herbs in a manner similar to digestion, **cayenne** will remain pungent, while **ginger** will take on a sweet taste. Therefore, the still-pungent **pepper** can aggravate an acidic intestinal condition if you eat too much of it, while **ginger's** anti-inflammatory properties can soothe the same condition. Several herbs exhibit a pronounced effect that increases therapeutic options. For example, **ginger** can be used to strengthen stomach digestion in a patient with inflammation further down the intestinal tract, while **cayenne** cannot.

- Herbs that change to a sweet taste after digestion will, like other inherently sweet herbs, stimulate evacuation, nourish the tissues, and reduce inflammation. According to Ayurvedic theory this will increase Kapha and decrease Pitta. Onions do this.

- Herbs that change to a sour taste after digestion will increase metabolism, warm the body, and stimulate bile flow. Such herbs will increase Pitta and calm Vata. Horse gram *(Polichos biflorus)* does this.

- Herbs that change to a pungent taste after digestion will dry the stool. In excess they cause dryness, constipation, and gas and reduce nutrient absorption. These herbs increase Vata and decrease Kapha. Vacha root *(Acorus calamus)* does this.

Ayurvedic doctors have lists that describe such actions for each of their herbs, but no such lists are available for Western or TCM herbs. Therefore, we must use our powers of deduction to identify these actions. For example, in the clinic, I know that **haritaki fruit** has a laxative action, yet is highly nourishing due to its sweet postdigestive effect. Since most laxative herbs tend to be weakening, this herb is a good choice for treating a case such as a weak elderly patient with chronic constipation.

Understanding Herbs by Their Chemical Components

Following are simplified descriptions of some of the more important nutrients and chemical components of plants, as understood by plant biochemists and botanists. Plants are potpourris of many chemicals, and when we describe a particular chemical we are always talking in general terms, because the chemical mentioned may undergo numerous variations in nature. If we mention that a plant contains a particular compound, you can take it as an indication that the compound exists in a significant concentration, while numerous other plants not mentioned may contain insignificant amounts of said compound.

The important thing to remember is that this basic knowledge can help you understand what herbs do and can therefore assist you in navigating the herbal marketplace. You may find this information helpful when attempting to interpret marketing claims. Remember, just because a chemical found in a plant is capable of a certain action, this does *not* mean that any herb containing that specific chemical will have the same effect or exhibit the same action. The chemical may not exist in sufficient quantity in the herb, or other chemicals within the product may modify its action.

Chemicals Found in Herbs

Alkaloids are a diverse group of chemicals, generally alkaline in nature, that have powerful biological effects. Morphine was the first alkaloid isolated, back in 1806. Some of the best-known alkaloids are atropine, caffeine, pilocarpine, lobeline, quinine, berberine, strychnine, nicotine, codeine, and ephedrine. Common uses of alkaloids include painkillers, narcotics, hypotensives, hypertensives, bronchodilators, stimulants, antimicrobials, and anti-inflammatories. **Coffee bean** *(Coffea arabica)* and **ephedra** (ma huang / *Ephedra sinica)* contain alkaloids.

Anthraquinones are laxative chemicals found in plants like **rhubarb root** *(Rheum emodi),* **cascara sagrada bark** *(Rhamnus purshiana),* and **senna leaf** *(Senna* species / *Casia tora).* These chemicals have topical effects on the large intestine and are not absorbed well. Anthraquinones can be very potent, and overuse can cause acute pain (called griping) and eventual tolerance and habituation.

Bitter principles are chemical characteristics unique to a diverse class of plant chemicals that includes the monoterpenes, and specifically, iridoids, sesquiterpenes, and alkaloids. Generally, these chemicals stimulate taste receptors in the mouth, which signal nerves in the stomach to trigger the release of digestive enzymes, which stimulates bile flow. Over a period of time, overuse of bitters may result in overstimulation, producing a reverse effect and dampening appetite. **Coptis rhizome** (huang lian /*Coptis chinensis)* is very bitter. Some bitters have antibiotic, antifungal, liver-protecting, and antitumor activities. Others are relaxing nervines, such as **valerian root** *(Valeriana officinalis)* and **hops** *(Humulus lupulus).*

Cardiac glycosides represent a specific class of steroidal saponins that have a marked action on the heart, strengthening the force and speed of systolic contraction. Herbs that contain them must be used with extreme caution under professional guidance, as the therapeutic dose is very close to the toxic one. **Foxglove** *(Digitalis purpurea)* contains cardiac glycosides.

Carotenoid pigments (coloring matter) are found in carrots, red and yellow vegetables, and dark leafy green vegetables. Carotenoids include carotenes and xanthophylls (oxygenated carotenoids). Carrots, squash, tomatoes, and spinach are good sources of carotenoids. Carotenoids have an affinity for fatty tissues in the body and help maintain healthy epithelial tissue and mucous membranes. Some carotenoids can be converted into vitamin A in the human body. (However, the problem of liver toxicity from excess vitamin A is not caused by carotenoids.) There are more than 600 different kinds of carotenoids, but only 30 to 50 varieties, particularly beta-carotenes, exhibit specific vitamin A activity.

Carotenoids offer many benefits to the body. They aid growth and repair of body tissue and protect the eyes from dryness. Lutein (a xanthophyll) is particularly important to the health of the eyes because it concentrates in the macula and protects against degeneration. Carotenoids help our bodies fight bacteria and infection, and aid in the formation of bones and teeth.

They also assist the regulation of cell differentiation, helping us to form healthy and mature cells as opposed to immature and undifferentiated cells. This is an important factor in cancer prevention. Carotenoids quench oxygen-free radicals, improve fertility, and enhance thymus function.

Carotenoid deficiency can prevent a mucus coating from forming on your trachca, lungs, rectum, and digestive system. Other problems include night blindness; rough, dry, scaly skin; and increased susceptibility to infections, as well as fatigue, insomnia, depression, loss of smell and appetite, dull hair, brittle nails, and inflamed eyelids.

Chlorophyll is the pigment found in all green plants which gives plants the ability to capture light energy from the sun. As a medicinal agent, it is known for its purifying and blood-building properties. It aids in liver function and has antiseptic properties. A 2% solution of chlorophyll taken as a dose of 1 tablespoon per day is very healing to the intestinal membranes of the digestive system. It is also an excellent intestinal deodorant.

Plant **fixed oils** contain high levels of essential fatty acids, the ones your body cannot manufacture by itself. These oils are important components of many herbal treatments. **Flaxseed oil** *(Linum usitatissimum)* and **evening primrose oil** *(Oenothera biennis)* are very high in omega-3 fatty acids, the ones most often missing in the diet, and are beneficial in reducing inflammation.

Flavonoids are a diverse set of chemicals which include many brilliant plant pigments that, like carotenoids, are responsible for many of the attractive colors you see in fruits and vegetables (though some are colorless). More than 4,000 flavonoid compounds have been isolated from plants so far. One notable medicinal effect of some flavonoids is their ability to strengthen blood vessel integrity and reduce inflammation. They also have antiviral and antimicrobial effects.

Flavonoids are extremely potent antioxidants and are often found in plants containing vitamin C. Dark-colored fruits are loaded with flavonoids. High concentrations of flavonoids are found in red and black grapes, red wine, **black elderberries** *(Sambucus canadensis),* **hawthorn fruit** (shan zha / *Crataegus pinnatifida),* **blueberries** *(Vaccinium myrtilloides)* and **bilberries** *(V. myrtillus),* **ginkgo leaf** *(Ginkgo biloba),* and **green** and **black teas** *(Camellia sinensis).*

These chemicals have potent antioxidant activity. Their presence in the basement membranes and surrounding collagen structures is responsible for maintaining proper permeability and stability in capillaries by neutralizing free radical poisons that break down blood vessel walls. Healthy and resilient capillary vessels are able to maintain their shape and function for normal, efficient microcirculation, which prevents water accumulation in the surrounding tissues.

This next one is a mouthful. The class of related flavonoid pigments responsible for the red, blue, and violet colors you see in many plants is known by several names, including **anthocyans, anthocyanins, anthocyanidins, proanthocyanins,** and **proanthocyanidins**. One subgroup, known as **oligomeric proanthocyanidins (OPSs),** represents a type of condensed tannin. These pigments are most notably found in grape seeds and French maritime pine trees. They include the chemicals **cyanidin, procyanidin, malvadin, petunidin, and delphinidin**. Whew! You can breathe now.

Gum resins are excreted when a plant is injured. Examples include **gum arabic** from *Acacia* species and seaweed gums such as **kelp fronds** *(Nereocystis luetkeana)* and **Irish moss** *(Chondrus crispus* / carrageenan). Some gums, like those found in **guggul gum** *(Commiphora mukul / Balsamodendron mukul),* stimulate the liver cells to burn cholesterol by promoting uptake of LDL (bad) cholesterol from the blood.

Indoles are found in cruciferous vegetables like broccoli, cabbage, cauliflower, brussels sprouts, and turnips. "Dithiolthione" is an indole that assists in the cells' release and subsequent replacement of peroxidase, an important component in the body's detoxification processes. Therefore, vegetables containing indoles can help remove pesticides, herbicides, heavy metals, and other chemicals from your body. Recent evidence indicates that, when eaten in sufficient quantities, these vegetables may play a key role in cancer prevention. Indoles also help to inactivate excess estrogens such as isoflavones.

Lectins are plant proteins that bind to glycoproteins on the surface of human cells causing agglutination, the clumping of cells together with each other or with other particles or bacteria. They often serve as growth factors.

Lignans (not to be confused with lignin) are plant chemicals commonly found in pulses and grains. Those found in **schisandra berries** (wu wei zi /*Schisandra chinensis)* and **milk thistle seed** *(Silybum marianum)* are very important for protecting and repairing liver cells. Other lignans have been shown to exhibit antiviral, antioxidant, and anticancer activities.

Mucilages are slimy, amorphous, carbohydrate substances (polysaccharides) found in plants like **slippery elm inner bark** *(Ulmus rubra),* **comfrey leaf** *(Symphytum officinalis),* and **psyllium seeds** *(Plantago* species). Mucilaginous herbs are used to coat and soothe the digestive tract.

Phytosterols and sterolins, such as beta-sitosterol, are ubiquitous steroidlike molecules found in plant cell walls. They are relatives of the carotenoids. Some of them are known to be generally energizing and may help inhibit the growth of tumors, stimulate the immune system, and regulate cholesterol levels. **Ashwagandha root** *(Withania somnifera)* and **guggul gum** contain phytosterols. These compounds have a history of safe use and do not cause any of the side effects associated with the more dangerous animal steroids.

Phytoestrogens are generally classified as steroidal compounds and as members of the isoflavone group of flavonoids (including genistein, daidzein, biochanin, and formononetin). These compounds are found in the legume family, especially in soybeans. They are also found in **red clover blossom** *(Trifolium pratense),* **licorice root** *(Glycyrrhiza glabra),* and **alfalfa leaf** *(Medicago sativa).*

Isoflavones are good antioxidants and anti-inflammatories. They have structural similarities to estrogens and have been found to bind to estrogen receptors while only weakly activating them. They seem to aid in the prevention of breast and other tumors, reduce hot flashes, prevent bone loss, and strengthen cardiovascular health in menopausal women. Overuse may weaken thyroid function if there is inadequate iodine in the diet.

Phytoprogesterones are plant chemicals that bind to intracellular progesterone receptors. They are found in several herbs, including **oregano leaf, turmeric root,** and **red clover blossom,** but have not yet been studied nearly as much as phytoestrogens. One study found that these compounds tended to be either neutral or antagonistic after binding to receptors, meaning that they blocked cell response.

Plant coumarins are chemicals that have anticoagulant, antimicrobial, and antispasmodic properties. Dicoumarol, derived from improperly cured **sweet clover,** is a component of the blood-thinning drug warfarin. Many coumarins are photoreactive and can cause skin rashes similar to those caused by members of the umbel family such as celery. Coumarins are used in doses up to 1 gram to treat edema. Though not all coumarins thin the blood, I still suggest exercising caution with patients taking blood-thinning medication. **Red clover blossoms** *(Trifolium pratense)* contain coumarins.

Plant enzymes are catalytic proteins that make possible many complex chemical reactions in the body. **Bromelain** *(Ananas comusus* / pineapple enzymes) and **papaya fruit** *(Carica papaya)* contain these protein-digesting enzymes, useful for digestion and reduction of inflammation and edema. Malt extract from barley is an easily digestible nutritive for improving carbohydrate digestion.

Polyphenols are naturally occurring plant phenol compounds that have antioxidant and anti-inflammatory actions, which contribute to their chemopreventive or anticancer activity. **Green tea leaves** have polyphenols.

Polysaccharides are complex starch molecules found in all plants. Some have been shown to help restore depressed immune response, perhaps by feeding and energizing white blood cells or by mimicking the bacterial cell walls to which they are naturally primed to respond. They do not seem to overstimulate normal immune systems. Scientists determine their effectiveness by measuring the extent to which they stimulate natural killer cells to attack tumors, and by their effect on the proliferation of immune cells.

Ganoderma mushroom (ling zhi / *Ganoderma lucidum)* and the maitake d-fraction (beta-glucan) derived from **maitake mushroom** *(Grifola frondosa)* are among the best examples of polysaccharides studied to date. The results are dose dependent, and it takes several weeks for them to reach peak levels of response in the blood cells.

Salicylates and salicins are aspirinlike compounds found in plants. They are generally pain-relieving and anti-inflammatory in action and are used to treat headaches and arthritis. In herbal terms, they reduce heat and dampness, mostly from the blood and joints. Plants containing salicin, like **willow bark** *(Salix* species) and **meadowsweet herb** *(Filipendula ulmaria),* work more slowly and do not cause the stomach irritation or bleeding sometimes seen with over-the-counter pain relievers.

Saponins are chemicals whose name is derived from the Latin *sapo,* meaning "soap." When plants containing saponins are placed in water and shaken, they tend to froth up and form a lather. When acting on internal surfaces of membranes and blood vessels, they lower surface tension and have a mildly irritating effect that helps break up oils and fats.

Their mechanism varies from herb to herb, but saponins generally exhibit anti-inflammatory and antiallergy properties, improve circulation and digestion, and reduce mucus. Once absorbed, they seem to have important beneficial effects on arterial and venous walls, with the ability to rupture red blood cells and perhaps to help with the removal of cellular debris. Saponins inhibit the formation of lipid peroxides; they decrease blood coagulation, cholesterol, and sugar levels in blood; and they stimulate the immune system. Some saponins are beneficial to the liver. **Yucca root** *(Yucca* species), **bupleurum root** *(Bupleurum* species), and **ginseng root** (ren shen / *Panax ginseng)* contain significant amounts of saponins.

Tannins are condensed flavonoids responsible for the astringent taste of certain herbs. The chemicals bind with proteins and form a protective layer on the skin and mucous membranes. In sufficient doses tannins can reduce diarrhea or intestinal bleeding. Externally, they can be used to treat burns or seal wounds. They are antimicrobial and can be used to inhibit infections of the eye, mouth, vagina, and rectum. They also have antioxidant effects. **Black tea** and **green tea** *(Camellia sinensis)* contain tannins.

Triterpenoid saponins represent a particular class of saponins, some of which have a strengthening effect on the adrenal gland where they mimic the activity of adrenocorticotropic hormone (ACTH). This is an important action for relieving many stress problems. They are also reputed to promote blood circulation and improve oxygen utilization. **Ginseng root** (ren shen / *Panax ginseng),* **licorice root** *(Glycyrrhiza glabra),* and **bupleurum root** (chai hu /*B. chinensis)* contain triterpenoid saponins.

Volatile oils are compounds that evaporate at room temperature, thereby allowing us to enjoy their odors as they turn to gas. They are generally antiseptic and antioxidant. Some of them also exhibit antifungal and insect-repellent actions. Volatile oils are easily transported throughout the body. Some can increase white blood cell formation, in turn increasing resistance to infection. Others act on the whole nervous system and are antispasmodic and relaxing. When applied externally, some volatile oils are warming and anti-inflammatory, while others will reduce itching. **Garlic** *(Allium sativum),* **oregano** *(Origanum* species), and **tea tree** *(Melaleuca* species) contain volatile oils.

Understanding Herbs by Their Physical Properties

Ayurvedic doctors have classified all their herbs based on their physical properties. Some herbal properties that are easy to identify and understand include heavy (to digest) and light (to digest), dry and greasy, and the previously discussed hot and cold. Physical properties can sometimes be very important when prescribing herbs. Some examples:

- Herbs that are heavy in property (heavy to digest) should not be used if digestion is sluggish. Bananas are heavy to digest.

- Herbs that are drying in property should not be used when the body is dehydrated. Adding a drying herb to dry skin will make it worse. **Tea tree oil** and **acorus root** (vacha) are drying.

- Herbs that are light in quality can be used in the presence of solid accumulations, such as cysts or plagues. **Acorus root** and **pinellia tuber** can lighten the body by dispersing heavy accumulations of mucus.

Understanding Herbs by Their Colors

Color is as fundamental to life as light. In plants, color represents the way the pigments bend and reflect visible light. Animals select their foods by color and visual appearance.

In primate studies, researchers have shown that the color of a leaf is an important indicator of its nutritive value. As leaves mature, they change color and toughen. Leaf lightness and yellowness have a strong negative correlation with toughness. We therefore choose the softest leaves—those highest in protein yet easy to digest. Consumers prefer egg yolks with the darkest golden yellow color, indicating pigment levels. By the way, this doesn't work as well in supermarkets, where bright colors and lights are used to fool us into buying things.

Basically, we need to eat lots of colorful fruits and vegetables, and we want to know more about which ones are best for our health. Therefore, the study of color in herbal medicine focuses primarily on the plant pigments—the colorful chemicals generated by plant metabolism—and how they affect the basic life processes. We discussed them in the previous section, where we learned that they are generally anti-inflammatory and helpful in detoxification.

However, we can gain more insight by dividing them up a bit:

Carotenoids are found primarily in red, orange, and yellow fruits and vegetables and, to a lesser extent, in dark leafy green vegetables. They protect plants from the free radicals (especially singlet oxygen) generated by the metabolic process of photosynthesis. Animals depend completely on dietary sources for carotenoids. They are fat-soluble and most closely related to Yin. Carotenes have an affinity for, and thus help neutralize, poisons found in the fat cells and soft fatty tissues and membranes, including the intestinal membranes, lungs, and even the membranes around cells and organelles. For these reasons, humans are classified as yellow-fat organisms.

> In one interesting case, a 20-year-old Japanese woman who wanted to lose weight ate almost nothing except carotene-rich pumpkins for 2 years. Her skin, of course, turned bright yellow, and she sustained some liver damage. Fortunately, she was able to regain her health quickly after adjusting her diet. It seems it takes a very large amount of carotenoids to hurt you.

Many carotenoids transform into vitamin A, which is necessary for maintaining healthy membranes and plays an integral role in the formation of the coating on your trachea, lungs, rectum, digestive system, and even the inside of your skin. Yellow xanthophylls such as lutein, a type of carotenoid found in such foods as egg yolks and yellow squash, help protect the delicate retinal membrane from ultraviolet (UV) radiation damage. Interestingly, carotenoid deficiency leads to a reduction in fertility, a classic Yin deficiency disease.

Various carotenoid supplements, especially red lycopene, have shown benefit in double-blind studies against oral lesions. They are also beneficial to general membrane integrity and act as protection against epithelial cancers, including breast, cervical, colon, esophageal, oral, pancreatic, and rectal. Scientists now theorize that each of the different carotenoids is capable of antioxidant and singlet-oxygen-quenching activity, with varying degrees of strength for each function.

Flavonoids are found in dark yet luminous blue, black, red, and violet fruits and vegetables. They generally relate most closely to Yang (within this overall cooling group) and help maintain immune function and neutralize poisons. Thus, they act to strengthen blood vessels and capillaries, regulate inflammatory cells, and even modulate gene expression. They have a number of functions related to circulation, including vasodilation and reduction of platelet stickiness and edema. Flavonoids also work in concert with vitamin C to help fight germs and viruses and reduce inflammation.

The anthocyanins and related flavonoids found in berries are strong enough to protect against vessel-related diseases such as diabetic retinopathy, Alzheimer's disease, and cardiac artery disease. Various flavonoids have been shown effective in double-blind studies against prostatitis, progressive pigmented purpurea, peripheral arterial occlusive disease, and chronic venous insufficiency.

Green **chlorophyll** is the main coloring matter in all green plants, and it relates most closely to Qi, the life force. The chlorophyll in plants traps photons of light and uses them to produce ATP, the basic energy used by all our human cells. Green plants and algae are high in chlorophyll, including **spirulina** and **chlorella,** and have developed a reputation as energy-boosting medicines as well as detoxification aids. However, scientific evidence on humans is sparse. One study showed that **spirulina** supplementation resulted in significantly higher iron storage and increased hemoglobin content in the blood of pregnant rats. Foods and herbs that contain high levels of chlorophyll show pharmacological evidence of cancer prevention, perhaps because pigments in green vegetables such as spinach, kale, broccoli, and lettuce bind with and thus stimulate excretion of cancer-causing chemicals. Even more interesting is a report from one researcher that "Given their exclusive dietary origin, . . . chlorophyll metabolites may represent essential nutrients that coordinate cellular metabolism (through nuclear receptors)."

Understanding Herbs by Their Tissue Affinities

One of the more useful concepts to grasp in herbal medicine is the idea that while many herbs have general systemic effects, certain herbs can also have affinities for specific organs or tissues. Further, tissues store specific nutrients and, just like your bank account, your stores can be high or low. This is called "pharmacokinetics."

Some examples:

- Carotenoids can be stored in adipose tissue, skin, liver, adrenals, testes, and ovaries. When you eat **carrots,** the carotenes first saturate the blood fats and then go to the tissues.

- The carotenoid called lutein has an affinity for the macula of the eye. Eating **spinach** can increase macular lutein levels, so it can be said that the healing nutrients in **spinach** "go to the eyes."

- The flavonoids in **milk thistle seed** *(Silybum marianum)* have an affinity for and are stored in the liver.

- **Ginkgo leaves** *(Ginkgo biloba)* exhibit numerous membrane-stabilizing and antioxidant effects on neural tissue, as well as increasing the transport of glucose and oxygen into nerve cells.

Pathologists look for disease by examining specific tissue changes and accumulations of toxic materials such as proteins, fats, and other substances. When the concentration of a necessary nutrient in tissues is low, the body cannot fight certain disease-causing processes, and the toxic substances accumulate. Diagnosis rests on establishing the nature of the accumulated materials and their topographic distribution.

These findings lend credence to the long-held contention of TCM practitioners that one can assign specific effects or actions (e.g., "nourishing" or "warming") to herbs used to treat designated areas of the body (upper or lower, for example), or specific organs or groups of organs. Thus a TCM practitioner will not use just any heat-reducing (anti-inflammatory) herb to treat liver inflammation, but will choose an herb known specifically to "cool the liver."

TCM doctors also make the following generalizations:

- Flower medicines tend to go to the upper areas of the body, especially the lungs, nose, and throat.

- Seed medicines tend to go to the TCM kidney system, loosely related to the reproductive, adrenal, and urinary systems.

- Root medicines tend to go to all the internal organs, heart, liver, lungs, intestines.

- Branches tend to go to the external meridians in the limbs (arms and legs).

Understanding Herbs with Intuition

It is often said that medicine is an art and not a science. This is meant to highlight the fact that factors unbeholden to scientific scrutiny, such as friendship, love, attention, and "gut feelings," are not only real but sometimes crucial to successful medical outcomes. Intuition could be defined as direct knowledge without recourse to ordinary thought. Intuition comes in the form of feelings, mental pictures, or an "inner voice." It requires a heart free of fear. Such insights are personal and generally should not be discussed, only acted upon.

In Section Three we will be discussing a wide variety of medical concepts when we discuss choosing herbs to treat different health problems. Let's remember this quote from one of Nai-shing's teachers in China, a fifth generation herbalist:

If you use cooling herbs for hot diseases, warming herbs for cold diseases, and tonics for diseases of deficiency, you will never be far from the truth.

—*Professor Li Bo-ning, former director of the Sichuan Acupuncture Research Institute*

CHAPTER 7

Understanding Herbs

The eye sees only what the mind is prepared to comprehend.
—Henri Bergson

You now have enough background in the history of herbal medicine and the language of herbs to go to the next level of understanding. If you are like most of us, the next thing you want to know is what the "best" herbs are for treating your particular health condition. I had to laugh at myself when I tried to define the word *best* for use in this book, as the field of herbal medicine is so vast. At our clinic, my wife Nai-shing and I keep over 1,000 herbs from all parts of the world in stock. This stock includes herbs from the three systems of herbal medicine we have both studied: TAM (Traditional Ayurvedic Medicine) from India and Nepal, TCM (Traditional Chinese Medicine) from China, and Western herbal medicine.

Nonetheless, when you watch doctors from each of these systems at work, as I have, you notice very quickly that they choose certain herbs most frequently, based on their high levels of safety and effectiveness. Many of these herbs are already famous. One cannot imagine TCM without **ginseng root** and **astragalus root,** TAM without **ashwagandha root** and **guggul gum,** or Western herbalism without **echinacea** and **dandelion root**. These are among the herbs I will discuss. I have chosen more than 80 herbs that Nai-shing and I consider to be among the most useful available to us in effectively treating the common diseases we see every day. About a dozen or so less commonly used herbs have also been included.

How do you know which herbs are best?

I draw my knowledge of herbal use from numerous sources:

- Traditional teachings (the wisdom handed down from the past)
- Scientific reports from around the world

- My personal experience

- Clinical experiences of my patients

- Reports from other professional herbalists and their patients

- Intuition

Of these, the traditional teachings of the past and the clinical results experienced by my patients have the greatest influence on my herbal choices. However, scientific findings often bring fascinating new insights into sharp focus, and I rely on them as well.

What are the premier herbs used by Ayurvedic doctors?

In Traditional Ayurvedic Medicine (TAM), the Sanskrit word **rasayana** is assigned to herbs that, although powerful in their results, can be used safely and indefinitely with complete confidence and without side effects. *Rasayana* describes an herbal preparation that promotes a youthful state of physical and mental health and expands happiness. Rasayana herbs have high levels of both safety and effectiveness. They are given to small children in India as tonics by their parents and are also taken by the middle-aged and elderly to increase longevity. Several of these herbs have been administered to animals to determine toxicity, and in some cases no toxicity is seen even when the herb comprises very high percentages of the fortunate mammal's diet. Such herbs do indeed exist. You may have heard of many of them already, as they are quite popular. They are as safe to consume as ordinary vegetables such as carrots and beets. I hope to expand your knowledge of some of these herbs and introduce you to a few jewels you have not encountered yet.

Are these the herbs used most often by Ayurvedic doctors to treat diseases?

Yes and no. Rasayana herbs can be found everywhere in India and Nepal, and they can be and are used by people of all ages and states of health. Ayurvedic doctors rely on them heavily in their tonic formulas for longevity and to treat chronic diseases. However, these herbs form only a moderate part of the expert herb doctor's repertoire. A good doctor from any tradition must know how to use many, many other herbs. For example, **niche herbs** are uncommon herbs that do only one thing well but are essential for treating certain conditions. I have included some of the more important ones, such as **ephedra**. Some herbs, as simple as **black pepper** or **ginger root,** are indispensable for helping to make an herbal formula work properly.

What are the premier herbs used by Western and European herbalists?

The premier herbs used by Western and European herbalists generally fall into a category known as **adaptogens,** herbs that bring balance back to the body no matter what the direction of imbalance. Some adaptogens will bring your blood pressure down if it is high, or bring it up if it is low. Others will regulate your thyroid whether its function is high or low. Soy products are good examples of these substances because they can be used beneficially whether estrogen levels are high or low. If the body's estrogen levels are low, the mild concentration of plant estrogens in soy will stimulate cell receptor sites (the on/off switches for cellular func-

> The word *adaptogen* describes an agent that:
>
> 1. Has a normalizing effect on a wide range of body functions.
> 2. Has a nonspecific action that helps the body overcome stress regardless of the direction of stress.
> 3. Is nontoxic when used in normal dosage.

tion). Conversely, if the body's estrogen levels are high, the same mild plant estrogens will compete with the more powerful human estrogens for the same sites. Thus, soybeans are hormonal adaptogens.

What are the best Chinese herbs?

You must remember that even the best Chinese herbs, such as **ginseng root** and **dang gui root,** cannot be used without some basic diagnostic information. Herbal choices must be made based upon individual needs. Following the Taoist philosophy of Yin and Yang—the balance and union of opposites—we achieve health by balancing and harmonizing the conflicts we hold within ourselves.

Over a thousand years ago, the ancient *Shennong Bencao Jing* (Pharmacopoeia of Herbs) included a category of herbs suggested for use every day to strengthen vitality, increase energy, and lengthen life span. Traditionally, such herbs are established tonics that are safe to use over a long period of time because they are balanced in terms of Yin and Yang. Many of them improve digestive function. Such herbs are commonly used for "fu zheng" (immune tonification) therapy, discussed in Chapter 19.

You've said that some herbs are very safe for long-term use, but what about all the others?

Truthfully, few herbs can meet the highest standard of an adaptogen or a rasayana herb, scoring high on scales of both safety and effectiveness for general daily use. In this book I will classify such herbs as **gold standard**.

There are many other herbs that are of great importance but must be used with a certain level of knowledge and caution. These herbs, which have excellent results with no side effects when used properly, still harbor a slight potential for misuse. Some are very safe, but are not particularly powerful or broad in effect. Some herbs are very useful and very safe but should not be used all the time. Throughout the book, I will classify such herbs as **silver standard**.

There are other herbs that, although extremely beneficial and important in the treatment of certain conditions, have a limited range of action or must be used with caution. Mild or moderate diuretics, for example, may be very useful for a few weeks or months, but I do not see the sense in taking them for long periods of time. I will classify these herbs as **yellow standard**.

The final group of herbs will be classified as **red standard**. These red standard herbs have certain essential properties that make them beneficial to many patients in states of poor health, but they also pose clearly defined dangers which must be known. Such herbs should be used only under the guidance of a trained professional.

There's one more thing. I'm not sure any particular herb should be used continuously without a break, unless dictated by medical necessity. The constant intake of the same foods is, I believe, a major cause of food allergy and other problems such as nutrient overload or deficiency. TAM doctors place strong emphasis on eating foods during the correct season, which causes a natural change in dietary items during the year. By the same token, I think it makes more sense to rotate even the best tonic herbs. Don't get stuck in the philosophy of using one herb for everything or using one herb forever.

CHAPTER 8

Important Herbs from Around the World

Knowledge is one. Its division into subjects is a concession to human weakness.

—Halford John Mackinder

I have more than 900 books in my herbal library, and I've learned that any fact you find about an herb may be somehow useful. However, the way a writer selects, filters, and presents information sometimes reveals more about the writer than the herb. As a clinician, there are certain books that I have always found myself going back to again and again. It took me a while to figure out why they stood out from the rest. The best ones are not all the same, because describing herbs is an art, unique to each plant and its characteristics. In many ways an herb is like a person. Descriptions are useful, but you have to get more intimate to really know the deeper truth. With people this means meeting them to see if your personalities are compatible, and with herbs it means taking them to see if they "work for you." I am going to offer the herbs from a variety of angles here, while at the same time trying to present the essence of each herb's usefulness in clinical situations.

Let's take a look at the layout I have chosen for the herbal descriptions that follow.

COMMON NAME

Latin: *Genus* species

WHAT IT DOES: Here I will give the broad properties of the herb including its taste, its heating and cooling properties, and specifically what it does to the body.

RATING: Here you will find the "color" categories as explained on pages 89–90.

SAFETY ISSUES: Any warnings about contraindications—possible adverse effects caused by misuse, overuse, or use by persons with certain medical conditions.

STARTING DOSAGE: Recommended starting adult dosage and preferred form.

DISCUSSION: One or more paragraphs.

As discussed in Chapter 6, **Latin names** are the most exact identification method, pretty much assuring that we know which herb we are talking about. For our purposes, however, I will provide the **common name** first, in **CAPITALIZED BOLD LETTERS.** This will be followed by the Latin name, and subsequently the name of the herb as it is known in Chinese, Sanskrit, or another foreign language, indicating that the herb is used by those cultures. This is important to avoid misidentification.

In the section called **"WHAT IT DOES,"** I will explain my understanding of the essence of the herb's action. Here I rely on traditional energetic descriptions that, in my opinion, are essential to realistic understanding. Years ago, I received quite a shock when reading an early British author's writings about Ayurvedic herbs. This chap decided to leave out all references to Vata, Pitta, and Kapha, which he decided had nothing to do with the "scientific" actions of the herbs. I'm here to tell you that nothing could be further from the truth. The energetic attributes of each herb are time-tested global descriptions that are among the most important tools we have in herbal medicine. It is these descriptions, more than anything else, that allow herbalists to select appropriate treatments in clinical situations.

Each herb's **"RATING"** provides a designated color value for that herb, determined according to values of safety and usefulness, as discussed on pages 89–90. This results in a color value for each herb—**gold, silver, yellow,** or **red**.

Following the safety rating you will find **"SAFETY ISSUES,"** highlighting any warnings, contraindications, or special precautions. Contraindications are specific cautions that provide reasons why certain people, such as pregnant women or persons taking certain drugs, should not use the herb. **Note that it is possible to have a gold standard herb which, while safe for use by most people, may still be contraindicated for some, such as pregnant women or people taking certain drugs.**

Children's dosages can be calculated using **Clark's rule**. Divide the child's weight in pounds by 150 to give the approximate fraction of the adult dose to be used by that child. For example, for a 75-pound child, use 75/150 or one half of the adult dosage to start.

I have also provided a **"STARTING DOSAGE"** for each herb. This offers the suggested starting dosage for an adult, as well as different available forms of preparation for the herb. Some herbs can be used in several different forms, while some work only as tinctures or in dry form or after undergoing special preparation. **Remember that the dosages listed are the approximate starting dosage when using the herb by itself. When the herb is used as part of a combination, the dosage will always be reduced.** In formulas, a single herb typically represents from about 5% up to as much as 50% or more of a formula.

My final section in each herbal description is the **"DISCUSSION,"** consisting of one or more paragraphs intended to provide you with additional details, research findings, and any other information which can round out your understanding of the herb. **For more information about any of the products, manufacturers, or distributors mentioned in this section, refer to the Resource Guide.**

AGASTACHE

Latin: *Agastache rugosa*   **Chinese:** Huo xiang
        Pogostemon cablin

WHAT IT DOES: Agastache is aromatic, pungent in taste, and slightly warming in action. It stops nausea and vomiting by dissolving mucus in the stomach.

RATING: Yellow, due to limitations in use

SAFETY ISSUES: Avoid contact with eyes due to volatile oil content.

STARTING DOSAGE:

- Dried powder: 4½ to 9 grams per day

- Concentrated powder: 1 to 3 grams per day

TCM doctors have discovered that **agastache** has a strong ability to stop nausea and vomiting. We use it in our clinic to treat cases of nausea that do not respond to the milder **ginger root.** In addition, this herb inhibits the actions of common fungi and bacteria that cause nausea and intestinal problems. You can find it in Chinese grocery stores as a major ingredient in various antinausea medicines, available in both pill and liquid forms. It is very valuable for treating the nausea of pregnancy or chemotherapy.

Research Highlights

- *Bacteroides* is a strain of bacteria that ferments carbohydrates in the intestinal, respiratory, and urogenital tracts and oral cavity linings, causing toxic gas formation. In a study of several pathogenic bacteria, terpenoids isolated from **agastache** exhibited marked antibacterial activity. This activity proved strongest against *Bacteroides* spp. (Osawa et al., 1990).

- The antiemetic activity of agastache was demonstrated in a recent experiment using young chicks (Yong Y et al., 1999).

AGURU WOOD

Latin: *Aquilaria agollocha*   **Sanskrit:** Aguru / Agaru   **English:** Aloewood
Eaglewood

WHAT IT DOES: Aguru wood is bitter in taste and hot in action. It increases blood circulation to the lungs and head area and tonifies and warms the entire body.

RATING: Silver, due to limited applications

SAFETY ISSUES: None known

STARTING DOSAGE:

- Crude powder: 2 grams two times per day

Aguru is a large tropical and subtropical, fragrant evergreen tree. The resinous wood strongly catalyzes circulation in the cranial organs and chest. This makes it a very effective treatment for bronchial asthma. It warms the lungs, causing a reduction in the spasms and mucus exudation (Vata and Kapha). It also relaxes tension in the muscles surrounding the lungs, so it is indicated specifically for spasmodic asthma. **Aguru wood** is also used as a tonic for improving mental function. It is often prescribed for this purpose in the form of incense, or as an herbal cigarette.

Research Highlights

- **Aguru wood** has been shown to reduce allergy reactions by inhibiting histamine release from immune cells (Kim et al., 1997).

- Studies in mice show that extracts of **aguru wood** possess potent central-nervous-system depressant activities (Okugawa et al., 1993). Since it doesn't contain any ephedrine, this herb can be used when **ma huang** is contraindicated.

ALFALFA

Latin: *Medicago sativa*

WHAT IT DOES: Alfalfa is sweet and slightly bitter in taste and cooling in action. It nourishes the blood.

RATING: Gold

SAFETY ISSUES: Alfalfa seeds and alfalfa sprouts have induced lupus in primates and should be avoided by everyone due to the presence of an amino acid, L-canavanine. Patients with lupus or other connective tissue diseases should not ingest alfalfa in any form.

STARTING DOSAGE:

- 1:5 tincture (with minerals retained): 20–40 drops two to three times per day

- Capsules or tablets: one to four 500-mg pills two to three times per day

Alfalfa is a classic nutritive tonic herb, rich in chlorophyll, protein, calcium, trace minerals, folic acid, and vitamins B_6, E, and K. The strong nutrient effects seen with clinical use may be credited to either of two attributes unique to this particular herb. First, the plant has an extraordinarily strong root system that penetrates up to 60 feet into the soil, allowing the herb to mine out precious nutrients. Second, the herb contains specified plant enzymes which enhance nutrient assimilation. **Alfalfa** is also a rich source of plant phytoestrogens, useful in balancing the hormones during menopause. The vitamin K content may also be useful for maintaining bone density.

I use **alfalfa** in a sweet liquid extract form as a nutrient tonic to stimulate gentle healing of the digestive tract membranes. The tonic effects become apparent after 1 or 2 weeks of use, often causing a sense of mild euphoria in the weakened. I frequently prescribe it for children and the elderly, especially when there are signs of emaciation and weakness. The tincture has a distinct root beer flavor, so I tell parents to add a tablespoon of it to cola-flavored natural sodas (actually made with juice and mineral water) from their local health food store. This is usually the easiest way to get kids to take it. Several weeks of use often imparts a general feeling of well-being in such cases. It is also a good tonic base for other herbs.

Several companies make **alfalfa** in tablets, although I prefer to use it in tincture form when possible. Boericke & Tafel offers a good, inexpensive product—**Alfalco**—in 32-ounce bottles. Herbalist & Alchemist offers a superior product that undergoes an extra step before packaging to replace the minerals usually lost during tincturing.

ALOE VERA GEL

Latin: *Aloe barbadensis*   **Sanskrit:** Kumari   **Chinese:** Lu hui
Aloe vera

WHAT IT DOES: Aloe vera gel is bitter in taste, cold in action, and mucilaginous. It heals and soothes skin irritations.

RATING: Gold (external use)

SAFETY ISSUES: Not for internal use when pregnant, if suffering from any intestinal or kidney disease, or during menstruation. Do not use in children under the age of 12, and internal use is not recommended in excess of 8–10 consecutive days. Completely safe when used externally.

STARTING DOSAGE:

- External use: apply liberal quantities of fresh gel from plant leaves topically.

I will only be talking here about the external use of **aloe vera gel**. (I believe there are other safer, more effective herbs that have the same internal applications.) **Aloe vera** is a plant that should be kept in every home, affording instant access to the fresh gel from its leaves for treating sunburn, minor burns, skin wounds, insect bites, acne, and bruises. It is one of the best household items for parents to keep on hand to educate children about using plants safely as medicine.

Aloe vera gel can benefit patients suffering from severe skin disorders such as psoriasis, frostbite, and radiation burns. The healing effects of this plant result from a complex set of antioxidant, anti-inflammatory, moisturizing, emollient, and antibacterial properties.

AMERICAN GINSENG ROOT

Latin: *Panax quinquefolius*   **Chinese:** Xi yang shen

WHAT IT DOES: American ginseng root is sweet and slightly bitter in taste and cooling in action. It is an adaptogenic (balancing) tonic that nourishes, moistens, and cools the body; strengthens the lungs; reduces weakness and fatigue; and strengthens and calms the nervous system.

RATING: Gold

SAFETY ISSUES: None known. Use cautiously with nausea and weak digestion.   .

STARTING DOSAGE:

- Dried powder: 3 to 6 grams per day

- 4:1 concentrated dried decoction extract: 1 to 2 grams per day

- 1:5 tincture: 30–60 drops 20 times per day

TCM doctors use **American ginseng root** as a Yin tonic and a Qi tonic. To see the benefits for yourself, use it after you've endured a severely weakening bout of fever or food poisoning, followed by signs of irritability and heat. It will greatly speed your recovery time. Though not as immediately energizing as **Chinese ginseng root, American ginseng root** gradually strengthens neurological force and is effective in slowly fighting off chronic fatigue, colds, coughs, and bronchitis. In our clinic we frequently add it to formulas where the patient has signs of fatigue and dryness in addition to the primary problem. I've noticed it often seems to strengthen the effects of other herbs. Perhaps this is due to the herb's numerous effects on the gut and the brain. Some scientists discount differences between **Chinese** and **American ginseng root,** noting they differ little in the lab. It is clear, however, that both are strongly tonic.

Research Highlights

- Animal studies show that a component, found in **American ginseng root** facilitates the uptake of choline into nerve endings, which suggests benefit for memory deficits (Salim, 1997). It also alters brain chemistry in a way that may improve sexual performance in animals (Murphy et al., 1998).

- Various pharmacological studies done on animals have shown heart-strengthening (cardiotonic) benefits of **American ginseng root,** a calming effect on the cerebral cortex of the brain, and memory-enhancing effects (Beninshin et al., 1991; Chen X et al., 1994; Yuan CS, 1998).

AMLA FRUIT

Latin: *Emblica officinalis*   **Sanskrit:** Amalaki   **English:** Indian gooseberry

WHAT IT DOES: Amla fruit is sour, sweet, and astringent in taste and cooling in action. It is a rasayana tonic that promotes longevity and is especially good for the heart. It fights upper respiratory infections.

RATING: Gold

SAFETY ISSUES: None known

STARTING DOSAGE:

- Dried powder: 2 grams two times per day

- 4:1 concentrated powder extract: 1 gram two times per day

Amla fruit comes from *Emblica officinalis,* a tropical and subtropical medium-sized tree that grows in arid areas. It is very highly regarded for traditional use as a heart tonic and as a rasayana for long life. Its tonic qualities are very strong, lending it medicinal value in the treatment of numerous diseases, including fever, cough, asthma, anemia, hemorrhage, and alcoholism. **Amla** is one of three ingredients in the famous Ayurvedic balancing tonic formula called **triphala** (three-fruit compound). It also comprises about 80% of the famous medicine called **Chyavanaprasha**, an ancient tonic made in the form of a jam that improves mental and physical well-being in people of all ages.

Modern research shows **amla** to contain an extremely high concentration of bioflavonoids and a stable form of vitamin C, and this may partially account for its reputation. TAM doctors called this herb "tridosaghna," meaning "an agent that stimulates the brain to subdue overbalance in the three controlling systems called Vata, Pitta, and Kapha." At our clinic we often add **amla fruit** to formulas when a gentle cleansing action is needed, especially in sensitive and weakened patients.

Research Highlights

- Tannin compounds found in **amla fruit** were tested for their effects in the brains of rats on three important free-radical-scavenging enzymes. Levels of all three increased, and there was a parallel decrease of oxidative stress (Bhattacharya et al., 1999). This illustrates that the antioxidant activity of **amla** is due to more than its high vitamin C content, a common misconception.

- Daily administration of a water extract of **amla fruit** protected laboratory mice from arsenic damage (Biswas et al., 1999), while another study confirmed that **amla fruit** strengthened bodily defense mechanisms against stress-induced free radical damage. The researchers reported that the **amla** appeared to cause an increase in the ability of target tissues to synthesize prostaglandins, which are essential to a host of important regulatory health functions (Rege et al., 1999).

- **Amla** may also possess cancer-fighting properties, as illustrated by several studies. Extracts of three Ayurvedic herbs, **amla fruit**, **tamalaki** *(Phyllanthus amarus),* and **katuki rhizome** *(Picrorrhiza kurroa),* significantly inhibited the ability of carcinogenic chemicals to induce liver cancer. Without the herbs, the incidence of tumors was 100% (Jeena et al., 1999).

- In another study, a group of mice that received dietary supplementation of **amla fruit** along with a known carcinogen experienced a significant reduction in cell poisoning when compared to mice that received only the carcinogen (Nandi et al., 1997).

- Studies have also indicated an ability to protect against elevated cholesterol levels and the resultant arterial damage. Fresh juice of **amla fruit** reduced the atherosclerotic effects of a high-fat, high-cholesterol diet in rabbits, as illustrated by the regression of aortic plaques (Mathur et al., 1996). An earlier human study also showed a decrease in cholesterol with **amla**. However, 2 weeks after **amla fruit** was discontinued, cholesterol levels rose again (Jacob et al., 1988). Also, all three fruits in **triphala** were shown to lower cholesterol significantly, although **vibhitaki fruit** *(Terminalia belerica)* proved slightly stronger than **amla** (Thakur et al., 1988).

ARJUNA BARK

Latin: *Terminalia arjuna*   **Sanskrit:** Arjuna

WHAT IT DOES: Arjuna bark is astringent in taste, cooling in action, and light and dry in property. It is an antipoison agent that tonifies, strengthens, and protects the heart and musculoskeletal system.

RATING: Gold

SAFETY ISSUES: None known

STARTING DOSAGE:

- Dried powder: 2 grams two to three times per day

- 4:1 concentrated powder extract: 1 gram two times per day

- 1:2 tincture: 20–40 drops two to three times per day

Arjuna bark is one of the most important heart tonics in Ayurvedic medicine, used to treat all forms of heart disease. It reduces the heart-damaging culprits of inflammation (Pitta) and mucus (Kapha) and is strong enough to protect against scorpion stings. **Arjuna bark** contains a fair amount of triterpenoid saponins, and cooking tends to activate these chemicals (which is why saponin-rich **Chinese ginseng root** is always cooked). Looking at the traditional literature, we see that for more than 1,500 years TAM doctors have boiled **arjuna bark** in milk or ghee to make medicine, having patients ingest it daily for up to a year.

I read an interesting report in the *Journal of Ethnopharmacology* about the tribes of the Maasai and Batemi in East Africa. It seems these people had the world's highest-cholesterol diet, consisting of basically nothing but milk and animal blood, yet they exhibited low incidences of heart disease and elevated cholesterol. Scientists finally figured out the reason. They prepared their blood and milk as a mouth-watering soup containing tree barks known to be rich in **saponins.**

Research Highlights

- The Indian Central Council for Research on Ayurveda and Siddha, citing 20 studies, reported that **arjuna bark** is valuable in treating angina pectoris, hypercholesterolemia, cardiac artery disease (CAD), and hypertension (Pandey et al., 1996; Dwivedi and Jauhari, 1997).

- Animal studies have also demonstrated its ability to improve liver mitochondrial function (Pandey et al., 1996).

- According to long-term outpatient evaluation, 500 mg of **arjuna bark,** taken three times per day in addition to standard medicines (diuretics, vasodilators, and digitalis) for 20–28 months (mean 24 months), contributed to improvement in symptoms, signs, effort, tolerance, and New York Heart Association Class, with improvement in quality of life (Bharani, 1995).

ASHWAGANDHA ROOT

Latin: *Convolvulus* species   **Sanskrit:** Ashwagandha
Withania somnifera

WHAT IT DOES: Ashwagandha root is bitter in taste, warming in action, and a strong rasayana tonic. It calms and strengthens the nervous system (Vata); reduces stress; strengthens immunity and vitality; increases sexual energy; and improves cognition and memory.

RATING: Gold

SAFETY ISSUES: Not to be used during pregnancy. Do not use *Withania somnifera* with barbiturates due to potentiation effects. The Nepalese *Convolvulus* species, has no known safety issues, but Western relatives such as bindweeds are associated with severe toxicity in animals (Todd FG et al., 1995).

STARTING DOSAGE:

- Dried powder: 2 grams two to three times per day

- 4:1 concentrated powder extract: 1 gram two to three times per day

- 1:5 tincture: 20–40 drops two to three times per day

There are two different plants known by the Sanskrit name **ashwagandha**. Both are effective. It is almost certain that the *Convolvulus* Himalayan mountain species found in Nepal is the original one described in Sanskrit texts, and that *Withania somnifera* was discovered and used later by doctors in India. In our clinic we use both of these plants to strengthen the immunity and vital force of weakened patients showing signs of anxiety or nervousness. **Ginseng root,** commonly used as a tonic, would not be a good choice in such case due to its excitatory action.

The *Convolvulus* species of **ashwagandha root** is a perennial bushy plant with white roots that is usually found in tropical areas. It commonly grows at the base of wheat, spiraling around the stems, and Dr. Mana and I located specimens within minutes when we searched wheat farms in Nepal. The root is an aphrodisiac and can be used to treat any nervous system disease. It is used to treat nervous exhaustion, poor memory, muscle weakness, and impotence. The strength of **ashwagandha root** seems to penetrate into the core of one's being. This species may be unique to the Himalayan regions, and *Convolvulus* species found in India is used as a purgative. The upper portions of the bindweeds found in North America are toxic.

Withania somnifera has now taken over the common name of **ashwagandha root** throughout the world. Also an excellent plant, it seems to impart overall energy to the system, with a marked calming effect. It is commonly called the "ginseng of India." The traditional way of preparing

Andrew Weil, M.D., reported in a Public Broadcasting System (PBS) special the case of a woman with multiple sclerosis who saw marked improvement in her overall health using this herb.

it for nerve diseases (Vataja) is to mix it into an approximate 50/50 ratio with ghee, and take 1 teaspoon two to three times per day. This tonic can be given to feeble children to increase their weight. It imparts a sense of well-being and strength as well as improved memory. In the interest of comparison, I have taken both forms of the herb. They are very similar in their calming effects, but the Nepalese variety has a much stronger aphrodisiac effect similar to that of **muira puama balsam.**

Research Highlights

- Investigators have demonstrated **ashwagandha root** is a true adaptogen, showing its effectiveness in animal models against a wide variety of biological, physical, and chemical stressors (Pandley et al., 1996; Rege et al., 1999; Archana et al., 1999; Dhuley, 1998).

- Pharmacological studies show it can prevent immunosuppression caused by exposure to strong chemical agents and may be valuable in restoring immunity after exposure to or treatment with such drugs (Ziauddin M et al., 1996). It also provides protection against some side effects of chemotherapy (Pandey et al., 1996).

- The alcohol extract of **ashwagandha root** has significant anti-inflammatory action in both acute and chronic types of inflammation, as demonstrated in rabbit, guinea pig, rat, and frog animal models (Pandey et al., 1996).

- Citing a total of 31 studies, the Indian Central Council for Research on Ayurveda and Siddha tells us that **ashwagandha root** exerts its most powerful pharmacological influence on the reproductive system, neuropharmacological disorders, cardiovascular system, respiratory system, bacteria, fungi, inflammation, and gastric acidity (Pandey et al., 1996).

ASTRAGALUS ROOT

Latin: *Astragalus membranaceus*   **Chinese:** Huang qi

WHAT IT DOES: Astragalus root is sweet in taste and slightly warming in action. It strengthens the vital force (Qi), nourishes the immune system, and strengthens the heart and lungs.

RATING: Yellow, due to limitations in usage

SAFETY ISSUES: Should not be used to treat acute infections. Use cautiously in patients with hypertension or heat signs.

STARTING DOSAGE:

- Dried powder: 1–3 grams per day for long-term use

Astragalus root is a very important vital energy (Qi) in TCM, as important as **ginseng root**. It has long been used to treat immune deficiency and fatigue, to heal wounds, to improve digestion, and to reduce edema caused by cardiac weakness. It is also very useful for chronic or acute low blood pressure. **Astragalus root** and **rehmannia root** are key herbs in most TCM prescriptions for treating chronic nephritis. **Astragalus** is noticeably stimulating, and its action is described as being able to "push the blood" and "bring energy up to the head." I wholeheartedly agree with the latter statement—I get a headache if I take it myself.

To determine whether a patient should take **astragalus** for immune tonification, the simple key sign I look for is weakness. It is also useful for patients who complain of catching every bug that comes around. It is best used in small doses over a long period of time for prevention of infections, in contradistinction to **echinacea** and **chrysanthemum flower,** which are best used with acute infections.

TCM doctors also use **astragalus root** for treating prolapse syndromes of the uterus, stomach, and anus, and to help stop uterine bleeding. I urge caution when using **astragalus** unless under the care of a qualified health care practitioner, because while it works very well in weak patients with signs of coldness, **it can create nervousness and headache and even raise blood pressure in patients with heat signs or hypertension.**

Research Highlights

- In a study of the effects of **astragalus** on strength and endurance in mice, the group that received **astragalus decoction** exhibited greater weight gain and greater endurance in swimming tests in comparison to the control group (reported in Bensky and Gamble, 1986).

- In various pharmacological and animal studies, **astragalus root** showed considerable immune-enhancing activity. Oral doses of the whole root or root extracts have been shown to increase phagocytic activity (cellular debris gobbling), enhance production of interferon (an important immune chemical), and activate natural killer (NK) cell activity. **Astragalus** also excites the central nervous system, strengthens heart contraction in fatigued patients, decreases protein in the urine, and conserves liver glycogen (Ma et al., 1998; Liang et al., 1995; Hong et al., 1994; Hong et al., 1992; Zhao et al., 1990; reported in Yeung, 1983).

- **Astragalus** has been studied in vitro for its effects on ischemic heart disease, heart failure, angina pain, and liver protection against poisonous agents (endotoxin). In one study of patients with ischemic heart disease, **astragalus root** relieved angina symptoms and improved EKG results (Li et al., 1995).

- A review of live animal research has indicated that it affords a cardioprotective benefit in cases of ischemic heart disease, heart failure, angina pain, and liver poisoning by endotoxin. An in vitro antioxidant mechanism allows the herb to offer this protection (Miller, 1998). Other researchers have come to the same conclusion with regard to liver protection (Wang and Han, 1992).

- In one interesting study that tested the ability of **astragalus root** to increase vital energy (Qi), researchers inserted microcomputers into the stomachs of healthy dogs after they received a concentrated **astragalus** solution. The readings indicated that the solution strengthened the movement and muscle tone in the intestine, especially the jejunum (Yang, 1993).

- Several studies have confirmed the ability of **astragalus root** to prevent heart damage caused by viral myocarditis. Researchers used a formula composed primarily of **astragalus root, ophiopogon root,** and **honeysuckle flower** in a randomized controlled cross-over clinical study of viral myocarditis in mice. They compared left ventricular function in the test group to the same function in a control group that received coenzyme Q_{10}. The researchers concluded that the formula could directly inactivate the Coxsackie B3 virus, protect the heart cells, and increase interferon and NK immune cell activity (Yan, 1991).

- Another group concluded, "it is a rational choice to treat patients with **astragalus** in viral myocarditis" (Guo et al., 1995; Peng et al., 1995).

- Two weeks after receiving injections of **astragalus fraction**, 15 of 19 patients with congestive heart failure experienced relief from chest distress and dyspnea, and improved capability to exercise (Luo et al., 1995).

- In a study of rats with acute brain edema caused by pertussis vaccine, a TCM formula called **bu yang huan wu tang** that contains 84% **astragalus root** was shown to raise declining levels of the important cellular antioxidants SOD (superoxide dismutase) and glutathione peroxidase. Researchers concluded that the formula protected the blood-brain barrier and certain brain cells from damage (Zhou et al., 1994).

- A controlled study to test the ability of TCM formulas to improve the quality of life of persons with chronic renal failure treated 36 patients with a decoction containing **ginseng root, astragalus root, licorice root, rhubarb root,** and **cinnamon twigs**. Researchers studied the effects on six symptoms: fatigue, lassitude in loin and legs, aversion to cold, anorexia, sexual dysfunction, and mental depression. Five patients improved markedly in symptom scores, and their creatine levels approached normal readings (Sheng et al., 1994).

BALA

Latin: *Sida cordifolia*   **Sanskrit:** Bala   **English:** Country mallow

WHAT IT DOES: Bala is sweet in taste and hot in action. It nourishes and strengthens immunity, heals the nerves, reduces pain, and stimulates formation of healthy new tissue.

RATING: Silver, due to minor limitations in usage

SAFETY ISSUES: Contains small amounts of ephedrine alkaloids. The amount of total alkaloids in **bala plant** by average dry weight is $\frac{1}{15}$ of that found in **ephedra**. **Bala seeds,** usually not commercially available, contain about four times as much of the alkaloids, about $\frac{1}{4}$ of that found in **ephedra,** and so should not be used unless under the care of a professional health care provider.

STARTING DOSAGE:

- Dried powder: 2 grams two times per day

- 4:1 concentrated powder extract: 1 gram two times per day

Bala is used as a tonic and to activate the function of the nervous system (Vata) by increasing blood circulation. As a tonic, it increases the vital properties of the serum (plasma), which is very important for the nourishment of the cells, the strength of healing power, and the maintenance of immunity. Following this effect, it has medicinal value in treating neuropathy related to any organ including the heart, brain, spinal cord, facial nerves, and inner ear. There is a gradual tissue-strengthening effect, most noticeable with increased wound healing after injury. It is used to stimulate healing of dry painful joints in osteoarthritis. TAM doctors also use it to heal the lung in tuberculosis, as well as for chronic bronchitis and chronic hemoptysis (spitting of blood).

The low level of ephedrine in **bala** does not warrant its substitution for **ephedra** in over-the-counter weight-loss formulas, though it probably lowers risk factors. It is possible that unscrupulous manufacturers may attempt to hide the presence of **ephedra** alkaloids by adding **bala** to their weight-loss products.

TAM doctors use **bala root** to make various complex oil preparations. These oils are used as external applications for various nervous sytem diseases, such as neuropathies, facial paralysis, spasmodic coughing or asthma, vertigo, seizures, and menstrual cramps. The oils are also used for rheumatic and arthritis pain. **Bala root** is a major ingredient in the famous medicinal oil called **narayana taila**.

Research Highlights

- Although it is a major Ayurvedic herb, there is still little scientific research available on **bala**. Test tube research has confirmed the presence of analgesic and anti-inflammatory activities in the aerial portions and roots (Kanth and Diwan, 1999).

- Pharmacological studies have shown the presence of mucins, fatty oils, and resins, as well as plant sterols, which may partially account for the tonic actions of the herb (reported in Kapoor, 1990).

BEET ROOT

Latin: *Beta vulgaris*

WHAT IT DOES: Beet root is sweet in taste and detoxifying in action. It nourishes the liver, intestines, and other internal organs and protects them from toxins.

RATING: Silver, due to limitations of medicinal potency

SAFETY ISSUES: None known

STARTING DOSAGE:

- Vegetable: ingest freely

- Dried powder: 2 to 3 grams two times per day

Beets are cultivated worldwide as both a food and a source of sugar. I personally think they are also a very effective herbal medicine. Remember that all fresh foods are medicinal, but only those with a unique composition that creates a higher-than-normal activity level qualify as medicines. The dark red color of the **beet root** is due to an intensely crimson pigment called "betanin," which bleeds out if the skin is pierced before cooking. For this reason experienced cooks usually bake, steam, or boil them with the skins intact. It also contains sugars (up to

A news report from the Czech Republic reported that villagers who ate **beets** along with their sausages were able to lower the usual increases in colon cancer found in that country due to diet. Research seems to be backing this up and giving us the reasons why.

22%), valuable fiber, anthocyans, and betaine. All by-products of beet production are sold for use in livestock feeds.

Betaine is important because it can help the body regenerate a key cellular antioxidant enzyme (methionine reductase), which in turn is used by the body to prevent the buildup of homocysteine, a very harmful chemical. Toxins such as alcohol and environmental chemicals work in the opposite direction, damaging our liver, blood vessels, kidneys, and intestines if we are low in this protective enzyme. Although medical research on **beet root** is presently sparse, I suspect that more evidence of its medicinal powers will emerge. I often mix **beet root powder** into herbal formulas to make them more palatable, especially to children.

Research Highlights

- Researchers tested the inhibitory effect of **beet root** extract against both the Epstein-Barr virus and mouse skin and lung cancers, revealing a higher order of activity compared to other red-pigment vegetables and fruits such as **cranberry, red onion skin,** and short and long **red bell peppers.** Researchers concluded that "the combined findings suggest that beet root ingestion can be one of the useful means to prevent cancer" (Kapadia et al., 1996).

- A controlled study done in Greece of patients with colorectal cancer showed they ate significantly more lamb and beef and less **beets,** spinach, lettuce, and cabbage (Manousos et al., 1983).

- A rat study suggested that **beet fiber** could help eliminate abnormal cells from an irradiated colon by initiating apoptosis (programmed cell death) (Ishizuka et al., 1999).

BILBERRY AND BLUEBERRY

Latin: *Vaccinium myrtillus*
Vaccinium myrtilloides

WHAT THEY DO: Bilberries and **blueberries** are sour in taste and cooling in action. They remove inflammation and congestion from tiny blood vessels, strengthening vessel integrity and microcirculation; they prevent oxidative stress damage to the eye and to neuronal cells.

RATING: Gold

SAFETY ISSUES: None known

STARTING DOSAGE:

- Blueberries: eat fresh berries freely in season; use frozen berries during the off-season

- Bilberry extract: 60–180 mg anthocyanosides per day

The colorful anthocyanoside pigment compounds in **bilberries** and (to a slightly lesser extent) **blueberries** find their way to the capillary vessel basement membranes and the surrounding collagen structures, where they neutralize free radicals which can weaken these tiny structures. Healthy and resilient capillary vessels are able to maintain their shape and function for normal, efficient microcirculation to prevent swelling in the surrounding tissues. This is very useful in the prevention of vascular complications of diabetes, and the improvement of night vision and overall visual acuity. For the same reasons, **bilberries** or **blueberries** can be used to treat intestinal inflammation, hemorrhoids, macular degeneration, rheumatoid arthritis, and varicose veins.

High doses of **bilberry extract** (and other flavonoids) act to strengthen the blood-brain barrier by acting on collagen fibers to protect sensitive peptide bonds from attack and actually restoring degraded basement membranes. Since weakness of

> A 1-pound bag of frozen **blueberries** eaten over a week's time provides approximately 400 mg of anthocyanosides, or about 60 mg per day.

the blood-brain barrier is a suspected component in diseases such as multiple sclerosis and chronic fatigue syndrome, I often tell patients with nervous system weakness to use **blueberries** in fairly large quantities over a long period of time.

Typically, I suggest that they eat one bag of frozen **blueberries** (this form seems to be the most convenient to obtain year-round) once or twice per week, pretty much forever. Most patients love this prescription. The stronger concentrated **bilberry extracts** are needed with more serious diseases such as MS and macular degeneration, unless you love to eat **blueberries**. The best thing about them is that, like **raspberries** and **blackberries,** they contain less sugar than most other fruits.

Research Highlights

- The antioxidant action of **bilberry extracts** can help prevent the problems caused by elevated LDL (bad) cholesterol levels (Laplaud et al., 1997).

- Other reported benefits based upon pharmacological studies include wound healing, antiulcer action (Martin A et al., 1998), and protection against damage to tendons, ligaments, and cartilage (Monboisse et al., 1984).

- Of great interest to me was a 1997 study showing that **bilberry extract** in high dosage (equivalent to 180 mg anthocyanosides per day) helped animals maintain normal permeability of the blood-brain barrier during induced hypertension. The same research group was able to demonstrate this over a series of experiments done over the next two decades (Robert et al., 1977a; Robert et al., 1997b).

BOSWELLIA GUM

Latin: *Boswellia serrata*   **Sanskrit:** Shallaki   **Hindi:** Salai guggul *(B. serrata)*
Boswellia carterii   **Chinese:** Ru xiang *(B. carterii)*   **English:** Frankincense

WHAT IT DOES: Boswellia gum is pungent and bitter in taste and warm in action. It reduces pain, swelling, and inflammation in the lungs, intestines, and joints.

RATING: Yellow, due to limitations in usage due to strong cooling action

SAFETY ISSUES: None known. Long-term use may damp appetite.

STARTING DOSAGE:

- Dried powder: 2 to 3 grams two to three times per day

- 4:1 concentrated powder extract: 250–750 mg two to three times per day

Boswellia gum is used as an effective pain-relieving anti-inflammatory in the treatment of osteoarthritis, rheumatoid arthritis, diarrhea, lung diseases (including asthma), boils, edema, pain, psoriasis, ulcerative colitis, bronchial asthma, and Crohn's disease. It works by affecting one of two classes of mediators of inflammation along the leukotriene pathway. Prostaglandins and leukotrienes are known collectively as "eicosanoids," and they ease pain and edema. TCM doctors use the related *B. carterii* species to remove blood stasis and reduce pain. What makes this herb stand out is its specificity and strength of effect.

Boswellia gum can often (but not always) be used as an alternative to NSAIDs (nonsteroidal anti-inflammatory drugs) and steroids, causing none of the common side effects such as stomach bleeding, ulceration, weakened heart, and even death seen with these

Western remedies. At our clinic we usually use **boswellia gum** in formulas for pain and inflammation. I have also used it successfully to reduce asthma symptoms in many patients. No plant works for all types of inflammation, so the best thing to do is test it out for a few weeks if using it by itself. Studies of **boswellia** toxicity in rats, mice, and monkeys have shown it to be safe, even at high doses.

Research Highlights

- A double-blind, placebo-controlled study done on 40 asthma patients in Germany showed marked improvement in the treated patients compared to the control group (Gupta et al., 1998). Another study, done on ulcerative colitis patients using a standardized extract for 6 weeks, reported improvement in 82% of patients (Gupta et al.,1997).

- **Boswellia** may even be useful in treating leukemia; one Chinese study showed that it stimulated leukemic cells to kill themselves, a phenomenon known as programmed cell death (Jing et al., 1999).

Note: The Chinese *Boswellia carterii* is sometimes called **mastic** and should not be confused with *Pistacia lentiscus*, also called **mastic,** which is used to treat ulcers.

BROMELAIN

Latin: *Ananas comosus* (source)

WHAT IT DOES: Bromelain is pungent and slightly sweet in taste, with a strong, long-lasting penetrating quality. It reduces inflammation and mucus, improves digestion and absorption, speeds wound healing, and helps fight tumors.

RATING: Silver, due to minor limitations in usage

SAFETY ISSUES: Do not use if taking anticoagulant (blood-thinning) medicines. Do not exceed suggested dosage unless prescribed by a physician. Overuse may weaken intestinal membranes.

STARTING DOSAGE:

- Enzyme pill: one to two 500-mg pills standardized to 2,000 GDUs (a measure of protein-digesting capacity) twice per day between meals

Bromelain is an herbal compound of digestive-enhancing enzymes derived from the stem of pineapple and has been used as a medicine since 1957. Several hundred scientific papers have appeared in the medical literature supporting its use for various problems

(Murray and Pizzorno, 1989). It is important to understand that **bromelain**'s digestive action takes place both in the digestive system and in the blood.

Your blood coagulates when a special protein named fibrinogen converts to the more elastic fibrin. **Bromelain** inhibits blood coagulation by both inhibiting fibrinogen and breaking down fibrin (Lotz-Winter H, 1990). It also blocks the formation of several inflammatory compounds and exhibits strong mucolytic (mucus-reducing) activity (Taussig and Batkin, 1988). When I see patients who cannot overcome chronic infections and are on antibiotics continuously, I give them **bromelain** to enhance the antibiotic's effectiveness and cross this impasse.

Because of its unique group of actions, we use **bromelain** at our clinic as an all-purpose anti-inflammatory and to speed wound healing, especially in patients with poor digestion or those recovering from recent trauma, surgical or otherwise. It is useful in angina, arthritis, athletic injury, connective tissue inflammation, bronchitis, burns, cellulitis, dysmenorrhea, edema, bruising, poor digestion, pancreatic insufficiency, pancreatitis, pneumonia, scleroderma, sinusitis, staph infections, postsurgical trauma, and thrombophlebitis. I consider **bromelain** second only to **tien chi root** for speeding recovery from trauma. Both can be used together as an effective combination.

Research Highlights

- **Bromelain** reduces edema, bruising, wound-healing time, and pain following surgery (Howat RC et al., 1972, reported in Murray and Pizzorno, 1989).

- **Bromelain** has direct anticancer effects, originally attributed to its ability to digest the protein coatings surrounding tumors. However, recent evidence indicates it may also strengthen the ability of monocytes to attack target cancer cells (Eckert K et al., 1999).

- **Bromelain's** digestion-enhancing quality increases the serum levels and effectiveness of several antibiotics (Smyth RD et al., 1968; Zimmermann I et al., 1978) and is almost as effective by itself as an antibiotic treatment for sinusitis, bronchitis, pneumonia, and staph infections (Seltzer, 1967; Weiss S et al., 1972).

BUPLEURUM ROOT

Latin: *Bupleurum chinensis*   **Chinese:** Chai hu   **English:** Chinese thoroughwax
Bupleurum falcatum

WHAT IT DOES: Bupleurum root is bitter and pungent in taste and cooling (anti-inflammatory) in action. It releases internal tension and lowers mental stress and anxiety, reduces dizziness and vertigo, warms cold hands and feet caused by tension, stimulates the immune system, reduces fever and liver inflammation, stimulates bile flow, protects the liver, and improves digestion.

RATING: Silver, due to minor limitations in usage (can generate wind)

SAFETY ISSUES: None known

STARTING DOSAGE:

- Crude herb: 3 to 12 grams per day

- Concentrated powder: 1 to 4 grams per day

Bupleurum is a very important silver standard herb, critically valuable for some patients. Its scientifically investigated actions are as diverse as our Chinese animal example in the text box. TCM doctors note that when you look at this plant, its branches splay outward in a free and unrestricted manner. This is the "Doctrine of Signatures" or traditional way of seeing the plant's main action—in this case, the removal of blockages from the free flow of the body's vital energy. (The "Doctrine of Signatures," or "Signature of God," is the idea that the shape, form, or color of a plant can tell you how to use it.) All the TCM clinical uses for this herb flow from this idea, because as the energy flows without blockage, the hands warm, the digestion eases, the mind calms, and irritation and heat decrease. Once when I took this herb myself, I was amazed to feel my hands begin to warm until they were actually buzzing in a pleasant way for over an hour.

Bupleurum root is a main ingredient in a formula called "Rambling without a Destination," which is a great formula name,

> **Bupleurum** is a good illustration of the problems we face when trying to translate Chinese thinking into Western words. We recall the story of the ancient Chinese dictionary, in which a Westerner looked up the word *animal* and found the following definition: "There are eight types of animals: (1) Cows (2) Pigs (3) Big animals (4) Animals that bite (5) Animals that live in holes (6) Animals that float (7) Mythical animals (8) Animals that belong to the emperor."
>
> Though this seems funny at first, it is actually a quite practical if not logical grouping. In ancient times, cows and pigs were the most important domesticated food sources, large animals and animals that bit were dangerous, animals that lived in holes and floated were good secondary food sources, mythical animals were a necessary part of religious observances, and messing with the emperor's animals got you killed.

isn't it? The formula is used to treat the same conditions as the root, but in persons with additional signs of weakness and nutrient deficiency. Drs. Dan Bensky and Randall Barolet, in their excellent 1990 professional TCM textbook *Formulas and Strategies*, quote an ancient text that recommends this formula for "girls with weak blood and Yin deficiency."

Research Highlights

- Numerous components of **bupleurum root** have shown anti-inflammatory activity in a wide variety of animal models (Just et al., 1998; Bergema et al., 1998; Tagaki et al., 1969).

- In a screening of 232 plants for anti-cell-adhesiveness activity, important for tumor cell and cancer metastasis inhibition, researchers found **bupleurum root saponins** to be one of the six most active (Ahn et al., 1998).

- **Bupleurum root extracts** protected rat livers from chemical insults, leading researchers to conclude that members of this species "have potential as broad spectrum antihepatic agents" (Chin et al., 1996).

- **Bupleurum root saponins**, like other saponin-rich herbs, show potent heart- and blood-vessel-protective effects. They have been shown to "inhibit the formation of lipid peroxides in the cardiac muscle or in the liver, influence the function of enzymes contained in them, decrease blood coagulation, cholesterol and sugar levels in blood, [and] stimulate the immunity system" (Purmova et al., 1995).

- In a series of experiments to determine the mechanism by which **bupleurum root saponins** inhibit kidney inflammation, researchers concluded that they reduced platelet sticking (blood stickiness), protected against loss of antioxidant capacity, and enhanced blood and kidney corticosterone levels (Hattori et al., 1991).

- Researchers have also determined that **bupleurum root** enhances macrophage cell activity (Matsumoto et al., 1995).

- Various clinical studies on humans have shown liver enzyme reduction in hepatitis, fever reduction in infection, and diuretic effects (reported in Bone, 1996).

- One of the most famous **bupleurum root**-based formulas is **minor bupleurum decoction,** which contains **bupleurum root, scute root, pinellia tuber, ginger root, ginseng root, honey-fried licorice root,** and **ziziphus fruit.** This formula was able to promote clearance of hepatitis B antigen from the blood of 14 chronically ill children (reported in Bone, 1996).

BURDOCK ROOT

Latin: *Arctium lappa*   **Chinese:** Niu bang zi

WHAT IT DOES: **Burdock root** is bitter and slightly pungent in taste and cooling in action. It improves digestive, liver, and bowel functions, reduces heat and inflammation, and helps detoxify poisons. It also heals the skin.

RATING: Gold

SAFETY ISSUES: None known

STARTING DOSAGE:

- Fresh vegetable: eat freely

- Decoction: 1 teaspoon of the root simmered in 1 cup of water for 10–15 minutes, taken three times per day

- Dried powder: 2 to 6 grams per day

- 1:5 tincture (dry root): 20–40 drops three times per day

Burdock root is available as a common vegetable, and it may be eaten freely in this form. As is common with many bitter herbs, **burdock** stimulates digestion, increases bile secretion, and reduces inflammation, which may account for its reputation as a liver detoxifier.

Burdock contains an abundance of inulin, a compound that feeds the friendly bacteria in the intestine. It is also mildly antibacterial and antifungal. Japanese scientists have shown that **burdock** contains **desmutagens**, a word coined for substances that inactivate mutagens (cancer-causing agents) such as pesticides and toxic compounds that are created in some meats during the cooking process.

These findings help explain why **burdock root** has traditionally been a first choice in treating frustrating skin conditions like eczema, boils, acne, and psoriasis. Herbalists believe that imbalances or toxins in the bowels carry through to the liver and blood, and if the liver or bowels are slow in getting rid of them, they are eventually "thrown out" to the skin. TCM doctors also use **burdock root** to treat fevers, cough, and swollen red throat.

Research Highlights

- Animal studies show that **burdock root** has liver protective anti-inflammatory and free-radical-scavenging activity, and in vitro studies suggest it has the ability to neutralize mutation-causing chemicals (Lin CC et al., 1996; Morita K et al., 1984).

CARTHAMUS FLOWER

Latin: *Carthamus tinctorius*   **Chinese:** Hong hua   **English:** Safflower flower

WHAT IT DOES: Carthamus flower is pungent in taste and warming in action. It promotes blood circulation and helps reduce pain.

RATING: Silver, due to minor limitations in usage

SAFETY ISSUES: Should not be used during pregnancy. Use with caution if taking anti-coagulant medications. Do not take during menstruation if bleeding is heavy.

STARTING DOSAGE:

- Dried powder: 3 to 9 grams per day

Note: To make a wine preparation add 9 grams of concentrated powder to 4 ounces of wine and take in 1-ounce doses throughout the day.

Carthamus flower has a beautiful red color. It is one of my favorite herbs for promoting blood circulation, and it stops pain and can be used safely to treat poor circulation, dysmenorrhea, and amenorrhea. At our clinic we also include it in formulas for treating angina pectoris and other serious cerebrovascular diseases. **However, in such cases we treat with carthamus only in coordination with a cardiologist to ensure patient safety.** TCM doctors also use it to reduce spleen and liver enlargement. A rare special form of this flower from Tibet called **tsang hong hua** is considered to be the highest quality. TCM doctors believe taking **carthamus flower** with wine strengthens the herb's ability to break down blood stasis.

Research Highlights

- Chinese laboratory studies have shown that **carthamus flower** can improve coronary blood flow and increase the time necessary for the blood to clot. Clinical trials with a tablet made from an alcohol extract of **carthamus** resulted in reduced angina pain, improved endurance, and improved EEG. Intravenous infusion also proved very effective (reported in Dharmananda, 1994).

- Decoctions of **carthamus flower** with other blood-moving and Qi-invigorating herbs have also proven beneficial in patients with coronary artery disease. In one study, patients reported significant reduction in symptoms, and 41% had an improvement in ECG after 1 month of treatment. Following the 4-month study, 90% of the patients were able to stop using nitroglycerin (reported in Bensky and Gamble, 1993).

- **Carthamus flower** has shown pharmacological actions in animal and in vitro experiments including dilation of the coronary artery, constriction on the kidney blood vessels, protection against brain injury from ischemia (lack of blood flow), and lowering of cholesterol (reported in Yeung, 1983).

CASTOR OIL

Latin: *Ricinus communis*   **Sanskrit:** Eranda

WHAT IT DOES: Externally, **castor oil** stimulates lymph drainage. Internally, it is used as a laxative.

RATING: Yellow, due to specific limitations in usage

SAFETY ISSUES: Castor oil is bitter and slightly sweet in taste. There are no known safety issues for external use. However, do not use for internal purposes with intestinal obstruction. Do not use internally for more than 10 days consecutively. **Warning: Do not ingest seeds—they are poisonous.**

STARTING DOSAGE:

- Oil—internal laxative use: ingest 1 to 2 tablespoons at bedtime

- Oil—external use: soak cotton or flannel pads in the oil and apply as a moist pack for ½ to 1 hour, using a heating pad to stimulate absorption.

Castor oil is used externally to stimulate movement and elimination in the lymphatic system, and internally as a laxative. I never use **castor oil** internally as a laxative for more than 1 or 2 days per month due to its potency and bad taste. However, like other laxatives, it can be used to cleanse the bowels in cases of chronic or acute skin eruptions. Following the Ayurvedic tradition, short-term use of a potent laxative like **castor oil** is recommended if the patient suffers from heart disease, severe hypertension (to quickly reduce elevated blood pressure), or chronic fever.

Use **castor oil** packs as follows:

1. Purchase a good-quality **castor oil,** preferably in organic form free of chemicals and pesticides.
2. Wash cotton or flannel cloth in clean, hot water to remove poisons.
3. Saturate cloth in **castor oil** and place over area of treatment.
4. Cover with plastic and apply heat—medium setting on heating pad—to increase penetration.
5. Leave on for 30 to 60 minutes.
6. Repeat every day or every other day for six days.

Dr. William McGarey tells us in his book *Edgar Cayce and the Palma Christi* that a Dr. Arthur Schoch treated 10 cases of severe skin eruption successfully with a few doses of **castor oil**. One patient reported to me that she could get pimples to disappear quickly by applying a single drop of **castor oil** to them a few times a day.

At our clinic, we use **castor oil** primarily as an external preparation, as packs placed over swollen glands, cancers, cysts, hard swellings, and other abnormal growths. The oil seems to stimulate the lymphatic system to draw away poisons. We usually place the packs over the lymph glands near the shoulders, groin, upper back, and neck; over the abdomen or liver; or over the kidneys.

I remember in particular a woman with chronically swollen lymph glands in the neck who had seen several doctors to no avail. **Castor oil packs** rid her of the problem in 2 weeks.

CHAGA MUSHROOM

Latin: *Inonotus obliquus*

WHAT IT DOES: Chaga mushroom has a bitter, coffeelike flavor. It stimulates the immune system and draws the life force out of tumors.

RATING: Silver, due to high concentration of nutrients

SAFETY ISSUES: None known

STARTING DOSAGE:

- 1:5 tincture: 40–60 drops two to three times per day

- Tea: dissolve 1 teaspoon dried mushroom in 1 cup of water several times per day

Chaga mushroom grows on birch trees in the colder northern climates. There have been 150 species of medicinal mushrooms found to inhibit the growth of different kinds of tumors, especially cancers of the stomach, esophagus, and lungs, but **chaga** seems to stand out from the rest. I learned about this mushroom from herbalist David Winston, who told me it has been used traditionally to treat different forms of cancer in Siberia, Canada, Scandinavia, the United States, and Russia.

Chaga is a fungal parasite that draws its nutrients out of living trees, rather than from the ground. Fungi digest food outside their bodies by releasing enzymes into the surrounding environment, breaking down organic matter into a form the fungus can then absorb. A look at the research on **chaga** shows a similar pattern with respect to its effect on tumors.

The anticancer properties of betulin or betulinic acid, a chemical isolated from birch trees, are now being studied for use as a chemotherapeutic agent. **Chaga** contains large amounts of betulinic acid in a form that can be ingested orally, and it also contains the full spectrum of immune-stimulating phytochemicals found in other medicinal mushrooms such as **maitake mushroom** and **shiitake mushroom**. Currently, **chaga** is available only from Herbalist & Alchemist (see Resource Guide).

Research Highlights

- Studies done in Poland have demonstrated **chaga's** inhibiting effects on tumor growth (Rzymowska, 1998).

- Betulin seems to work highly selectively on tumor cells because the interior pH of tumor tissues is generally lower than that of normal tissues, and betulinic acid is only active at those lower levels (Noda et al., 1997).

- Once inside the cells, betulinic acid induces apoptosis (programmed cell death) in the tumors (Fulda et al., 1997).

CHASTE TREE BERRY

Latin: *Vitex agnus-castus*

WHAT IT DOES: Chaste tree berry is bitter and pungent in taste and cooling in action. It relieves symptoms associated with PMS and menopause.

RATING: Yellow, due to limitations in usage

SAFETY ISSUES: Do not use when pregnant or nursing. Use with caution if taking hormones or birth control pills.

STARTING DOSAGE:

- Tincture: 15–35 drops three times per day

- Dried berry: 1–2 grams two times per day (chew slowly)

Chaste tree berry has risen in popularity over the past 10 years because of its effect on the female hormone system. It has the ability to increase progesterone production, inhibit FSH (follicle-stimulating hormone or follitropin), and inhibit prolactin. Research has shown these effects to be nontoxic and attributes them to dopamine-receptor-site binding. FSH assists in follicle maturation in females, encouraging progesterone production. Additionally, it increases the secretion of estradiol, one of the female estrogens. Simply put, **chaste tree berry** helps increase both estrogen and progesterone, with a stronger effect on progesterone. This explains its traditional use as a remedy for PMS, menopausal symptoms, and breast pain (mastodynia).

At our clinic we often use **chaste tree berry** to treat simple PMS symptoms before resorting to more complex formulas.

> In men, inhibition of prolactin causes a decrease in sperm production. Since **chaste tree berry** inhibits prolactin, monks used it in medieval times to reduce male sexual desire.

Although we usually use stronger herbs like **lycium bark, red clover blossoms,** and **soy extracts** to treat hot flashes, sometimes adding **chaste tree berry tincture** can improve results.

There is a commercial German **chaste tree** product (Agnolyt) that is beneficial for amenorrhea, PMS-related water retention, mouth ulceration, and severe constipation. However, for best results when treating amenorrhea it needs to be taken for up to a year. Elevated prolactin levels are often found in people with celiac disease. Therefore, it may be wise to undergo a trial withdrawal of gluten before using **chaste tree berry**.

Research Highlights

- In a double-blind, placebo-controlled study of 100 patients, extract of **chaste tree berry** was found effective in the treatment of breast pain related to the menstrual cycle (Halaska et al., 1998).

- In a randomized controlled clinical trial involving 52 women with menstrual problems due to elevated production of prolactin, **chaste tree berry** capsules reduced prolactin levels significantly and restored the menstrual cycles to normal without side effects (Milewicz et al., 1993).

- In a series of animal studies, **chaste tree berry extract** proved as effective as a synthetic dopamine agonist (Lisuride) in inhibiting prolactin secretion (Silutz et al., 1993).

CHRYSANTHEMUM FLOWER

Latin: *Chrysanthemum parthenium*   **Chinese:** Ju hua   **English:** Chrysanthemum

WHAT IT DOES: Chrysanthemum flower is sweet and slightly bitter in taste and slightly cold in action. It reduces heat and congestion in the liver, lungs, and eyes, eases coughs and colds, fights viral illness and infection, and prevents headaches and dizziness.

RATING: Yellow, due to minor limitations in usage

SAFETY ISSUES: Should not be used during pregnancy, as it is a uterine stimulant. Occasional minor side effects such as mouth and gastric disturbance have been reported. Some scientists voice concerns about potential allergic reactions or cross-reactivity with blood-thinning agents such as warfarin and Ticlopidine.

STARTING DOSAGE:

- Fresh leaves: one to three per day

- Standardized capsules (600 mcg parthenolide): one to three capsules per day

- Concentrated powder: 1 to 3 grams per day

Chrysanthemum flower is used extensively in TCM formulas to treat upper respiratory infections, allergies, headaches, red eyes, and hypertension. It effectively reduces irritation and inflammation in the lungs, nasal passageways, and throat, and scientific studies have shown it to be antibacterial, antifungal, and antiviral.

It also has a calming antihypertensive effect. The Chinese use it for the same purposes **echinacea** is used in the West, and it is commonly found in various cold and sinus remedies such as the famous **Yin Chiao,** available in many Chinese grocery stores.

TCM doctors rate **chrysanthemum** according to its colors and place of origin. **White chrysanthemum** (bai ju hua) is considered slightly superior to other forms for nourishing the liver, and so is used to treat diminished vision. **Yellow chrysanthemum** (huang ju hua) has a greater wind- and heat-clearing activity, and is used most often to treat eye redness and headache. The best-quality **yellow chrysanthemum** comes from the Chinese city of Hangzhou. This type, in addition to its other uses, is strong enough to reduce dizziness caused by elevated blood pressure.

> We keep Yin Chiao pills on hand at our clinic and give patients three pills three times per day at the first sign of a cold. It will often stop the cold within 24–48 hours, or at least shorten the duration by a few days. I have one elderly patient who calls me every year and asks for a big supply of what she calls her "Yin Choo cold pills." I think she's hawking them on the side at her retirement home.

Chrysanthemum flowers have become popular in the West, under the name **feverfew,** as a remedy for migraine headaches. The two names are considered interchangeable in this country, but Nai-shing notes that the **chrysanthemum flowers** she has seen growing in America are smaller and exhibit different coloring than the wild flowers she collected in the fields in China. Large differences have been found in various commercial preparations, and there are concerns about processing methods, so be sure to purchase **chrysanthemum** from a reliable supplier.

Research Highlights

- **Chrysanthemum flowers** have shown in vitro antibiotic effects and have reduced blood pressure, headache, and dizziness in hypertensive patients (reported in Bensky and Gamble, 1993).

COCOA BEAN

Latin: *Theobroma cacao*   **Chinese:** Cha ku li

WHAT IT DOES: Cocoa bean is bitter in taste and warming in action. It stimulates the mind and elevates mood.

RATING: Yellow, due to minor limitations in usage (contains caffeine)

SAFETY ISSUES: None known

STARTING DOSAGE:

- Dried powder: 1 to 2 grams two times per day. May be used sweetened or unsweetened.

The Latin *Theobroma* means "Food of the Gods." **Cocoa bean** and its derivative, **chocolate,** can help digestion, increase blood flow to the heart, and ease chest congestion. It is high in antioxidants and happens to taste better than most other herbs. In Central America, **cocoa bean** has long been used to treat pregnancy problems and ease childbirth, coughs, chest congestion, and fever. Its use in the Western world took off in 1876 with the invention of **milk chocolate**.

Cocoa bean contains caffeine, tryptophan (a serotonin precursor), theobromine (a substance similar to caffeine), and amandamides (substances that activate the same receptor in the brain as marijuana). Of course, commercial **cocoa** products are loaded with sugar, so I prefer to make my own hot cocoa with **soy milk,** sweetened with a mixture of **honey** and **stevia leaf.** Sugar-free **cocoa powder** can be a good choice in formulas for patients in need of mild mood elevation. By the way, the amandamides are present in very, very small amounts, so if you want to get high from **chocolate,** you have to get fat, too.

A recent Harvard School of Public Health study that received national attention in the popular press revealed that males who eat **chocolate** once or twice per week live, on average, 1 year longer than those who do not indulge. Unfortunately, the same result has not been demonstrated in women.

Cocoa bean and **chocolate,** like **coffee bean** and **tea leaves,** contain xanthines, chemicals that help relax bronchial spasms and can be useful for treating allergies and asthma, especially in emergencies where no other medication is available.

The xanthines include caffeine, theobromine, and theophylline. People may actually use **chocolate** instinctively as a form of self-medication for dietary deficiencies, or to increase low levels of neurotransmitters such as serotonin and dopamine. Additionally, many Americans are deficient in magnesium, and **chocolate** craving may be a sign of magnesium deficiency.

Research Highlights

- A placebo-controlled crossover study at the Institute of Sports Medicine at Beijing Medical University looked at the effect of **chocolate** on exercise recovery rates. **Chocolate bar** supplementation before exercise improved recovery by keeping blood sugars and other blood chemicals at good levels for up to 30 minutes after completion of 1 hour of running (Chen et al., 1996).

- Researchers have found that the episodic nature of **chocolate** cravings fluctuates with hormonal changes in women just before and during the menses, suggesting a hormonal link (Bruinsma and Taren, 1999).

- One cup of **cocoa** has about half as much caffeine as one cup of coffee, and it has a slower onset and longer course of action. Contrary to popular belief, and contradicting some earlier studies, caffeine in normal doses does not appear harmful to the heart and does not increase risks of heart attack or arrhythmia (Chou and Benowitz, 1994).

- Animal studies have shown that **chocolate** supplementation seems to correct magnesium deficiency, but in the interest of calorie-counting and overall dietary sensibility it probably makes sense to correct this problem with dietary adjustments or supplementation rather than a **chocolate** feast (Planells et al., 1999).

- Surprisingly, **milk chocolate** does not seem to elevate blood fats such as cholesterol in spite of its high saturated fat content. Controlled studies indicate repeatedly that this is due to the unique effect of a saturated fatty acid called stearic acid (Kris-Etherton and Mustad, 1994).

CORDYCEPS MUSHROOM

Latin: *Cordyceps sinensis*   **Chinese:** Dong chong xia cao   **English:** Winter worm summer flower

WHAT IT DOES: Cordyceps mushroom is sweet and bland in taste and warming in action. It strengthens immunity and fortifies and heals the lungs and kidneys.

RATING: Gold

SAFETY ISSUES: None known

STARTING DOSAGE:

- Dried powder: 2 grams two to three times per day
- 1:5 tincture: 10–15 drops two to three times per day

   Winter worm summer flower is the direct translation from Chinese of this amazing mushroom that grows out of caterpillar larvae in the Himalayas. TCM doctors use it medicinally to treat chronic cough, wheezing from deficiency, emphysema, and consumptive cough. Because it tonifies both Yin and Yang, it is very safe and can be taken over a long period of time to stimulate endocrine function, reduce fatigue, and calm nervousness. **Cordyceps** was reportedly used at the Olympics by Chinese women's track and field teams to enhance performance when they set nine world records. From the scientific point of view, attention has focused on **chaga**'s immune-enhancing and cancer-fighting properties. At our clinic, we find **cordyceps** most useful for treating lung and kidney weakness of any variety. We also use it with other medicinal mushrooms after cancer therapy to strengthen the immune system. Although it is clear that similar nutrients in most medicinal mushrooms are generally found to stimulate immunity, it is also obvious that various mushrooms have different actions when given to living beings.

Research Highlights

- **Cordyceps,** like many other medicinal mushrooms, contains complex sugars (especially beta 1,3 glucan) and other nutrients (nucleosides, triterpenoids) which seem to strongly nourish and activate various components of the immune system, useful in treating cancer, chronic fatigue, and other immune disorders (Borchers et al., 1999; Nakamura et al., 1999).

- It also seems to have value in treating nephritis (Lin et al., 1999; Li et al., 1996).

- **Cordyceps** may help the immune system recognize tumors that otherwise might escape immune surveillance (Chiu et al., 1998).

- Other benefits include positive effects on the cardiovascular and nervous systems and an antiaging effect (Zhu et al., 1998).

DANDELION ROOT AND LEAF

Latin: *Taraxacum officinale*   **Sanskrit:** Atirasa   **Chinese:** Pu gong ying

WHAT IT DOES: Dandelion is bitter, slightly pungent, and sweet in taste. It speeds removal of inflammation and dampness from the liver, intestines, and gallbladder and detoxifies the blood. The leaves promote urination.

RATING: Gold

SAFETY ISSUES: None known. Excessive dosage may dampen appetite in some individuals.

STARTING DOSAGE:

- Crude herb: 2 to 6 grams per day

- Tea: one cup two to four times per day

- 1:5 tincture: 30–60 drops two to three times per day

Dandelion is receiving a bit less press than it used to, due to the publicity surrounding newer and more glamorous herbs. It has a worldwide reputation among traditional healers for its beneficial and safe effects on the liver, and its gentle nature allows it to be used safely over long periods of time. Most people are familiar with **dandelion**, and we know its leaves make a fine, mildly bitter salad green, delicious when tossed with sea salt, lemon juice, and olive oil.

> **Dandelion's** long milky taproot is well known to gardeners, who waste countless hours trying to eradicate it from their lawns. I have a clear memory of an elderly neighbor painstakingly removing **dandelion roots** and **chickweed** from his lawn, while suffering from health conditions that could have been treated with both herbs.

Dandelion is rich in minerals like iron, phosphorus, calcium, potassium, and boron and vitamins A, B, and C. It contains up to 25% inulin, a phytochemical also found in high levels in **burdock root** and **echinacea**. It seems to selectively nourish and increase the body's supply of favorable intestinal bacteria such as bifidobacteria.

Other components of the herb, including triterpenoid saponins, have been found to stimulate macrophage activity in animals and prevent tumor growth (Takasaki et al., 1999).

In the 1898 classic *King's American Dispensatory* Felter and Lloyd tell us, "Dandelion has long been supposed to exert an influence on the biliary organs, removing torpor and engorgement of the liver as well as of the spleen . . . [and is useful for] chronic diseases of the skin and impairment of the digestive functions."

Because it gently improves bile flow, many people find it useful as a mild laxative. I've used it myself for this purpose. Its bitter components stimulate the nerves in the stomach to secrete more acid, gently stimulating appetite and improving nutrient absorption. Improvement in the clearance of bile has a general anti-inflammatory action, and this is most likely responsible for its reputation for improving skin disorders.

Dandelion is also known by Western herbalists to be a valuable nonirritating di-

> Professor Weiss, author of the standard German medical school textbook on herbal medicine, tells us that scientists in his country have reported the definitive value of regular use of **dandelion** in preventing the formation of gallstones. I usually have my patients drink one or two cups of **dandelion tea** per day (tea bags are widely available) when they have existing gallstones and want to avoid surgery. This often puts them into a latent, symptom-free stage of the disease.

uretic. Because it is rich in potassium, a vital mineral often lost when the kidneys are over-stimulated by drugs, it can be used safely to treat water retention even when caused by weakness of the heart. The leaf is more effective than the root as a diuretic, and at our clinic we use it as a safer alternative to the popular diuretic Lasix. **Check with your doctor before making this substitution.**

TCM doctors value **dandelion** highly, using it to reduce fire in the liver, especially when accompanied by red, swollen eyes. They also use it for detoxification, hepatitis, acute infections, flu, and skin ulcers. TAM doctors consider it to be an antipoison. They use it for dysentery, fevers and, vomiting.

DANG GUI ROOT

Latin: *Angelica sinensis*   **Chinese:** Dang gui   **English:** Dong quai
                                                              Tang kuei

WHAT IT DOES: Dang gui root is sweet, pungent, and bitter in taste and warming in action. It nourishes the female essence, tonifies blood, helps form healthy new blood, and catalyzes circulation (moves the blood).

RATING: Gold/silver, due to minor limitations in usage

SAFETY ISSUES: Do not use during pregnancy without consulting a qualified medical practitioner. Do not use with heavy menstrual bleeding. Do not use if taking blood-thinning medications such as Coumadin.

STARTING DOSAGE:

- Dried root: 2 to 4 grams two to three times per day

- 4:1 dried decoction: 1 to 2 grams two times per day

- 1:5 tincture: 30–60 drops in water or juice two to three times per day

The first thing you may notice when you encounter **dang gui root** is its strong but pleasant musky odor. According to Chinese theory, this odor indicates that the herb not only will nourish, but also will disperse the blood through the body, penetrating the tissues and making the skin glow, the hair luxuriant, and the mind serene (qualities seen in young women in their prime). Similar effects are reported for **shatavari,** the Ayurvedic **wild asparagus root,** which also has a strong musky odor.

Dang gui root is among the most important of Chinese blood tonics, perhaps sharing the stage only with **shou wu root. Dang gui root** is used to treat dysmenorrhea, amenorrhea, female infertility, anemia, tinnitus, hair loss, blurred vision, and heart palpitations.

Dang gui, as part of the **blood-moving group** (see Chapter 9), can be used for a wide variety of complaints. For example, at our clinic we were able to slow progression of severe lung fibrosis in one elderly patient for about 2 years.

Though **dang gui** is not estrogenic, it has a similar effect, binding to estrogen receptors in women. Western analysis might therefore say it would be useful for treating hot flashes and menopausal symptoms. However, TCM analysis points out that the root's warming action would make it a poor choice unless combined with other appropriate cooling herbs. At our clinic we use it only in menopausal patients with blood deficiency. **There are concerns about adulteration of this herb with related species, so try to purchase only from reliable and knowledgeable dealers.**

Research Highlights

- Pharmacological studies done on **dang gui's** reputed blood-forming properties show that its polysaccharides "could obviously promote the proliferation and differentiation" of various blood components, including blood growth factors (Wang et al., 1998).

- **Dang gui root** in animal models could also correct experimental atrial fibrillation induced by drugs (Chang and But, 1987).

- Combining **astragalus root** with **dang gui root** is a very potent method of improving blood parameters. A 1993 study showed the abiltiy of this combination to improve all measured blood indexes (Xue et al., 1993).

- In an amazing study, Chinese patients with ABO- and Rh-incompatible blood types were given tablets of a blood-moving formula containing **dang gui root, leonorus** (yi mu cao / *Leonorus heterophyllus*), **white peony root, banksia rose** *(Rosa banksia),* and **cnidium rhizome** (chuan xiong / *Ligusticum wallichii*). The preventative treatment significantly lowered the mortality rate in cases of Rh-type incompatibility (Bian et al., 1998). This study has not been replicated.

- In one study, the blood-moving qualities of both **dang gui root** and **cnidium rhizome** proved strong enough to prevent the formation of abnormal fibrous tissue in animal models of pulmonary fibrosis (Dai et al., 1996).

DEER ANTLER

Latin: *Cervus species*   **Chinese:** Lu rong

WHAT IT DOES: Deer antler is sweet and salty in taste and very warming in action. It tonifies and stimulates deficient Yang metabolic energy, increases sex drive, and strengthens the heart, bones, and blood. It increases the ability to work.

RATING: Yellow, due to highly stimulating nature

SAFETY ISSUES: Use cautiously with cases of severe emaciation and dryness.

STARTING DOSAGE:

- Velvet or tip of antler: 500 mg one to three times per day. Start with low dosage and increase slowly.

TCM doctors use the velvet and tip of young **deer antler** to treat fatigue, coldness, cold hands and feet, tinnitus, male impotence, hypothyroidism, and general metabolic weakness. It strengthens the tendons and bones, making it an effective treatment for osteoarthritis and osteoporosis. The Chinese believe that the tip of the antler contains the most nutrients, so it commands the highest price. It nourishes the bone marrow, stimulates red blood cell production, and increases cardiac energy output. It also speeds bone healing. We use it frequently in our clinic to strengthen cancer patients who have been weakened by chemotherapy or radiation. New Zealanders use it for children who fail to thrive.

Deer antlers are amazing structures. They demonstrate the incredible metabolic energy of these animals. Everyone knows that strong fingernail growth is a sign of good health, but consider the rapid annual growth of these bony structures, covered with living velvet and enriched by large blood vessels and nerves. The antlers of species such as the red deer develop each year in about 150 days, during early spring and summer. This is a tremendous metabolic achievement. Planetary Formulas makes a high-quality antler product (see Resource Guide).

Research Highlights

- Androgen hormones are substances that stimulate male sex organ function. These hormones and various growth factors are factors in **deer antler** formation (Li et al., 1999; Francis and Suttie, 1998).

- As **deer antlers** grow, supportive nerves must grow in tandem, at a rapid rate of up to 1 cm per day. This growth rate is related to the presence of neural and other growth factors (Garcia et al., 1997; Suttie et al., 1993; Suttie et al., 1995). This indicates that deer antlers may be beneficial in nerve regeneration.

- Chinese studies report that **deer antler** speeds healing of fractured bones, strengthens heart output in patients with severe fatigue (at moderate, not high dosage), and stimulates production of reticulocytes (young new red blood cells) and hemoglobin (reported in Yeung, 1983).

ECLIPTA

Latin: *Eclipta alba*   **Sanskrit:** Bhringaraja *(alba)*   **Chinese:** Han lian cao *(prostrata)*
Eclipta prostrata

WHAT IT DOES: Eclipta is cooling in action. Ayurvedic **eclipta** (bhringaraja) is bitter in taste, while Chinese **eclipta** (han lian cao) is sweet and sour in taste. Both reduce inflammation, obstructive swelling, and pain from the liver and blood. They also calm stress and nourish the hair roots.

RATING: Yellow, due to limited applications

SAFETY ISSUES: None known

STARTING DOSAGE:

- Dried powder: 2 grams two times per day

- 4:1 dried decoction: 500 mg two times per day

- Fresh leaf juice: 1 to 2 teaspoons three times per day

Two distinct species of **eclipta** are differentiated by my Ayurvedic teacher in Nepal, one with white flowers and one with yellow flowers. TAM doctors use **eclipta** to treat liver cirrhosis, infectious hepatitis, and liver and spleen enlargement. They boil the leaf juice with sesame or coconut oil and apply it topically, both to retard graying of the hair and to make the hair more luxuriant. Doctors in Nepal use **eclipta** drops dissolved in sesame oil to treat sinusitis, migraine headache, and inflammation of the eyes, nose, and ears.

TCM doctors use a similar species (milder in taste) internally to treat dizziness, blurred vision, vertigo, and premature graying of hair, especially in cases of Yin deficiency. The simple combination of **ligustrum fruit** (nu shen zi / *Ligustrum lucidum)* and **eclipta** is a well-known and effective Yin tonic.

In 1996, I created a treatment by adding Ayurvedic **eclipta** to some of the standard TCM herbs for hair loss. I soon had a regular clientele of men and women using the formula. After an average of 3 months of use (it takes time to grow hair), they reported better results than we had previously experienced with the TCM formula alone. I remember in particular a young African-American woman who was so ashamed of her severe hair loss (complete with bald patches) that she wore a cap at all times. After a year or so she came back to show me her lush hair, all in beautiful braids.

Research Highlights

- In one study, topical application of fresh **eclipta** leaf juice mixed with **neem oil** reportedly stimulated hair growth, and in some cases changed gray hair to black (Chandra K, 1985).

- Seven pharmacological and histological animal studies reported in India by the Central Council for Research on Ayurveda and Siddha have shown strong protective effects on the liver. Histopathological studies showed significant reduction in elevated liver enzymes and alkaline phosphate, and healing of liver tissues, within 4 weeks following chemical insults (reported in Pandey, 1996).

- The liver-protective effects of **eclipta** *(alba)* seem to result from its ability to regulate levels of drug-metabolizing enzymes in the liver (Saxena et al., 1993).

- Researchers have also reported a calming hypotensive effect (reported in Pandey, 1996; Gupta, 1976), as well as antibacterial and antiviral activity (reported in Pandey, 1996).

- Additionally, **eclipta** *(prostrata)* and some of its constituents were shown in animal experiments to neutralize toxicity and bleeding caused by snake venom and mushroom toxins (Melo et al., 1994; Mors, 1991).

For those of you out there who could use a little help with dull, thinning, or graying hair, here is my formula.

Using 4:1 concentrated dried decoction extract powders, combine:

2 parts **eclipta,** and 2 parts **shou wu root.**

1 part each of **cooked rehmannia root, raw rehmannia root, dang gui root, salvia root, schisandra berries, codonopsis root** (dang shen root or *C. pilosula),* **mu gua fruit** *(Chaenomelis lagenaria),* and **chiang huo rhizome** *(Notopterygium incisum).*

Dose: 2 grams twice a day. If the patient has poor circulation and coldness, we add 1 part **deer antler.**

ELDERBERRY

Latin: *Sambucus* species

WHAT IT DOES: Elderberry fruit is sour in taste and cooling in action. **Elderberry flower** is pungent and bitter in taste and has similar activity to the fruit. **Elderberry** reduces heat and inflammation and strengthens the immune system to fight viral infections, including influenza.

RATING: Gold

SAFETY ISSUES: None known. Unripe fruits may cause nausea.

STARTING DOSAGE:

- Dried berry or flower (ground): 2 to 4 grams two to three times per day

- 1:5 tincture: 35–60 drops three to five times per day for healing; 40–60 drops once per day for prevention

   Elderberry extracts or tinctures are used around the world to enhance immune function and increase antibody response during infections. Due to high concentrations of lignans and flavonoids, the berries have antiviral and anti-inflammatory activity (Yesilada, 1977). They work extremely well in the treatment of influenza and can also be used to treat upper respiratory tract infections including sinusitis and sore throat. Commercial extracts are now available, and most of them are sweetened sufficiently to please the children, a problem with bitter alternatives.

   I often use **elderberry tinctures** in children, often in combination with **echinacea** tinctures. I add ground **elderberries** to powdered formulas as a pleasant boost to otherwise bitter-tasting herbs whenever there is a need to strengthen immunity.

Research Highlights

- A report from Israel on the *Sambucus nigra* species of **elderberry** concluded, "Considering the efficacy of the extract in vitro on all strains of influenza virus tested, as well as the clinical results, low cost, and absence of side-effects, this preparation could offer a possibility for safe treatment for influenza A and B" (Zakay-Rones et al., 1995).

EPHEDRA

Latin: *Ephedra sinica*   **Chinese:** Ma huang

WHAT IT DOES: Ephedra is pungent and slightly bitter in taste and warming in action. It relaxes the muscles surrounding the lungs, dilates the surfaces vessels of the skin, and increases metabolism.

RATING: Red, due to high potential for misuse

SAFETY ISSUES: Use only under professional medical guidance. Do not use long term. Do not use during pregnancy or nursing. Do not exceed recommended dosage. Do not use with MAO-inhibiting drugs, blood-pressure-lowering drugs, steroids, beta-blockers, or antidepressants. Do not use if you have glaucoma, hypertension, heart disease, insomnia, cardiac asthma, adrenal weakness, prostate enlargement, arteriosclerosis, hyperthyroidism, diabetes, anorexia or bulimia, kidney disease, or a history of kidney stones. Do not use as a weight-loss agent unless under medical supervision.

Symptoms of ephedra overdose include rapid heartbeat, increased blood pressure, nervousness, insomnia, and sweating. Discontinue immediately if you experience any of these symptoms.

STARTING DOSAGE:

Adults
- Total alkaloids: 15–30 mg per dose, not to exceed 300 mg per day

- Crude herb: no more than 1.5–9 grams per day in divided doses as a tea

Children
- Total alkaloids: 0.5 mg per dose per weight kilogram, not to exceed 2.0 mg per kilogram per day

Note: Total alkaloids in crude herb can be as high as 3.3%.

Ephedra (ma huang) is a very useful herb that the Chinese use to disperse coldness, open the pores, and promote perspiration, which can be helpful in treating chills, fever, and headache. It also controls wheezing and relaxes the muscles around the lungs, which explains its wide use as a treatment for asthma and cough. This plant contains **ephedrine** and **pseudoephedrine,** powerful alkaloids found in many over-the-counter asthma medications (ephedrine) and nasal decongestants (pseudoephedrine). These components also stimulate the central nervous system.

If you have high blood pressure, ephedra can be deadly. TCM doctors do not generally consider **ephedra** to be dangerous, but they prescribe the whole plant, not the extracted alkaloids, to patients with specific symptoms, and usually as only 10% of a prescription. **Ephedra** is an essential herb of TCM that simply is not prescribed when there are signs of heat or hypertension.

It is possible for healthy people to safely use products containing **ephedra** when consumed in moderate amounts, and many people taking over-the-counter hay fever remedies do so with little or no trouble. Unfortunately, **ephedra** is now sold as a stimulant and a weight-loss product for its metabolism-stimulating and appetite-suppressing properties. Many people who are overweight also have hypertension—just imagine how dangerous **ephedra** can be in these particular cases. That's not to say the herb doesn't work for weight loss. In fact it does, and the result is even more powerful when combined with **green tea,** due to the additional action of caffeine. The combination of these two types of stimulants can be especially powerful. But again, this should be done under the guidance of a professional with experience about safety and dosage. Asthma and weight loss are both complex, serious problems. You can't treat them safely just by swallowing over-the-counter herbal pills.

Research Highlights

- When used over time, **ephedra** can weaken the adrenal glands. Michael Murray, N.D., faculty member at the John Bastyr Naturopathic Univeristy and best-selling author, recommends combining it with adrenal supportive herbs such as **licorice root, ginseng root,** and nutrients like vitamin C, magnesium, zinc, B$_6$ and pantothenic acid (Murray, 1991).

- There continue to be numerous reports of ephedrine-related toxicity and death. In a random study of nine commercially available supplements, only three contained the ephedrine content listed on the label, and the alkaloid content ranged from 1.08–13.54 mg per pill. There were also significant variations among different lots of the same product (Gurley et al., 1998a). In a second study, the same researcher concluded that **ephedra** toxicity "results from accidental overdose often prompted by exaggerated off-label claims and a belief that 'natural' medicinal agents are inherently safe" (Gurley et al., 1998b).

- **Ephedra** exhibits anti-inflammatory activity (Ling et al., 1995), which may enhance its usefulness for treating asthma.

- In the Canadian Forces Warrior Test, the combination of caffeine and ephedrine improved performance. Doses tested were 375 mg of caffeine and 75 mg of ephedrine, within safe levels for healthy subjects (Bell and Jacobs, 1999).

- In a study of obese monkeys, the combination of caffeine and ephedrine caused an increase in energy expenditure, a decrease in food intake, and weight loss (Ramsey et al., 1998).

- Although unsupervised use of **ephedra** or ephedrine can be dangerous, researchers conducted a controlled double-blind study on 136 obese and normal patients undergoing proper treatment with blood-pressure-lowering drugs as they attempted to lose weight. Subjects took 20 mg of ephedrine and 20 mg of caffeine. All groups lost weight, and the combination of ephedrine and caffeine did not reverse the effects of the blood pressure medications (Svendsen et al., 1998). An earlier clinical trial also found that ephedrine plus caffeine was as effective as dexfenfluramine (Astrup et al., 1995).

- A Harvard Medical School study found that the combination of ephedrine, caffeine, and aspirin was "well tolerated in otherwise healthy obese subjects, and supports modest, sustained weight loss even without prescribed caloric restriction (dieting)" (Daly et al., 1993).

EPIMEDIUM HERB

Latin: *Epimedium grandiflorum*   **Chinese:** Yin yang huo   **English:** Horny goat weed
E. species

WHAT IT DOES: Epimedium herb is pungent and sweet in taste and warming in action. It increases sperm production and motility, increases sex drive and fertility, enhances metabolism, and strengthens the bones.

RATING: Yellow, due to limitations in use

SAFETY ISSUES: Not for long-term use, which may induce vomiting and dizziness in some people due to warming effects.

STARTING DOSAGE:

- Dried powder: 3 to 12 grams per day

- 4:1 concentrated powder: 1 to 3 grams per day

The Chinese name for **epimedium herb** (yin yang huo, or horny goat weed) derives from folklore accounts that originated in the northern plains of China. It seems that goats in this region that grazed on this weed would—how can I say this gently—experience increased emissions spilling onto the grass. Farmers tend to notice this sort of thing. Recently, I've heard rumors that this herb is gaining increasing popularity in Hollywood, as one might expect. We use it as a frequent addition to formulas for treating impotence, low sex drive, and frequent urination. It works for both men and women. It is also useful for hypothyroid conditions. The concentrated powder can be dissolved in wine. Don't expect miracles.

Research Highlights

- Pharmacological and animal studies in China indicate that **epimedium** increases sperm production, increases sexual desire, and stimulates the sensory nerves. It also increases mating behavior in animals (reported in Yeung, 1983; reported in Bensky and Gamble, 1993; Dong et al., 1994; Kuang et al., 1989).

- **Epimedium extracts** (polysaccharides and glycosides) stimulate the immune system and have shown the ability to reverse suppressed immunity in animal models and clinical trials on humans. The glycosides increase coronary flow, reduce blood pressure slightly, and exhibit liver-protective effects (reported in Huang, 1999; Lee et al., 1995).

- In a study of rats with kidney disease, **epimedium** reduced the level of BUN and serum creatinine (Cheng et al., 1994).

- **Epimedium decoction** proved very effective in a controlled trial on patients with chronic kidney failure who required hemodialysis. The herb increased their sexual drive significantly and improved their immune function, as well as the overall quality of the patients' lives (Liao, 1995).

- Researchers have tested **epimedium** in vitro and in vivo for its effects on osteoporosis. In the test tube, it improves bone resorption (by osteoclasts), and in rats it increases mineral content and promotes bone formation (Yu et al., 1999).

- In a study on rats, water extract of **epimedium** reversed the side effects of long-term use of steroids, reducing adrenal atrophy and bone loss (Wu et al., 1996).

FENNEL SEED

Latin: *Foeniculum vulgare*   **Sanskrit:** Mahdurika   **Chinese:** Xiao hui xiang

WHAT IT DOES: Fennel seed is sweet in taste, carminative, and aromatic. It strengthens the digestion, freshens the breath, reduces gas, and relieves lower abdominal pain.

RATING: Silver, due to mild action

SAFETY ISSUES: None known

STARTING DOSAGE:

- Seed: 1 to 2 grams, two to three times per day

TCM doctors find **fennel seed** useful for relieving menstrual and lower abdominal pain. TAM doctors use it to strengthen digestion, which is helpful in the treatment of dysentery, colitis, and flatus. Fennel seeds should be kept in every kitchen and used according to the Indian custom of chewing a small handful of them after meals to aid digestion and freshen breath.

Try this if you want to impress your date when dining out. After the meal, rinse your mouth out with water three times. This will dilute the bacteria in your mouth enough to prevent tooth decay when you can't brush your teeth. Then chew some **fennel seeds** to freshen your breath and reduce post-meal flatulence. If you really want to go wild, carry a tiny vial of rose water and slap some onto your hands and face for a clean, fresh scent!

FEVERFEW

Latin: *Tanacetum parthenium*   **Sanskrit:** Atasi

WHAT IT DOES: Feverfew is sweet and slighty bitter in taste and slightly cold in action. It reduces heat and inflammation and prevents headaches and dizziness.

RATING: Yellow, due to limitations in usage

SAFETY ISSUES: Should not be used during pregnancy, as it stimulates the uterus. Occasional mild side effects such as mouth and gastric disturbances. Some concerns about potential allergic reactions or cross-reactivity with blood thinners such as warfarin and Ticlopidine.

STARTING DOSAGE:

- Standardized capsules (600 mcg parthenolide): one to three capsules daily
- Tincture (recently dried herb): 15–35 drops three times daily

Feverfew is now well known as a reliable remedy for migraine headaches. It also has a long history of use against arthritis. It prevents release of inflammatory chemicals from white blood cells and platelets, making it useful for rheumatoid arthritis.

Because of major differences in various commercial preparations, be sure to purchase from a reputable supplier.

Research Highlights

- Researchers assessed the ability of **feverfew** to prevent migraines in a randomized double-blind, placebo-controlled crossover study using 60 patients. They found a reduction in the mean number and severity of attacks in each 2-month period of the study. The duration of the attacks, however, was unchanged. There was also a decrease in degree of vomiting. There were no serious side effects (Murphey et al., 1988). A previous study of 17 patients showed similar results (Johnson et al., 1985). Many studies have shown **feverfew** effective for easing migraines (Volger et al., 1998).

FLAXSEED OIL

Latin: *Linum usitatissimum*   **Sanskrit:** Atasi

WHAT IT DOES: Flaxseed oil is sweet and sour in taste and warming in action. It nourishes and moistens cell membranes and reduces inflammation.

RATING: Gold

SAFETY ISSUES: None known. Whole seeds should be taken with sufficient fluids.

STARTING DOSAGE:

- Oil: 1 tablespoon per day
- Capsule: quantity equivalent to 1 tablespoon of oil per day

Flaxseed oil is one of nature's richest vegetable sources of omega-3 fatty acids, absolutely essential nutrients found insufficiently in most people's diets. **Flaxseed oil** helps the body produce hormones, energy, and moisture, while simultaneously slowing biochemical pathways that lead to inflammation. These oils end up in the membranes surrounding every cell in the body. This is why it is found in many, many natural medicine protocols.

Ayurvedic doctors use **flaxseed oil** in the form of cooking oil for treatment of urinary diseases and also as a massage oil to calm the nerves, or Vata. I use it whenever I see signs of dryness, inflammation, and fatigue pointing to a dietary-caused omega-3 deficiency. Some patients do better with fish oils, which are easier for the body to incorporate into the membranes, or with **evening primrose oil,** which seems to work better with diabetics. Some authorities suggest grinding fresh **flaxseed** to ensure purity and quality.

Research Highlights

- Dietary **flaxseed** has been shown to help lower HDL cholesterol levels (Jenkins et al., 1999).

- There is some evidence that lignans in the oil may be active in cancer prevention (Nesbitt et al., 1997).

GARLIC BULB

Latin: *Allium sativum*   **Sanskrit:** Lasunam   **Chinese:** Da suan

WHAT IT DOES: Garlic bulb is pungent in taste, and warming in action. It penetrates deeply into the system to protect the internal organs and vessels against infection and blockage. It moves the blood and aids in the digestion of fats and oils.

The Chinese add **garlic, onion,** or **ginger** to oils before cooking meats to reduce toxicity, perhaps because the antioxidants in these and other spices slow the degradation of oils during the cooking process.

RATING: Gold

SAFETY ISSUES: Use cautiously with sensitive stomach or gastrointestinal inflammation. May cause skin inflammation in some individuals. Check with your doctor if taking blood-thinning medications and using garlic in large daily amounts.

STARTING DOSAGE:

- Raw or cooked herb: one medium-size bulb two to three times per day

Garlic bulb is one of the most effective anti-microbial herbs, with antibacterial, anti-fungal, and antiviral properties. It acts on respiratory infections such as chronic bronchitis, respiratory catarrh, and recurrent colds and flu and is a powerful preventative for these conditions as well as for digestive infections. **Garlic** lowers blood pressure and blood cholesterol and triglyceride levels, prevents arteriosclerosis, and acts as a tonic on the cardiovascular system (Steiner et al., 1998). It also strengthens the immune system and has anticancer effects, causing lymphocyte proliferation, cytokine release, NK activity, and phagocytosis in both in vitro and in vivo studies. Aged **garlic** may be superior to the fresh herb in these aspects (Sumiyoshi, 1997). Ayurvedic doctors point out that excessive use can overbalance Pitta energy, causing inflammation.

> By now everybody knows about **garlic**'s medicinal powers. However, I am amazed that a multi-billion-dollar industry has grown out of concerns about the social effects of the odor. The odor is actually the release of volatile sulfur compounds through the lungs into the air. This is why it is very effective for treating chronic lung infections. I mean, if the stuff makes *people* go away, what do you think it does to germs? I tell patients to use **garlic** pills if necessary, but to use the real thing whenever possible.

TCM doctors report that garlic is useful for increasing sexual energy, and combating simple impotence, killing parasites such as hookworms and pinworms. It relieves intestinal toxicity and is used to treat diarrhea and dysentery caused by poor digestion or worms. It can be mixed with sesame oil and applied topically to the skin to reduce toxic swelling or fungal infections, or to the ear for fungal infections, but **remember that too strong a preparation may burn the skin.**

Research Highlights

- Thousands of years ago, TAM doctors reported **garlic** useful for combating worms, skin diseases, insanity, epilepsy, and abdominal and gastric tumors. Scientists at the National Cancer Institute confirmed the latter use when they reported that "infection with *H. pylori* is a risk factor, and **garlic** may be protective in the development and progression of advanced precancerous gastric lesions" (You et al., 1998).

- Pharmacological and animal experiments show that **garlic bulb** and **aged garlic extracts** have antiallergy effects (Kyo E et al., 1997), reduce intracellular oxidative stress (Ide and Lau, 1999), have antitumor activities (Kyo E et al., 1998; Lamm and Riggs, 2000; Lau BH et al., 1991), lower blood pressure (Pedraza-Chaverri J, et al.), prevent hypertension induced by chronic inhibition of nitric oxide synthesis (Life Sci. 1998;62(6):PL 71–7. PMID: 9464471; UI 98124118), strengthen immune response (Salman H et al., 1999; Gao YM et al., 1993), prevent cancer (Tang Z et al., 1997), and lower cholesterol (Morcos NC, 1997).

GINGER ROOT

Latin: *Zingiber officinalis*   **Sanskrit:** Ardrakam   **Chinese:** Gan jiang
                                                Sunthi

WHAT IT DOES: Ginger root is pungent in taste and is warming and mildly tonic in action. It improves digestion, reduces nausea, settles the stomach, and reduces inflammation.

RATING: Silver

SAFETY ISSUES: Ginger may increase absorption of pharmceuticals.

STARTING DOSAGE:

- Dried powder: 500–1,500 mg one to three times per day

- Tea: drink freely

Ginger acts as a digestive aid as well as a peripheral blood circulation stimulant, so it is useful for increasing poor circulation. Its pungent essential oils aid digestion by stimulating the activity of digestive enzymes (Platel K et al., 1998). However, despite its hot spicy taste, **ginger** inhibits the synthesis of the "bad guy" inflammatory chemicals prostaglandin and thromboxane (Kiuchi et al., 1992).

TCM doctors tell us that **fresh ginger** is better than dry ginger for easing nausea, indigestion, and stomach pain and for stopping diarrhea caused by poor digestion. Conversely, they tell us **dry ginger** is better for warming the body. The anti-inflammatory actions of **ginger,** noted cen-

Suggestions for using **ginger**:

- **Ginger tea** is a simple remedy for the common cold.
- When using fresh **ginger**, I tell patients to use a garlic press to extract the juice.
- I suggest adding **ginger, garlic,** or **onion** when cooking with oils, as they contain antioxidants that keep the oil from degrading as quickly from the heat.

turies ago by TAM doctors, are strong enough to reduce muscular discomfort and pain in osteoarthritis and rheumatoid arthritis (Srivastava et al., 1992). They explain this action in a pungent herb, as due to the vipaka (postdigestive action) being sweet and therefore nourishing and anti-inflammatory.

I sometimes mix **ginger** with honey to form a paste (occasionally adding ground black pepper), which is a very simple antiasthma formula suitable for young children in the early stages of the disease. Generally, this treatment needs to be kept up for several months to see its full effectiveness.

Research Highlights

- Because of its digestive and antinausea actions, **ginger** can be used to treat dyspepsia, nausea, and vomiting associated with pregnancy, vertigo, dizziness, and motion sickness (Schmid et al., 1994; Visalyaputra et al., 1998).

- It has also been shown to increase gastroduodenal motility (Micklefield et al., 1999).

- Pharmacological studies show that part of **ginger root's** anti-inflammatory action is due to inhibition of the formation of inflammatory prostaglandins (Kiuchi et al., 1992).

GINKGO LEAF

Latin: *Ginkgo biloba*   **English:** Maidenhair tree   **Chinese:** Bai guo ye / Yin guo ye

WHAT IT DOES: Purified **ginkgo leaf** is bitter and astringent in taste and stimulating and warming in action. It increases oxygen and blood flow to the brain and extremities and increases nutrient and oxygen absorption by nerve tissue.

RATING: Silver

SAFETY ISSUES: Use cautiously with anticoagulant drugs. Do not use with pharmaceutical MAO inhibitors. Avoid use prior to surgery, except as noted for bypass surgery.

STARTING DOSAGE:

- Standardized extract (6% terpene lactones and 24% flavone glycosides): 40–60 mg two times per day

- 1:2 tincture: 35 drops two to three times per day

The **ginkgo tree** is a fascinating and beautiful living entity, reputed to have survived the Ice Age. It is often planted along roadsides because of its ability to remain vibrant and alive in polluted city conditions. **Ginkgo leaf** has shown a powerful effect on various aspects of brain and nerve function and cerebral circulation in more than 500 studies. Some of its major uses include the treatment of vertigo and neurological disorders, memory and concentration problems, and diminished intellectual capacity due to poor circulation. It may also delay the onset of Alzheimer's disease.

When standardized in a 50:1 concentration, **ginkgo** belongs to a category of substances known as phytopharmaceuticals—halfway between crude herbs and pharmaceuticals. The herb is standardized because it is necessary to remove some slightly toxic phytochemicals from **ginkgo** before use, though the level of concentration does not need to be very strong. Naishing uses a 5:1 powder concentrate in her formulas, and I often use the 1:2 tincture. No adverse effects have ever been reported in these benign forms. I think these

> I remember one patient who experienced a sudden vision loss caused by optic ischemia. After prednisone treatment failed to prevent the loss of vision (down to 20/200) during the first week, three ophthalmology specialists insisted that nothing further could be done and that the damage was permanent. Dr. Abel and I intervened and, using a complex combination of TCM blood-moving herbs including **ginkgo** along with antioxidant nutrients, were able to restore this patient's vision to 20/80 within 3 weeks.

lower concentrations are best if you are creating a formula and want a milder medicine. I have found that well-prepared organic tinctures can often produce the desired results in very low dosage.

There have been limited reports of people developing bleeding or hemorrhage while taking **ginkgo** at the same time as anticoagulant or platelet-inhibiting drugs. However, when you consider a German survey of data on millions of patient-years of use (which means billions of **ginkgo pills** taken) without any reports of significant bleeding, I would think that the risks are very mild even in this area (DeFeudis, 1991). Caution is still wise, of course, and I do not suggest taking **ginkgo** if you are on blood-thinning medications, unless you consult a qualified health care practitioner.

I have found it very valuable for improving mental alertness and mood in some elderly patients, though I seldom use it alone. If taken in excess it can sometimes cause irritability. I have rarely found it to be an effective memory enhancer in younger persons with good circulation, though scientific reports do show some benefit to short-term memory. **Ginkgo** can be very useful in treating some cases of tinnitus, but you need to use it for a couple of months to see results. The high level of good scientific test results found with **ginkgo** is due to the fact that so much research has been done. Many, many others herbs will reach this level of proof in the coming years.

Research Highlights

- Researchers performed a meta-analysis of all studies of **ginkgo** treatments for cognitive function in Alzheimer's patients. They concluded that there was a "small but significant effect of 3- to 6-month treatment with 120 to 240 mg of **ginkgo biloba extract** on objective measures of cognitive function" (Oken et al., 1998).

- Among the most encouraging studies are those that show improvements in depression with the elderly. Clinically depressed patients taking standard medications improved significantly with the addition of **ginkgo** (Schubert and Halama, 1993).

- Equally encouraging was an open trial showing that treatment with **ginkgo** was 84% effective in neutralizing sexual dysfunction caused by antidepressant medicines, especially selective serotonin reuptake inhibitors (SSRIs) (Cohen and Bartlik, 1998).

- Animal studies have shown that **ginkgo's** effect on nerve cell membranes may possibly restore age-related declines in serotonin receptor sites (Huguet et al., 1994). If this also occurs in humans, it may explain some of the beneficial effects of **ginkgo** on mood in the elderly (reported in Murray, 1996).

- Controlled trials have shown effectiveness with tinnitus (Meyer, 1986), acute cochlear deafness (Dubreuil, 1986), senile macular degeneration (Lebuisson et al., 1986), and diabetic skin lesions (Pepe et al., 1999).

- Patients undergoing cardiopulmonary bypass often have severe problems during recovery, including tissue necrosis. In one randomized controlled trial testing **ginkgo extract** (EGb 761), patients were given either the extract or a placebo 5 days prior to surgery. Doctors collected blood samples at crucial stages of the operations and up to 8 days postsurgery. Researchers saw a reduction in free radical generation and a significant delay in leakage of oxygen-carrying muscle proteins. These results suggest that presurgical administration of **ginkgo extract** can help prevent complications (Pietri et al., 1997).

- In an animal study using **ginkgo** in combination with superoxide dismutase (SOD), **ginkgo's** inhibition of platelet-activating factor (PAF) significantly reduced oxidative damage to intestinal membranes after induced ischemia in rats (Droy-Lefaix et al., 1991). This is a convincing argument for the use of **ginkgo** with low temperature dried **wheat sprouts** (which provide SOD) as an important intervention after ischemic injury, such as optic neuritis.

- When administered to Chernobyl workers involved in the infamous nuclear accident, **ginkgo leaf extract** inhibited blood levels of radiation-induced chromosome-damaging factors by 83%. Researchers noted, however, that only the complete extract (as opposed to isolated components) exerted significant effects (Alaoui-Youssefi et al., 1999).

- **Ginkgo** increased pain-free walking distance more than 300% in diabetic and nondiabetic patients with arterial blockage disease (Li et al., 1998).

- In a randomized controlled trial, **ginkgo leaf oral liquor** was shown to significantly reduce clinical symptoms, airway hyperreactivity, as well as improve the pulmonary function of asthmatic patients (Li et al., 1997). It has also been shown to benefit in children's asthma (Keville, 1996).

- In a multicenter randomized controlled clinical trial of 545 schizophrenic patients receiving 120 mg of **ginkgo** three times a day in addition to their regular neuroleptic medication, researchers found a general reduction in negative symptoms including thought disturbance (Luo et al., 1997).

- A double-blind 3-month study of 70 patients with vertigo showed that **ginkgo** significantly reduced the intensity, frequency, and duration of the disorder. By the end of the trial, 47% of the patients taking **ginkgo** were symptom free, compared to 18% of those who received the placebo (Haguenauer et al., 1986).

- A randomized controlled study of **ginkgo extract** found it effective in treating breast and leg swelling and mood changes during PMS episodes (Tamborini and Taurelle, 1993).

- In a controlled blood flow study on 10 healthy subjects, **gingko** decreased red blood cell aggregation (clumping) by 15% and increased blood flow into the capillaries under the fingernails by 57% 2 hours after ingestion (Jung et al., 1990).

- Blood stasis can cause oxygen starvation of the venous lining tissue, leading to the development of varicose veins. In a randomized controlled clinical trial, **ginkgo extract** was one of four medicines shown to reduce circulating cells indicative of venous wall damage (Janssens et al., 1999).

- In a randomized, double-blind and placebo-controlled five-way crossover design study **ginkgo leaf extract** was shown to improve memory, the best results occurring at a dose of 120 mg per day. The benefits were more apparent in individuals over the age of 50 (Rigney et al., 1999).

- In a controlled crossover study, **ginkgo** was shown to benefit glaucoma patients by increasing ocular blood flow (Chung et al., 1999), and an earlier controlled study of blood flow to the retina showed similar results. Researchers concluded that "damage to the visual field by chronic lack of blood flow [is] significantly reversible" (Raabe et al., 1991).

GINSENG ROOT

Latin: *Panax ginseng*   **Chinese:** Ren shen   **English:** Essence of Man

WHAT IT DOES: Ginseng root is sweet and slightly bitter in taste and warming in action. It strengthens the vital force (Qi), tonifies the digestive and immune systems, reduces fatigue, sharpens the mind, and slows aging.

RATING: Gold

SAFETY ISSUES: Do not use during acute fevers. Do not use with hypoglycemia or hypertension. Overdose or taking late at night may cause nervousness and sleeplessness. May cause irritability in some sensitive individuals. Consult with your physician if you are taking cardiac glycosides.

STARTING DOSAGE:

- Dried powder: 3 to 9 grams per day

- Concentrated powder extract: 1 to 3 grams per day

Note: It is common to use a combination of the two forms.

Ginseng root can also be lifesaving for the elderly. My dad began to lose weight and feel weak after he passed the age of 80, and Nai-shing made him a **ginseng**-based formula that immediately turned this situation around. Our relatives visiting from China were amazed when, at the age of 81, he chopped down and removed a large tree single-handedly. I hear they still tell this story in China.

Wild ginseng root is collected in the mountains of northern China and in Korea. There are two common preparations of the cultivated root, sun-dried or roasted **ginseng** and sweet **red ginseng**.

Americans have known about the tonic effects of **ginseng** since colonial times. It is a strong tonic of the vital force (Qi) and is especially useful when there is extreme deficiency presenting with symptoms of cold limbs, anemia, weak respiration, weight loss, chronic fatigue, and a weak pulse. It strengthens the immune system, helps generate fluids, and strengthens the heart. In our practice, we find it indispensable for keeping cancer patients strong when undergoing chemotherapy.

Ginseng can be lifesaving if administered following sudden bodily trauma or shock, such as blood loss after an accident. In such cases, administer a large dose of **ginseng**—about 3 grams of dried powder every 2 or 3 hours, up to 30 grams per day. Doctors in Chinese hospitals use a formula called "Generate the Pulse" (shengmai san) for the same purpose, and it is more effective than **ginseng** alone. It is made from equal parts of **ginseng root, ophiopogon root** (mai men dong / *Ophiopogon japonica),* and **schisandra berries**.

Research Highlights

- **Ginseng's** antiaging effects are theorized to be a result of its ability to increase the body's synthesis of DNA, RNA, and protein, as well as synthesis of gonadotropins and ACTH, all of which can prolong cell life (reported in Huang, 1999).

- Healthy male volunteers given **ginseng root** showed cardiovascular benefits, indicated by a substantial decrease in heart rate 2 weeks after the end of a 9-week experiment (Kirchorfer, 1985).

- It may also improve muscular oxygen utilization (Pieralisi et al., 1991).

- **Ginseng** may be of benefit to non-insulin-dependent diabetic patients. Researchers in one study reported, **"Ginseng** therapy elevated mood, improved psychophysical performance, and reduced fasting blood glucose and body weight. The 200-mg dose of **ginseng** improved glycated hemoglobin and physical activity" (Sotaniemi et al., 1995).

- Russian studies have shown that **ginseng** increases mental activity, efficiency of concentration, and intelligence. This is accomplished partly through increased biosynthesis of neurotransmitters (reported in Huang, 1999).

GOTU KOLA LEAF

Latin: *Centella asiatica*   **Sanskrit:** Brahmi   **Chinese:** Luo de da
        Hydrocotyle asiatica   Mandukaparni   Ji xue cao

WHAT IT DOES: Gotu kola is bitter and astringent in taste and cooling in action. It is a brain and memory tonic and an anti-poison, also useful for wound and skin healing.

RATING: Gold

SAFETY ISSUES: None known

STARTING DOSAGE:

- Dried decoction: 2 grams two to three times per day

- 4:1 concentrated powder extract: 1 gram two times per day

- 1:5 tincture: 20–40 drops two to three times per day

Gotu kola is an annual small spreading plant found growing near rivers and ponds. TAM doctors use it as a brain and memory tonic and have found it especially useful in children. In Nepal, during the ceremony for the first day of spring, **gotu kola leaf** is given to schoolchildren to help them in their studies by improving memory and concentration. It is very safe and extremely effective.

TAM doctors also use it to cleanse the system of toxins and reduce inflammation. TCM doctors use **gotu kola** to clear up boils and toxic fevers.

Gotu kola is often confused with another plant, **bacopa** *(Bacopa monniera),* which is also named **brahmi**, found more in the south of India. **Gotu kola** is the original plant found in ancient Sanskrit texts, and bacopa was added much later. Both plants are used for memory and concentration, but their energies are different. **Gotu kola** is cooling and antipoison, while bacopa is warming and stimulating. Be sure to check the Latin name if you are purchasing these herbs to ensure you're getting the right one.

Gotu kola grows abundantly in India, China, Australia, Africa, Ceylon, Indonesia, and Madagascar, so plants are harvested and used freely in the markets. Unfortunately, the chemical profiles differ among these species, and quality varies significantly. If you drink two or three cups per day of *good-quality* **gotu kola,** you should notice the results quickly.

The primary effects of **gotu kola** include both wound healing and improvement of mental clarity and emotional balance. It doesn't surprise me that one herb can affect such seemingly unrelated physiologies. For one thing, the nervous system and skin both originate embryologically from the ectoderm, and the skin is a sense organ. I think further investigation is warranted to explore **gotu kola**'s effects on other sense organs such as the eye, as well as on neurotransmitters, immune status, and other nervous system parameters. At our clinic we sometimes find it useful in treating attention deficit disorder (ADD).

Research Highlights

- Western scientists have focused on the herb's wound- and skin-healing effects. Numerous studies from around the world have demonstrated its efficacy in treating keloids, leg ulcers, phlebitis, slow-healing wounds, leprosy, surgical lesions, cellulitis, burns, dermatitis, venous disorders, and even cirrhosis of the liver (Maquart et al., 1999; Shukla et al., 1999; Hausen, 1993; Cesarone et al., 1992). These studies illustrate the plant's numerous stimulating effects on the healing processes of the skin and connective tissue.

- The Indian Central Council for Research on Ayurveda and Siddha, citing more than 10 pharmacological and animal studies of **gotu kola**, also found evidence of the following characteristics: CNS depressant, memory enhancer, anticonvulsant, antispasmodic, behavior and intelligence enhancer, and blood sugar regulator (Pandey et al., eds., 1996).

GRAPEFRUIT SEED EXTRACT

Latin: *Citrus paradisi*

WHAT IT DOES: Grapefruit seed extract is sour and bitter in taste and cooling in action. It is a relatively nontoxic contact antimicrobial useful in chronic intestinal infections.

RATING: Yellow

SAFETY ISSUES: Avoid direct contact with skin or mucosal surfaces. Do not exceed recommended dosages.

STARTING DOSAGE:

- Topical wash: 4 to 5 drops in 4 to 8 ounces of water (this makes a strong wash for external use only)

- Internal dilution: 4 to 6 drops in ¼–½ cup water three times per day

- Pill (usually equivalent to 5 drops of GSE): 1 pill three times per day in most cases

Grapefruit seed extract (GSE) is an antifungal and antibiotic. It is used to treat bacterial and fungal intestinal infections, ear and sinus infections, and vaginal infections. It is relatively nontoxic to human tissues compared to other antimicrobials and can be used internally for fairly long periods of time (up to 6 months) with no apparent side effects.

Studies have found it effective in fighting a wide variety of pathogenic organisms, including candida (yeast), herpes, staph, salmonella, *E. coli*, influenza, and various parasites including protozoa. It works only on contact, so it is ineffective in the treatment of blood diseases. Moreover, studies done on it show that it is effective only when it contains preservatives added during manufacture, especially triclosan, an ingredient used in mouthwashes and toothpastes.

We use **GSE** in our clinic as part of a treatment for patients with chronic intestinal infections who exhibit symptoms such as severe chronic gastric gas, bloating, and pain. These types of infections, termed intestinal dysbiosis, can contribute to widespread system problems including mental confusion, chronic fatigue, chronic vaginal yeast infections, muscle pain, chronic constipation, and severely impaired immunity.

> Dr. William Crook brought one form of intestinal dysbiosis to the general public's attention in his classic book *The Yeast Connection*. I have seen many, many female patients enraged when their doctors refuse to even consider chronic intestinal yeast infections as a cause of the above-mentioned problems. Although I hope gastrointestinal specialists learn to accept and treat this simple syndrome, most currently treat the idea like kryptonite. One of my patients told her doctor that the symptoms she had experienced for 5 years went away after 2 months of herbal treatment and dietary modifications. He almost threw her out of his office, exclaiming, "Don't you think my dozen years of medical training taught me anything? I'm a specialist!"

Whenever using this herbal medicine, I advise patients to use a good broad-spectrum **acidophilus** product to ensure preservation of the "good guy" intestinal flora. I also advise them to avoid simple sugars like the plague, as they feed the "bad guy" infection-causing organisms. It is important to recognize that not all strains of "bad guys" respond to this extract, and other agents may be needed.

Effects similar to those of **GSE/triclosan** can be obtained with completely natural **neem** concentrate. However, **neem** contains very strong "natural" chemicals, some of which have insecticidelike properties. **Neem** is also clinically more difficult for some patients to tolerate than **GSE.**

You can use **GSE** when traveling to disinfect local water supplies. Use 10 drops of **GSE** per gallon of water, and let it sit for several hours. You can also disinfect toothbrushes by placing them in a water solution containing **GSE.**

As it turns out, **GSE** is not a completely natural product. Although very clinically effective, it is actually a combination product that essentially acts as a "mouthwash" for the intestines. Purists may want to avoid it, in spite of its clinical usefulness.

Research Highlights

- A team of researchers in 1999 confirmed earlier reports (Sakamoto et al., 1996) that the microbial-inhibiting effects of **GSE**, though quite effective, occurred only in samples containing the preservatives triclosan and methyl paraben (von Woedtke et al., 1999).

- Triclosan is an antimicrobial agent used in dentifrices, mouth rinses, and skin care products. It boasts a positive safety profile and is nontoxic with no long- or short-term carcinogenic, mutagenic, or teratogenic actions (Bhargava and Leonard, 1996; DeSalva et al., 1989).

GUGGUL GUM

Latin: *Commiphora mukul*   **Sanskrit:** Guggulu
Balsamodendron mukul

WHAT IT DOES: Guggul gum is bitter and pungent in taste and hot in action. It is a longevity tonic that stimulates the breakdown of mucus, tumors, fat, and cysts.

RATING: Gold

SAFETY ISSUES: Do not use during pregnancy. Excess use of concentrated **guggulipid** may cause headache, mild nausea, and vomiting and may cause reduced bioavailability of the drugs diltiazem (Cardizem) and propranolol.

STARTING DOSAGE:

- Concentrated dried extract: 1 to 2 grams two times per day

- Standardized lipid: 500 mg (yield = 25 mg guggulsterone) three times per day

  Note: Use only prepared extracts.

Guggul gum has been used in Ayurvedic medicine for centuries to treat abnormal growths, tumors, cysts, arthritis, glandular swelling, cancer, and inflammation and as a rasayana for promoting long life and health. It is so important in TAM healing that it has its own group of compound medicines listed in the TAM materia medica.

Two of the best-known medicines are **yogaraja guggulu** and **kaisara guggulu. Yogaraja guggulu** is used to treat enlargement of the abdomen, peritonitis, rheumatism, neurasthenia, sciatica, and nervous system (Vata) diseases in general. It also has significant anti-inflammatory properties. **Kaisara guggulu** is used to treat weak digestion, constipation, boils, diabetic ulcers, abdominal tumors, leprosy, leukemia, psoriasis, and inflammation-related (Pitta) diseases.

Guggul gum has been popular in the West since researchers discovered its significant cholesterol-lowering properties in human trials. The gum can be separated into base, acid, and neutral fractions. The neutral fraction contains most of the cholesterol-lowering activity, while the acid fraction contains some anti-inflammatory components.

Concentrated dried decoction extracts focusing on the cholesterol-lowering aspect are now being mixed with other cholesterol-lowering herbs and nutrients (such as **ginger root** and niacinamide) and sold as alternatives to Western drugs. I personally think this is probably a safer alternative to some of the Western cholesterol-lowering drugs.

Guggul gum in its traditional form is almost always used in combination with **triphala** and/or **guduchi stem** *(Tinospora cordifolia)*. Both of these have strong antipoison, antioxidant, and anti-inflammatory properties. TAM doctors also divide **guggul** into two types, new and aged, and prescribe them differently. The aged form has been considered a major anti-cancer herb since ancient times.

Research Highlights

- In human trials, a combination of **guggul gum** and **puskaram tuber** *(Inula race-mosa)* proved superior to nitroglycerin in reducing the chest pain and dyspnea associated with angina (Miller, 1998; Tripathi et al., 1988).

- **Guggul** may also have value in acne treatment. In one study, a majority of patients with serious nodulocystic acne experienced a progressive reduction (about 60–70%) in lesions when treated with **guggulipid,** results comparable to patients who received tetracycline (an antibiotic) treatment. The researchers noted that patients with very oily skin responded remarkably better to **guggulipid** than the antibiotic (Thappa et al., 1994).

- Clinical studies done in 1956 by Chopra showed **guggul's** ability to elicit significant improvement in psoriasis cases (Pandey et al., 1996).

- **Guggul gum** may also have mild thyroid-enhancing activity due to its effects on fats (Panda et al., 1999).

GUDUCHI STEM

Latin: *Tinospora cordifolia*   **Sanskrit:** Guduchi   **English:** Heart-leaved moonseed

WHAT IT DOES: Guduchi stem is bitter in taste and warming in action and is a rasayana tonic for good health and longevity. It has antitoxin and anti-inflammatory properties, reduces mucus, and has a calming, stabilizing effect on the nervous system (Vata).

RATING: Gold

SAFETY ISSUES: None known

STARTING DOSAGE:

- Dried powder: 2 grams two to three times per day

- 4:1 concentrated powder extract: 1 gram two times per day

The **guduchi** plant is a long creeper with a succulent stem that grows in temperate and subtropical forests. It is used to treat fevers, hepatitis, gout, toxemia, and urinary diseases. It is also often used by itself as a tonic tea.

Guduchi stem is a diuretic, helping expel toxins including uric acid through the urine. It is an aphrodisiac, useful in treating impotence and debility from chronic disease. Dr. Mana told me this herb has the special power (prabhava) of restoring balance without ever causing overbalance (samanam). In our clinic we use **guduchi stem** to treat infectious or chronic diseases where there is a need to detoxify and strengthen without disturbing the system further, such as with chronic hepatitis patients or those undergoing chemotherapy.

Research Highlights

- Studies have shown **guduchi** to have significant general anti-inflammatory effects as well as specific anti-inflammatory action in cases of rheumatoid arthritis and liver toxicity (Pandey et al., 1996).

- **Guduchi stem** was tested for its ability to handle changes in immune cells after rats were exposed to different types of toxins. It was found to normalize phagocytic function irrespective of the nature of change in the cells, complying with the definition of an adaptogen (Rege, 1999).

- Animals treated with the herb were able to significantly recover liver function in the weeks following experimentally inflicted damage. Their liver immune cells (Kupffer cells) were protected against the damage, while those animals not given the herb exhibited perpetuation of damage (Nagarkatti et al., 1994).

- **Guduchi**'s hepatoprotective and immunomodulatory properties were also shown to enhance the host defenses of a group of surgical patients, as indicated by the absence of postdrainage sepsis (Rege et al., 1993).

- Another group of researchers concluded that **guduchi stem** and **shatavari root** were potent immunostimulants, with value for patients receiving cytotoxic drugs, when they were found to protect mice against bone marrow suppression from cyclophosphamide, a chemotherapeutic agent (Thatte UM et al., 1988).

GYMNEMA

Latin: *Gymnema sylvestre*   **Sanskrit:** Gurmar

WHAT IT DOES: Gymnema is bitter in taste and cooling in action. It improves blood sugar control in diabetics, numbs the taste of sweet completely (for about 20 minutes), and decreases appetite (for about 90 minutes).

RATING: Yellow

SAFETY ISSUES: None reported. Should not be used by people with low blood sugars (hypoglycemia).

STARTING DOSAGE:

- 1:1 extract: 5 to 10 ml per day
- Pill: 500–1,000 mg three times per day

The Sanskrit word for **gymnema** (gurmar) means "sugar destroyer." It grows in the wild forests of central India, all the way to the Western Ghats and up to the Himalayas. Research indicates that **gymnema** stimulates insulin secretion. Japanese studies have shown that it improves glucose tolerance in animal models of diabetes, and other studies show that the effects can last for up to 2 months after discontinuation.

This herb is a good long-term tonic for Type 1 and 2 diabetics. Results are best seen after long-term administration, over 6 months to a year. I prefer to use it in combination with several other herbs for blood sugar control, because it affects only a few aspects of the imbalance.

In case you're curious, sugar tastes like sand for 20 minutes after you chew on a little **gymnema**.

Research Highlights

- Triterpenoid saponins in **gymnema** are responsible for its dramatic sweet-taste-blocking action (Baskaran et al., 1990).

- One animal study testing extracts of **gymnema** confirmed earlier conclusions of human studies that the herb stimulates insulin release, adding that it works by increasing permeability in the islets of Langerhans, allowing more insulin to escape into the blood (Persaud et al., 1999; Shanmugasundaram KR et al., 1990).

- In tests on diabetic rabbits, **gymnema dried leaf powder** not only helped control elevated blood sugars but also corrected metabolic derangements in the liver, kidney and muscles (Shanmugasundaram KR et al., 1983).

- **Gymnema** does *not* seem to improve insulin resistance in diabetic rats, although other herbs have been known to do so (Tominaga et al., 1995).

- **Gymnemic** acids found in **gymnema** have been found to bind cholesterol, causing it to be excreted in the stool of animals (Nakamura et al., 1999).

- **Gymnemic** acids also bind glucose and a common fatty acid (oleic acid) in the intestine, causing reduced uptake into the blood (Wang et al., 1998; Shimizu et al., 1997).

HARITAKI FRUIT

Latin: *Terminalia chebula*   **Sanskrit:** Haritaki   **English:** Chebulic myrobalan
Chinese: He zi

WHAT IT DOES: Haritaki fruit is sweet, sour, and astringent in taste, as well as slightly bitter and pungent. It is hot in action. It strengthens immunity while exerting a mild laxative effect.

RATING: Gold

SAFETY ISSUES: Not for use by pregnant women due to laxative effect.

STARTING DOSAGE:

- Dried powder: 2 grams two times per day

- 4:1 concentrated powder extract: 1 gram two times per day

Haritaki fruit embodies all tastes except salt, one of the many reasons it is designated in TAM as a rasayana tonic, good for health and long life. It is also tridosagna, meaning it can be used with any type of health imbalance. Furthermore, it is an anulomanum—a mild laxative that aids digestion. **Haritaki** is used to nourish the heart, liver, and kidney and to treat diseases of the eye, for which it is used both internally and externally.

There are seven types of **haritaki fruit**:

- **Vijaya** looks just a squash and can be used in any case.

- **Rohini** is round in shape and more effective for healing.

- **Putana** is small in size with big hard seeds and is useful for external plastering.

- **Amrita** is fleshier and good for body purification.

- **Abhaya** has five lobes and is more effective for ophthalmic use (external).

- **Jivanti** is yellow in color and good for all cases.

- **Chetaki** has three lobes, is good to use in the form of powder, and is more laxative than the others. Chetaki comes in two varieties—white and black.

The mature (ripe) **haritaki fruits** are harvested during the autumn season, when they have the strongest medicinal and laxative effect. Drying the fruit properly in the sun to make a powder reduces the laxative effect slightly, and cooking or steaming reduces it even further, due to oxidation of the laxative chemicals.

Traditional doctors disapprove of cooking the fruit when it should be sun-dried (a tedious process). The cooking process is thought to weaken the herb's medicinal effectiveness. However, TCM doctors often cook laxative herbs (such as **rhubarb root,** which is soaked in wine, then fried) in order to remove the laxative properties, so they can be used for other purposes without discomfort to the patient.

Haritaki fruit contains anthraquinonelike (laxative) chemicals as well as tannins and astringents. To bring out these opposing actions within a given product, Ayurvedic doctors administer it with warm water to strengthen the laxative action and with ice cold water to promote the astringent action. For example, the juice mixed with cold water can be used as a mouthwash to treat spongy gums.

The postdigestive or delayed reaction of **haritaki fruit** (vipaka) is very strongly nourishing, so this is an excellent choice as a laxative in weak or elderly patients.

Haritaki fruit is part of **triphala,** the three-fruit formula. It is generally administered in **triphala** form rather than by itself to draw upon the tonic effects. Each of the **triphala fruits** is tonic, and together they act to balance the three primary balancing forces, Vata, Pitta, and Kapha. At our clinic, following the Ayurvedic tradition, I add **triphala** to many, many combinations for this balanced tonic action. The wide variety of liver-protective, antioxidant, nutritive, and antimicrobial virtues found in these three fruits lends much credence to this traditional practice.

TCM doctors use dried or cooked **haritaki fruit** to tighten up the stool for chronic diarrhea and dysentery and to "tighten" the lungs in chronic cough. By stating that it can be used for both hot and cold patterns of disease, they are acknowledging the balanced action of this herb.

Research Highlights

- Researchers tested a 10% solution of **haritaki fruit** extract as a mouth rinse to study its effect on bacteria. The mouthwash significantly inhibited salivary bacterial count and total streptococcal *(S. mutans)* count for up to 3 hours compared to placebo, apparently by blocking their ability to utilize sugars (Jagtap and Karkera, 1999).

- **Haritaki fruit** was one of six Ayurvedic herbs administered to animals to test their adaptogenic potential. All six traditional rasayana plants were able to aid the animals against a variety of different stressors working in different ways (Rege, 1999).

- Alcohol extracts of 82 Indian medicinal plants were tested in vitro against several pathogenic and opportunistic microorganisms. Only five plants had a broad-spectrum as well as potent action, one of which was **haritaki fruit**. The others were **amla fruit, vibhitaki fruit, chitrakam** *(Plumbago zeylanica),* and **kutaja** *(Holarrhena antidysenterica).* Subsequent animal testing showed no cellular toxicity (Ahmad et al., 1998).

- Tests of alcohol extracts revealed gallic acid and its ethyl ester, two potent antimicrobial substances that acted against even resistant strains of *Staphylococcus aureus* (Sato et al., 1997). In an AIDS model with immunosuppressed mice, **haritaki fruit** was one of four herbs found to significantly reduce viral loads in a chronic lung infection (CMV) commonly found in AIDS patients (Yukawa et al., 1996).

- **Haritaki fruit** was one of four herbs screened out for potency to test for use with the antiviral drug acyclovir against herpes (HSV-1) in a study at the Toyama Medical and Pharmaceutical University in Japan. When acyclovir was combined with any one of the herbal extracts and ingested in oral doses similar to human use, the results were significantly stronger than the use of the drug or the herbs alone, especially reducing viral loads in the brains of the animals (Kurokawa et al., 1995).

- Rabbit studies of the cholesterol-lowering actions of each of the **triphala fruits** showed that **haritaki fruit** had the strongest effect. Although all three fruits reduced cholesterol, **haritaki fruit** significantly reduced cholesterol deposits in the liver and aorta compared to controls (Thakur et al., 1988).

HAWTHORN

Latin: *Crataegus pinnatifida*   **Chinese:** Shan zha
C. laevigata
Crataegus species

WHAT IT DOES: Hawthorn berries and **flower buds** are sour and sweet in taste and slightly warming in action. **Hawthorn** nourishes the heart, increases oxygen flow to the heart muscle, reduces blood vessel inflammation, and helps digest fats and oils.

RATING: Gold

SAFETY ISSUES: Patients taking cardiac glycosides such as digitalis should inform their physicians that **hawthorn** may potentiate the drug's effect, and dosage may need to be adjusted.

STARTING DOSAGE:

- Dried powder: 10–100 grams per day

- Concentrated powder extract: 2–15 grams

- Concentrated syrup: 1 to 4 teaspoons per day

- Fresh berries: consume as desired

Similar (but not identical) species of **hawthorn** are used by both Chinese and Western herbalists to benefit the heart. Western herbalists consider it to be "food for the heart." At our clinic we use it in formulas for all heart and cholesterol-related problems. It is safe and effective for long-term use. For serious heart conditions, it may be best to use concentrated dried decoction extracts and syrups, which contain more of the beneficial pigment compounds. The darker the syrup, the better. TCM herbalists use the fruit to help patients digest fats and other heavy foods. Because the species are not identical, it is best to use the Western variety *(C. oxycantha* and *C. laevigata)* to treat heart problems and the Chinese variety *(C. pinnatifida)* to treat digestion-related disorders. It is very common in China to see children eating candy-coated **hawthorn fruit** on a stick.

Hawthorn is used to treat hypertension, hypercholesterolemia, palpitations, tachycardia, angina, cardiomyopathy, coronary artery disease (CAD), and varicose veins. The fruit contains high levels of procyanidins, which are known to be cardiotonic (Rehwald, 1995). The mature flower buds and young leafy spring tips are quite high in flavonoids and proanthocyanins, which are useful for treating diabetes and arthritis, as well as for strengthening and repairing connective tissue (reported in Upton, 1999).

Some herbalists report that long-term use of **hawthorn**, 6 months to a year or more, can sometimes reverse essential hypertension. I have had two patients for whom this has been true, both able to go off their Western medication. This clinically observed effect may be due to gradual reduction of low-level inflammation affecting the inner walls of the vessels combined with **hawthorn's** numerous other heart-protecting activities.

Research Highlights

- German physicians combine **hawthorn** with digitalis in cases of rapid heartbeat with and without atrial fibrillation and report it can also be used for heart conditions for which digitalis is not yet indicated (Blesken, 1992).

- Studies have shown **hawthorn** to be sufficiently strong to benefit patients with NYHA (New York Heart Association) stage II cardiac insufficiency (Weikl et al., 1996) as well as patients in stage I and stage II congestive heart failure (Ammon et al., 1981).

- Chinese researchers have also reported a beneficial effect on angina symptoms (Weng et al., 1984).

ISATIS ROOT AND LEAF

Latin: *Isatis tinctoria*
I. indigotica

Chinese: Ban lan gen (root)
Da qing ye (leaves)

WHAT IT DOES: Isatis root and **leaf** are bitter in taste and cold in action. They reduce fever and heat, cool the throat, and kill microbes.

RATING: Red, due to safety issues

SAFETY ISSUES: Should not be used for extended periods of time or in patients with severe weakness. Long-term use can reduce beneficial intestinal bacteria. **Use only under the guidance of a trained professional.**

Note: In 1990, there were 38 reports in China and 16 in Taiwan of adverse reactions to **isatis**.

STARTING DOSAGE:

- Dried powder: 2 to 3 grams per day
- Concentrated dried decoction extract: 1 to 4 grams per day

Isatis is one of the most effective TCM herbs used as an herbal antibiotic, antiseptic, and antiviral. TCM doctors use it whenever there are signs of fever or toxic heat from viral illness, blood poisoning, leukemia, hepatitis, meningitis, scarlet fever, laryngitis, tonsillitis, mumps, and other similar ailments. It is an effective alternative to Western prescription antibiotics in some cases. Although the root is used most commonly, the leaves are useful as well. TCM doctors say **isatis leaves** "go to the upper part of the body" more than the root, so leaves are used for upper respiratory infections along with the root.

I find it very safe for short-term use, less than 3 weeks. Long-term use can weaken digestion and sometimes can induce a very interesting but reversible feeling of internal coldness, to the point of shivering. I have experienced this phenomenon, and it was a truly enlightening sensory introduction to the concept of "coldness." I always use this herb with caution, as it can induce nausea in sensitive individuals and weaken digestion over time. **Isatis** contains several potent dark pigments, including blue indigo and red-colored indirubin.

Research Highlights

- Indirubin binds to and blocks enzymes that govern cell division, thus stopping the proliferation of blood cancer cells. An article in *Nature Cell Biology* reported the results of a study examining the effects of indirubin extract on chronic myelocytic and chronic granulocytic leukemia. According to the report, 26% of the chronic myelocytic leukemia patients showed complete remission and 33% showed partial remission. Remissions lasted up to several years. The toxicity of the extract was relatively mild (Hoessel et al., 1999).

- The Experimental Pharmaceutical Factory at the Beijing College of TCM found alcohol to be superior to water for extracting indigotin and indirubin (Zhang et al., 1990). Additionally, meisoindigo, an indirubin derivative, seems to inhibit cancer cell replication more effectively due to its superior absorption (Ji et al., 1991). From an herbalist's point of view, these two studies might argue for the treatment of leukemia with alcohol extracts of herbs containing indigo and indirubin, such as **isatis**, combined with digestion improving herbs such as **black pepper** or **long pepper**. Other herbs which have shown antileukemic action in the laboratory include **boswellia gum** and **turmeric root**.

- In a controlled rat model of chronic *Pseudomonas aeruginosa* lung infection mimicking cystic fibrosis, **isatis** and **genkwa flower** *(Daphne giraldii /* yuan hua) were each able to reduce the incidence of lung abscess and to decrease the severity of lung pathology (Song et al., 1996). We now know that alterations in fatty acid metabolism are responsible for many of the symptoms of cystic fibrosis symptoms, and that DHA (docosahexaenoic acid) derived from marine algae or fish is effective therapy for reversing these symptoms (Freedman et al., 1999). Consequently, I wonder if the combination of these TCM herbs and DHA would provide even greater benefit for this disease.

- In laboratory studies of mice, **isatis root polysaccharides** increased the weight of the spleen and number of white blood cells and lymphocytes significantly, as well as neutralizing some of the immune suppression caused by hydrocortisone (Xu and Lu, 1991).

- A number of studies of acute viral respiratory tract infections and infections normally requiring antibiotic therapy have demonstrated the efficacy of a combination of **echinacea root, white cedar leaf tips,** and **wild indigo root,** which contains compounds similar to **isatis** (Wustenberg et al., 1999).

KAVA ROOT

Latin: *Piper methysticum*   **English:** Kava / Kava-kava

WHAT IT DOES: Kava root is bitter, pungent, and slightly astringent in taste and warming in action. It tranquilizes the mind, calms anxiety, and reduces skeletal and bladder muscle spasms and pain.

RATING: Yellow, due to limitations in usage

SAFETY ISSUES: Do not use during pregnancy or nursing. Do not exceed recommended dosage. Do not use when depressed. **Kava** potentiates the effects of barbiturates and of benzodiazepines such as Xanax. Do not use in patients with Parkinson's disease. Extreme excess dosage over time may cause a reversible scaly rash. In a single case, use of **kava root** with alprazolam resulted in a coma (Almeida and Grimsley, 1996).

STARTING DOSAGE:

- Standardized extract: 100–250 mg one to three times per day

  Note: When standardized, extracts contain 30% kavalactones, also called kavapyrones.

Kava root relaxes the central nervous system and can be used to treat conditions like irritable bladder syndrome, anger, anxiety, nervousness, and insomnia. It is a very effective treatment for irritable bladder because it numbs pain as well as relaxing spasms. According to written accounts, inhabitants of the Pacific Islands have used **kava root** as a mild intoxicant since the1772–75 voyages of Captain Cook. Typically, they would chew the root, then cover it with water. After it softened, they would strain it and drink the liquid. They now have more sophisticated uses for it, such as drinking the tea before marriage counseling sessions to prevent chair throwing. My experience with **kava** is that it induces a mild euphoria in the average person.

Kava root may be a good substitute for some prescription medications for anxiety. However, a qualified physician should supervise any changeover. It is important to distinguish between anxiety and depression, as **kava** should usually be used only in cases of anxiety and irritability. **It may exacerbate depression.**

For clarification purposes, depression is when you want to lie in bed forever and hide from the world, and nothing matters. Anxiety is when your mind races out of control with fears. I have seen many patients who were self-medicating with herbs and did not seem to understand the differences between these conditions or the differences between **kava root** and **St. John's wort**. There are several combination products on the mass market that contain combinations of **kava root** and **St. John's wort**. This may be of benefit for persons suffering from both anxiety and depression. However, if it makes you too calm or makes you more anxious, you may not know whether to discontinue the herbs or double the dosage! Your best bet is to try each herb individually for a short period of time and determine which one is more effective for your condition. Some people may benefit more from the combination.

Research Highlights

- **Kava** seems to work through a variety of biochemical mechanisms. The mood-elevating actions may be due to the activation of the mesolimbic dopaminergic neurones (Baum et al., 1998).

- In a clinical multicenter randomized double-blind controlled trial of 101 outpatients suffering from anxiety, **kava extract** demonstrated a clear superiority over placebos, according to the Hamilton Anxiety Scale. Adverse events were rare. The researchers reported these results as support for the use of **kava extract** "as a treatment alternative to tricyclic antidepressants and benzodiazepines in anxiety disorders, with proven long-term efficacy and none of the tolerance problems associated with tricyclics and benzodiazepines" (Voltz et al., 1997).

- A placebo-controlled randomized double-blind study tested the effect of a standardized **kava extract** on safety when taken with alcohol. Twenty males and females participated in seven skill-performance tests over several days. The **kava** did not cause any negative additive effects. However, the **kava**-and-alcohol group showed a "remarkable" advantage over the alcohol group on the concentration test (Herberg, 1993).

- In a controlled double-blind crossover study comparing the effects of oxazepam (a benzodiazepine antianxiety agent) and a **kava root extract** on recognition and memory tasks, subjects were asked to recognize and recall words. Oxazepam caused a reduction in memory for both old and new words, while **kava** showed a slight increase in recognition rate (Munte et al., 1993).

KUDZU ROOT AND FLOWER

Latin: *Pueraria lobata*　　**Sanskrit:** Bidari kand　　**Chinese:** Gao gen
P. tuberosa

WHAT IT DOES: Kudzu is sweet in taste and cooling in action. The root is a general tonic that calms the nerves and heart and relaxes tension and spasms in the upper body. The flower reduces alcohol cravings.

RATING: Silver

SAFETY ISSUES: None known

STARTING DOSAGE:

- Dried powder: 5 to 15 grams per day

- Tea: cut the fresh or dried tuber into small pieces (about ½ inch in diameter), and decoct for about 30 minutes.

> **Kudzu** vine is seen as a major ecological problem in the southern United States, where it is taking over and growing everywhere. Perhaps turning it into a cash crop would be of great benefit.

We use **kudzu root** in our clinic according to TCM tradition, in formulas whenever we see chronic upper body tension, stiffness, muscle spasm, and pain. It is also useful for reducing thirst and fever. **Kudzu root** may be mildly beneficial for treating heart conditions. Patients with angina and hypertension often report that they feel much better after using this herb for a period of time, confirming traditional Ayurvedic reports that it acts as a general tonic for health and long life. For the heart, it can be taken as a tea on a daily basis.

If you eat **kudzu** before you drink alcohol in excess, you will be overcome by hangover nausea almost immediately due to a chemical reaction involving a component called acetaldehyde. This will of course discourage alcohol use for a very long time. I suggest the government require manufacturers to put **kudzu root** right into all alcoholic drinks, along with some **milk thistle seed** to protect the liver, a little **white peony root** to aid in spatial coordination, and some B vitamins to reduce toxicity. This would serve as an instant solution to most alcohol-related problems, including overconsumption, liver damage, morning-after hangovers, and drunk driving.

Research Highlights

- Compounds in **kudzu root** have been shown to suppress voluntary alcohol consumption in alcohol-preferring rats (Lin and Li, 1998).

- Individual saponins isolated from **kudzu root** have shown liver-protective activity in vitro with cultured rat liver cells (Arao et al., 1998; Arao et al., 1997).

- **Kudzu** contains phytoestrogenic compounds, including daidzin and daidzein (Lin and Li, 1998).

- Women of the Bhil tribe of Madhya Pradesh use **kudzu tubers** to increase milk production, and it is also used on farm animals for the same purpose (reported in Pandey, 1996).

- In several Indian studies, extracts of **kudzu tubers** caused 100% postcoital anti-implantation activity in rats, hamsters, and guinea pigs, leading to speculation that it might prove useful as a nontoxic abortifacient.

- In a study of 250 female patients, 50% of the pregnant participants taking **kudzu tuber** experienced pregnancy termination (Chandoke et al., 1981).

- Reviews of experimental studies and clinical application of **kudzu root** in China have also reported cardiovascular applications. The observed actions include increased blood circulation to the brain, antiarrythmia, increased blood flow in the coronary artery, mild antihypertensive actions, and mild blood-sugar-lowering effects (Lai and Tang, 1989; reported in Yeung, 1983).

LEMON

Latin: *Citrus limon*   **Sanskrit:** Nimbu

WHAT IT DOES: Lemon is sour in taste and cooling in action. It stimulates the internal organs and helps resolve kidney stones and gallstones.

RATING: Yellow

SAFETY ISSUES: None known

STARTING DOSAGE:

- Fresh fruit—use as described below

The **lemon** is one of our most common fruits, and TAM doctors draw our attention to its differences from other sour fruits. **Lemon** is unique in that its trees bear fruit continuously throughout the year, it has the ability to constrict the capillaries, and it exhibits a cooling rather than a warming action. (This cooling action makes it a stimulating summer beverage.) It has several interesting medicinal uses.

TAM doctors believe **lemon** has medicinal value in treating indigestion, nausea, and loss of appetite. To stop even severe nausea temporarily, chew or squeeze a piece of **lemon peel** and inhale the spray. It works only for a few minutes, but this

> I am very partial to organic **lemons** because the pesticides used on most citrus fruits are detrimental to your health.

can be important if you suffer from hepatitis or morning sickness. **Lemon** is one of several citrus products than can inhibit tumor formation. When administered with a chemical carcinogenic agent, oils of **orange, tangerine, lemon,** and **grapefruit** inhibited tumor formation in both the stomach and lungs of mice.

Perhaps most importantly, research performed at the University of California in San Francisco showed that patients with kidney stones who could not tolerate traditional pharmaceutical approaches benefited when they supplemented their diets with 4 ounces of reconstituted **lemon juice** per day. **Lemon juice** is a natural source of citrate, and 4 ounces provides about 6 grams of citrate. This level doubles urinary citrate levels and lowers urinary calcium excretion, which is required to prevent kidney stone formation. If it were up to me, I'd make sure patients always used the juice of organic fresh **lemons,** which contain limolene, a phytochemical that helps dissolve gallstones and is found mostly in the white parts on the inside of the rind.

LICORICE ROOT

Latin: *Glycyrrhiza glabra*   **Sanskrit:** Madhukam   **Chinese:** Gan cao
Zhi gan cao

WHAT IT DOES: Licorice root is sweet in taste and cooling in action. It detoxifies poisons from the blood and liver and reduces general inflammation and pain. It moistens and heals the lungs and digestive tract.

RATING: Silver

SAFETY ISSUES: Do not use during pregnancy. Do not use in high doses or for a prolonged period of time unless under the care of a qualified health care practitioner. Use cautiously with kidney disease and liver disorders or if taking thiazide diuretics, cortisone, or cardiac glycosides. **Licorice** prolongs the half-life of cortisone. **The DGL form of licorice is free of side effects.**

STARTING DOSAGE:

- Crude powder: 1 to 3 grams three times per day, up to 6 weeks

- Concentrated 4:1 granules: 150–250 mg three times per day

- Tincture (Make a strong decoction and then preserve with 22% grain alcohol): 15–25 drops two to three times per day

   Licorice root is one of the most widely used herbs in the world. Every major medical tradition uses it as medicine, usually describing its effects as cooling and tonifying. TCM doctors use it in two forms. Regular **licorice root** is considered to have an intrinsic harmonizing effect useful for reducing side effects from large combinations of other potent herbs, and for disguising their bitter or acrid flavors. **Licorice** is said to strengthen the digestion and the hormonal systems and moisten the lungs. TCM doctors also use a honey-fried form to warm digestion when indicated. TAM doctors use **licorice root** to reduce the pain of sore throat and ulcers, to subdue poisons, and as a major ingredient in cough syrups.

   Almost 50 years ago, a scientist by the name of Revers reported that **licorice paste** reduced abdominal symptoms and caused radiographic evidence of ulcer healing. However, about 20% of patients developed edema, headache, and other symptoms due to overdose, leading to a loss of enthusiasm (Schambelan, 1994). This led to the development of **DGL (deglycyrrhizinated licorice),** a form of **licorice** that does not contain the agents responsible for the side effects. The deacidified **DGL** tablet or capsule form used in Europe and America seems devoid of any side effects and is effective for healing the intestinal membranes.

Paul Bergner, editor of *Medical Herbalism*, wrote an article citing recent Japanese and Chinese research highlighting the numerous positive and protective effects **licorice root** exerts on the liver. Its antihepatotoxic effects make it useful in treating chronic hepatitis and possibly cirrhosis. **Licorice root** contains plant (phyto) estrogens similar to those found in **soy,** and has an estrogenlike effect, binding strongly to estrogen receptors. This makes it a good treatment for easing hot flashes, though I would do this only at recommended doses in a formula with other herbs.

Many patients express concerns about using **licorice** because they have seen negative press coverage of this herb. It is important to understand that these reported concerns are dose related. **Licorice** is traditionally used as approximately 5% of a formula, and that is what I usually do with it. If a patient takes the typical 6 to 9 grams of concentrated 4:1 powder per day, this works out to about 1.2–1.8 grams of licorice, well within recommended dosage levels. Personally, I've never seen any of the potassium depletion and sodium retention effects described in the literature, and the pharmacologists I've consulted with assure me that such effects are rare and easily reversible simply by stopping use.

The various components of **licorice root** act in a number of different ways in the test tube, on animals and on humans. It is important to keep in mind that specific results of scientific studies, such as the ones listed below, often relate to particular components of **licorice**. By examining these various reports you will be able to see the general pattern of cooling and detoxification noted by ancient doctors.

Research Highlights

- We now know that the negative effects of **licorice** overdose, such as blood pressure elevation and fluid retention, are caused primarily by its dose-dependent inhibition of a specific enzyme called 11-HSD. Analysis reveals that this inhibition occurs only after multiple doses of 1.5 grams per day of pure glycyrrhizic acid. Daily doses of 500 mg or less cause little or no problem (Krahenbuhl et al., 1994; Heilmann et al., 1999; White et al., 1997). In other words, **licorice root** is safe when used in proper dosage.

- According to several studies, **DGL licorice** is a very effective ulcer treatment (Morgan et al., 1985; Morgan et al., 1982; Morgan et al., 1987; Russell et al., 1984; Tewari and Wilson, 1973).

- Glycyrrhizin is a major anti-inflammatory compound found in **licorice.** Its anti-inflammatory action is due in part to the selective inhibition of thrombin (a clotting factor), which results in the removal of blood congestion. Glycyrrhizin was the first such compound to be isolated from a plant (Francischetti et al., 1997).

- Glycyrrhizic acid, a component of **licorice root,** was found to inhibit the growth and cytopathology of several unrelated DNA and RNA viruses without affecting cell activity and ability to replicate. Glycyrrhizic acid irreversibly inactivates herpes simplex virus particles (Pompei et al., 1979). For this reason, **licorice** tincture or paste can be applied directly to lesions.

- In animal studies, **licorice root** has been shown to enhance liver detoxification of poisons, causing significant increases in liver and urinary excretion of acetaminophen (Moon and Kim, 1997).

- The complex sugars found in **licorice root** and many other herbs stimulate macrophages (immune cells), but some scientists have expressed concerns that the effects seen in laboratory experiments might have been overstated and due solely or in part to bacterial contamination. However, additional studies determined that macrophage stimulation by **licorice root** still occurred in plants grown in aseptic conditions (Nose et al., 1998).

- A compound in **licorice root** called beta-glycyrrhetinic acid has been identified as a potent inhibitor of a certain cascade of inflammatory immune system chemicals (Kroes et al., 1997).

- **Licorice extract**, along with glutathione and the bioflavonoids, belongs to a class of substances known as "desmutagens." Scientists Kada and Shimoi categorized these molecules according to their unique ability to bind to toxic chemicals and cancer-causing agents (Shankel et al., 1993).

- **DGL** can be used as a mouthwash for small mouth ulcers (Das et al., 1989) and may reduce stomach bleeding caused by aspirin (Rees et al., 1979).

- **Licorice alcohol extract** contains a subclass of polyphenol flavonoids called isoflavones that may reduce the negative effects of LDL cholesterol and reduce atherosclerotic lesion areas in mice (Fuhrman et al., 1997; Aviram, 1996). This effect was later shown to be similar to that of the bioflavonoid **quercetin** (Belinky et al., 1998).

- **Licorice root** has an effect on corticosteroid metabolism that links it to certain receptors in the brain and may eventually lead to applications in studies of mood, neuronal survival, and feedback related to blood pressure. Researchers hope to develop useful means to target specific action sites on the brain (Seckl, 1997).

- A **licorice root extract,** mostly glycyrrhizin (a saponin extracted from **licorice),** has been shown pharmacologically to stimulate interferon (Eisenburg, 1992), suggesting that a combination might be more effective than either alone. A clinical test on humans showed results for hepatitis C (a reduction in viral load and ALT, which is a liver enzyme that is released into the blood when liver cells are damaged), but results failed to achieve significance (Abe et al., 1994).

LONG PEPPER

Latin: *Piper longum*   **Sanskrit:** Pippali

WHAT IT DOES: Long pepper is pungent in taste and hot in action and is tonic. It improves appetite and digestion, helps control coughs and asthma, and increases absorption of other nutrients and herbs.

RATING: Silver, as it contains both tonic effects as well as some restrictions

SAFETY ISSUES: Use cautiously with stomach weakness or hyperacidity. Do not use continuously in high dose for longer than 2 weeks. Low dosage (as a spice) is safe for long-term use.

STARTING DOSAGE:

- Dried powder: 200-mg concentration, 1½ grams two to three times per day (larger amounts—up to 30 grams per day—may be used if cooked for 2 hours)

Long pepper is an interesting medicine. It is one of three parts of the famous Ayurvedic digestive formula called **trikatu** (the other two are **black pepper** and **ginger root). Long pepper** is pungent and stimulating to the appetite and can be added to the diet to improve nutrient absorption. TAM doctors use it for bronchitis, asthma, cough, and fever and to stimulate the medicinal effects of other herbs.

Scientific attention has focused on piperine, an alkaloid found in **long pepper** and **black pepper,** which stimulates an enzyme that promotes amino acid uptake from the digestive tract and increases heat in the GI tract. Piperine appears to increase blood concentrations of **turmeric root.** Therefore, instead of using the more expensive and perhaps slightly dangerous **turmeric** extract called curcumin, all you may need to do is add either of the **peppers** to ordinary **turmeric root,** about 5% by weight, for short periods of time (perhaps a few weeks at most).

Numerous studies of **long pepper** show blood levels of various vitamins and nutrients to increase by as much as 30% when ingested concurrently. Nonetheless, I do not recommend long-term continual use due to the herb's strongly spicy quality. Atal (1985) estimated that the inhibition effect lasts only 1–6 hours in animals, and this makes it very useful with ingested nutrients. However, if **long pepper** is taken continuously or in excess, it could also keep toxic molecules from being metabolized and excreted. I add **long pepper** or **trikatu** to herbal formulas for short periods of use to aid digestion when weak, especially if the patient has signs of mucus. TAM doctors report that **long pepper** reduces colic pain and mucus and can be used for cough and asthma. It stimulates the medicinal effects of other herbs. Unlike **black pepper, long pepper** is reputed to have tonic qualities—good for long life.

Research Highlights

- Piperine has an affinity for fatty tissue, where it interacts with the cell membranes. Its components are absorbed very quickly across the intestinal barrier, increasing permeability (Johri et al., 1992), so researchers theorize that it attaches to various molecules and helps them across (Khajuria et al., 1998).

- Piperine's most important action may be the inhibition of liver and intestinal glucuronidation, which allows molecules to flow into the blood without being excreted (Atal et al., 1985).

- Especially interesting to me was one study published in *Planta Medica* showing how piperine dramatically increased blood concentrations of **turmeric root,** one of my favorite anti-inflammatories (Shoba et al., 1998).

- **Long pepper** also has some mild liver-protective activity (Koul and Kapil, 1993).

MAITAKE MUSHROOM

Latin: *Grifola frondosa*   **Japanese:** Mushikusa   **English:** Hen-of-the-Woods

WHAT IT DOES: Maitake mushroom is sweet in taste and neutral in energy. It is a nourishing adaptogenic tonic that helps nourish the immune system and identify, target, and destroy invaders, including cancer cells.

RATING: Gold

SAFETY ISSUES: None known

STARTING DOSAGE:

- Fresh mushroom: ½ cup cooked, two to three times per week

- Dried fruiting body capsules: two 500-mg capsules two to three times per day

- Extract tincture (1 gram mushroom = 30 drops): 15–30 drops two to three times per day

- Proprietary D-fraction liquid: 5 to 25 drops two times per day

Maitake mushrooms are a wonderful food tonic, illustrating Nature's ability to harness her magic. They have been harvested in eastern North America for years and sold to restaurants as a delicacy. The Japanese retrieve them from the mountains of Northeast Japan. Now that they are becoming available commercially as foods, make sure to include them in your diet. When eaten whole, they tonify the body, increase energy, keep the immune system healthy, and increase longevity. We use **maitake extracts** as a staple in our treatment of immune-compromised cancer patients. The extracts contain high levels of beta-glucan, a well-researched immune-system-activating agent.

Research Highlights

- Extracts of **maitake** show antitumor action by directly activating various immune system components, including macrophages, complement, cytokines, natural killer (NK) cells, and tumor necrosis factor (Borchers et al., 1999; Nanba et al., 1997; Kurashige et al., 1997).

- Beta-glucan seems to override the normal resistance of tumor cells to the cytotoxic activation of phagocytes and NK cells. This allows the complement part of the immune system to function against tumor cells in the same way that it normally functions against bacteria and yeast (Kubo et al., 1999).

- **Maitake mushroom** has demonstrated an ability to alter fat metabolism in animal studies by inhibiting both the accumulation of liver lipids and the elevation of serum lipids (Kubo et al., 1996).

- The fruiting body of **maitake** was confirmed to contain substances that exhibit antidiabetic activity, as illustrated by its ability to lower blood glucose levels (Kubo et al., 1994).

- Feeding studies show that **maitake mushroom** can lower blood pressure in hypertensive rats (Kabir and Kimura, 1989).

- It is important to note that despite the similarities of the anticancer substances (including glucans) found in various mushrooms, they differ in their effectiveness against specific tumors and in their ability to elicit immune responses (Borchers et al., 1999).

MILK THISTLE SEED

Latin: *Silybum marianum*

WHAT IT DOES: Milk thistle seed is sweet in taste and cooling in action. It strongly protects, repairs, and nourishes the liver, stomach, and intestines.

RATING: Silver

SAFETY ISSUES: Milk thistle may speed clearance of pharmaceutical drugs. Use cautiously (consult your physician) if taking drugs that require adequate blood levels, such as cardiac glycosides or cyclosporine.

STARTING DOSAGE:

- Concentrated standardized silymarin capsules (70–210 mg): 1 to 2 pills, two to three times per day

- 1:5 tincture: (grind seeds before adding alcohol): 20–40 drops three times per day

When I was growing up in the 1950s and '60s, it was commonly believed among Western physicians that nothing could repair a severely damaged liver. This changed with the emergence of **milk thistle**. However, in TAM and TCM there are numerous liver herbs, some perhaps stronger than **milk thistle,** and there is a wide breadth of knowledge concerning how to use them to benefit the liver. Some of them described in this chapter include **bupleurum root, eclipta, guduchi stem, white peony root, scute root, shilajatu, turmeric root, and schisandra berries.**

Milk thistle is a true liver tonic, useful for treating numerous liver and gall-bladder conditions including hepatitis and cirrhosis. **Milk thistle seed** is especially useful whenever chemicals, alcohol, chemotherapy, or medicines compromise the liver. It reverses toxic liver damage and protects against hepatotoxic agents, including the **deathcap toadstool** *(Amanita phalloides).* It is used for this purpose in European hospitals. It also stimulates protein synthesis in the liver, helping with the formation and growth of healthy new liver cells by selectively inhibiting certain inflammatory chemicals in liver cells. At our clinic, I like to combine **milk thistle seed** with **dandelion root** and **turmeric root** to create a simple liver tonic that heals, repairs, detoxifies, and gently stimulates the liver.

The benefits of **milk thistle** and other liver agents were well known before 1919, when Dr. Finley Ellingwood's classic, *American Materia Medica, Therapeutics and Pharmacognosy,* described in detail how **milk thistle** improves "general bilious conditions" such as jaundice, hepatic pain, and swelling. Early physicians also used it to treat congestion in the spleen, kidneys, and veins. Its range of action is very wide.

Research Highlights

- **Milk thistle** "has been shown to have clinical applications in the treatment of toxic hepatitis, fatty liver, cirrhosis, ischemic injury, radiation toxicity, and viral hepatitis via its anti-oxidative, anti-lipid peroxidative, antifibrotic, anti-inflammatory, immuno-modulating, and liver regenerating effects" (Luper, 1998).

- In a unique application of this herb, Russian scientists have studied the addition of **milk thistle** to bread to observe its effects on health and metabolism. They reported that the addition of *Silybum marianum* to bread products exerted a general restorative influence, increasing internal protection resources, capacity for work, and vital activity (Gil'miiarov et al., 1998).

- In a double-blind study examining patients with liver cirrhosis due to alcohol, after 5 years there were almost three times as many deaths in the control group as in the group taking **milk thistle** (Benda et al., 1980). A later study illustrated similar results (Ferenci P et al., 1989).

- In a model designed to examine the effect of alcohol on pregnant women, a group of rat pups that received a diet consisting of 35% ethanol exhibited marked mental deficits, including poor social memory. The group that received silymarin (the active ingredient in **milk thistle seed**) in addition to the ethanol scored much better, indicating a protective effect (Reid C et al., 1999).

- Because it contains polyphenolic antioxidants, **milk thistle** may also have potential as a cancer preventative agent (Zhao et al., 1999). Noting that most antioxidants afford protection against tumor promotion, in a complex study measuring several parameters, researchers reported the protective effect of silymarin, indicating that it exhibited highly protective effects against tumor promotion (Lahiri-Chatterjee et al., 1999).

- **Milk thistle** was found to have an anticancer effect on both breast and prostate cancer (Zi X et al., 1998). It also protects the kidneys against toxicity from the chemotherapeutic agent cisplatin in animal models, without reducing its effectiveness against cancer (Bokemeyer et al., 1996; Gaedeke et al., 1996). It also protects against the kidney toxicity of cyclosporine, an antirejection drug (Zima et al., 1998).

- Studies have shown a protective effect of silymarin on stomach and intestinal membranes (Alarcon de la Lastra et al., 1995). This may be due to a selective increase in total glutathione content in the liver, intestine, and stomach found in animal studies (Valenzuela A et al., 1989).

MILKY OAT SEED

Latin: *Avena sativa*

WHAT IT DOES: Milky oat seed is sweet in taste and mildly stimulating and cooling in action. It restores strength to the nervous system when exhausted and reduces craving for tobacco and drugs.

RATING: Gold

SAFETY ISSUES: None known

STARTING DOSAGE:

- Tincture (fresh seed, 1:2): 20–40 drops three to four times per day

Milky oat seed is a mild but reliable remedy for strengthening the entire nervous system after periods of prolonged stress. The seed is harvested when it becomes milky. Growers must squeeze the seeds each day until the milky juice oozes out, which occurs only for 5–8 days. Once collected, the juice must immediately be turned into a tincture. It is used to treat nervous debility, stress, weak nerve force, anxiety, depression, and the accompanying exhaustion and general fatigue. A chief virtue of **milky oat seed** is its extreme tolerability by otherwise highly sensitive patients who have difficulty withstanding treatment with stronger tonic herbs. It seems to exert an immediate effect (necessary when patients exhibit extreme anxiety and nervousness) as well as a long-term strengthening benefit.

I often combine it with **skullcap,** which has stronger sedative action. Good alternatives include "Avena-Scullcap compound" made by Herb Pharm and "Phytocalm formula" made by Herbalist & Alchemist. These formulas have seen many of our patients through severely stressful periods and have helped many more avoid resorting to stronger Western medications. It is safe for use by everyone, even infants.

> Dr. John Christopher, a well-known herb doctor of the last generation, tells the story of a patient who brewed a tea of **skullcap, milky oat seed,** and a few other nervines and left it to cool on the stove. Her infant child climbed up on the counter and drank about 5 or 10 times the adult dose, prompting her to call Dr. Christopher in hysterics. He calmed her down and told her the child would be fine. After a very long sleep, the mischievous infant awoke well rested and in good spirits.

Herbalist David Winston, who maintains an extensive private herbal medicine library, reports that **milky oat seed** was used extensively by early physicians, and he mentions finding a pamphlet detailing its use for treating morphine addiction as far back as the 1880s. European herbalists have also traditionally used it to treat opium addiction. Numerous studies serve to substantiate, at least partially, claims of the herb's usefulness in addiction control, including its effectiveness as an aid for smoking cessation. Although the research done so far is sparse, the clinical results I have seen remain impressive.

Research Highlights

- In a placebo-controlled study, researchers gave a fresh alcohol extract of **mature oat plant** to heavy smokers. The extract was found to reduce cigarette usage significantly more than the placebo (Anand, 1971).

- In another study, a tincture of **oat seed** taken with malic acid and apple juice for 4 weeks led to a 67% reduction in cigarette consumption (Raffalt and Andersen, 1975).

- Chemical studies have revealed that the addition of water to **milky oat seed** causes a significant loss of potency. Water extracts have not been significantly more effective than placebos in studies of its ability to control addictions (Gabrynowicz 1974; Bye et al., 1974)

- Pharmaceutically prepared fresh alcohol extracts of both **fresh oat plants** and **oat**

seeds have exhibited activity as nicotine and morphine antagonists (Connor et al., 1975).

- Additionally, out of a group of 10 male chronic opium addicts taking a 2-mL dose (about 30 drops) three times per day of **oat tincture,** 6 gave up opium without serious withdrawal symptoms. During a follow-up period of 3 to 19 months, the 6 successful participants were able to stay off opium completely (Anand, 1971).

MILLETTIA STEM

Latin: *Millettia* species   **Chinese:** Ji xue teng   **English:** Chicken blood vine
Spatholobus suberectus

WHAT IT DOES: Millettia stem is sweet in taste and warming in action. It nourishes the blood and bone marrow, moves the blood, and reduces muscle and joint pain in deficiency syndromes.

RATING: Silver. Use cautiously if taking blood-thinning medication.

SAFETY ISSUES: None known

STARTING DOSAGE:

- Dried crude powder: 9 to 15 grams per day
- 4:1 concentrated dried decoction: 3 to 6 grams per day

Millettia stem is another of the TCM "moving blood" and "supply blood" herbs used normally to treat problems such as anemia, dysmenorrhea, irregular menstruation, and amenorrhea. Because it is a stem, TCM doctors say it is useful to treat muscle and joint pain by opening obstructions to Qi flow in the meridians. Because it both nourishes and moves the blood, it is a good choice for patients with deficiency.

We always include it in formulas for cancer patients suffering from leukopenia due to radiation or chemotherapy, along with other herbs from the same category such as **dang gui root, carthamus flower, white peony root, salvia root,** and **cooked rehmannia root.** In severe cases of anemia, it is useful to dissolve concentrated granules of these herbs into molasses to form a paste and spoon-feed it to the patient. I would use up to 1 tablespoon every 2 to 3 hours, adding some **ginger root** if there is a digestive problem.

Research Highlights

- Pharmacological studies in China show that the blood-forming effects take place in the bone marrow, significantly stimulating hematopoiesis while exerting a beneficial effect on the marrow microenvironment. Microscopic examination has shown a reduction in hyperplasia and an increase in the proliferation of microvessels (Su et al., 1997).

- In clinical studies in China on cancer patients with impaired immune function, various compound formulas using **millettia stem** have shown increases in white blood cell function, hemoglobin, and platelets (reported in Dharmananda, 1999).

MUIRA PUAMA

Latin: *Ptychopetalum* species   **Spanish:** Muira puama   **English:** Potency bark

WHAT IT DOES: Muira puama is sweet in taste and warming in action. It increases sex drive and stimulates nervous system energy.

RATING: Yellow, due to limited mode of action

SAFETY ISSUES: None known

STARTING DOSAGE:

- 1:4 tincture: 20–40 drops two to four times per day, up to 60 drops for a single dose

  Note: Muira puama must be used in tincture extracted form.

Muira puama is a Brazilian rain forest herb traditionally used as an aphrodisiac, as is obvious from the English translation of its name. It is used to treat male impotence, low sex drive, and female frigidity. Researchers in Europe and Japan have studied the balsam, an aromatic oily extract of the herb, since 1969. According to Italian research reports in the popular press, **muira puama** produces an androgenic effect similar to **yohimbe bark** (an alkaloid of which is now a prescription medicine), but without its side effects. It is reputed to exert an awakening effect on sexual desire in both sexes, as well as an increase in the production of sperm in men. The exact mechanism of action is currently unknown.

At our clinic, we find **muira puama** quite effective as a short-term remedy. However, good holistic medicine dictates the additional need to identify underlying causes of the problem that should be treated long term. Fortunately, the quick results this herb produces in many cases give the patients confidence to pursue further treatment.

Research Highlights

- The Institute of Sexology in Paris, France, did a clinical study of **muira puama** with male patients complaining of low sex drive and the inability to maintain an erection. In many cases, the herb proved effective within 2 weeks. At a daily dose of about

30–90 drops of the 1:4 tincture extract, 62% of patients with loss of libido claimed that the treatment had "a dynamic effect," and 51% of patients with erection failure also reported improvement (Waynsberg, 1990).

MYRRH GUM

Latin: *Commiphora myrrha* **Sanskrit:** Daindhava **Chinese:** Mo yao
Commiphora molmol

WHAT IT DOES: Myrrh gum is bitter in taste, aromatic, and cooling in action. It invigorates the blood and reduces pain and swelling caused by blood stasis.

RATING: Red

SAFETY ISSUES: Do not use if pregnant. Do not use with excessive uterine bleeding. Do not use with evidence of kidney dysfunction or stomach pain.

STARTING DOSAGE:

- Dried gum powder: 1 to 3 grams per day
- Concentrated dried decoction extract: 250–750 mg per day

Myrrh gum has an intense dark color, reflecting its medicinal potency. It exerts a strong and certain action against specific types of pain and swelling, such as that of rheumatoid arthritis. It is strong enough to soften hard swellings and carbuncles. Like all plant resins, **myrrh** can also lower blood cholesterol levels by binding to lipids.

Biblical references to "frankincense and **myrrh**" refer to this herb along with **boswellia gum**, which is another useful resinous anti-inflammatory. Early physicians considered **myrrh tincture** to be the most effective topical medicine for treating sore and spongy gums. The tincture is diluted down to 10–15% with water and applied directly to the gums. It is also useful as a gargle for spongy enlarged tonsils. In India, it is used for similar applications, with the addition of honey and **rose petals** to the solution.

At our clinic we use both of these plants frequently when there is painful swelling in the joints. The action is often broader and more satisfying than that of aspirin and other NSAID compounds alone. I do not use **myrrh** by itself. It's simply too strong. I prefer to use it as a smaller part of a formula, perhaps 5%, and just for a month or two.

The practice of using single strong anti-inflammatories, which block chemical actions, can often create side effects. We are now beginning to gain a scientific understanding of why the common practice of mixing anti-inflammatory herbs, found in all herbal cultures, is so effective.

If you completely block a chemical pathway the body is using for some purpose, like ridding itself of a toxin, it will often express its displeasure by creating a side effect, a chain of chemical events. The different herbs work in a myriad of ways, with actions on many different chemical pathways. If you gently moderate several of these pathways, the result will often be a significant reduction of pain and swelling without side effects. Hopefully, then, by working in concert with changes in diet and lifestyle, the body can overcome the original imbalance or causative factors and come to a more complete resolution.

Research Highlights

- In an attempt to determine the cause of its effectiveness, researchers examined the individual ingredients of an herbal formula used traditionally by Kuwaiti diabetics to lower blood glucose. Only **myrrh** and **aloe gums** effectively improved glucose tolerance in both normal and diabetic rats (Al-Awadi and Gumaa, 1987).

- Mixing **myrrh gum** into vinegar increases its ability to remove blood congestion and relieve pain (reported in Yeung, 1983).

NEEM LEAF AND OIL

Latin: *Azadirachta indica*   **Sanskrit:** Nimba

WHAT IT DOES: Neem leaf is bitter in taste and cold in action. It reduces fever and inflammation, reduces itching, and kills microbes and fungus. **Neem oil** is used externally to heal wounds and boils.

RATING: Red

SAFETY ISSUES: Do not use for longer than 3 weeks due to damping effect on digestive, sexual, and reproductive functions. Do not use this product unless under the guidance of a properly trained professional.

STARTING DOSAGE:

- Dried powder: 1 to 2 grams two times per day
- 1:5 tincture: 10–20 drops two times per day
- Concentrated powder extract: 150–250 mg two to three times per day

Ayurvedic doctors use **neem leaves** for skin diseases, itching, and fever, especially malarial fever. They also use it internally and externally for all forms of fungal and other infections. We use concentrated **neem leaves** at our clinic to treat skin diseases with severe itching and intestinal problems related to candidiasis or other fungal infections. We often combine **neem** in formulas with other antifungal plants and tell patients to restrict sugar intake and take acidophilus capsules. This helps kill the "bad guy" intestinal bacteria, restricts their favorite fuel (sugar), and adds "good guy" acidophilus back into the intestine. A few weeks on this sort of antifungal program can work wonders with these types of infections, even in persistent cases.

Neem oil is used in India in numerous varieties of hair lotion, medicated soap, and toothpaste. It is considered to be effective as a topical treatment for chronic skin conditions, ulcers, and leprosy. The warm oil is also useful when applied to treat ear infections. **Traditionally used to treat malaria, neem is a very bitter and potent plant, so it should be used only when other methods have failed.**

Research Highlights

- Oral administration of dry **neem leaf** for 24 days resulted in a reduction in the weight of the seminal vesicles and prostate of albino rats, showing an antiandrogen effect (Kasutri et al., 1997). However, it is important to note that the dosage—20–60 mg per day—was much higher than the recommended human dose. A review of the toxicity data by the pharmacognosy department at the University of Utrecht in the Netherlands concluded, "reported toxicity of preparations and isolated compounds are low, except for the seed oil" (Van der Nat et al., 1991).

- Test tube studies of **neem seed extract** on the human malaria parasite showed a strong inhibitory effect by way of a different mechanism of action than other antimalaria drugs. **Neem seed** is active not only against the parasite stages that cause the initial clinical infection but also against the stages responsible for malaria transmission (Dhar et al., 1998).

- When applied to the skin, solutions of 1–4% **neem oil** in 96–99% coconut oil afforded 81–91% protection against mosquito bites for 12 hours (Mishra et al., 1995; Sharma et al., 1993).

- When applied with urea to rice crops, **lipid neem extracts** slowed mosquito breeding, reduced incidence of Japanese encephalitis, and significantly increased grain yield in a cost-effective manner (Rao et al., 1995).

- In a study of 814 people with scabies, topical application of a skin paste made of **neem leaves** (4 parts) and **turmeric root** (1 part) cured 97% of the cases within 3 to 15 days of treatment (Charles and Charles, 1992).

- The insecticide activity of **neem extract** seems to come from its ability to reduce appetite and disrupt growth in certain insects, including mosquitoes (Ley, 1990).

- Application of **neem oil** appears to induce a strong blockage of fertility. In a controlled study of fertile female Wistar rats, a single intrauterine dose of **neem oil** caused a 100% infertility rate for periods of 100 to 180 days, while all the control animals became pregnant. Within 5 months, more than 50% of the test females regained fertility. There was no visible effect on ovarian function (Upadhyay et al., 1990).

- In a related study, the researchers discovered that **neem oil** acts as an alternative to vasectomy. As with females, a single-dose injection of **neem oil** in male rats caused infertility for 8 months, blocking sperm production without affecting testosterone (there did appear to be a reduction in testicular size). The effects may be due to a local immune response against the sperm (Upadhyay et al., 1993).

- In an unrelated study, oral administration of **neem extract** for 10 weeks caused a significant decrease in total testosterone in male rats. There were no cytotoxic effects (Parshad et al., 1994).

- The antifertility effect of **neem oil** was also reported in rhesus monkeys (Bardhan et al., 1991).

- Oral administration of **neem seed extract** (Praneem) caused abortion early on in the pregnant female baboons and bonnet monkeys. The treatment was tolerated well, and tests of blood chemistry and liver function were normal. The primates regained fertility subsequent to treatment (Mukherjee et al., 1996).

- As a result of the aforementioned effects, researchers investigated **neem oil** for hormonal properties. They found that it had no estrogenic, antiestrogenic, or progesterone-related activity. They concluded that since the postcoital contraceptive effect of **neem oil** seems to be nonhormonal, it is less likely to elicit side effects than steroidal contraceptives (Prakesh et al., 1988).

OREGANO OIL AND LEAF

Latin: *Origanum vulgare*
　　　　O. species

WHAT IT DOES: Oregano oil is pungent in taste, aromatic, and warming. It penetrates into the system, breaks up congestion, and kills microbes. **Oregano leaf** stimulates appetite and detoxifies food.

RATING:

- **Leaf:** Gold

- **Oil:** Red

SAFETY ISSUES: Do not use oil without diluting it. Do not exceed recommended dosage. Direct contact with oil to sensitive areas of skin, eye, or mouth can cause severe burns.

STARTING DOSAGE:

- Sinus drops with essential oil: 1 to 5 drops of oil diluted in 1 ounce of water or olive oil

- Internal use of essential oil: 1 to 3 drops of oil diluted in 1 ounce of water, several times per day; shake well before using

- Leaf: add fresh or dried leaf freely to foods

The Greek name for this useful herb spice is *origanos,* or "delight of the mountains." **Oregano** can and should be used freely as a spice in salads and soups, as it lowers the concentration of microbes in food. The essential oil contains volatile oils, complex chemicals that are known for the odor they emit as they turn to gas. These gases generally have antiseptic, antimicrobial, and antioxidant effects as they disperse aggressively throughout the body. Carvacrol and thymol, two volatile oils found in **oregano**, are known to thin mucus, relieve coughing, and relax muscle spasms. These actions make the herb a very useful treatment for lung disorders, including pneumonia, sinus congestion, hay fever, chronic bronchitis, and rhinitis.

In our clinic, we add **oregano oil** to water or olive oil to make sinus drops and have patients snort 2 or 3 drops as often as desired to open congestion and kill microbes. Those who are plagued by frequent sinus infections (accompanied by gunky green mucus) find that keeping these drops around the house can stop these infections before they take hold. To kill stubborn toenail fungus, put 2 or 3 drops of undiluted **oregano oil** on a cotton pad and tape it directly to the toenail. You may need to do this twice per day for a couple of months. The penetrating quality of the vapors permeates deeply enough to root out and kill fungus lurking below the nail bed. For a stronger effect, soak the toenails in vinegar every day to make them more porous, and add some **neem leaf extract** to the **oregano oil**.

> My friend Bob Klezics came to me complaining of chronic chest congestion. He had found some relief with herbs but found that he had to keep taking the herbs or the problem would return. He finally discovered Oregamax, a commercial product made from a particularly potent form of Greek **oregano,** and his congestion disappeared in 2 or 3 days, never to return.

Research Highlights

- In a test of **oregano, mint, basil, sage,** and **coriander** essential oils for activity against yeast and fungi, **oregano** proved to be the strongest, inhibiting the yeast broth completely at 1,000 parts per million (Basilico and Basilico, 1999).

- In studies against food-borne pathogens, **oregano oil** proved effective against numerous species, including *Bacillus cereus* (Ultee et al., 1999); *Salmonella enteritidis* (Koutsoumanis et al., 1999); *Acinetobacter baumanii, Aeromonas veronii* biogroup sobria, *Candida albicans, Enterococcus faecalis, Escherichia coli, Klebsiella pneumoniae, Pseudomonas aeruginosa, Salmonella enterica* subspecies enterica serotype typhimurium, *Serratia marcescens,* and *Staphylococcus aureus* (Hammer et al., 1999); and *Giardia duodenalis* (Ponce-Macotela et al., 1994).

- **Oregano leaf** is one of six herbs found in a particular screening to contain a high concentration of phytoprogesterones (Zava et al., 1998).

- Food studies on **oregano leaf** indicate that it stimulates appetite when added to pasta in tomato sauce (Yeomans et al., 1997) and has the same effect when added to animal feed (Villalba and Provenza, 1997). In an interesting show of instinctive intelligence, 250 pregnant women reported aversion to meats, poultry, and sauces flavored with **oregano** (Hook, 1978).

- In an investigation of 60 plants, Dr. James Duke, author of *The Green Pharmacy* and one of the world's leading experts on medicinal plant chemicals, reported that **wild oregano** contained the highest levels of antioxidants (reported in Duke, 1997). It is especially high in vitamin E compounds, especially gamma-tocopherol (Lagouri and Boskou, 1996).

PEPPERMINT LEAF AND OIL

Latin: *Mentha piperita*   **Chinese:** Bo he *(M. haplocalyx)*   **Sanskrit:** Putani *(M. arvensis)*

WHAT IT DOES: Peppermint leaf is sweet, and **peppermint oil** is sweet and slightly pungent in taste. Both are aromatic and cooling in action. **Peppermint leaf** cools and soothes the throat, lungs, stomach, and mind. **Peppermint oil** reduces intestinal spasms internally and calms itching externally.

RATING: Silver

SAFETY ISSUES: None known

STARTING DOSAGE:

- Tea: 1 to 2 teaspoons of leaf per cup of water

- Enteric-coated oil capsule: 2 milliliters (mL) two times per day between meals

Herb Pharm makes an almost magical **peppermint** remedy called Grindelia-Sassafras compound that our patients love. It relieves the unbearable itch associated with poison oak, ivy, and sumac.

The wonderful aroma of **peppermint tea** comes from the release of soothing volatile oils into the air. The immediate pleasurable reaction everyone has to this scent speaks volumes about what this plant can do. It has a mild anesthetic action on the intestine, so it is useful for treating nausea, morning sickness, vomiting, and stomach pain, especially when combined with **ginger root**. It also exhibits a mild anti-inflammatory action and can be used with **honey** or **ginger** as a simple remedy for colds, fevers, and flu.

Peppermint tea is good for bad breath, and TCM doctors use similar mint species to treat sore throat, red eyes, headache, and cough. Because it has a soothing effect on the mind, it is also helpful in easing painful periods and lessening general anxiety.

Peppermint oil is prescribed specifically to treat irritable bowel syndrome (IBS), a problem which accounts for 50% of all visits to gastrointestinal doctors. Studies show **peppermint oil** directly relieves intestinal smooth muscle spasms and promotes rhythmic peristaltic movement, usually working within a few weeks. Before using the oil, make sure that you truly are suffering from intestinal spasms, and not a more serious inflammatory colitis.

Menthol crystals can be extracted from mint oils, which have a wonderful anesthetic action on the skin, due to a stimulation of the nerves that perceive coldness. You can apply a few drops of **peppermint oil** to a cloth and wipe down the body to cool down a fever.

PHELLODENDRON BARK

Latin: *Phellodendron amurense*   **Chinese:** Huang bai

WHAT IT DOES: Phellodendron bark is bitter in taste and cold in action. It reduces inflammation and dampness, especially from the lower parts of the body. It has broad-spectrum antibacterial and antiviral activity.

RATING: Yellow, due to limitations of use

SAFETY ISSUES: Do not use during pregnancy. Avoid long-term use due to alkaloid content.

STARTING DOSAGE:

- Dried powder: 3 to 10 grams per day
- 4:1 dried decoction: 1 to 3 grams per day

Huang means yellow in Chinese, and **phellodendron bark** is one of the "three huangs," or bright yellow plants used for treating inflammation and infection (the other two are **scute root** and **coptis rhizome).** The yellow color comes from an alkaloid called berberine, a substance that is slightly to mildly toxic in pure form, which is why it is not recommended for use in pregnancy. Berberine is also found in **goldenseal root** *(Hydrastis canadensis),* **Oregon grape root** *(Mahonia aquifolium)* and several other well-known herbs.

The clinical differentiation among these three yellow TCM plants serves as an excellent argument against concentrating on a single chemical or group of chemical compounds in a plant. TCM doctors tell us that **scute root** is most useful for treating inflammation in the lungs and upper respiratory tract, including allergies.

TCM doctors offer the insight that **phellodendron bark** can be used when there is weakness and nutrient deficiency present, while **coptis rhizome** should be avoided in such cases. In 1999, a member of the herbalists' Internet group in which I participate was suffering from a persistent lower leg inflammation. A formula containing **coptis rhizome** proved ineffective, so Nai-shing substituted **phellodendron bark,** which resolved the problem within a few weeks.

On the other hand, **coptis rhizome** is useful for treating upper body inflammation, but not allergy. Rather, it is most effective when there is strong heat in the heart and other organs, high fever, and sore throat.

Phellodendron bark is more appropriate for treating inflammation in the lower parts of the body and for heat caused by deficiency. For menopause, a deficiency condition, it can be used to control hot flashes. In the lower parts of the body it is used to control thick yellow vaginal discharges, hemorrhoids, foul-smelling diarrhea, and dysentery. It is also used to treat dampness and heat in the legs, such as red, swollen, and painful knees, legs, or feet.

Research Highlights

- Berberine comprises only about 0.6–2.5% of the plant's material, so researchers decided to study the rest of the plant without this compound. The berberine-free fraction of **phellodendron bark** exhibited antiulcer activity, anti-inflammatory properties, reduction of gastric acid secretion, and anti-cholera-toxin effects (Uchiyama et al., 1989).

- Chinese studies on **phellodendron bark** show a broad-spectrum antibiotic effect against organisms that cause diphtheria, dysentery, typhoid fever, staph infections, pneumonia, conjunctivitis, trachoma, and meningitis. It is often used in injectable form (reported in Huang, 1999; reported in Yeung, 1983).

- Others have shown action against various forms of candida, as well as viruses (Park et al., 1999).

- In tests examining eight different herbs, **phellodendron bark** proved to be the most potent suppressor of immune inflammation in animal graft-versus-host reactions (Mori et al., 1994). In a later study, the same researcher discovered that unlike cortisonelike drugs, **phellodendron bark** did not suppress antibody production (Mori et al., 1995).

- Studies also indicate a possible application in cataract prevention. A water extract of **phellodendron bark** and **aralia cortex** applied to the eye lenses of diabetic rats "dramatically" reduced high sorbitol levels as well as other cataract-causing chemicals (Lee et al., 1999).

- Many herbalists believe that berberine-containing herbs work only topically, not internally. Dr. Duke reports that there is increasing evidence of systemic antimicrobial effects (Brennan M, 2000).

PINELLIA TUBER

Latin: *Pinellia ternata*   **Chinese:** Fa ban xia

WHAT IT DOES: Pinellia tuber is pungent in taste and warming in action. It dries up and dissolves mucus in the lungs, stomach, and intestines and stops nausea and vomiting.

RATING: Yellow, due to limitations in use and potential minor toxicity

SAFETY ISSUES: Pinellia must be processed prior to use, to remove toxic elements. The traditional method is to cook it with ginger, vinegar, and/or alum. Do not use during pregnancy. Do not use long term. Do not use with bleeding disorders. Use only under the guidance of a trained professional.

STARTING DOSAGE:

- Dried powder (purified): 2 to 6 grams per day
- 4:1 dried decoction: 500–1,000 mg per day

Pinellia tuber is perhaps the strongest TCM herb for removing phlegm. We use it frequently at our clinic to treat coughs and upper respiratory infections with thick and tenacious phlegm. It is useful in the digestive system when there are signs of nausea, poor digestion, and overall sluggishness, with a thick white coating on the tongue.

It can also be used to stop chronic diarrhea due to poor digestion. It is almost always prescribed in formulas along with **tangerine peel** and/or **ginger root** to promote a more effective action (synergy).

A classic formula considerd the best one for mucus reduction anywhere in the lungs or digestive tract is called **two-cured decoction.** It consists of **pinellia tuber, tangerine peel, poria mushroom,** and **honey-fried licorice root**.

Research Highlights

- In animal experiments, taste stimulation by **pinellia tuber** caused suppression of gastric vagus nerve activity, while stimulation with **ginger root** caused an increase in nerve activity. The mixture of the two herbs had a neutral effect. This demonstrates the rationale behind traditional use of the two herbs together (Niijima et al., 1998).

- The reticuloendothelial system (RES) consists of phagocytic immune cells (those that eat foreign materials and particles). The RES exists primarily in the liver, and it helps attack cancer cells (Baas et al., 1994). In pharmacological studies of pinellian G, a complex sugar extracted from **pinellia tuber**, researchers recorded significant RES-stimulating activity and a reduction in inflammation (Tomoda et al., 1994). This may partially explain the herb's antiphlegm activity.

PORIA MUSHROOM

Latin: *Poria cocos*　　　**Chinese:** Fu ling

WHAT IT DOES: Poria mushroom, actually the sclerotium (hardened mass enveloping the mushroom), is bland and sweet in taste and neutral in action. It promotes fluid discharge and strengthens digestion.

RATING: Silver

SAFETY ISSUES: None known. Use cautiously in dehydrated patients.

STARTING DOSAGE:

- Dried powder: 6 to 18 grams per day
- 4:1 concentrated dried decoction: 1½ to 4½ grams per day

Poria mushroom is commonly used in TCM because it is a gentle and safe aid for removing stagnant fluids (dampness) from the digestive system. In our clinical practice, perhaps as many as 40% of our patients have impaired or sluggish digestion, and many of them cannot tolerate strong herbs at first. **Poria** is an excellent choice in these cases, as it safely improves digestion and can be used freely. It is also used for urinary difficulty and edema. Recently, studies have shown it to have immune system benefits similar to those of other medicinal mushrooms, though perhaps milder. The inner part of the sclerotium found near the root is called **poria spirit** (fu shen) and is used to calm anxiety.

Research Highlights

- Japanese scientists reported that **poria mushroom** stimulated various immune system chemicals (interleukins and tumor necrosis factor), while suppressing a growth factor (Yu et al., 1996).

- It has also been shown to slow tumor growth in mice (Kaminaga T et al., 1996) and to prevent pathological changes to the kidneys of mice with nephritis (Hattori et al., 1992).

- The saponins found in **poria mushroom** possess a calming effect on digestion that proved strong enough to prevent vomiting in frogs who were given an emetic agent (Tai T et al., 1995).

PRICKLY ASH BARK

Latin: *Xanthoxylum* species   **African:** Fagara/Yeah/Igi-ata
         Zanthoxylum species

WHAT IT DOES: Prickly ash bark is pungent in taste and hot in action. It stimulates the circulation and breaks up blood congestion.

RATING: Yellow, due to limitations in use

SAFETY ISSUES: Do not use during pregnancy or if taking blood-thinning medications. Use with caution if you have stomach or intestinal inflammation.

STARTING DOSAGE:

- Powder: 250–750 mg two to three times per day

- Decoction: 1 teaspoon of bark in 1 cup of water two to three times per day

- 1:5 tincture: 10–20 drops two to three times per day

  Note: Tincture is the preferred form due to ease of use.

Prickly ash bark stimulates the circulation, lymphatic system, and mucous membranes. It is effective in treating chilblains (constriction of small arteries), leg cramps, varicose veins, ulcers, and other problems resulting from blood congestion and cold. Various related species can be found around the world, but they contain different amounts and types of phytochemicals. In Nigeria, people use the root of **fagara** (related to prickly ash) as a chewing stick to aid in oral hygiene. And in Nigeria and Ghana, a decoction of the root bark is a common treatment for toothache pain, childbirth pain, and trauma and is also used as a general tonic.

Doctors in Nigeria use **fagara** *(F. zanthosyloides)* to reduce the painful crisis of the genetic disease sickle cell anemia. This herb has a variety of unusual properties that reduce platelet and blood cell sticking.

After reading the reports from Nigeria, I decided to try **fagara's** relative **prickly ash bark** for the same indication. I gave some to a young African-American girl in the first grade who constantly missed school and needed to be hospitalized three to four times per

In 1995 I wrote the following letter, which was printed in my local paper.

February 10, 1995
News Journal (Wilmington, DE)

To the editor:

This is in response to your article Tuesday Jan. 31, 1995 reporting on the use of the cancer drug hydroxyurea for reducing the crisis of sickle cell anemia in adults. The article is noteworthy not for what it says, which is quite accurate, but for what it omits. For instance, it omits the fact that this treatment is currently not recommended for children due to its severe side effects. According to the PDR, it requires close physician supervision (weekly blood tests), because it "causes bone marrow depression, leukopenia, anemia, . . . affects DNA synthesis . . . may be mutagenic," and is a "known teratogenic agent in animals." This risk is balanced against a 50% reduction in sickle cell crisis episodes. It might be interesting to ponder why our scientists have not heard of the fagara chewing stick *(Zanthoxylum* ssp.), a widespread plant species found in the forest savanna mosaic of the lowland rain forest in west tropical Africa. It has been reported since as early as 1975 that "the root extract and the aromatic acids have been shown to significantly reduce the painful crisis of sickle-cell patients." In fact, the crude extract is currently dispensed by the Nigerian health service for the management of sickle cell anemia. Far from having side effects, it is used freely in Africa as a chewing stick to prevent tooth decay, a tea for pain during childbirth, and as a tonic for general body weakness. It is considered quite safe for use by children.

Sincerely,

Alan Tillotson

year due to the painful sickle cell crisis. I gave her about 25 drops three times a day. She immediately stopped having serious problems, her thinking was no longer fuzzy, the frequency of her attacks went down to about one per year, and the severity of the attacks decreased appreciably. She has blossomed into a beautiful junior high school student, the sickle cell disease now only a bit-player in the background of her life.

Another of my patients had lived with the disease his entire life, with almost constant pain and bimonthly crises. I gave him 35 drops three times per day, and he immediately improved in the same way as the young girl. This improvement in both frequency of attacks and level of pain has persisted in three of my long-term patients over many years. The wholesale cost of this medicine is less than $20 per month at full dosage. My biggest fear is that this knowledge will be co-opted by a pharmaceutical company and made available to the many suffering children only at an exorbitant cost.

Research Highlights

- We do not know the full extent or the cause of the antisickling activity of **prickly ash, fagara** and other *Zanthoxylum* species plants. Researchers have identified several types of coumarins (blood-thinning chemicals) (Chen et al., 1995), as well as various alkaloids that reduce platelet sticking (Sheen et al., 1996; Ko et al., 1990).

- Among the agents known to possess antisickling inhibitory activity at low concentrations are the aqueous extract of the roots of *Zanthoxylum xanthoxyloides* (antisickling ether fraction), vanillic acid, parahydroxybenzoic acid, and paraflurobenzoic acid (Osoba et al., 1989).

- In vitro testing of 43 African plants traditionally used to treat malaria have shown strong antimalarial action in 4 of the plants, including the *Zanthoxylum chalybeum* species of **prickly ash.** The other plants that demonstrated this action against malaria were *Cissampelos mucronata, Maytenus senegalensis,* and *Salacia madagascariensis* (Gessler et al., 1994).

RASPBERRY/BLACKBERRY

Latin: *Rubus* species   **Chinese:** Fu pen zi

WHAT IT DOES: Raspberry and its relative, **blackberry,** are gentle astringents and blood-nourishing tonics that are good for the immune system and the eyes.

RATING: Yellow

> If you think of vitamin C as Pavarotti (the opera singer), then flavonoids act like the supporting orchestra. The big guy sounds great by himself, but he's even better with a good orchestra in the background.

SAFETY ISSUES: Do not use in high dosage with restricted urination.

STARTING DOSAGE:

- Fresh or frozen whole berry: for therapeutic benefit, eat 1 to 2 pounds per week.

Berries are my favorite fruits. They are low in calories and high in colorful flavonoid nutrients. Flavonoids aid in the body's absorption and utilization of vitamin C, which is synthesized from plant and yeast sugars.

Modern scientists now agree that chemical waste products (secondary metabolites) produced by plants, including plant pigments, can act as protective agents which can repel insect herbivores through a variety of mechanisms.

TAM doctors, however, knew of the benefits of fruit and plant pigments long ago. More than 24 years ago, my Ayurvedic teacher told me that colorful or strong-smelling plant waste products would neutralize poisons in animals. That is, eating colorful fruits and herbs would neutralize poisons found in human blood and tissues. We now know that flavonoid pigments increase blood vessel integrity and have antiviral, antimicrobial, antiallergy, and even liver-protective effects. In addition to their benefit to immune function (as potent antioxidants), they also improve capillary and cerebral blood flow, reduce platelet aggregation (blood stickiness), and affect cholesterol, histamine, and prostaglandin metabolism. All of these actions make them especially valuable for the heart and blood vessels.

The astringency of **raspberries** and **blackberries** (caused by their condensed tannins) explains their traditional use for treating bedwetting and simple diarrhea. The Chinese tell us that their **raspberry** (fu pen zi) is very effective for this. These berries protect inflamed mucous membranes, reduce excess secretions, and inhibit viruses and other pathogens. Though not quite as high in tannin concentration as **green tea** or **oak bark, raspberries** and **blackberries** are usually much more enjoyable for both children and adults.

> You can purchase frozen berries and process them in a blender. Taste the unsweetened juice and you will realize how little natural sugar **raspberries** actually contain—about 75% less than strawberries. Simply add some **stevia leaf** for sweetness, and you have a delicious low-calorie fruit juice that is safe and helps inhibit microbes. This juice is also good for diabetics and people trying to lose weight.

When treating chronic intestinal infections (including yeast infections) it is beneficial to restrict all simple sugars, including fruit sugars. The only exceptions are **blackberries** and **raspberries,** due to their low sugar and high tannin content.

Phytonutrients called "furanones" are important natural flavoring and aroma agents found in **raspberries, strawberries, pineapples, tomatoes,** and some other foods. The colors and aromas act to attract animals (and people) to the fruits, ensuring seed dispersal via defecation at a new location. In addition, they have been found to be very effective anticancer components of the animal diet, protecting against carcinogenic chemicals. Researchers have identified two food-derived furanones that exhibit antioxidant activity comparable to that of vitamin C. They are also sometimes mutagenic (destructive) to bacteria (Colin-Slaughter, 1999).

Raspberry leaf tea is well known for its ability to facilitate childbirth by relaxing the uterus, ligaments, and tendons. It should be consumed freely (several cups per day) beginning about 4 to 6 weeks before delivery. A kennel owner once told me that ever since she started using it with pregnant dogs, the pups just "popped out."

RAUWOLFIA ROOT

Latin: *Rauwolfia serpentina*   **Sanskrit:** Sarpagandha
African: Numerous *(R. vomitoria* species)   **Chinese:** Lu fu mu (various species)
English: Rauwolfia / Indian snake root

WHAT IT DOES: Rauwolfia root is bitter in taste and cooling in action. It lowers blood pressure, tranquilizes the mind, and promotes sleep.

RATING: Red, due to safety issues

SAFETY ISSUES: Use only under the guidance of a trained physician or herbalist in proper dosage. Do not use in pregnancy, breast-feeding, or depression. May exacerbate symptoms of Parkinson's disease. Do not combine with alcohol, barbiturates (Pfeifer et al., 1976), SSRIs, or blood-pressure-lowering agents such as beta-blockers, unless under guidance.

STARTING DOSAGE:

- Tincture (standardized to 1.0% weight/volume total alkaloids): 2 to 12 drops three times per day

Rauwolfia is a reliable blood-pressure-lowering and tranquilizing agent when used properly. It is used in traditional medicine in India, China, Africa, and many other countries. In India and Nepal, it is a common treatment for hypertension and insomnia. Gandhi took it frequently at night for its calming actions. It warrants a red rating because of its ability to cause severe reactions in overdose, including trembling and collapse.

Reserpine, the chief alkaloid in **rauwolfia root,** seems to be the component responsible for its blood-pressure-lowering activity. Doctors began using reserpine-based hypertension medicines in the 1950s, but they went out of favor because of the side effects, chiefly depression. Consequently, **rauwolfia** can be acquired only from a licensed health care professional.

During the scientific controversy in the 1950s surrounding the question of whether reserpine by itself was superior to the whole **rauwolfia root,** an Indian physician named Dr. Vakil reviewed all 151 studies available at the time. He came to the conclusion that the combined action of the whole root improves tolerance and reduces the risk of side effects that occur with the use of isolated alkaloids.

In collaboration with Western doctors, I have used a **rauwolfia tincture** safely to treat dozens of patients with mild to moderate hypertension. We combine 30–50% of a standardized whole root tincture with other mild herbal tinctures known to lower blood pressure, such as **linden flowers** and **mistletoe**. In mild cases, we start with two drops three times per day and perform regular blood pressure checks, instructing the patient to increase the dosage until the blood pressure normalizes or they reach the limit in dosage. Patients marvel at how effectively they can control their pressure drop by drop and control the dosage to manage day-to-day variations. We stop dosing at well below the levels where side effects usually develop. If it does not sufficiently lower the patient's pressure, the doctors will prescribe mild Western medication at a lower-than-normal dosage. This combination treatment will often work.

Rauwolfia root is not curative. Following traditional Ayurvedic procedure, once we have controlled the blood pressure we employ other herbal agents, especially **hawthorn,** and lifestyle changes to resolve the underlying problem.

Research Highlights

- The mechanism of action of **rauwolfia root** differs from most other blood-pressure-lowering agents, acting on the central nervous system. This may explain why it works when other medicines fail (Weiss, 1988; Shibuya and Sato, 1985).

- In doses higher than those used for hypertension, **rauwolfia alkaloids** cause a depletion of norepinephrine, resulting in a tranquilizing effect. Very high doses can cause a loss of coordination (reported in Huang, 1999).

- Many patients who take medication to control hypertension still have problems with balance, due to difficulties in circulatory regulation. Upon examination of blood-pressure-lowering agents available up to 1980, researchers discovered that only **rauwolfia** alkaloids and clonidin do not have an undesirable influence on balance (Teichmann and Vogel, 1980).

- In a Chinese study on 200 patients with moderate hypertension, **rauwolfia alkaloids** lowered blood pressure by as much as 30–40% with minimal side effects (reported in Huang, 1999).

- **Rauwolfia root** has proven highly effective (89%) in cases of chronic hives (reported in Huang, 1999).

- The pharmacological effects of resperpine were formerly cause for concern that it might promote breast cancer. However, in epidemiological studies, **rauwolfia alkaloids** did not increase the risk of breast cancer (Shapiro et al., 1984; von Poser et al., 1990).

- **Rauwolfia root** has occasionally proven effective in cases of malnutrition that were unresponsive to high-protein or high-energy diets (reported in Huang, 1999).

RED CLOVER BLOSSOM

Latin: *Trifolium pratense*

WHAT IT DOES: Red clover blossom is sweet and slightly salty in taste and cooling in action. It thins, cools, nourishes, and detoxifies the blood and reduces respiratory irritability.

RATING: Yellow

SAFETY ISSUES: Do not use during pregnancy. Use cautiously with blood-thinning pharmaceuticals.

STARTING DOSAGE:

- Tincture (dried 1:5): 10–30 drops two to six times per day

Red clover blossoms can be used as part of a safe treatment for chronic skin problems such as eczema, eruptions, and psoriasis. In our clinic, we have sometimes found that addition of this gentle herb to our treatment protocol for childhood eczema can improve results in difficult cases. Perhaps the mild blood-thinning chemicals (coumarins) and the herb's hormonelike nourishing qualities improve microcirculation and bring more moisture and nutrition to the skin cells.

It also exhibits mild antibacterial activity against gram-positive organisms and was used by early physicians for dry, irritable, or spasmodic cough, including whooping cough. They also reported that it retarded cancers.

Red clover contains a broader spectrum of beneficial plant estrogens (isoflavones including genistein, daidzein, biochanin, and formononetin) than the more commonly used **soybean extracts**. This may account for its usefulness in reducing hot flashes and maintaining bone health after menopause, and may also explain its repuation as a cancer fighter.

> Much of the **red clover** found in capsule form or as dried blossoms is brown and basically inert. During harvesting, wildcrafters must collect it with plastic gloves to avoid contamination, then carefully dry it to keep its deep colors intact. Therefore, I use it only in tincture form from companies like Herbalist & Alchemist or Herb Pharm.

It is important to note that the use of phytoestrogens in herbal therapy should be guided by the philosophy of treating the whole person. For example, we often use liver herbs such as **dandelion root** *(Taraxacum officinale),* **burdock root** *(Arctium lappa),* and **white peony root** *(Paeonia lactiflora)* to improve the liver's conjugation of estrogenic compounds to enhance their elimination from the body.

Research Highlights

- A recent randomized controlled trial indicated that **red clover** helps maintain the elasticity of large arteries such as the thoracic aorta, reducing cardiac risk (Nestel et al., 1999).

- Of the 150 herbs and spices tested for estrogen and progesterone activity, only **red clover, thyme,** and **turmeric** were found to exhibit high levels of both (Zava et al., 1998). This indicates that the herbs are more beneficial (balanced) than herbs that exhibit only estrogenic activity, as progesterone deficiency is as much a problem for menopausal women as estrogen deficiency.

REHMANNIA ROOT

Latin: *Rehmannia glutinosa*   **Chinese:** Shu di huang (cooked)   **English:** Chinese foxglove
Sheng di huang (raw)

WHAT IT DOES: Rehmannia root strengthens and nourishes the blood and Yin, reduces inflammation, and strengthens the kidneys.

RATING: Gold

SAFETY ISSUES: Do not use with indigestion, poor appetite, or diarrhea.

STARTING DOSAGE:

- Dried powder: 9–30 grams per day

- 4:1 dried decoction: 3 to 9 grams per day

In the thick black roots of **rehmannia,** TCM doctors see a strong reservoir of nutrients beneficial to the kidneys and blood and capable of removing heat and inflammation. The cooked form of **rehmannia** is sweet in taste and warm in action, while the raw form is sweet and bitter in taste and cold in action. The raw form, being cold in action, is used more frequently to remove inflammation. Conversely, when you cure the root by cooking it with wine it becomes more nourishing and warm in action. Both forms are used in the treatment of deficiency diseases where the presence of heat (look for a red tongue) causes symptoms such as fever, menopausal hot flashes, and thirst. **Rehmannia** can be used when there is a need to generate fluids—especially with the weakness that results from prolonged low-grade fevers.

Rehmannia root is very thick and gummy, so it can impair digestion, which explains the contraindications listed above. It is one of the base herbs included in the highly valued **six-flavored rehmannia pill** (liu wei di huang wan), also called **rehmannia six formula,** used as a primary treatment for Yin deficiency. Scientific studies have shown a number of interesting actions of this herb.

We use **rehmannia root** in our clinic routinely to treat problems related with Yin deficiency, such as fatigue with heat signs, irritability, and low-grade fevers. Herbs useful for Yin deficiency are those that increase the body's ability to absorb or use nutrients necessary for protection, regeneration, and repair. For the treatment of nephritis, we often combine **rehmannia root** with **astragalus root, shilajatu,** and **triphala. Rehmannia root** is also very useful in treating autoimmune diseases in general.

Research Highlights

- Its anti-inflammatory action has been shown in animal models to reduce inflammation in the central nervous system by affecting astrocytes—CNS immune cells (Kim et al., 1999).

- **Rehmannia-** and **astragalus-root-**based formulas may also help reduce nephritis and its complications. In one study of 100 patients, researchers reported that their formula "was markedly effective for proteinuria, hematuria, improvement and recovery of renal functions, edema, anemia, anorexia, etc. in comparison with the control group" (Su et al., 1993).

- **Rehmannia six formula** has been shown effective for protecting white and red blood cells, as well as heart, liver, and kidney function during chemotherapy (Xu, 1992).

- One interesting study done on guinea pigs showed an ability to protect against chemical-induced deafness, verified by scanning electron microscope of the inner ear (Zhuang et al., 1992).

- In one study performed in China, when Yin-deficient animals were pretreated with **Rehmannia six formula,** they sustained less damage to their periodontal tissues from outside trauma than nontreated animals (Cai et al., 1990).

REISHI MUSHROOM

Latin: *Ganoderma lucidum*   **Chinese:** Ling zhi   **English:** Spirit plant

WHAT IT DOES: The fruiting body of **reishi mushroom** is sweet in taste and neutral to slightly warming in action. It calms the spirit; strengthens immunity; slows aging; strengthens the heart, lungs, and liver; and relaxes spasms.

RATING: Gold

SAFETY ISSUES: None known

STARTING DOSAGE:

- Syrup: 4 to 6 milliliters (mL) per day
- 1:5 tincture: 10 mL three times per day
- Concentrated 5:1 tablet: 500 mg two to three times per day
- Dried powder: 3 to 15 grams per day

The once extremely rare and precious **reishi mushroom** is now cultivated and widely available. It is a very potent immune system and longevity tonic. Traditionally used to "nourish the heart and pacify the spirit," it has also been found to have numerous other health benefits.

At our clinic we use several mushrooms to strengthen the immune system to prevent and treat cancer, including the **royal agaricus mushroom** and **chaga mushroom**. Each mushroom has its own unique energy that gives us clues about when to use it clinically. **Reishi** is the most calming of the medicinal mushrooms, so I use it when there is immune deficiency with signs of nerve (Vata) weakness. It can also be used in formulas for insomnia and general nervousness. According to medicinal mushroom expert Terry Willard, Ph.D., it combines well with **maitake mushroom**.

Reishi calms the central nervous system, exerting a blood-pressure-lowering effect beneficial to the heart. It is now employed in China for treatment of autoimmune diseases and to calm hypersensitivity. Like many other medicinal mushrooms, **reishi mushroom** can be used to treat cancer patients due to its ability to activate NK cells, macrophages, T-lymphocytes, and cytokines, all important immune system components. Kee Chang Huang reports that **reishi** "exerts a synergistic effect with other anticancer chemotherapeutic agents or radiotherapy, to augment the clinical therapeutic effect in the treatment of cancer patients."

Research Highlights

- **Reishi** has been shown in several studies to lower cholesterol levels, helping to prevent atherosclerotic changes in the blood vessel walls (reported in Huang, 1999).

- Clinical studies on over 2,000 patients in China have shown a very high (60–90%) effectiveness in the treatment of chronic bronchitis (reported in Huang, 1999; Tasaka et al., 1988).

RHUBARB ROOT

Latin: *Rheum palmatum*   **Sanskrit:** Amlavetasa   **Chinese:** Da huang
R. officinale
R. species

WHAT IT DOES: Rhubarb root is sour and bitter in taste and cooling in action. It is a stimulant laxative that drains inflammation from the liver, large intestine, and kidney.

RATING: Yellow, due to problems with long-term usage

SAFETY ISSUES: Do not use during pregnancy or nursing. Do not use with bowel obstruction or gout. Do not use in cases of severe deficiency. Do not use long term. Use only under supervision with inflammatory bowel disease. Long-term use can cause hypertrophy of the liver, thyroid, and stomach, as well as nausea, griping, abdominal pain, vomiting, and diarrhea. Short-term or occasional use is safe in appropriate dosage unless otherwise contraindicated.

STARTING DOSAGE:

- Dried powder: 1 to 6 grams per day, usually taken at night

- 4:1 dried decoction extract: 1 to 3 grams per day, at night

- 1:5 tincture: 20–80 drops once per day, at night

In spite of the contraindications (which are common to most laxatives), **rhubarb root** is still my favorite of the readily available laxatives. Of course with simple constipation, it is always better to try basic remedies first, like increasing dietary fiber and fluid intake. TCM doctors use **rhubarb root** to treat constipation, high fever, abdominal distension, gallstones, jaundice, and, surprisingly, acute dysentery, due to the herb's antibacterial activity. They stir-fry **rhubarb root** with wine to reduce the laxative effect when it is used for diseases other than constipation. TAM doctors use it in formulas to treat cirrhosis of the liver, alcoholism, neurasthenia, and asthma. Recent experimental discoveries offer important evidence of **rhubarb's** effect on kidney failure.

The major concern with herbs containing "anthraquinones"—natural laxative chemicals such as emodin and sennidin—is that long-term use can lead to dependence.

Anthraquinones stimulate peristalsis approximately 6–8 hours after ingestion. The effects on the gut are largely topical, and the substances flush out of the system without being absorbed. It seems that **rhubarb root** has an advantage over other laxatives like the more powerful **senna** and **cascara sagrada.** Its higher tannin levels tend to tighten the bowel after 14–18 hours, somewhat limiting the possibility of the flaccid condition that can re-

> **Glyconda,** a formulation of pharmacist John Uri Lloyd, was one of the most famous of the Eclectic remedies. He combined glycerin, a nonsugar sweetening agent, with **rhubarb root, goldenseal,** and **cinnamon bark,** occasionally adding **ginger root** and **peppermint oil**. He adjusted the amount of **rhubarb** to make sure it would not purge, and the amount of **goldenseal** to make sure it was not too bitter. When made properly, it had a pleasant sweet taste, agreeable even to most children. Doctors administered it by the teaspoon or tablespoon to clear the stomach and intestine of "fermentive and irritative conditions."

sult from laxative overuse. In fact, the tannins are the reason that small doses of **rhubarb** (.03 to .3 gram) can actually cause constipation.

In our clinic, we treat constipation with lifestyle changes and supportive formulas containing small amounts of **rhubarb root** mixed with other herbs that strengthen the digestion, improve liver function, and lubricate the bowel. The **rhubarb** dosage can be reduced with improvements in bowel and liver health.

Research Highlights

- In a 3-month clinical trial, alcohol extracts of **rhubarb** made into tablets reduced obesity complicated with hypertension, menstrual irregularities, and elevated blood lipids (Chen, 1995).

- Test tube studies of emodin, an active component of **rhubarb root,** demonstrated inhibition of *Trichomonas vaginalis* (Wang, 1993).

- Oral administration of emodin cured intravaginal infections in mice (Wang, 1993).

- A 10-year controlled clinical double-blind trial at the Xiang Shan TCM Hospital in Shanghai tracked all patients using three types of alcohol-extracted **rhubarb** tablets to treat chronic upper digestive bleeding. All three types were shown to stop bleeding within 56 hours at an effectiveness rate greater than 90% (Zhou and Jiao, 1990).

- Researcher Deng Wenlong, of the Sichuan Provincial Institute of Chinese Materia Medica, presented a paper at Chengdu University of TCM in China explaining **rhubarb's** traditional reputation for treating fevers and inflammatory diseases. He began by describing endotoxins, chemicals that are released into the host as a result of the breakdown of the cell walls of gram-negative bacteria. He demonstrated that endotoxin content in the blood increased greatly in the presence of severe stress, inflammation, or infection and that the bowel was the greatest repository of endotoxin. With the use of **rhubarb** (and other herbs) to remove endotoxin from the bowel, animals infected with a variety of febrile diseases experienced faster resolution (Deng, 1994).

- A controlled randomized clinical trial on rats evaluated the effects of **rhubarb extract** on uremia—the collection of nitrogenous wastes in the blood due to kidney diseases. The uremia symptoms decreased and other blood markers improved, prompting the researchers to conclude, "both the in vivo and in vitro studies have proved the effectiveness of **rhubarb** in preventing the progression of chronic renal failure" (Li and Liu, 1991).

- A randomized controlled clinical trial examined the effect of **rhubarb extract** on patients with terminal end-stage kidney failure. Blood tests showed a decrease in negative blood markers and an improvement in positive blood markers (albumin, lipoprotein, apolipoproteins) in the test group subjects (Ji et al., 1993).

- According to animal studies, the beneficial effect of **rhubarb extract** is dose dependent and due partially to suppression of swelling in kidney tubular cells (Zheng, 1993). In a study on diabetic rats with nephropathy, **rhubarb extract** stopped the swelling (renal hypertrophy) at an early stage, and so may be useful in the early stages of human diabetic kidney disease (Yang and Li, 1993).

SALVIA ROOT

Latin: *Salvia miltiorrhiza*   **Chinese:** Dan shen   **English:** Asian red sage

WHAT IT DOES: Salvia root is bitter in taste and slightly cold in action. It promotes blood circulation while reducing inflammation.

RATING: Gold

SAFETY ISSUES: Should not be used while taking anticoagulant medications such as warfarin unless under the direction of a qualified health care practitioner. Bleeding may result. Do not use internally in tincture form.

STARTING DOSAGE:

- Crude herb: 3 to 15 grams per day

- Concentrated 4:1 dried decoction: 1 to 4 grams per day

TCM doctors use **salvia root** to invigorate and move the blood. In animal experiments it has been shown to increase coronary blood flow, lower blood pressure slightly, improve microcirculation, and mitigate injury and accelerate recovery from ischemic attack (stroke). Human experiments illustrate numerous circulation benefits, including dilation of the coronary arteries and increased capillary action. Because it has a strong cooling action,

> According to TCM theory, herbs that increase circulation to the roots of the hair can prevent hair loss and slow the graying process. The related **garden sage** *(Salvia officinalis)* has been used for the same purpose. An African-American dockworker once told me his grandfather had a great head of hair into his 90s, which he attributed to the use of sage tea to "keep the water off the brain."

salvia has a distinct advantage in certain medical conditions over warming herbs such as **prickly ash bark**. It is especially useful in coronary artery disease, where there is almost always a combination of inflammation and blockage. It is the most commonly used "blood-moving" herb in our clinic. A popular **salvia**-based formula in China called Tanshinone IIA is used frequently to treat various cardiovascular problems. A similar formula is available in the U.S.A. from a company called ITM.

Research Highlights

- In one experiment, 81% of patients with coronary artery disease (CAD) who were given a **salvia**-based formula reported benefits, while 57% experienced normalization of EEG (reported in Dharmananda, 1994).

- A controlled trial of patients who had developed adhesive intestinal obstruction (a common post-surgery complication) was done by giving them an injection of **salvia**

root extract before closing the abdominal cavity. The patients were then given an oral blood-moving formula and were followed for 2 to 9 years. They demonstrated a 100% effectiveness rate, with no adhesions developing, while more than one-quarter of the control group patients (given antibiotics) experienced continued problems (Wang et al., 1994).

- A series of four animal experiments done in Italy showed that **salvia root extract** reduced alcohol absorption from the gastrointestinal tract, reduced alcohol craving, reduced blood alcohol levels, and even affected the animal's ability to discriminate between alcohol and water. Researchers concluded that the use of **salvia**like medicines "may constitute a novel strategy for controlling excessive alcohol consumption in human alcoholics" (Colombo et al., 1999).

- **Salvia root** has been shown to inhibit fibrosis (formation of scar tissue) in animal wound-healing models (Liu M et al., 1998), while similar protective effects were found against chemically induced liver fibrosis in rats. In fact, histological examination showed that **salvia** could actually reverse the fibrosis (Wasser et al., 1998). These studies demonstrate that **salvia root** shows promise in prevention and treatment of cirrhosis of the liver.

- **Salvia root** has also been indicated in the prevention of memory and learning deficits caused by aging in animal models (Nomura et al., 1997).

- Restenosis (arterial blockage) occurring after angioplasty is a major surgical problem. In a study of air-injured carotid arteries in rats, the **salvia**-treated group experienced less thickening of the arteries. These results indicate that **salvia root** may be used to prevent arterial restenosis after angioplasty (Zhou et al., 1996).

- There is even evidence that **salvia root** may protect against structural damage to the optic nerve in cases of ocular stress and induced intraocular hypertension. In a glaucoma study on rabbits, researchers concluded that the protective effect of **salvia root** was due to improved microcirculation in the retinal ganglion cells and the optic nerve (Zhu et al., 1993).

SARSAPARILLA ROOT

Latin: *Smilax* species   **Chinese:** Tu fu ling

WHAT IT DOES: Sarsaparilla root is sweet and bland in taste and neutral in action. It removes toxins from the bowel and reduces inflammation and dampness from the blood, liver, urinary system, and skin.

RATING: Yellow, due to limitations in usage

SAFETY ISSUES: None known

STARTING DOSAGE:

- Dried root: 3 to 12 grams per day

- 4:1 dried decoction: 1 to 4 grams per day

- 1:5 tincture: 2 to 4 milliliters (mL) in water or juice three times per day

Sarsaparilla root has been famous in the West since 1574, when a French physician described its use in treating syphilis. Various *Smilax* species are used to treat infections and inflammation—especially those affecting the skin and intestines—in many countries including India, China, Europe, the United States, Brazil, Guatemala, and Saudi Arabia. Because of the historical use for syphilis, many herbalists now use **sarsaparilla root** for Lyme disease, also caused by a spirochete organism.

Naturopaths believe that **sarsaparilla root** binds and removes endotoxin from the bowel, perhaps by stimulating liver clearance. I have found **sarsaparilla root** to be very useful in treating various skin diseases, especially psoriasis. Interestingly, psoriasis has been linked with higher circulating levels of endotoxin. When the patient shows serious signs of toxicity—greasy yellow tongue, rapid pulse—I sometimes start with a laxative (which also removes endotoxin) for a few days, then follow with pure **sarsaparilla** powder for a week or so. I usually follow this with a longer-term formula designed to restore balance to the whole system. I find it difficult to completely eradicate psoriasis, but we have helped several patients achieve semiremission for several years.

Research Highlights

- In 1942, the *New England Journal of Medicine* published a controlled study showing that an endotoxin-binding saponin extract of **sarsaparilla** was effective in reducing psoriasis symptoms (Thurman, 1942; reported in Murray and Pizzorno, 1989).

- Clinical tests in China demonstrated that the Chinese species called **tu fu ling rhizome** *(Smilax glabra)* is effective for treating syphilis in about 90% of acute cases and 50% of chronic cases (Bensky and Gamble, 1986). Since Lyme disease is also caused by spirochete organisms, it may prove beneficial in the treatment of this disease as well. TCM doctors use **tu fu ling rhizome** to treat joint pain, turbid urine, and jaundice caused by heat and dampness.

- Deng (1994) tells us that endotoxin—chemicals released into the host after breakdown of the cell walls of gram-negative organisms—accords closely with the idea of "pathogenic toxins" in TCM. His studies have shown that the removal of endotoxin helps control many inflammatory and febrile diseases.

SCHISANDRA BERRY

Latin: *Schisandra chinensis*   **Chinese:** Wu wei zi   **English:** Five-flavored fruit

WHAT IT DOES: Schisandra berry is sour in taste, astringent, and warming. It calms the mind and nerves, nourishes the Yin, generates fluids, strengthens general vitality, and tonifies and protects the heart, liver, and lungs.

RATING: Gold

SAFETY ISSUES: Use with caution if pregnant. Avoid if you have elevated intracranial pressure or epilepsy. May increase stomach acidity. May potentiate barbituates.

STARTING DOSAGE:

- Dried powder: 3 to 9 grams per day

- 4:1 dried decoction: 1 to 3 grams per day

- 1:4 tincture (dried berries, soaked overnight before preparation): 25–35 drops three times per day

Note: For treatment of hepatitis, administer 3 grams three times per day.

Schisandra berry is one of my first choices in the treatment of neurasthenia, along with **milky oat seed** tincture, **skullcap tincture,** and **ashwagandha root**. Neurasthenia—nerve weakness, fatigue, and pallor—is a condition that has reemerged as a synonym for chronic fatigue or other stress-related disorders. Historically, TCM doctors have always considered this fruit to be a superior medicine, able to prolong life. One reason for its reputation is that it contains five tastes. Interestingly, Ayurvedic herbs that are said to contain multiple tastes—**haritaki fruit, vibhitaki fruit,** and **amla fruit**—are also revered as life-prolonging (rasayana) tonics.

Medicinally TCM doctors use the tonic and astringent actions of **schisandra berries** to treat chronic cough and wheezing due to lung deficiency, as well as for chronic diarrhea. They are also used to quiet the spirit and calm the heart and to treat irritability, palpitations, night sweats, disturbed dreams, and insomnia. The modern Chinese understanding states that these clinical effects result from an amphoteric (balancing) effect on the sympathetic and parasympathetic nervous systems. The way I understand it, **schisandra berries** stabilize the nervous system.

Schisandra berry is one of the three ingredients in "Generate the Pulse" powder, along with **ginseng root** and **ophiopogon root,** routinely used in Japanese and Chinese hospitals to treat coronary artery disease. Animal studies have shown it effective to protect against and to treat cerebral ischemia (stroke or blockage of blood flow to the brain). None of the three individual herbs was able to prevent damage when administered alone, an impressive demonstration of herbal synergy.

Research Highlights

- Pharmacological studies have demonstrated the liver-protective effects of **schisandra berry extracts.** Rat livers were "remarkably" protected by an extract of **schisandra berries** against deadly poisons (Mizoguchi et al., 1991).

- Male mice that received diets containing 5% **schisandra berries** exhibited a threefold increase in the important liver cytochrome P-450 antioxidant system (Hendrich et al., 1983). Equally important is the enhancing effect of **schisandra** on the status of liver mitochondria in rats (Ip et al., 1998).

- **Schisandra berries** were shown to lower elevated liver enzyme levels in patients with chronic viral hepatitis (Chang and But, 1986; Liu et al., 1982).

- **Schisandra berries** have been shown to promote heightened learning ability in animals and increased antidepressant effects and endurance in humans (reported in Bone, 1996).

- The combination of **ginseng root** and **schisandra berries** reportedly improves memory (reported in Huang, 1999).

- Human clinical studies have shown anti-inflammatory actions of **schisandra seed powder** (reported in Upton, 1999).

- Human studies in Russia indicate that **schisandra** has an adaptogenic activity, prompting telegraph operators to transmit messages more accurately, increasing recovery after exercise, and improving blood levels of nitric oxide after heavy exercise. It was also shown to promote recuperation in racehorses after exercise (reported in Upton, 1999).

SKULLCAP

Latin: *Scutellaria lateriflora*

WHAT IT DOES: Skullcap is bitter in taste and cooling in action. It calms the nerves.

RATING: Silver, as not everyone needs to be calmed

SAFETY ISSUES: None known

STARTING DOSAGE:

- 1:2 tincture (fresh plant): 20–40 drops, two to six times per day

Note: Use only in tincture form.

Skullcap tincture is an excellent and reliable nervine. It relaxes and strengthens the nervous system in a manner that can be felt within 30 minutes. It is reliable and safe for treating premenstrual syndrome (PMS) symptoms as they occur. The highly respected English herbalist David Hoffman tells the story of how he found **skullcap** the best remedy for PMS when he lived on a commune as the only male with dozens of women. It is strong enough to calm anxiety in fairly serious situations, such as alcohol or drug withdrawal and hysteria. In these cases it needs to be taken every 2 to 3 hours, increasing the dosage until you see results. Based upon a recommendation from herbalist David Winston, I gave **skullcap tincture** to a patient with Parkinson's disease, and she experienced a moderate reduction of tremors, improving her quality of life.

Herbalist David Winston suggests using 60–120 drops four times per day to help control the tremors associated with Parkinson's disease.

According to *King's American Dispensatory,* **skullcap** "is tonic, nervine, and antispasmodic," and "it has proved especially useful in chorea, convulsions, tremors, intermittent fever, neuralgia, and many nervous affections. In all cases of nervous excitability, restlessness, or wakefulness, attending or following acute or chronic disease, from physical or mental overwork, or from other causes, it may be drunk freely with every expectation of beneficial results. When its soothing effects have ceased, it does not leave an excitable, irritable condition of the system, as is the case with some other nervines" (Felter and Lloyd, 1898).

Dried **skullcap**, commonly found in over-the-counter herbal preparations, is basically inert and therefore useless. The related Chinese herb **scute root** is more anti-inflammatory and less calming in action.

SCUTE ROOT

Latin: *Scutellaria baicalensis*　　**Chinese:** Huang qin

WHAT IT DOES: Scute root is bitter in taste and cold in action. It drains heat and inflammation from the liver, lungs, blood, and intestines. It also reduces allergy symptoms.

RATING: Yellow, due to limitations in usage

SAFETY ISSUES: Not to be used as a general tonic. Use for the indications listed below.

STARTING DOSAGE:

- Dried powder: 3 to 10 grams per day

- Concentrated dried decoction extract: 1 to 4 grams per day

Scute root is a broad-spectrum, antimicrobial, antipyretic, and anti-inflammatory herb that is especially useful for treating lung infections. It is used for treating high fever, flu, pneumonia, and the accompanying irritability, thirst, cough, and mucus. It also acts on the digestive system, easing diarrhea and dysenterylike disorders. TCM doctors use it in formulas for treating chronic allergy and inflammation. In mild doses, about 10% of a formula, it can be used safely over a long period of time.

Scute root contains a yellow flavone called "baicalein." Its structure is very similar to that of quercetin, a bioflavonoid frequently used by naturopathic physicians to treat allergy. **Scute root** is very reliable, and we use it more frequently in our office than perhaps any other anti-inflammatory. I find it an especially effective treatment for asthma and digestive system inflammation.

Research Highlights

- According to numerous in vitro and animal studies, the flavonoids in **scute root** possess arteriosclerosis-preventative and chemoprotective actions (Gao et al., 1999; Shao et al., 1999; Lim et al., 1999; Kim et al., 1999; Yabu et al., 1998; Park et al., 1998; Amosova, 1998; Kimura et al., 1997; Lin et al., 1980).

- Several animal studies have demonstrated a hypotensive (blood-vessel-relaxing) effect (reported in Bone, 1996).

- **Scute root** dry extracts and flavonoids can restore normal blood cell production depressed by sleep deprivation or other psychoemotional stress (Dygai et al., 1998).

- Researchers in Russia administered **scute root** preparations to lung cancer patients undergoing chemotherapy. The herb helped restore depressed T-lymphocytes and other immunoglobulins (Smol'ianinov, 1997).

- Baicalein partially but significantly ameliorated kidney damage in rats receiving intravenous injections of a toxic serum (Wu et al., 1985).

- Research indicates that **scute root** offers neural benefits as well. Oxygen deprivation leads to rapid mitochondrial-related energy loss and cell destruction. In rat studies, **scute root** has been shown to prevent energy loss in the brain mitochondria and preserve mitochondrial membranes (Saifutdinov and Khazanov, 1998).

- Glial cells help to protect and maintain nerve cell integrity. When tested on rat glioma cells, two major flavonoids found in **scute root** (baicalin and baicalein) were shown to protect against histamine-related damage by inhibiting inflammatory phospholipase (Kyo et al., 1998).

- It has also shown some success in China as a treatment for chronic hepatitis, as indicated by the results of one study that reported a 70% success rate (reported in Bone, 1996).

SHALAPARNI

Latin: *Desmodium gangeticum*   **Sanskrit:** Shalaparni

WHAT IT DOES: Shalaparni is sweet in taste and mildly warming in action. It is calming, strengthening, and anti-inflammatory. It restores balance to the system when other herbs fail.

RATING: Gold

SAFETY ISSUES: None known

STARTING DOSAGE:

- Crude powder: 2 grams two times per day

Shalaparni is a subtropical perennial spreading herb that grows in dry hilly areas. It is a general tonic and aphrodisiac, has a calming, sedative effect, and is also used to control inflammation, fever, and neurological imbalances. This plant has unique medicinal value to regulate the function of the nervous system (Vata), venous system (Pitta) and arterial system (Kapha). These three regulatory systems balance each other to restore health. However there are several very serious diseases where herbal medicines fail to work, such as typhoid fever and tuberculosis. **Shalaparni** is often effective in restoring balance to the system when the other herbs fail.

Research Highlights

- The leaves and stem of **shalaparni** are used in African countries for fevers, skin diseases, and anxiety states (Iwu, 1993).

- **Shalaparni** was one of five Nigerian herbs tested by a Walter Reed Army Institute research team for alkaloids active against serious parasitic protozoal diseases (Iwu et al., 1994). Although Dr. Iwu's group found promising results, the diseases treated by these herbs (malaria, leishmaniasis, and trypanosomiasis) are found primarily in poor countries, so drug companies have shown no interest in developing them. Therefore, Dr. Iwu plans to encourage local companies and herbal practitioners to develop these plant extracts as phytomedicines.

- Other species of *Desmodium* have shown very interesting effects. TCM doctors use **guang jin qian** *(Desmodium styracifolium)* to remove heat and dampness from the liver and gallblader, to treat stones (Hirayama et al., 1993), and for jaundice. They use **pai chien cao** *(D. pulchellum)* for fevers and malaria (reported in Huang, 1999). African *D. adscendens* is analgesic and supresses convulsions, seizures, and mortality in mice when induced by chemical poisons (N'gouemo et al., 1996).

- Traditionally used for asthma, crude extracts of *D. adscendens* have also been shown to be "the most potent potassium channel openers known." This means the plant extracts are able to both regulate the tone of the airway smooth muscle and inhibit the release of allergic and inflammatory bronchoconstrictive chemicals from nerves in the lung (McManus et al., 1993; Addy and Burka, 1988).

- In light of the potent regulatory effects reported for various *Desmodium* species plants, I found it fascinating that chronobiologists are studying the movements of *D. gyrans* leaflets. It seems the leaflets show strong up-and-down rhythmical movements due to swelling and shrinking of motor cells in special organs caused by ion pumping followed by depolarization (Engelmann and Antkowiak, 1998). The movements are circadian, meaning that they follow 24-hour cycles, and can be altered by electromagnetic radiation (Ellingsrud and Johnsson, 1993).

SHILAJATU

English: Bitumen   **Sanskrit:** Silajit / Shilajatu   **Hindi:** Silajit / Shilajeet
Mineral pitch

WHAT IT DOES: Shilajatu is bitter and slightly pungent in taste and mildly warming in action. It has the distinct odor of cow urine. **Shilajatu** strengthens immunity, reduces fatigue, slows aging, tonifies the brain, cleanses the blood, and strengthens the liver and kidneys.

RATING: Gold

SAFETY ISSUES: None known

STARTING DOSAGE:

- Purified sediment: combined with 50% **triphala,** use 1 to 2 grams two times per day

Shilajatu is an exudation gathered off Himalayan mountain faces. In the heat of summer it can be found on the southern slopes. It is a black, gummy substance that hardens easily into a solid rocklike mass. It is a complex but completely natural mixture of minerals with organic and inorganic compounds and is one of the most important rasayana tonics in Ayurveda.

Shilajatu contains aluminum, antimony, calcium, cobalt, copper, iron, lithium, magnesium, manganese, molybdenum, phosphorus, silica, sodium, strontium, zinc,

In 1976 I was traveling through Afghanistan, contracted severe dysentery in the 110-degree heat, and lost almost 60 pounds during the following few weeks. I was so weak I could hardly stand. I was transported quickly by my tour guide's bus to Kathmandu, where I first met the eminent Ayurvedic healer Dr. Mana Bajra Bajracharya. Dr. Mana gave me anti-dysentery herbs, some **deer musk** to revive me, and a **shilajatu**-based formula to restore my energy. I still remember the strong odor of the **shilajatu** and the amazing effect it had, restoring my energy so quickly. I know that Dr. Mana's emergency treatment saved my life.

fatty acids, hippuric acid, benzoic acid, fulvic acid, chebulic acid, tannic acid, resin and waxy matter, gums, albuminoids, glycosides, and an ichthyol oil. The substance must be purified before use. It is mixed with water and filtered, then slowly evaporated in the sun. Then the sediment is again mixed with water, filtered and evaporated. This process is repeated a total of seven times. It is then combined with other herbs, most frequently with **triphala** (three-fruit compound).

Shilajatu is a precious resource in the mountain kingdom of Nepal, and unscrupulous traders extract it and transfer it across borders into India, where it is sold as an expensive commodity. It is believed that hundreds of tons are secreted away, while local doctors have difficulty finding it at a reasonable cost. It is currently illegal to export **shilajatu** from Nepal, and the only legal sources in America come from India.

Shilajatu can be used with benefit for long periods of time and is a true tonic. It increases the potency of other herbs. Ayurvedic doctors use it to strengthen immunity and cleanse the blood, noting that it benefits the liver and kidneys, our two most important blood-filtering organs. They use it to treat diabetes, anemia, aging, bronchitis, skin diseases, acne and boils, liver diseases, constipation, dyspepsia, allergies, fatigue, cancer, and all urinary diseases. It also speeds wound healing. It is the first treatment given to people suffering from kidney failure and various chronic nerve diseases. The native peoples of the northern regions of Russia and Afghanistan collect and use a similar rock secretion (mumiyo) from their mountains.

Research Highlights

- The Indian Central Council for Research on Ayurveda and Siddha cited a series of experiments showing significant anti-inflammatory activity as well as cardiotonic action (Pandley et al., 1996; Frotan and Acharya, 1984).

- Laboratory experiments have shown that **shilajatu** is antiulcerogenic, stabilizes mast cells, and has protective effects on the liver and pancreas (Tiwari et al., 1973; Ghosal et al., 1989; Acharya, 1988; Vaishwanar et al., 1976; Mitra et al., 1996).

- A clinical study done in Russia on 38 patients with swollen prostate (BPH) showed a reduction in subjective and objective symptoms (reported by Sodhi, 2000).

SHOU WU ROOT

Latin: *Polygonum multiflorum*   **Chinese:** Ho shou wu
                                       Hé shou wu
                                       Shou wu

WHAT IT DOES: Shou wu root is bitter, sweet, and astringent in taste and slightly warming in action. It nourishes the blood, protects the liver and heart, reduces heat, and fertilizes the hair roots. It promotes longevity.

RATING: Gold

SAFETY ISSUES: Do not use with diarrhea, as it is mildly laxative. Use in combination with digestive tonics if there is weak digestion.

STARTING DOSAGE:

- Prepared powder (parboiled and dried): 9 to 15 grams per day

- 4:1 concentrated dried decoction extract: 2 to 4 grams per day

Shou wu translates as "black hair." It is one of the strongest TCM blood tonics and is an ingredient in many tonic formulas. Blood tonics are used in TCM when there are signs of pallor, dizziness, lethargy, dry skin, menstrual disorders, or pale tongue. It is the main ingredient in a TCM base formula we use to delay or reverse balding and premature graying of hair, which can be purchased commercially in Chinese grocery stores under the name "Alopecia pills." One popular way of preparing this herb is to cook it in black bean gravy.

Research Highlights

- **Shou wu root** has been shown to reduce blood cholesterol levels (reported in Huang, 1999).

- Pretreatment with **shou wu root** was proven more effective than treatment with vitamin E in preventing heart injury in mice (Yim TK et al., 1998).

- Extracts of **shou wu root** also significantly reduced tumor incidence in animals exposed to mutagenic chemicals (Horikawa et al., 1994).

- In a study on rats, **shou wu root** and **astragalus root** inhibited lipid peroxidation damage against the cardiac mitrochondria (Hong et al., 1994). In another study it exhibited similar effects when it extended the lives of quails (Wang, 1988; reported in Bone, 1996).

SIBERIAN GINSENG ROOT BARK

Latin: *Eleutherococcus senticosus*

WHAT IT DOES: Siberian ginseng is sweet and slightly pungent in taste and neutral in action. It nourishes the adrenal glands, supports liver metabolism, and increases energy and endurance against stress and pollution.

RATING: Gold

SAFETY ISSUES: None known. In rare instances it may raise blood pressure. There is a remote possibility that its mild anti-platelet-aggregation effects might interact with blood-thinning medications.

STARTING DOSAGE:

- Powdered 5:1 extract: 500–1,000 mg two to three times per day

- 1:2 tincture: 30 drops three times per day

Siberian ginseng is the herb for which the word *adaptogen* was coined. It is one of the medicines we use most frequently in the clinic, because it really helps fight stress-induced fatigue. It increases general vitality, strength, endurance, and the ability to overcome the effects of long-term illness. We prefer it to **ginseng root** in sensitive individuals who may find the stronger herb too hot or overly stimulating to the nervous system.

Siberian ginseng has been shown to delay stress reactions during the alarm phase of stress. When we are alarmed, our adrenal glands release corticosteroids and adrenaline that trigger the fight-or-flight reaction. If these hormones are depleted by short- or long-term stress, we develop adrenal exhaustion. **Siberian ginseng** delays the onset of the exhaustive phase by causing a more efficient release of these hormones into our system.

Several negative studies have been published since the original Russian research. However, my own personal experience and that of my patients shows **Siberian ginseng** to be very effective in a majority of those who take it. I have spoken with suppliers, and they tell me that much of the **Siberian ginseng** used in America is made from the whole root, while the original Russian studies were performed using the root bark. If you find a good supply, the results should be immediately obvious.

Research Highlights

- In a placebo-controlled study of the effects of a **Siberian ginseng** extract on the immune system of healthy individuals, researchers reported "a drastic increase in the absolute number of immunocompetent cells, with an especially pronounced effect on T lymphocytes." In addition, they observed a general enhancement of the activation state in T-lymphocytes (Bohn et al., 1987).

- According to translations of original Russian research, **Siberian ginseng** has the ability to increase our endurance and capacity to work by improving the ability of the liver and adrenals to regulate hormonal levels, dispose of lactic acid, and regulate blood sugar (reported in Farnsworth et al., 1989).

- Russian telegraph operators were able to increase the number of messages they could handle by taking about 60 drops of a **Siberian ginseng** tincture daily (reported in Farnsworth et al., 1989).

- Factory workers taking about 60 drops of a **Siberian ginseng** tincture daily recorded a 50% reduction in illness and a 40% reduction in lost work days (reported in Farnsworth et al., 1989).

SLIPPERY ELM INNER BARK

Latin: *Ulmus rubra*

WHAT IT DOES: Slippery elm inner bark is sweet in taste and neutral in action. It coats and soothes the intestines and kidneys.

RATING: Silver, due to mild action

SAFETY ISSUES: None known

STARTING DOSAGE:

- Powder: 2 to 4 teaspoons, two to three times per day

I make use of its soothing action by finely grinding about 60% **slippery elm** with 40% anti-inflammatory herbs like **licorice root** or **boswellia gum**, giving about 1 teaspoon two or three times per day. This attaches the herbs to the surface mucosa a little longer than normal, promoting the healing process. We have had perhaps a hundred patients over the years with various forms of chronic intestinal inflammation who have found this simple prescription a vital intermediate step in their healing process.

Slippery elm contains abundant vegetable mucilage, which has a coating action useful in treating digestive conditions with inflamed mucous membrane linings such as gastritis, gastric or duodenal ulcer, enteritis, and colitis. It also soothes bladder and kidney inflammation.

The powder can be prepared in gruel form: mix warm water and honey to make a paste, add 2 to 4 teaspoons of the powder, and take with water two to three times per day. The soothing action is quick and direct, which helps with patient compliance. **Slippery elm** is also known for its nutritive qualities. Eclectic doctors used to boil a teaspoon of it with milk to alleviate bowel complaints in recently weaned children.

Research Highlights

- Herbalist John Heinerman reported on a laboratory study done in India where researchers fed a similar highly mucilaginous herb **(comfrey root)** to cats. They demonstrated upon autopsy that the mucilage formed a smooth coating over the entire digestive tract which lasted for over 24 hours (Heinerman, 1979).

ST. JOHN'S WORT

Latin: *Hypericum perforatum*

WHAT IT DOES: St. John's wort is bitter and astringent in taste and cooling in action. It elevates the mood, stimulates the nerves, and strengthens immunity.

RATING: Silver, due to action on other medications

SAFETY ISSUES: Do not use if pregnant. Use cautiously with anxiety. May potentiate MAO inhibitors. High doses may lead to photosensitivity. Do not take with protease inhibitors (used for HIV and AIDS) or cyclosporine. Because this herb can strengthen liver detoxification causing quicker drug clearance, use cautiously with all pharmaceutical drugs.

STARTING DOSAGE:

- Crude herb: 2 to 4 grams per day

- Standardized extract pills containing 300 mg of hypericin: 1 pill three times per day

- 1:2 tincture (recently dried): 25–35 drops three times per day

St. John's wort is a nervine stimulant useful in treating neuralgia, depression, and irritability due to menopausal changes. It is prescribed throughout the world as a mild antidepressant, sold seven times as frequently for that purpose as Prozac, and it has an impressive safety profile. Long-term use can improve sleep quality, and it is helpful in easing minor nerve-related pains such as sciatica and neuritis.

Originally, one of the compounds in **St. John's wort**, "hypericin," was thought to be the "active ingredient." This turned out to be false, though it can still be used as a marker to measure the strength of a particular batch. Another chemical called

> Standardized extracts are usually advertised as superior to other products. However, **St. John's wort** has been used for centuries in Europe, and seeing the beautiful blood-red liquid tincture, one can't help thinking it must be potent. A good 1:2 tincture will give you sufficient concentrations of the required components with 4–5 ml per day, or approximately 25–35 drops three times per day.

"hyperforin" is now considered to be the important marker compound. Scientists have determined a method to ensure that the fragile active compound (hyperforin) in **St. John's wort** is preserved and stable in the finished product. From an energetic standpoint, the bitter and astringent tastes of **St. John's wort** stimulates the nerves, while the cooling effect reduces irritation and inflammation, and the red color nourishes the heart.

I use **St. John's wort** whenever I see a patient with mild depression or depressed immunity due to mental causes, and especially if they have a viral illness or signs of nervous irritation. I find it useful for chronic hepatitis, not only for its antiviral qualities, but to help lift the black cloud that appears when patients are told they have an incurable illness that will lead to cirrhosis and liver cancer in 10 or 20 years. In one case, a patient of mine with hepatitis C compounded by depression had this lift within a few days of beginning treatment with **St. John's wort.**

Hypericin and pseudohypericin are antiviral, so **St. John's wort** can be used externally when brewed as a tea to dab onto herpes sores (though I prefer to use Earl Grey tea bags). **St. John's wort** also contains several other antiviral, antibacterial, and anti-inflammatory phytochemicals, including xanthones, phloroglucinol derivatives, and flavonols.

Because **St. John's wort** is able to induce a liver detoxification enzyme (CYP3A4), it can lower drug and toxin levels in the blood. This is positive in most cases, and may account for why it clears the mind. However, in the case of drugs where maintaining blood levels is critical, as with in HIV protease inhibitors and organ rejection drugs, the same effect can be deadly. Dr. Duke points out that broccoli, brussels sprouts, and tobacco also induce similar liver detoxification of drugs.

Research Highlights

- The antidepressant activity of **St. John's wort** has been shown in a number of studies to act on three major biochemical pathways, inhibiting the synaptic reuptake system for serotonin, norepinephrine, and dopamine with rough equality of action. It is the only antidepressant than can act in this way (Nathan, 1999).

- A controlled human clinical study showed **St. John's wort** effective in reducing symptoms of depression, anxiety, and sleep disturbance ((Muldner and Zoller, 1984).

STEVIA LEAF

Latin: *Stevia rebaudiana*

WHAT IT DOES: Stevia leaf is sweet in taste and neutral in action. It sweetens without adding calories.

RATING: Yellow, due to limitations in use

SAFETY ISSUES: None known. **Do not use in excess.**

STARTING DOSAGE:

- Drops or powder: add to food and drink as a sweetener, to taste

Stevia leaf is a natural sweetener that comes from the rain forests in Paraguay and Brazil. Per weight gram, the purified white dried leaf extract of **stevia** is up to several hundred times as sweet as sugar—almost as sweet as saccharine. Unlike white sugar, **stevia leaf** is calorie-free and nondisruptive to blood sugar levels. So far, there have been no recorded side effects from **stevia** consumption. It has passed strict Japanese health trials and is used in Japan to sweeten diet sodas. Several drops take the place of several teaspoons of sugar. Although **stevia** in its sweetening dosage does not have medicinal effects, it is an important tool in helping patients manage their sugar intake.

Many people working to improve their health discover that it is difficult to stay away from excess sugar in foods and drinks. For example, it is difficult to find drinks other than spring water that are beneficial to your health and low in sugar among the typical offerings of sodas, milk products, alcohol, sugared drinks, and various hybrids containing things you can't pronounce. Commercial sugared sodas are loaded with chemical additives like caffeine and phosphoric acid. They have little nutritional value and cause health problems, including calcium loss in children. The few natural choices, such as juices, contain natural sugars in amounts too high for persons with diseases such as diabetes or intestinal infections.

For a natural, low-calorie soda, add some **stevia leaf** and **lemon**, **lime, black cherry** or other flavoring to carbonated mineral water. Spring-water-based sparkling waters such as Perrier (available in most supermarkets) offer the benefit of additional healthful minerals. To make a low-calorie fruit drink, use about 10–20% pure juice and the rest water, along with several drops of **stevia**. A glass of this kind of beverage 1 hour before meals can actually assist in weight reduction by decreasing hunger. For those people who aren't on a no-sugar diet, about 20% fruit juice of any kind mixed with **stevia** works well. You should experiment to find the flavors you like best.

Though safety concerns about saccharine seem to be overblown (Elcock and Morgan, 1993; Chappel, 1992), there are still many concerns associated with aspartame. There is actually a large consumer movement behind these questions—you can follow this ongoing controversy on the Internet. For these reasons, **stevia leaf** is a good addition to our natural pharmacy.

Research Highlights

- In animal models, **stevia** exhibits a mild diuretic effect at high doses (Melis, 1996; Melis, 1995).

- When given to fasting rats, it causes an increase in stored sugars (glycogen) in the liver. This effect has not been shown in humans, but the results offer promising implications for hypoglycemics and Type 1 diabetics, both of whom have problems with storage of glycogen. **Stevia** may have a beneficial effect beyond replacing sugar (Hubler et al., 1994).

- In another study of human subjects in good health, water extracts of **stevia leaf** caused a decrease in blood sugars and an increase in glucose tolerance (Curi et al., 1986).

- **Stevia** has shown very little, if any, significant toxicity in both human and animal studies. In an experiment with cultured human lymphocytes, there was no evidence of mutagenic activity until dosage reached very high levels (Suttajit et al., 1993).

- Studies have also confirmed that **stevia** does not possess any cancer-causing potential in animals (Das et al., 1992) and has no effect on growth or reproduction in hamsters (Yodyingyuad and Bunyawong, 1991).

STINGING NETTLE

Latin: *Urtica dioica*   **Sanskrit:** Vrishchikali

WHAT IT DOES: Stinging nettle leaf is bitter in taste and cooling in action. It cleanses the blood. **Nettle seed** nourishes and removes toxins from the kidneys.

RATING: Yellow, due to strong action

SAFETY ISSUES: Do not touch or ingest fresh plant.

STARTING DOSAGE:

- Dried leaf powder: 2 grams two to three times per day as an infusion (10–15 minutes)

- 1:5 leaf tincture: 20–40 drops two to five times per day

- Standardized leaf extract: 250–350 mg two times per day

- 1:5 seed tincture: 20–40 drops two to five times per day

Stinging nettle is well known for its poisonous hairs that contain formic acid and histamine. Both of these chemicals can cause severe stinging and inflammation upon contact. Consequently, it makes sense that the rest of the plant contains a number of materials that protect its interior structures from its own poisons. Scientific studies show that **stinging nettle** has a number of very interesting, wide-ranging, and unique compounds that block inflammation. *This herb is a good example of how different parts and preparations of the same plant can have quite different actions and uses.*

Herbalist David Winston reported in 1999 that he had successfully used **nettle seed** to reduce creatinine levels in six cases of severely diminished kidney function, including glomerulonephritis and other degenerative kidney diseases. He believes this seed is a kidney "food," useful for treating severely diminished kidney function, glomerulonephritis, and other degenerative kidney diseases. Following his lead, I was able to stabilize a severe case using this preparation. Thanks to **nettle seed**, the patient showed marked and completely unexpected improvement in creatinine levels (a marker for disease progression). The general improvement stopped after 2 years, and she began to slowly decline, but at a much slower rate than normal for this stage, apparently buying a few precious years for this elderly woman.

Nephritis is a debilitating and very expensive disease to treat. A group of doctors from Washington contacted me looking for natural medicine treatments, and I referred them to David. A study is currently underway. If the results are positive, **nettle seed** will prove to be a very important herbal medicine.

Cultures in many different parts of the world prepare the tender parts of **stinging nettle** by cooking them as vegetables. The dried form of **nettle leaf** is prepared as a tonic useful for nourishing the blood and can be used to treat anemia. Both Western and TAM herbalists use it for this same purpose.

Stinging nettle leaf is traditionally used to cleanse the blood by removing toxins. It can be a beneficial treatment for eczema, particularly in children. It can also be used to treat lower back pain caused by chronic low-grade infection—it is best prepared as an infusion for this purpose. **Nettle leaf** can also be used to reduce prostate swelling.

Research Highlights

- **Nettle leaf extracts** reduce inflammation, in part, by suppressing the release of inflammatory cytokines. They do this by blocking a chemical inducer known as NF-kappaB, which alters gene expression. This may be one explanation for the beneficial effects this herb has exhibited in rheumatoid arthritis (Riehemann et al., 1999).

- One set of in vitro experiments on live blood using extracts of **stinging nettle leaf** exhibited its ability to slow down the inflammatory cytokine response caused by endotoxins. In the same experiments, when there was no endotoxin present, the **nettle leaf** actually stimulated an immune response. Researchers believed these results could explain the positive effects of this extract in the treatment of rheumatic diseases (Obertreis B et al., 1996).

- The herb has also been indicated as a treatment for prostate diseases. Lignans obtained from **stinging nettle roots** attach to and alter prostate membranes (Schottner et al., 1997). This in turn leads to less prostate tissue stimulation, and a reduction in prostate swelling (Lichius et al., 1997).

- **Stinging nettle** is an approved medicine for the treatment of prostate diseases in Germany (Vahlensieck Jr. et al., 1996).

- **Nettle leaf** contains a lectin called UDA that has been shown to stimulate the production of a protein-digesting enzyme called gelatinase B. Low levels of UDA concentration reduce sticky proteins in the blood and reduce inflammation, but high levels can cause shock. Researchers from the Pasteur Institute have said that UDA "is an unusual plant lectin that differs from all other known plant lectins . . . [due to] its ability to discriminate a particular population of CD4+ and CD8+ T cells." Such unique and extremely specific actions are beginning to give herbalists and physicians new tools for fine-tuning the immune system and may play important roles in development of therapies against very serious diseases (Galelli et al., 1993). Other plants that share this action include **bindweed** *(Convolvulus arvensis)* and **meadow saffron** *(Colchicum autumnale),* both of which exhibit some toxicity (Dubois et al., 1998).

STONEROOT

Latin: *Collinsonia canadensis*

WHAT IT DOES: Stoneroot is sour and spicy in taste and warming in action. It relaxes constriction and clears venous congestion and inflammation from the mouth, throat, and lungs, down through the lower bowel and anus.

RATING: Silver, due to limitations in usage.

SAFETY ISSUES: None known

STARTING DOSAGE:

- 1:2 tincture (fresh whole root): 30–40 drops three to five times per day

Stoneroot is very useful for treating various types of venous congestion associated with constriction and lack of venous tone, including hemorrhoids, varicose veins, benign prostatic hypertrophy (BPH), and chronic laryngitis. The whole plant is used as a tincture, and it can be used in formulas treating gastritis and colitis. Eclectic physicians used stoneroot as an effective gargle for "minister's throat," a condition of scratchy congestion that results from talking too much. Used over time, this herb strengthens the veins.

At our clinic, we combine **stoneroot** with **gotu kola** and **butcher's broom** to make a very effective formula. In addition to prescribing this for internal use, we instruct patients to use cotton to apply the combination topically over spider veins twice a day. Before I was married I suggested this to a girlfriend, and the treatment made her spider veins disappear within 2 months. I got lots of points for that one.

TANGERINE PEEL

Latin: *Citrus reticulata*   **Chinese:** Chen pi

WHAT IT DOES: Tangerine peel is aromatic, warm, and pungent in taste and warming in action. It aids digestion, dries up mucus, and reduces nausea.

RATING: Yellow, due to limitations in usage

SAFETY ISSUES: None known

STARTING DOSAGE:

- Dried powder: 3 to 9 grams per day

- Dried peel: 1 to 2 teaspoons per day

- Whole fruit: one or more per day while in season, including the juice and the white rind

Doctors use aromatic **tangerine peel** to dry up mucus in the lungs and stomach. It helps regulate and strengthen digestion and is a component of many TCM formulas used to treat diarrhea, nausea, dyspepsia, and cough, especially when accompanied by copious sticky sputum. Chinese pharmacological studies show that it increases the secretion of gastric juices and relaxes the smooth muscles in the gastrointestinal (GI) tract. It also stimulates secretion and expectoration in the lungs. TCM doctors say it moves the Qi downward, so it also is useful for treating hiccups and vomiting. Immature **tangerine peel** (zhi shi) has similar properties but shows a stronger unblocking action and is most often used to treat digestive and mucus problems with constipation.

The herbal concept of heat is a much more palpable experience with **tangerines** than with **oranges**. Both fruits are similar in taste, though **tangerines** are a bit sweeter. However, if you eat several **tangerines** in one sitting, the next day you can often feel the effects of the heat they produce, sometimes causing dryness and a burning sensation in the digestive system and mouth. This effect does occur nearly as frequently or as powerfully with **oranges**.

Tangeritin, a bioflavonoid found in **tangerine peel,** has been shown to strengthen epithelial cells in a manner that inhibits the metastasis of cancer cells. Naturopath Bill Mitchell explained in a lecture that the compound increases the functional integrity of E-cadherin, which is a cell-to-cell adhesive protein found to be deficient in tissue samples of most cancer patients. Based on these results, we can deduce that **tangeritin,** and its source, **tangerine,** might be useful as a cancer preventative. The reasoning is simple—about 80% of breast cancers start in the epithelial tissue lining the breast ducts, and this bioflavonoid makes the tissue tougher and more resistant. In order to get this benefit you must eat quite a bit of fruit, so the body will have enough left over to store in the tissue. I suggest eating at least one **tangerine** pretty much every day while the fruit is in season (but not year-round).

Research Highlights

- An extract of **tangeritin** (not **tangerines** per se) blocked the cancer-inhibiting action of tamoxifen in female mice. It takes quite a large number of **tangerines** to extract the amount of **tangeritin** used in the experiments, and mice may not metabolize it in the same way as humans. However, researchers caution against excessive use of **tangerine** products during tamoxifen therapy until we know more (Bracke et al., 1999).

- Chinese clinical trials have shown decoctions of **tangerine peel** and **licorice root** to be 70% effective within a few days for treatment of mastitis when treatment began in early stages of the disease. However, the treatment was not effective in chronic or purulent cases (reported in Bensky and Gamble, 1993).

TEA LEAVES

Latin: *Camellia sinensis*   **Sanskrit:** Chai   **Chinese:** Hong cha

WHAT IT DOES: Tea leaves are bitter and astringent in taste and stimulating in action. There are two different types of medicinal tea. **Black tea** directly neutralizes external viral outbreaks, while **green tea** prevents cancer, strengthens immunity, stimulates the nerves, and neutralizes bacterial, chemical, and radiation poisons.

RATING: Gold **(green tea)**, Silver **(black tea)**

SAFETY ISSUES: Excessive long-term internal use of black tea is not recommended because it may weaken digestion.

STARTING DOSAGE:

- Topical application of tea bag: apply externally as directed below for lesions
- Tea: drink 1 to 2 cups per day for general protective benefits

Green tea and **black tea** both come from the same plant. **Black tea leaves** are fermented, which elevates the tannin content, while **green tea** is steamed to preserve important medicinal constituents. The caffeine, theobromine, and theophylline found in **tea leaves** can help relax bronchial spasms and may be used to treat asthma attacks in emergencies when no other medicine is available.

Herpes sores are very ugly and embarrassing, and getting rid of them quickly is a high priority. According to a report in the journal *New Scientist,* external application of **black tea bags** is a simple cure for viral infections like herpes. It works better than the common treatment acyclovir, costs less, and has fewer side effects. You can apply cooled liquid from brewed **black teas** such as Earl Grey to lesions, including cold sores, genital herpes, and shingles. Simply put a tea bag in boiling water for a few minutes, cool it, and apply it to the skin for 5 minutes two or three times per day. The tannins in the tea calm the lesions, dry them up more quickly, and keep them from recurring for longer periods of time than usual. At the first warning tingle that typically precedes a herpes eruption, I tell patients to apply ice to the area for a few minutes, for as long as they can stand the cold. Then they use the tea bag cure for about 3 days. I capitalize on the success of this simple symptomatic treatment to get patients to trust me so they will work seriously with me to treat the real cause of the breakouts—usually an underlying problem of weakened immunity. Fast symptomatic cures are an important part of herbalism.

Research Highlights

- In a study of rats with chemically induced gastric ulcers, hot water extract of **black tea** significantly reduced gastric lining erosion (ulcer formation). The results suggested that the tea helped preserve the cellular antioxidant glutathione peroxidase (Maity et al., 1998).

- Both **green** and **black tea** show the ability to prevent various kinds of bacterial infections (Chosa et al., 1992), and in one study, **green tea** inhibited the growth of various bacteria species that cause diarrhea (Toda et al., 1989).

- Promising experimental results on **green tea** continue to accumulate. Researchers have identified a wide variety of benefits, including the existence of a polyphenol (epigallocatechin-3-gallate or EGCG) that encourages cancer cells to kill themselves (apoptosis). There are approximately 200 mg of this compound in a single cup of tea (Hirose et al., 1994; Wang et al., 1994).

- According to one study, long-term administration of EGCG to mice via their drinking water significantly prolonged their life span after lethal whole-body X-irradiation (Uchid et al., 1992).

- Another group of researchers concluded, "the main constituent of Japanese **green tea,** EGCG, is a practical cancer chemopreventive agent available in everyday life" (Fujiki et al., 1992).

- **Green tea extract** (EGCG and caffeine) is known to stimulate thermogenesis, the natural heat production process in the body that aids weight loss. In a recent double-blind study, subjects experienced an increase in daily energy expenditure and fat oxidation, concurrent with increases in the concentration of the extract (Dulloo et al., 1999).

- Clinical studies indicate that increased consumption of **green tea** lowers cholesterol levels, even when subject rankings are adjusted based on smoking, alcohol use, physical activity, and body mass index (Kono et al., 1992).

- **Green tea** has also been shown to prevent the formation of dental caries in animals by inhibiting the attachment of bacteria to teeth (Otake et al., 1991).

TEA TREE OIL

Latin: *Melaleuca alternifolia*

WHAT IT DOES: Tea tree oil is sweet and pungent in taste, with a penetrating and drying action. It is an effective topical antibacterial and antifungal.

RATING: Silver

SAFETY ISSUES: For external use only. Poisonous when taken internally. Avoid contact with eyes or mucous membranes. Dilute with olive or other oil if skin irritation occurs.

STARTING DOSAGE:

- Standardized oil (full-strength or diluted): apply directly to the affected skin

Tea tree oil derives from the **tea tree,** native to New South Wales, Australia. In 1930, a surgeon from Sydney reported that **tea tree oil** dissolved pus, leaving surgical wounds clean without any apparent damage to the tissues. During World War II it was issued to soldiers for use as a topical disinfectant (reported in Murray, 1991). **Tea tree oil** can be applied externally to treat fungal infections, athlete's foot, and abscesses. It is also used for bruises and insect bites. It has several qualities that make it more valuable than other antimicrobial oils. It has a complex chemical structure, making it difficult for microorganisms to develop immunity against it. It penetrates deeply into the tissue, and does not seem to injure healthy tissue at therapeutic dosage.

Olive oil has a soothing quality that neutralizes the drying effect of **tea tree oil.** The old adage for skin conditions is to dry if moist, and moisten if dry. With moist conditions, use **tea tree oil** by itself, and for dry conditions, mix it with **olive oil.** The best way to get rid of toenail fungus is to mix

> My office manager, Mary, uses **tea tree oil** to effectively soothe her minor psoriasis problem.

tea tree oil with **oregano oil, thyme oil,** or pure **neem leaf,** put it on a cotton pad, and tape it right to the toenail. Change the pad twice daily, and keep it up for a couple of months. To improve results, soak your toenails in vinegar for 20 minutes each night. The vinegar also kills fungus and makes the nail more permeable. Use vinegar and **tea tree oil** at different times of day.

Research Highlights

- The antiseptic action of **tea tree oil** is partially due to its ability to activate immune system white blood cells (Budhiraja et al., 1999).

- In a randomized, double-blind, placebo-controlled study, patients with a 6- to 36- month history of toenail fungal infections were treated with a cream containing 2%

butenafine hydrochloride and 5% **tea tree oil**. After 16 weeks, 80% of the test group patients (those who used the cream) were cured. None of the patients in the placebo group were cured. In a follow-up, none of the test group patients had experienced any relapse, and none of the placebo patients had improved (Syed et al., 1999).

- In another double-blind study, 60% of patients with toenail fungus who used 100% **tea tree oil** had partial or full resolution (Buck et al., 1994).

- In tests of intravaginal **tea tree oil** suppository products used to treat yeast infections, all three products exhibited sufficient fungicidal action to be effective (Hammer et al., 1998).

- Patch tests on 28 patients for sensitivity to **tea tree oil** resulted in three (about 11%) strong reactions (Rubel et al., 1998), indicating a need for caution when first applying the oil.

- **Tea tree oil** demonstrated effective activity against *Candida albicans, Trichophyton rubrum, T. mentagrophytes, T. tonsurans, Aspergillus niger, Penicillium* species, *Epidermophyton floccosum,* and *Microsporum gypsum* (Concha et al., 1998).

- A study at an inner city HIV/AIDS clinic evaluated the effectiveness of **oral tea tree oil solution** on AIDS patients with persistent mouth and throat yeast infections resistant to fluconazole (an antifungal agent). After 4 weeks, 8 of 12 patients demonstrated a positive response, and 2 were cured (Jandourek et al., 1998).

- One very interesting study tested **tea tree oil** against resident skin flora (the bacteria that are normally present on your skin) and transient flora (bacteria likely to cause disease). The results indicated that "**tea tree oil** may be useful in removing transient skin flora while suppressing but maintaining resident flora" (Hammer et al., 1996).

- A single-blind randomized trial tested a 5% **tea tree oil** gel on 124 patients with mild to moderate acne. Results showed a significant reduction in the number of inflamed and noninflamed lesions with fewer side effects than benzoyl peroxide lotion (Bassett et al., 1990).

TIEN CHI ROOT

Latin: *Panax pseudoginseng*   **Chinese:** Tien chi / San qi / Tian qi
Panax notoginseng

WHAT IT DOES: Tien chi root is sweet and slightly bitter in taste and warming in action. It stops bleeding while simultaneously reducing blood congestion and clotting. It also relaxes, detoxifies, and repairs blood vessels and speeds wound healing. It is a mild tonic.

RATING: Gold

SAFETY ISSUES: Do not use during pregnancy.

STARTING DOSAGE:

- Crude powder from Yunnan Province: 2 to 3 500-mg pills two times per day for 3 weeks following traumatic injury

Note: May be used up to 3 months or longer for chronic conditions.

Tien chi root is very popular among martial artists because of its unusual ability to simultaneously stop bleeding and reduce blood stagnation. This makes it the premier Chinese herb for wound healing. It reduces swelling and pain and is used to treat traumatic injury, diabetic retinopathy, optic neuritis, hemorrhage, surgical wounds, blood clots, sprains, and fractures.

The root from Yunnan Province is considered to be the best quality, harvested from remote mountains in the autumn or winter of the third or seventh year before its flowers bloom.

Tien chi root is the main ingredient in **Yunnan Paiyao capsules,** known throughout the world for their unparalleled ability to heal wounds, stop hemorrhage, and repair tissue. I often prescribe **tien chi root** for 2 or 3 weeks to speed healing from surgery. The use of pure **tien chi tablets** can usually stop retinal bleeding within 2 days, and over 3 months, it can heal the capillaries and basement membranes at the back of the eye. I use it myself several

I recall a particular case referred to us by Dr. Abel. The patient was a diabetic woman who had undergone more than four emergency surgical operations for bleeding diabetic retinopathy. Thanks to the hemostatic action of **tien chi tablets** she stabilized within days, and continued use over the next 3 years stabilized her vision loss and prevented the need for further surgical intervention.

months per year to prevent retinopathy, and so far I have never had a problem (40 years and counting). In addition to the herb's benefits on diabetic retinopathy, one of the components of **tien chi root** has been indicated for lowering glucose-induced increases in blood sugar.

Research Highlights

- Studies from China show that it speeds recovery from wounds by over 50% (reported in Dharmananda, 1994).

- Studies have shown that this action is strengthened by repeated administration and tends to be dose dependent (Gong YH et al., 1991).

- In mouse studies, **tien chi root extract** has shown significant antitumor activity on skin tumors induced by chemical toxins (Konoshima et al., 1999).

- In a study of patients with essential hypertension, **tien chi root saponins** were shown to precipitate remarkable improvement in left ventricular diastolic function. The researchers concluded that the herb could improve heart muscle relaxation by enhancing calcium pump activity, inhibiting intracellular calcium overload, and lightening left ventricular muscle mass (Feng et al., 1997). In spite of this positive effect, however, the herb is not a reliable blood-pressure-lowering agent by itself, though it may be a useful addition to a treatment protocol (Lei XL et al., 1986).

- The development of cardiac dysfunction and weakness immediately following traumatic burns is a serious problem, one that is very difficult to treat. In a placebo-controlled trial performed on rats at the Institute of Burn Research in Chongqing, China, researchers determined that **tien chi root** was effective in improving early postburn cardiac function (Huang et al., 1999).

- The actions of this herb on the cardiovascular system are complex, involving multiple mechanisms. Studies done at the Chinese Academy of Medical Science in Beijing have shown that the saponins in **tien chi root** act as calcium channel blockers in neurons (Ma et al., 1997).

- The protection the whole root affords against hypoxic damage is attributed to the improvement of energy metabolism, preserving the structural integrity of neurons (Jiang KY et al., 1995).

- Other effects include lipid-lowering activity (Xu et al., 1993), increased outflow of coronary vessels and relaxed constriction of ileum smooth muscles (Hu Y et al., 1992), and antiarrhythmic activity (Gao BY et al., 1992).

- A study on rabbits suffering from hemorrhagic shock examined the effects of various combinations of **salvia root, tien chi root,** and **chuan xiong rhizome** *(Ligusticum wallichii)*. Blood tests showed that all three herbs were effective for relieving blood pressure and heart rate reduction but that the combination of any two herbs was superior to using a single herb, improving results and lowering the required dosage (Wang et al., 1997).

TULSI

Latin: *Ocimum sanctum*   **Sanskrit:** Tulsi   **English:** Holy basil

WHAT IT DOES: Tulsi is bitter in taste and cold in action. It reduces fever and affords potent short-term protection against toxins and stress.

RATING: Yellow, due to limitations in use

SAFETY ISSUES: Do not use if pregnant or nursing. Do not use for extended periods of time.

STARTING DOSAGE:

- Dried powder decoction: 2 grams two to three times per day

- 4:1 concentrated powder extract: 500–1,000 mg two to three times per day

Tulsi is a very effective treatment for certain types of fevers, flus, and colds, including typhoid and malarial fevers. In our clinic we use it to treat tough fevers, especially when there is lung constriction. It is effective as a tea mixed with honey and taken twice a day. Its action is narrow, so it may work only against specific organisms such as *Aspergillus* fungi and *E. coli*. Traditional doctors do not use strongly cooling herbs for extended periods—I would recommend the same caution here.

Ayurvedic doctor and naturopathic physician Virender Sodhi mentioned in a lecture that **tulsi** is considered sacred in India, and many households will keep a plant near the center of the home for purification purposes. It seems the plant gives off small amounts of ozone, an unstable form of oxygen that helps break down toxic chemical compounds into their elemental forms. This reaction is completely harmless to humans, but it irritates the heck out of viruses, bacteria, and small insects, chasing them away.

I was once giving a lecture on herbs at a Yoga ashram in upstate New York, and one of the guru's disciples came in and said he was experiencing a conflict. He was trying to complete his cleaning duties and still spare the lives of insects. It seems capturing and carrying the little guys outside took up too much time. If it was up to me, I would have voted for helping them along into their next lives, but the guru suggested putting **tulsi** plants in the rooms.

Research Highlights

- Recent evidence suggests that ocimum flavonoids in **tulsi tea** may offer protection against radiation damage via antioxidant action and by inhibiting radiation-induced lipid peroxidation (Devi, 1998; Uma, 1999). The researchers concluded that the low dose needed for protection, and the high margin between the effective and toxic doses, made the ocimum flavonoids promising for human radiation protection.

- **Tulsi** has shown effectiveness against *Aspergillus niger* and other fungi, as well as the bacteria *E. coli* and *S. aureus* (reported in Pandey, 1996).

- **Tulsi** has shown strong anti-inflammatory activity via both the cyclooxygenase and lipoxygenase pathways (Singh, 1998), and ulcer-protective activity against aspirin, alcohol, and other ulcerogenic chemicals (Singh and Majumdar, 1999).

- It has also demonstrated cellular protection against the early events when cells become cancerous (Karthikeyan et al., 1999; Prashar et al., 1998).

- The cooling action of **tulsi** has been found strong enough to lower T_4 concentrations in the blood of mice (Panda and Kar, 1998) and to lower sperm counts in animals (Seth et al., 1981; Kasinanthan et al., 1972).

- In an interesting study of albino rats exposed to noise in single episodes (100dB), the animals showed significant elevation of corticosterone levels. When exposed to the noise repeatedly (4 hours daily for 30 days) the rats had depleted hormone levels, indicating chronic stress. **Tulsi alcohol extract** prevented these hormone changes, illustrating its stress-protective action (Sembulingam et al., 1997).

- This action was also demonstrated against pentobarbital, electroshock- and pentylene-tetrazole-induced convulsions, and forced swimming in rats and mice (Sakina et al., 1990).

TURMERIC ROOT

Latin: *Curcuma longa*   **Sanskrit:** Haridra   **Chinese:** Jiang huang / Yu jin

WHAT IT DOES: Turmeric root is bitter in taste and warming in action. It strongly reduces inflammation and mucus in all parts of the body, protects the liver, lungs, and intestines, and helps prevent and treat cancer.

RATING: Gold

SAFETY ISSUES: Due to mucin-reducing effects, do not use the concentrated extract (curcumin) or oil in high doses, especially if you have bile duct obstruction, gallstones, or stomach ulcers. Use **turmeric** as a spice freely.

STARTING DOSAGE:

- Crude powder: 500 mg two to three times per day

Turmeric is a common tuberous vegetable spice used all over the world. It stimulates gastric juices, and it is used in Indian households in most vegetable dishes as an anti-food-poisoning agent that also reduces mucus formation.

Turmeric root is used externally by TAM doctors to treat skin diseases and as a plaster to reduce swelling. It is a valuable anti-inflammatory. Modern research has shown it to be a powerful antioxidant, anti-inflammatory, and antihepatotoxic herb, useful in the treatment of many inflammation-related conditions such as diabetes, hepatitis, arthritis, diarrhea, psoriasis, eczema, asthma, and smoking-related lung inflammation.

Turmeric rhizome is yellow in color and egg-shaped (called jiang huang), with numerous secondary garlic-bulb-like projections (called yu jin). TCM doctors report that these two parts have different medicinal properties. Though similar in action, the larger **jiang huang** is used to invigorate the blood, relieve menstrual cramps, and treat the pain and swelling associated with trauma. The smaller **yu jin** is cooler in action and used more to break up blood stasis and relieve constrained liver energy with symptoms of internal tension.

Turmeric root can be rendered more effective in treating inflammation by adding a small amount of **trikatu** (three-pepper compound). Piperine, an alkaloid found in **black pepper** and **long pepper,** enhances the bioavailability of **turmeric** considerably. For patients low on funds who suffer from arthritis, I suggest purchasing a pound of **turmeric** from an Indian grocery store, and then adding about 3% **trikatu**. This can be taken in half-teaspoon doses three times per day at a cost of less than $10 for a 6-month supply. Based upon traditional use patterns, I think it is better to use this formula for periods of 3 to 4 weeks, with a 1- or 2-week rest in between.

Research Highlights

- The anti-inflammatory action of **turmeric root extract** is partially based on its ability to strongly inhibit arachidonic acid (AA) metabolism, which affects the inflammatory enzymes 5-lipoxygenase and cyclooxygenase. This gives it a lower side effect profile than aspirin (reported in Bone, 1991).

- Various pharmacological and animal models have shown curcumin and **turmeric root** to possess cancer, radiation, and chemical toxin protective effects (Chun et al., 1999; Singhal et al., 1999; Kang et al., 1999; Bhaumik et al., 1999; Navis et al., 1999; Choudhary et al., 1999; Khar et al., 1999; Kawamori et al., 1999; Lee et al., 1998; Huang et al., 1997).

- In a study of 32 patients with chronic eye inflammation (anterior chamber uveitis), a 375-mg dose of curcumin three times per day for 3 months showed improvement comparable to the effects seen with a similar cortisone dose (Lal et al., 1999).

- Several studies suggest that **turmeric root** also has a mild to moderate cholesterol-lowering action (Ramirez-Tortosa et al., 1999; Pandey et al., 1996; Deshpande et al., 1998).

- Because it has low toxicity as well as antiplatelet, anti-inflammatory, and antioxidant activities, it appears to be a good addition to the diet for long-term prevention and treatment of cardiovascular diseases (reported in Bone, 1991).

- Slow tissue repair and wound healing are difficult problems for diabetics. In an animal study done at the Center for Combat Casualty and Life Sustainment Research in Bethesda, Maryland, curcumin was shown to enhance wound repair in diabetes-impaired healing (Sidhu GS et al., 1999).

- It has also been shown to reduce diabetic kidney damage (Suresh et al., 1998).

VALERIAN ROOT

Latin: *Valeriana officinalis*

WHAT IT DOES: Valerian root is bitter, slightly sweet, and pungent in taste. It is warming in action with a strong odor. It calms the nerves and muscles and helps induce restful sleep.

RATING: Yellow, due to limitation in use

SAFETY ISSUES: None known. Use cautiously when driving. May potentiate the effects of benzodiazepine drugs.

STARTING DOSAGE:

- 1:2 tincture (fresh herb): 15–30 drops two to three times per day, and up to 60–120 drops 1 hour before bedtime

- Concentrated 4:1 powder: 250–750 mg one to three times per day

Valerian root is an excellent nonnarcotic nervine for treating certain forms of anxiety and tension. It is best known as a gentle, safe sleep aid and is most often used to treat insomnia, stress, and anxiety. It has an additional antispasmodic action that makes it useful for easing muscle tension and menstrual cramping. **Valerian root** is easily identified by its strong, unpleasant odor. Every herbalist knows that there are patients for whom it works quite well, and others for whom it does not work at all.

Valerian occasionally has an excitatory effect, making insomnia worse. There are three possible reasons for this. First, as **valerian root** ages, the odor worsens due to the degradation of chemicals called valepotriates. As this degradation occurs, the herb becomes less effective at inducing sleep. Therefore, I use only tinctures made from fresh plants (as opposed to dried). Second, the Eclectic doctors classified **valerian** as a warming cerebral stimulant, more effective "when brain circulation is feeble." If your system is irritated and hot, the warming and stimulating qualities of **valerian** may exacerbate the problem.

Finally, pharmacological studies show that **valerian** has a dual action depending on dosage. It's still worth trying. You will know after 3 or 4 nights of use whether or not it has value for you. If it does work, it induces a calm, restful sleep, and you awaken the next morning with no sense of a "drug hangover."

Research Highlights

- **Valerian root** interacts with GABA (gamma-aminobutyric acid) and benzodiazepine sites. At low concentrations **valerian extracts** enhance activity at specific sites, but at higher concentrations they inhibit the same sites (Ortiz et al., 1999).

- Based on reports from animal experiments demonstrating the ability of **valerian root** to cause vasodilation and relieve smooth muscle spasms (Hazelhoff et al., 1982), researchers performed a controlled clinical trial on 82 chronic heart disease patients with angina pectoris. The total effective rate in reducing symptoms was greater than 87%. **Valerian** was significantly superior to **salvia root** in short-term symptom reduction (Yang and Wang, 1994).

- In a randomized controlled clinical trial on 128 subjects, an aqueous extract of **valerian root** caused a significant improvement in sleep quality, most notably for people who were poor or irregular sleepers, smokers, and those who reported difficulty in falling asleep quickly (Leathwood et al., 1982). A follow-up study showed that **valerian root** is as effective at improving the ability to fall asleep quickly as barbiturates and benzodiazepine (Leathwood and Chauffard, 1985).

- In a controlled clinical trial, **valerian root** did not cause the side effect of morning-after sleepiness seen commonly with pharmacological sleep agents (Lindahl O and Lindwall, 1989).

- In a controlled double-blind clinical trial, **valerian root** in combination with **St. John's wort** was reported to be more effective than Valium (diazepam) (Newall et al., 1996).

VIBHITAKI FRUIT

Latin: *Terminalia belerica*   **Sanskrit:** Vibhitaki   **English:** Beleric myrobalan
Bibhitaki

WHAT IT DOES: Vibhitaki fruit is sour and astringent in taste and warming in action. It combines tonic qualities with action as a mild laxative that reduces inflammation and fever (Pitta), cough, and mucus (Kapha).

RATING:

- Sun-dried: gold
- Ripe: silver, due to laxative effect

SAFETY ISSUES: None known

STARTING DOSAGE:

- Dried powder: 2 grams two times per day
- 4:1 concentrated powder extract: 1 gram two times per day

Vibhitaki fruit comes from a large tree that grows in the subtropical mountainous climates of the Himalayas. **Vibhitaki fruit** is widely used in formulas for fevers, productive coughs, and general inflammation. It is part of the famous three-fruit tonic **triphala,** along with **amla fruit** and **haritaki fruit.** The fresh ripe fruit has a stronger laxative effect, while the sun-dried fruit is less laxative. The cooked or steamed fruit loses laxative action and becomes more astringent and binding.

Dr. A. Lakshmapathi applied **triphala powder** to a cut he sustained from a dirty razor, and covered it with a bandage. The cut completely healed within 72 hours with no evidence of a scar. After that, he used it for healing fresh surgical wounds with great success for many years. The tonic qualities of **vibhitaki fruit** are also used to aid in hair growth in parts of India. The fruit pulp can be applied directly over nontraumatic corneal ulcers.

Research Highlights

- The high level of tannins (17%) may partially account for its healing actions (reported in Kapoor, 1990).

- Alcohol extracts of 82 Indian medicinal plants were tested in vitro against several pathogenic and opportunistic microorganisms. Only five plants had a broad spectum as well as potent action, three of which were the fruits of **triphala**. Subsequent animal testing showed no cellular toxicity (Ahmad et al., 1998).

- Pharmacological studies show **vibhitaki fruit** lowers cholesterol in rabbits fed a high-cholesterol diet (Shaila et al., 1995).

- **Vibhitaki lignans** have demonstrated activity against malaria and fungal strains (Valsaraj et al., 1997).

- **Vibhitaki fruit** has shown antihistamine action against experimental asthma in animals (reported in Pandey, 1996).

- The Gerontology Research Center at the National Institutes of Health screened numerous Ayurvedic plants looking for new psychotherapeutic compounds active against various cellular receptors related to mental health. **Vibhitaki fruit** stood out, and was found to contain several active compounds which affected receptor sites which would tend to calm nervousness (Misra, 1998).

- It has shown antihistamine action against asthma in human clinical trials (Trivedi et al., 1982).

VILWA FRUIT

Latin: *Aegle marmelos*   **Sanskrit:** Vilwa / Bilwa   **English:** Vilwa tree

WHAT IT DOES: Vilwa fruit is sweet and astringent in taste and warming in action. It slowly heals difficult-to-cure chronic diarrhea.

RATING: Yellow, due to limitations in usage

SAFETY ISSUES: None known

STARTING DOSAGE:

- Dried powder: 2 grams two to three times per day
- 4:1 concentrated powder extract: 1 gram two times per day

Vilwa is a tropical and subtropical medium-sized thorny tree that produces fruit year-round. **Vilwa fruit** is one of those niche herbs that tend to work when nothing else does, in this case for the treatment of subacute and chronic intestinal malfunction. The raw, unripe fruit pulp is sweet and astringent in taste, and TAM doctors use it alone or in formulas to treat diarrhea, dysentery, chronic sprue, and amoebic dysentery.

I use it to treat cases of chronic diarrhea that don't respond to conventional or alternative treatments within a reasonable period of time. I don't usually use it right away, because it is important to try to correct underlying digestive system weakness, dietary errors, and other contributing factors. **Vilwa root bark and leaves** are bitter and astringent in taste and can be used in nerve disorders (to reduce Vata). It is also added to medicinal compounds used to treat and reduce colic pain and swelling.

> I once treated a very motivated and intelligent young patient who was going to the bathroom 10 times a day. She had consulted numerous doctors and had done everything possible to control the problem. She was taking more than two dozen different herbal and vitamin supplements, followed a sensible diet, exercised religiously, and corrected other metabolic problems. Nonetheless, she had daily episodes of diarrhea that resisted every remedy. I had her cut out all but the most essential of her dozens of daily pills and gave her a simple **vilwa fruit** prescription—4 500-mg capsules three times per day of the concentrated powder. After 2 weeks, the frequency of her diarrhea episodes decreased to every other day.

Research Highlights

- In a randomized double-blind controlled study of patients with irritable bowel syndrome (IBS), researchers administered a combination of **vilwa fruit** and **bacopa** that proved effective in 64.9% of patients, compared to only 32.7% in the placebo group.

The researchers concluded that this Ayurvedic therapy was "particularly beneficial in diarrhea predominant form as compared to placebo" (Yadav et al., 1989).

- **Vilwa fruit** is also selectively effective against hookworm and Raniket disease virus (reported in Pandey, 1996) but ineffective against shigellosis (Haider et al., 1991).

WHEAT SPROUTS

Latin: *Triticum* species   **English:** Wheat sprouts

WHAT IT DOES: Wheat sprouts are sweet in taste and cooling in action. They boost cellular antioxidants for detoxification.

RATING: Silver

SAFETY ISSUES: None known. Use cautiously if constipated.

STARTING DOSAGE:

- Dried sprouts: 2 to 3 grams twice per day on an empty stomach, taken with several glasses of water

Note: Use for periods of 3 to 6 weeks, then take a break.

The popularity of products known today as low-temperature-dried **wheat sprouts** began decades ago when Ann Wigmore of the Hippocrates Institute used **"wheat grass"** juice to treat numerous diseases, to all accounts with great success. It turns out that in their early stages of growth, **wheat sprouts** contain high levels of several important cellular antioxidants—glutathione peroxidase, catalase, methionine reductase, and superoxide dismutase. The scientific community was initially skeptical of this claim, as it was believed these nutrients were destroyed in the intestinal tract. Studies have subsequently shown that a small but significant portion of the antioxidants can be absorbed in the digestive tract.

> Sprouting is widely used in various cultures to improve the nutritional value of grain seeds. The practice appears to selectively increase the uptake of various trace elements.

I have used **wheat sprouts** with great success for rapid yet safe detoxification when patients show signs of accumulated inflammation due to long-term poor diet or exposure to chemicals. I usually treat them with 3 900-mg tablets twice per day for periods of 3 to 6 weeks. I instruct patients to drink a large volume of water, as the poisons seem to be flushed out through the urine. In some cases, patients will experience flulike symptoms for a period of 3 or 4 days, and often there is also a strong odor in the urine. After this inconvenience passes, seemingly intractable inflammations seem to melt away.

I have treated myself with various forms of **wheat grass** or **wheat sprouts** and I can verify that they have a fairly rapid (3–4 weeks) and noticeable detoxification effect. I felt a definite looseness and freedom of movement in my joints after treatment.

A close friend of mine had a severe plantar fasciitis (foot pad inflammation) which was resistant to a slew of different anti-inflammatory preparations, both natural and prescription. Six weeks on **wheat sprouts** decreased his pain by about 75%. I also saw a patient who enjoyed a temporary (1-year) but quite dramatic partial reversal of his graying hair using **wheat grass juice.** TCM doctors use **immature wheat seed** (fu xiao mai) to nourish the heart and calm the spirit when accompanied by symptoms of heart palpitations, irritability, and emotional instability.

WHITE ATRACTYLODES RHIZOME

Latin: *Atractylodes macrocephala*   **Chinese:** Bai zhu

WHAT IT DOES: White atractylodes rhizome is sweet and bitter in taste and warming in action. It strengthens the vital force, improves digestion, and aids in recovery from chronic illness or fatigue.

RATING: Gold

SAFETY ISSUES: None known

STARTING DOSAGE:

- Dried powder: 9 to 24 grams per day

- Concentrated powder: 1 to 4 grams per day

White atractylodes is perhaps the most commonly prescribed TCM herb for treating poor appetite and indigestion with signs of fatigue and/or diarrhea—the condition TCM doctors call spleen Qi deficiency. We use it in our clinic as a first-line digestive treatment. In Western countries, it is not as well known as other digestive herbs such as **bromelain, black pepper, ginger,** or pancreatic digestive enzymes.

> The related species called **black atractylodes** (cang zhu /*Atractylodes lancea* rhizome) is drier, excellent for drying digestive system dampness. It is often combined with **magnolia bark** (hou po) for epigastric fullness, reduced appetite, and vomiting.

According to TCM theory, **white atractylodes** directly enables the digestive system to do its job of transporting nutrients. Doctors often prescribed it with **ginseng root, pinellia tuber, tangerine peel, poria mushroom,** and **licorice root** in a classic digestive formula called "Six Gentlemen Decoction." Considering how many illnesses are related to digestive weakness, this herb is an important addition to the modern herbalist's repertoire.

Research Highlights

- In an experimental attempt to scientifically define the TCM concept called Spleen Qi deficiency, researchers examined the gastric mucosae of 247 patients. They reported "retrograded degeneration" of all kinds of antrum gastric mucosa cells, with 82.3% showing sparse, broken, and swollen mitochondria. The severity of the damage was more intense with patients who had additional Yang deficiency, as indicated by inflammation and vacuolation—holes in the tissue (Ren and Niu, 1992).

- Pharmacological and animal testing shows that **white atractylodes** increases secretion of gastric juices in the stomach and intestines, promotes urination, prevents glycogen loss in the liver, and increases body weight and muscle strength over time (reported in Bensky and Gamble, 1986; reported in Yeung, 1983).

- One clinical trial looked at patients with severe gastric disease caused by *Campylobacter pyloridis*. Patients in one group received one of two TCM medicines, either a combination of **astragalus root, white atractylodes,** and **white peony root** or **dandelion root** and **oldenlandia**. The other group received an antibiotic. The effective improvement rate was the same for both groups—about 80%. Pathology, endoscopic, and bacteriology tests showed differences between the two groups to be statistically insignificant (Fang, 1991).

WHITE PEONY ROOT

Latin: *Paeonia lactiflora*   **Chinese:** Bai shao

WHAT IT DOES: White peony root is bitter and sour in taste and cooling in action. It nourishes the blood of the liver, reduces pain, and soothes and clears the mind.

RATING: Gold

SAFETY ISSUES: Do not use if you have diarrhea.

STARTING DOSAGE:

- Dried powder: 2 grams two to three times per day

- Concentrated 4:1 dried decoction: 1 to 4 grams per day

White peony root is one of Nai-shing's favorite herbs. TCM herbalists rely on its nourishing and calming actions to treat nervousness, skin eruptions, anemia, painful menstruation, muscle spasms, and mental depression. The fact that this herb calms while enhancing cognition and reducing pain makes it very useful at our clinic. Nai-shing has often used the simple combination of **white peony root** and **licorice root** to reduce nerve pain, especially trigeminal neuralgia.

Research Highlights

- **White peony root** has been shown to lower testosterone levels in women but not men. In a study of seven infertile women, a simple combination of **white peony root** and **licorice root** induced regular ovulation in six of the subjects, two of whom subsequently conceived (reported in Bone, 1996).

- Several animal studies have demonstrated the muscle-relaxing effects of **white peony root** (reported in Bone, 1996).

- Animal studies have also demonstrated the cognition-enhancing effects of paeoniflorin, a major component of **white peony.** It has been shown to block chemically induced mental deficits in rats, allowing them to run mazes more quickly (Ohta et al., 1993), and to slow learning impairment in aged rats (Bone, 1996).

- Studies have identified **white peony root** as one of several Chinese herbs with the ability to improve memory by inhibiting prolyl endopeptidase (PEP), an enzyme that metabolizes several neurotransmitters (Tezuka et al., 1999).

- High-fat diets produce lipid peroxides, which inflame the linings of blood vessels and contribute to arteriosclerosis. In a 1991 study on rabbits, **white peony root** inhibited formation of the peroxides, correlating with a 74.2% reduction in aortic lesion size (Jia and Tang, 1991).

- A later study of rats on a high cholesterol diet showed a protective effect on the endothelial cells lining blood vessels. **White peony** caused an increase in vessel lining relaxation and a reduction in free radical damage (Goto et al., 1999).

- The combination of **salvia root** and **white peony root** has also been shown to protect rats against acute chemically induced liver damage (Qi, 1991).

WHITE SANDALWOOD

Latin: *Santalum album*   **Sanskrit:** Chandanam   **Chinese:** Tan xiang

WHAT IT DOES: White sandalwood is bitter in taste, aromatic, and cooling in action. It reduces fever, heat sensations, and dizziness. It also promotes the flow of vital energy (Qi) and relieves pain.

RATING: Silver

SAFETY ISSUES: Contraindicated in diseases involving the kidney parenchyma, due to its high volatile oil content. Do not use at full dose for longer than 6 weeks. Use cautiously with blood-thinning medication.

STARTING DOSAGE:

- Powdered heartwood: 1 to 2 grams two times per day

The highly fragrant heartwood of **white sandalwood** is burned as incense in Oriental temples as well as on funeral pyres. It contains volatile oils, dark resins, and tannic acid. It is a slow-growing parasitic tree that attaches its roots to those of other trees and draws water and minerals through a specialized structure called a haustorium.

Ayurvedic doctors use **white sandalwood** medicinally to treat fever, dizziness, heat sensation, and menopausal hot flashes. It is also used as an antipoison (visaghna) to reduce Pitta (inflammation) in various types of poisoning. TCM doctors use **white sandalwood** to promote the movement of Qi and to relieve pain. They also use it to treat stomach, chest, and abdominal pain and for vomiting.

> Following the TAM indications, I have used **white sandalwood** powder in the clinic successfully for hot flashes. I have also found the nose drops very effective for nasal inflammation. I often combine it with **red sandalwood** (rakta chandanam *Pterocarpus santalinus),* which aids its cooling action. Nai-shing uses it for the TCM indications, including stomach pain and painful menstruation.

White sandalwood incense is useful for relieving anxiety and depression and as a meditative aid. The oil can be applied as a cooling massage. The tea is a useful treatment for bladder and urinary tract infections. Make a tea by simmering 1 teaspoon of the powdered heartwood in water for 10 to 20 minutes. Drink 1 cup three or four times per day. When added to **sesame oil,** a few drops of **sandalwood oil** can be used as anti-inflammatory nose drops. Drop 2 or 3 drops in each nostril two to five times per day.

Research Highlights

- Chinese scientists have found **white sandalwood** useful for treating coronary artery disease (reported in Bensky and Gamble, 1993).

- Researchers have also found that oil from the wood enhances liver function in mice, increasing glutathione S-transferase (GST) activity and acid soluble sulphydryl (SH) levels. This suggests a possible internal protective action against chemicals (Bannerjee et al., 1993).

- Other studies have indicated **white sandalwood** as a potentially effective chemopreventive agent against skin cancer when used topically (Dwivedi and Abu-Ghazaleh, 1997).

WILD ASPARAGUS ROOT

Latin: *Asparagus racemosus*   **Sanskrit:** Shatavari   **Chinese:** Tian men dong
Asparagus lucidus

WHAT IT DOES: Wild asparagus root is sweet and slightly bitter in taste and cold in action. It calms the nerves, reduces inflammation, and protects and moistens the intestinal and lung membranes. It also promotes fertility and lactation.

RATING: Gold

SAFETY ISSUES: None known

STARTING DOSAGE:

- Crude powder: 1 to 2 grams two times per day
- Concentrated dried decoction: 500–1,000 mg two to three times per day

Wild asparagus root is a tropical and subtropical thorny, perennial, and tuberous shrub, sometimes growing as high as 20 feet. TAM doctors say the *racemosus* species calms the nerves, reduces inflammation, and strengthens the heart, brain, and mind. In our clinic we have found it quite effective for increasing breast milk production in nursing women and also for promoting fertility and nourishing the female reproductive system. We also use it whenever we see chronic inflammation combined with dryness and fatigue. It works well when administered with healthy oils such as those from **flaxseed** and fish in cases of dryness.

A simple Ayurvedic "mental clarity tonic" combines **wild asparagus** with eggs (preferably organic). I have made omelettes with the much milder grocery store asparagus, and I almost always note a mild increase in mental clarity over the next few hours (not that my brain isn't plenty clear already).

TCM doctors use a similar form of **wild asparagus root** *(lucidus* species) as a Yin tonic to replenish the vital essence, promote the secretion of body fluids, and moisten and nourish the lungs. They also mix it with honey to soothe the lungs and relieve coughs and bronchitis.

Research Highlights

- After exposing mice to the carcinogen ochratoxin A (OTA), researchers reported a significant decrease in the activity of their immune system macrophage cells, especially interleukins (activating chemicals) and tumor necrosis factor (TNF, a group of cancer-killing chemicals secreted by macrophages). Treatment with **wild asparagus root** significantly inhibited this suppression, as illustrated by increased production of TNF-alpha (Dhuley, 1997).

- Indian researchers performed a series of tests on six Ayurvedic tonic (rasayana) plants. They discovered that **wild asparagus root** exhibits adaptogenic and protective activities against a variety of chemical and environmental stressors. The effects were equivalent to those of **amla fruit, guduchi stem, ashwagandha root, long pepper,** and **vibhitaki fruit** (Rege et al., 1999).

- Pharmacological studies in China and India have shown **wild asparagus** to possess various anticancer, cardioprotective, and immune stimulating effects (reported in Pandey, 1996; reported in Yeung, 1983; Thatte and Dahanukar, 1998).

- **Wild asparagus root** also has shown a mild antacid effect on the stomach in humans and contains fat and carbohydrate digestive enzymes (Dalvi et al., 1990; Dange et al., 1969).

- Adhesions are a very problematic aftereffect of surgery. Based on its immunostimulant properties, researchers tested **wild asparagus root** for its ability to modulate this problem. Animals treated with the herb showed a significant increase in macrophages and, 15 days after surgery, a significant decrease in adhesion scores (Rege et al., 1989).

- Numerous human and animal studies, including randomized controlled trials, have confirmed the stimulating effect of **wild asparagus root** on breast milk production (Sharma et al., 1996; Pandey et al., 1996; Patel and Kanitkar, 1969; Sabnis et al., 1968; Joglekar et al., 1967).

- Interestingly, the *International Journal of Cancer* also reported an inhibitory effect on chemically induced breast cancer in rats (Rao, 1981).

SECTION

THREE

HERBS TO TREAT
THE WHOLE BODY

CHAPTER 9

Herbal Treatment: The Big Picture

Make everything as simple as possible, but not simpler.
—Albert Einstein

Every day, Nai-shing and I formulate treatment protocols specific to the individual needs of our patients. In this section I want to show you how we go about putting our knowledge to use in the clinic. In earlier chapters, I introduced you to how herbalists around the world solve real medical problems with scientific reliability. To do that, it was necessary for me to give you background information and basic vocabulary.

In Section One, we covered the basic herbal traditions, herb growth and preparation, safety issues, and some essential language tools. In Section Two, I introduced you to the most important and trusted herbs my wife and I use in our practice. This section may be a bit more technical, but you are now ready to understand it, so let's begin.

First of all, to treat real diseases, it is not enough to know what the individual herbs do. You must also incorporate diagnostic information, physiological knowledge, problem-solving skills, and guiding philosophical principles. We will explore a few of the main diagnostic and conceptual tools used by the three different medical systems I work with, all the while recognizing that we are navigating one small tributary of a wide herbal sea.

Now, let's examine some facets of our major herbal traditions.

- Our discussion of Traditional Chinese Medicine (TCM) will explore some of the concepts regarding causative factors, which are clinically very useful and are simple enough to begin to apply right away.

- Our discussion of Western medicine will examine blood testing, a practice of great value in understanding your health.

- Our discussion of Ayurveda will show you how these ancient truths are still relevant and valuable to modern medicine. I will go out on a limb here and reveal some evidence that may shock you into seeing the world in a different light.

• We will also examine how these three systems work together, including a simplified tongue and pulse diagnosis system appropriate for beginning and intermediate students.

Creating Herbal Solutions to Health Problems

When you are ready for herbal treatment, whether for yourself or for others, your first step is to examine the individual's health and identify problem areas. Most people could stand to make at least a few dietary and lifestyle changes to improve their health. Once you have identified the areas that need improvement, you can begin to develop a treatment protocol. Remember, you can always make adjustments along the way as you determine which therapies or regimens work best.

When it comes to the world of herbal therapy there are several levels of knowledge and expertise, beginning with the novice and ending with the skilled practitioner. It is important to identify your level so you know how to proceed.

Level 1: Rank Beginner. If you are completely clueless, but smart enough to know that you don't know, the best thing you can do is find a good natural medicine therapist and follow the advice you're given. Do some research on your own before choosing a practitioner. Get recommendations from people you trust. After working with a good herbal practitioner, your understanding will mature. See the Resource Guide for information on how to locate a practitioner.

Level 2: Educated Consumer. If you have already educated yourself in the basics of holistic medicine, you may want to get a good diagnosis from your doctor and research over-the-counter treatments as well. Once you are familiar with all the available options, you can make a choice whether to see a professional or begin to develop your own herbal protocol using the guidelines I've provided. When you have completed this book, you will be better equipped to sort through the wealth of information available. Don't fall into the trap of using a remedy that is "good for the liver" or "good for diabetes."

Most of the herbs I list are readily available in the consumer marketplace, but you may have difficulty tracking down a select few. If you're not sure how to obtain some of the herbs and preparations I've discussed, refer to the Resource Guide at the end of the book—you may find the answers there. If not, ask the manager or owner of your local natural foods store.

I would suggest starting slowly, incorporating just a few well-chosen single herbal or nutritional products along with the necessary and appropriate lifestyle changes. Depending on the results you want to achieve, it is possible that a combination product or formula already exists for your particular needs. Write out a list of the herbs I have recommended for your particular needs, and take it with you to the store. You may find a prepackaged formula (tincture or pills) that contains at least some if not all of the herbs you're looking for. Do not hesitate to seek out professional help if the problem is more complicated.

Level 3: Budding Herbalist. If you are a budding herbalist, you not only are self-educated, but may also have amassed a solid base of experience using various herbal medicine therapies. You may not feel limited to pills and capsules. You may want to try combining a group of herbs in a formula after studying each one carefully. This will require you to find reliable sources for some of the more exotic Chinese and Ayurvedic herbs. (See the Resource Guide for sources of most of the herbs I use.) The herbs may not all be available in the same form, so be creative.

For example, if you compile a list of 10 herbs you want to use, and find that 7 are available as crude powders and 3 as tinctures, it may be necessary to make a tea from the crude herbs and add the tinctures to the tea before drinking. If you have a serious health problem, consult with a qualified health care practitioner; don't trick yourself into thinking you can treat nephritis compounded by liver disease at home.

> Let's say you've determined that you are suffering from nervous exhaustion. You read that my favorite "nerve tonics" include **ashwagandha root** (both forms), **milky oat seed, skullcap,** and **American ginseng root.** Before you go out and buy all the crude herbs and prepare each one separately, see if you can find one or more of the herbs either by themselves (as tinctures or pills) or in combination products. For example, you might come across an "Herbal Relax" tincture that contains **milky oat seed** *(Avena)* and **skullcap** along with four or five others. You could use any of the herbs alone or in combination to treat nervous exhaustion.

Level 4: Skilled Therapist or Physician. If you are a skilled therapist or physician looking for solutions to health problems faced by your patients, you may recognize the inherent difficulties in trying to match herbs with patients in the real world. You probably already have good sources for herbal materials and utilize a system of clinical and differential diagnosis. Either you have already explored the patient's health condition and understand the underlying causative factors, or you're in the process of working this out.

Now, you can read about my personal approach to each specific disease process and note the herbs I recommend for treatment. Then you can do your own supplemental research to identify and select only those herbs that match your patient's particular needs.

Skilled practitioners entering from a scientific discipline background must also recognize the philosophy of herbal medicine, which includes attention to your patients' emotional and spiritual needs, in addition to their physical and dietary requirements. Herbal medicine is more than herbs.

Please note that within the discussion of each disease, I have identified important causative factors, as well as possible herb choices, if those factors are relevant in a particular case.

Diagnosis: Signs, Symptoms, and Specifics

Classification and Diagnosis

The general public is most accustomed to approaching health conditions by diagnostic category or name, such as *asthma, diabetes,* or *arthritis.* This is often the standard approach of Western medicine, and it is important. In fact, a specific and clear diagnosis based upon physiology is very, very important. If someone has eye pain, for example, it is important to make sure a hidden tumor or chemical poisoning is not the cause.

However, although diagnostic terms offer us important information about the problem, it is often not enough to help us determine the proper herbal treatment. In fact, although we do not usually realize it, each of us is bound by often-unexamined beliefs about the nature and meaning of disease drawn from our culture and upbringing.

For example, a diagnosis of asthma seems to clearly tell us that the patient has trouble breathing. However, it does not tell us the level of inflammation in the lungs, the amount of mucus in the lungs, the amount of tension in the surrounding muscles, the level of diaphragm use or disuse, or anything about contributing causes such as exposure to toxins or cigarette smoke. Therefore, you cannot simply take "asthma" herbs and expect good results.

To understand how an herbalist or trained holistic doctor thinks, you must first recognize that diseases can be examined, diagnosed, and treated from different points of view. When a practitioner draws ideas from a system of thought, whether Western, naturopathic, Ayurvedic, or Chinese, we say the prescribed treatment is based upon **signs** and **symptoms.**

We define a **symptom** as any departure from normal structure, function, or sensation experienced by the patient. The most important part of this definition is the phrase "experienced by the patient."

We define a **sign** as a change in the normal structure or function of the body that can be discovered by examination. The focus of this definition is the idea that a sign is "discoverable by examination."

Symptoms are subjective, while signs are objective and usually more physiologically specific. Symptoms and signs do not quantify the disease. Rather, they should lead to an accurate understanding of the underlying cause.

Causative Factors

In Western medicine, causation is related to morbid changes in the biochemical or physical structure and function of the body. Determining the cause requires data collection (urine, stool, images, subjective and objective findings, etc.) and systematic comparison and contrast of the findings until a diagnosis can be made.

In TCM, causation *(bing yin)* is related to "patterns of imbalance" which are discovered by the signs and symptoms as understood in this system. Determining the pattern requires a questioning process along with pulse and tongue observation to define the nature or mechanism of the imbalance (e.g., deficient, excess, cold, hot, wind), and the location (e.g., internal organs, blood, energy meridians) of the imbalance.

In TAM, causation (hetu) is related to aggravating agents (foods, behaviors, emotional changes, seasonal influences, physical injuries, etc.) that cause either direct physical damage or an imbalance in **Vata, Pitta,** and/or **Kapha** which leads to the emergence of **doshas** *(pathogenic defects)*. Determining the imbalance requires questioning, observation, and testing to define the prognosis, symptoms, and anatomical dysfunction. Diseases are defined both by specific name (as in Western medicine) and by the nature and location of the doshas.

Understanding the TCM Causative Factors

TCM doctors use several basic ideas beyond **Yin, Yang,** and **Qi** (discussed in Chapter 6) to assist in their diagnoses and herb choices. As I mentioned earlier, these terms are effectively used to describe the external world we live in, as well as conditions that can penetrate and reside in the body.

Deficiency and **excess** are basic TCM medical terms. In diseases of deficiency, there is a preexisting weakness in the tissues or immune system that creates a hypersensitivity to normal conditions. In excess conditions, the disease is due to causative factors like stress or toxins that congest or overcome normal resistance.

> **Yang** diseases tend to be external, excessive, hot, and dry in nature. **Yin** diseases tend to be internal, deficient, cold, and damp in nature.

For example, a high cholesterol level is a disease of deficiency if caused by a weak thyroid (which slows down the metabolism). Conversely, the same condition is a disease of excess if caused by a dietary excess of poor-quality fats.

One well-known health problem that can help us understand how deficiency can cause what appears to be a feverlike condition are the hot flashes that often accompany menopause. Everyone recognizes that you cannot effectively use anti-inflammatory Western medicines or strongly cooling herbs to stop hot flashes. This is a deficiency problem—it is actually the hormonal decreases occurring during menopause that create this problem. Hence, it is necessary to use estrogen replacements or herbs that supplement and nourish the deficiency.

The different way each person's body responds to illness has important implications for diagnosis and treatment. For example, just because two patients suffer from hypertension doesn't mean you can prescribe the same herbs to treat both of them! If one is a 96-pound, 80-year-old grandmother, and the other looks like Arnold Schwarzenegger, you obviously need to account for differences in their body size, strength, and general state of health before recommending a treatment.

- Diseases of deficiency are usually treated with nourishing tonics.

- Diseases of excess are usually treated with herbs that remove the excess or stimulate the excretory organs to do so.

Heat and **cold** have already been described in terms of the herbal energetics, or the actions of herbs. Some herbs are described as heating and some as cooling. Similarly, diseases can be hot (inflammatory) and hypermetabolic in nature, or cold and hypometabolic.

TCM doctors explain the difference between internal and external heat and cold. External heat results from an influence outside of the body, as when the skin is inflamed by the sun. Internal heat results from internal disturbance, fever, or toxins. External cold results from an outside influence, as when the body gets chilled due to low air temperature. Internal cold results from a metabolic weakness inside the body, as when the thyroid is underactive.

- Hot conditions are treated with cooling herbs.

- Cold conditions are treated with warming herbs.

Dampness refers to an accumulation of fluids in the body. When the dampness resides in the outer muscles and tissues, you feel stiff and swollen, often with dull pain and edema. If the dampness resides in the digestive system, you might feel nausea and sluggish digestion. If the dampness resides in the lungs, you will feel heaviness and air hunger. Dampness has three basic levels in Chinese thinking. The first is simple fluid accumulation. Second is thicker, partially congealed dampness. Third is a thicker, viscous accumulation of mucus.

- Dampness is treated with herbs that remove dampness or break up mucus, or herbs that increase metabolism to drive out the dampness. TCM doctors also use herbs that stimulate Qi to drive out the dampness.

Dryness is the opposite of dampness and can be caused when heat and inflammation dry out the bodily fluids, or when blood supply to the tissue(s) is poor.

- Dryness is treated with herbs that moisten, or herbs that nourish the blood.

Wind refers to disturbances of the nervous system, which result in symptoms like spasms, paralysis, dizziness, shaking, convulsions, and nervous tension and/or irregular functioning in individual organs or systems. Pains or tensions that quickly move from one area to another are also attributed to wind by TCM doctors, as well as certain skin and liver problems. TAM doctors look for signs of gas or swelling in tissues or in the abdomen that yield to external pressure and bounce back.

Basic Treatment Guidelines

- If you are treating a deficiency condition, choose herbs that are nourishing and tonifying.
- If you are treating a condition of excess, choose herbs that are detoxifying.
- If you are treating a hot condition, use herbs that are cooling.
- If you are treating a cold condition, use herbs that are stimulating and warming.
- If you are treating a damp condition, use herbs that reduce mucus and swelling.
- If you are treating a dry condition, use herbs that are moistening and nourishing.
- If you are treating a windy condition, use herbs that are calming and antispasmodic.

These ideas show that the TCM, Western, and TAM conceptualization of "wind" are a bit different. I consider the Ayurvedic approach the clearest, so I use it in my practice. However, if I am reading about or using TCM herbs, I defer to their understanding to fully grasp how and why they would choose a particular herb. The same is true when I am choosing Western herbs.

- Wind is treated in TAM with herbs that calm, warm, and nourish. They also reduce Vata dosha. In TCM, wind is heated with herbs that nourish the blood, herbs that remove heat from the liver, or herbs that nourish the Liver Yin. Western herbalists treat wind with antispasmodic and nervine herbs.

Making TCM Causative Factors Real and Useful

It is easiest to understand how causative factors "exist" during most disease processes when we combine them to describe a problem. For example, if you have a fever and a chest cold with thin green phlegm, this is a heat-and-mucus condition. If you have a fever and a spasmodic cough, this is a wind-and-heat condition. I use this simple system of classification not only to help me prescribe herbs, but also to aid in selecting appropriate diets during illness.

- For a spasmodic cough with fever, a TCM doctor would use herbs that remove wind and heat from the lungs.

- For knee and ankle swelling that "bounces back" when pressed, indicating trapped gas, the TAM doctor would use an appropriate swelling treatment (Kapha-reducing diuretic herbs) along with herbs that reduce Vata.

- For painful urination with a "funny smell," a Western holistic doctor or a naturopath would order a urinalysis to culture for infectious organisms, do blood tests to check for metabolic problems, and prescribe herbs or antibiotics based upon results.

The Importance of Scientific Diagnostics

As mystified as people are with Oriental medical concepts, I have seen just as many if not more people mystified by Western diagnostic concepts and tests. Blood tests, for example, are windows into your health, because your blood interacts with just about every cell in your body. Equally important as Yin or Yang, these tests are excellent ways to measure the benefits or failure of herbal treatment, providing—in conjunction with symptom changes—guidance to your caretakers.

Over the past 70 years, scientists have made tremendous progress in disease diagnosis and in our understanding of pathological processes. Good diagnostics are a vital part of holistic medicine. At our clinic we see many patients after they have received a diagnosis from Western-trained doctors, and we also send patients out to Western specialists when we find a need for further diagnosis. Oftentimes, using specific scientific diagnostics in conjunction with herbal signs and symptoms can be critically useful for choosing the correct treatment protocol, herbal or otherwise.

I remember a particular case where a patient came to Nai-shing for acupuncture and herbal treatment for severe spinal pain. Nai-shing recognized there was something seriously wrong and immediately referred the patient to one of the physicians with whom we work. He discovered a tumor on the patient's spine. In this case, the doctor's specialized skill was instrumental in saving the patient's life.

Today, as the study of herbs continues, we know much more about the specific biochemical actions of herbs. Therefore, if someone has, for example, a deficiency of a particular blood component, such as platelets or red blood cells, we can choose herbs that have been shown to improve those blood parameters. I discuss this in more detail in Chapters 12 and 19.

The following is a simplified explanation of the most common blood tests that your doctor may run. Good physicians will explain these tests to you, and as a patient you have the right to get copies for your own edification. Normally you will find reference ranges next to your test results in each category, so you can see if your numbers fall within normal values.

Complete Blood Count (CBC). This test measures the total number of red and white blood cells. It works with percentages and analyzes them in different ways. The CBC includes a number of different tests and measures your numbers against average values in each area to determine if they are high or low.

1. *RBC test.* Measures the number of red blood cells in a given volume of blood. Your red blood cells carry oxygen to your tissues. A low count of red blood cells can indicate blood loss, reduced RBC production (often due to nutritional deficiencies), or increased RBC destruction.

2. *WBC test.* Measures the number of white blood cells. A low white cell count can often

be attributed to the same general causes as for RBCs and may indicate immune system deficiency. An increased white count may indicate that the body is fighting an infection.

3. *HGB test.* Measures your RBC hemoglobin, a protein that carries oxygen and carbon dioxide. A low level of hemoglobin indicates a reduced ability to carry oxygen, which can be caused by many chemical factors such as auto fumes, toxic gases, cigarette smoke, and blood loss. Elevated levels can indicate vitamin B_{12} deficiency.

4. *HCT test.* Measures hematocrit, the proportion of RBCs in your blood. A low hematocrit count indicates anemia, possibly due to nutritional deficiencies.

5. *MCV test.* Measures the average size of your RBCs (mean corpuscular volume). The RBCs can swell up in response to inflammation, liver disease, or even abnormal production problems in the bone marrow. This increased MCV often causes them to die off faster, leading to anemia. When cells are too small (low MCV), it can often indicate nutritional deficiencies.

Individual White Blood Cell Tests. The segmented neutrophil test, lymphocyte test, monocyte test, eosinophil test, and basophil test are all different types of WBC tests. These cells are easily depleted by infections or chemical stress, so if these numbers are low, or imbalanced with too many of any one type and not enough of another, it usually indicates some type of physical or chemical stress. This phenomenon is directly related to immune system deficiency, which we will discuss in more detail in our discussion of the immune system in Chapter 19.

Platelet Test. Platelets are small corpuscles that participate in the blood-clotting process. Low numbers may indicate bone marrow or autoimmune problems. High numbers may indicate poor spleen function.

Blood Chemistries. Blood chemistry tests look for different substances normally found in your blood serum.

1. *TC (total cholesterol) test.* There are several different types of lipids (fats) in your blood. This test measures the blood level of a particular lipid called cholesterol. Elevated levels may increase your risk of arteriosclerosis, stroke, and heart attack.

2. *HDL (high-density lipoprotein) test.* The high-density lipoprotein is a good and important fat. I tell people to remember this as "Happy DL." If levels are low, it indicates a greater risk of cardiac artery disease. Things that can lower HDL include lack of exercise, genetic factors, and chemical drugs.

3. *LDL (low-density lipoprotein) test.* LDL is bad cholesterol, which I tell patients to

remember by calling it "Lousy DL." People with LDL levels that are too high are at greater risk of developing heart disease.

4. *Glucose test.* This test measures the amount of sugar in your blood. Elevated levels indicate poor glycemic control or diabetes, and low levels can indicate the presence of hypoglycemia.

5. *Triglyceride test.* This test measures a type of blood fat that is usually elevated due to a dietary sugar excess.

6. *Uric acid test.* Uric acid is a waste product from nucleotide metabolism. Uric acid is actually an antioxidant, produced by your body in response to inflammation. High levels indicate the presence of gout or arthritis, and occasionally kidney disease or leukemia.

7. *Total protein test.* Proteins are manufactured and used by your body for innumerable processes related to growth, repair, and defense. Elevated levels can indicate problems in the liver, kidneys, or general metabolism, while low levels often indicate nutritional deficiency conditions.

7a. *Albumin test.* Elevated levels of this protein relate to dehydration, while lowered levels relate to malnutrition, poor absorption, liver and kidney disease, and metastatic cancers.

7b. *Globulin test.* Elevated levels indicate lupus, melanoma, liver disease, and sarcoidosis. Lowered levels indicate immune system deficiency.

7c. *A/G ratio.* This is the ratio between albumin and globulin. A lowered ratio is indicated in severe inflammation or infection, liver disease, colitis, kidney disease, diabetes, and metastatic cancers.

8. *Calcium test.* Calcium in your blood is necessary to maintain bone metabolism and numerous other metabolic processes. Deficiency can relate to heart palpitations, muscle spasms, bone loss or bone diseases, inflammation, vitamin D deficiency, and so on.

9. *Inorganic phosphorus test.* Elevated levels of phosphorus are found in parathyroid problems, bone and calcium metabolism problems, diabetic acidosis, and some forms of kidney disease.

10. *Bilirubin total test.* This test measures the ability of the liver and spleen to break down and eliminate dead red blood cells. Elevated levels indicate liver disease or certain types of anemia.

10a. *Bilirubin direct.* Elevated levels are related to obstructions, such as obstructive jaundice, gallstones, and tumors.

10b. ***Bilirubin indirect.*** Elevated levels indicate liver diseases, anemia, or gallbladder disease.

11. ***BUN (Blood urea nitrogen) test.*** This test measures the ability of the liver and kidneys to eliminate the by-products of protein metabolism. Elevated levels are seen in adrenal, liver, thyroid, and anterior pituitary dysfunction. Low levels are seen in posterior pituitary dysfunction.

12. ***Creatinine test.*** This test measures the ability of your kidneys to excrete a by-product of muscle metabolism. Increased levels are seen in kidney failure, urinary obstruction, dehydration, muscle diseases, and hyperthyroidism.

13. ***BUN/creatinine ratio.*** This test is a measure of kidney function. Elevated levels can mean kidney disease, excess protein, insufficient fluid intake, and prostate swelling (BPH).

14. ***Sodium test.*** Sodium is related to maintenance of calcium-phosphorus ratios and acid-alkaline balance. Elevated levels are related to dehydration, excess salt intake, and kidney diseases. Low levels are related to low adrenal function, heart failure, and vomiting.

15. ***Potassium test.*** Potassium is essential to heart and kidney function. Elevated levels are related to acidosis, adrenal deficiency, pharmaceutical side effects, and kidney disease. Decreased levels are found in liver cirrhosis, malnutrition, alkalosis, diarrhea, fatigue, irregular heartbeat, and kidney diseases.

16. ***Carbon dioxide test.*** CO_2 levels are related to blood acid and alkaline balance. As levels rise, hemoglobin decreases leading to oxygen starvation. Elevated levels are found in lung disease and alkalosis, and low levels are found in acidosis, inflammation, or hyperventilation.

17. ***Magnesium test.*** Magnesium is an important mineral for many metabolic processes. Low levels can indicate diarrhea, muscle or other spasms, poor nutrition, heart irregularity, and diabetes.

18. ***SED rate.*** The sedimentation rate test measures clumping of red blood cells. It elevates when there is an infection or inflammation anywhere in the body. It does not indicate where the inflammation is, only its existence.

Blood Enzymes. Enzyme levels in your blood act as markers for damage to various tissues. Elevated levels indicate problems in specific areas, especially with your liver.

1. ***LDH test.*** This test measures lactate dehydrogenase, an enzyme that is widely distributed in the body. Elevated levels indicate heart tissue destruction (heart attack), anemia, leukemia, malignancies, brain or muscle damage, seizure activity, and liver damage.

2. *ALT (SGPT) test.* This enzyme (alanine aminotransferase) is related to liver metabolism, and elevates in liver congestion, hepatitis, cirrhosis, liver cancer, severe inflammation, chemical or drug exposure, and pancreatitis.

3. *AST (SGPT) test.* This enzyme (aspartate aminotransferase) elevates in heart inflammation, heart attack, liver diseases, trauma, pericarditis, pancreatitis, seizures, and chemical or drug exposure.

4. *Alk Phos test.* This enzyme (alkaline phosphatase) measures metabolism in bone, liver, and tumor cells. It elevates in prostate cancer, prostatitis, heart attack, excessive platelet destruction, and liver or bone diseases.

In our practice we use these blood tests extensively to monitor the progress of our patients. If a patient has hepatitis, we monitor their liver enzymes. If a patient has an immune system deficiency, we monitor the white blood cell counts. Because herbs are so effective at lowering elevated liver enzymes and raising WBC counts, this is a perfect example of the integration of systems.

Ayurveda Made "Real"

Vata, Pitta, and Kapha in Diagnosis and Treatment

I remember attending a conference with a budding holistic M.D. many years ago. As I talked to him about Vata, Pitta, and Kapha, I could see him growing impatient. Finally he said, "I'm trying to remain open-minded. But, frankly, I'm fed up with ethers, auras, Yin, Yang, Kapha, and Qi. Let's get real."

I understand his dilemma. The modern mind finds these terms primitive. We feel more comfortable calling confusion "cognitive dissonance." The word "ulcer" sounds better to us than "fire in the stomach." However, our primary interest is in the meaning behind the terms. The job of a good translator is to change the words without altering the underlying meaning, and to find ways to make unfamiliar concepts clear.

The question I want to tackle here is, "Do the concepts behind Ayurveda's divisions have a basis in physical reality?" I think that they do, and this becomes clear when we change the words a bit and examine some lesser-known areas of biology. When we examine large patterns, we must by necessity lose a certain amount of detail. However, it is a mistake to think that these simplified concepts can completely grasp the complexity of life. They cannot.

They can, however, at the clinical level, help us find order within the complexity and see relationships that are otherwise hidden.

In other words, we need some background before we can understand the Ayurvedic divisions as more than folklore or contrived religious concepts. My teacher, Dr. Mana, like all Ayurvedic physicians, firmly believes that the ancient ideas are based in philosophy (actually spiritual knowledge discovered by sages) but exist in harmony with physical realities. Like TCM and Western herbology, the concepts lead to successful prescriptions and cures. Essentially, Vata, Pitta, and Kapha as well as Yin, Yang, and Qi are methods that allow you to see what is out of balance.

However, to remain truly universal, and to avoid materializing these ancient concepts, we have to consider a few more ideas. Can we find Vata, Pitta, and Kapha elsewhere in the world of biology? Can these terms help us to see things that we could not see before? Remember first that the concepts behind Vata, Pitta, and Kapha describe three elemental processes or energies understood since ancient times as regulatory, destructive (transformation or energy), and creative (growth), respectively. The organism is a whole that lives in dynamic relationship to these processes, and thus itself is arguably a regulated process, and not a "thing." In time this translates as processes of absorption, transformation, and production. For example, the eye can absorb a photon of light and transform it into a molecular cascade of reactions, which result in the production of a neural electrical impulse. The digestive system absorbs nutrients and transforms them through a different cascade into our physical structures.

The same three aspects can also be identified in the spatial organization of an embryo. Consider that in the early stages of embryonic development, human cells divide into three primary germ layers, called ectoderm, mesoderm and endoderm. The ectoderm develops into our entire nervous system (Vata). Our metabolic heart, muscle, bone, urogenital, and vascular (blood and lymph) systems (Pitta) arise from the mesoderm. Our nutrient-absorbing digestive tract (Kapha) develops from the endoderm. All (and I mean all) organs and cells in our body develop out of these three layers. Is it not possible to consider these three primary germ cells as progenitors of three large metasystems that maintain a systemic integrity throughout life? What we normally consider to be organs are actually subsystems within these three. In this way of thinking, might we consider these germ layers to be our metaorgans? Further, might they not maintain a systemic integrity throughout our life spans?

The prefixes *endo-*, *ecto-*, and *meso-* refer to locations. *Endo-* means inner, *ecto-* means outer, and *meso-* means intermediate. As we move inwardly into the organism we see the same divisions in the form of an almost infinite hierarchy of nested compartments, all with insides, outsides, and middles. Thus, our individual cells have smaller organelles within them, such as the nucleus and the mitochondria. Some physicists believe (and offer mathematical proof) that this pattern of nesting is necessary to maintain thermodynamic and biochemical equilibrium within living organisms (Ho, 1998).

What happens if we move outward? Let's consider the work of Wolfgang Schad, the brilliant German zoologist. (Allow the *Twilight Zone* theme song to play through your head as you read this.) In his book *Man and Mammals: Toward a Biology of Form,* Schad describes how relative differences in these three primary systems explain much about mammalian physiology. Schad notes that not only are there three primary organic systems operating *within* mammalian organisms, but these "systems" can also be seen *without,* in the three largest external groupings of Western Hemisphere mammals—the rodents (Vata), the carnivores (Pitta), and the ungulates (Kapha), which together comprise more than 70% of mammals in this area.

- **Vata animals.** Rodent physiology (mice, squirrels, beavers, etc.) emphasizes nervous system development. Small in size, they are known to have *restless* and *highly sensitive* natures.

- **Kapha animals.** Ungulate physiology (cows, horses, pigs, deer, etc.) emphasizes digestive processes. They are large in size, with *passive* temperaments. The multiple stomachs of the cow constitute a striking example.

- **Pitta animals.** Carnivore physiology (lions, tigers, weasels, etc.) emphasizes metabolic and energetic processes. *Predatory* and *aggressive* in nature, these animals epitomize energy and power.

The late Sufi writer Indres Shah was once questioned by a disgruntled critic who was offended that a story Shah told led him to challenge his own beliefs. He asked why, in his stories, the Sufis (sages) always win, implying that Shah's examples were selectively chosen to distort. In essence, Shah replied, "For the same reason that, although in real life people do make math mistakes, and mathematical theories can be disproved, the calculation examples in math books always add up correctly to help the students learn." He then pointed out that the questioner's challenging emotional attitude and form of questioning served as an effective block to the learning process.

Schad pointed out that cows' horns are actually teeth that have moved up (note that canines are nowhere to be found in cow dentition!). He then revealed that the tripartite divisions within and without all mammals could even be recognized within the subgroups.

Thus, within the large ungulates, we have divisions into the superdocile cows, the more aggressive swine, and the relatively nervous high-strung horses. And within the small nervous rodents, we have the more sensitive mice, the more docile squirrels, and the more aggressive porcupines. Finally, even within the sensitive mouse group, we have the supersensitive harvest and field mice (Vata), the larger, more docile hamsters (Kapha), and the obviously more aggressive rats (Pitta).

Ayurveda in Cell Biology

If my attempt to link ancient philosophy with modern science is to succeed, I must show that these basic patterns occur in other places, such as at the cellular level. It is easy to find Vata (regulation), Pitta (energy release), and Kapha (growth) in the individual cell. The nucleus, containing the master blueprint DNA, is obviously a regulatory (Vata) center. The cell membrane regulates the import and export of nutrient molecules—the raw materials for growth (Kapha). And in the cytoplasm of each cell we see the many organelles involved in a variety of energy and production processes, including hundreds of mitochondria, our ultimate energy (Pitta) source, providing cyclical energy to transform raw materials into useful ones.

When we look at cells from a structural point of view, we see that fatty acids (Kapha) are the major building blocks of the membranes, sugars called "nucleosides" are the building blocks of DNA and RNA (Vata), and amino acids are the building blocks of our worker bee proteins (Pitta). We will discuss the three main macronutrients, fats, carbohydrates, and proteins, in the next chapter.

One of the hottest areas in biology is research into "molecular cell signaling systems." Molecules travel through the body until they reach receptor sites on cells where they bind and regulate cell responses. The vast majority of signaling molecules (like mammals) belong to one of three large families. All signaling molecules start off as Vata or regulatory phenomena. It appears that cells respond to three types of basic signals.

- **Ion channel-linked receptors (Vata).** Stimulation of these sites alters the flow of ions, producing an electrical effect. They are the receptors that control voltage changes related to neurotransmission.

- **G-protein-linked receptors (Pitta).** Stimulation of these cell membrane sites generally causes increases in energy activation, including cyclic AMP (which energizes nerve cells as one function), sugar breakdown (which increases energy production), accelerated heartbeat, and activation of cellular response to light and smells.

- **Enzyme-linked receptors (Kapha).** Stimulation of these receptor sites causes activation of growth factors, proteins that regulate cell growth, proliferation, and differentiation in our tissues.

Ayurvedic Body Types

With the background information just provided, it should now be easier to recognize and understand the existence of the three Ayurvedic body types as one expression of the tripartite patterns found throughout mammalian physiology. My experience in learning to distinguish these body types has helped me greatly in my clinical practice. It was not easy at first; in fact, it took me more than 2 years to be able to identify a patient's body and energy type quickly at the time of first meeting. New clients are amazed when they hear their basic personality traits since childhood described in detail after you've met them only 5 minutes ago.

- **Vata** types are sensitive and restless in nature, generally high in intelligence, thinner (due to weaker digestion), and prone to nervousness and fatigue when ill.

- **Pitta** types are aggressive and strong-willed in nature, generally hot, highly energized and physically strong (due to strong metabolism), and prone to inflammatory conditions when ill.

- **Kapha** types are slow and stable in nature, generally heavy and solid physically (due to strong digestion), and prone to mucus and "sluggish" conditions when ill.

General Guidelines for Herb Use Based on Body Type

- Sensitive Vata types should use lower doses of herbs and should use warming, calming, and nourishing herbs.

- Strong-willed Pitta types should use higher doses of herbs and use more cooling and detoxifying herbs.

- Slow, stable Kapha types should use more warming, spicy, energizing, and mucus-reducing herbs.

It is difficult to use this theory properly unless you realize that everyone contains all three within themselves and that many people are **Vata-Pitta, Vata-Kapha,** and **Pitta-Kapha.** If you are not sure of your body type, use the process of elimination. If you need more help in figuring out your body type, see the book *Ayurvedic Healing* by Dr. David Frawley.

Ayurveda in the Clinic

Dr. Mana has taken the Ayurvedic concepts further, focusing on internal regulation. He points out that each organ and system in the body has arteries, nerves, and veins that regulate its health. Vata, as the regulator of movement, can be equated with nervous system control. Kapha, as regulator of creative processes, can be equated with (or seen in action within) the body's arterial supply of nutrients. Pitta, as regulator of destructive processes, can be equated with venous drainage of fiery metabolic wastes. These direct associations help us gain a practical clinical understanding of Ayurveda. Each organ can be discussed in terms of how well the nervous system is doing its job (Vata), whether or not the organ or body system has sufficient or excessive nutrient and fluid supply (Kapha), and whether or not it is efficiently producing energy and draining away inflammation and waste (Pitta).

Following Ayurvedic logic, destructive agents, such as unhealthful foods, germs, viruses, and toxins, enter the body or are internally generated during metabolism, after which they mix with normal gases, bile, and mucus. These bodily components then act as carriers for both pathogens (waste) and nutrients. When the effects of pathogens exceed the body's ability to detoxify and excrete (through urine, feces, sweat, exhalation, etc.) they begin to overpower their carriers.

Ayurvedic doctors monitor the health of the body through careful observation of these components. Any emergence of physical symptoms or changes in the organism as a whole indicates that a corruption, blockage, or alteration has occurred.

For example, if the liver cannot sufficiently detoxify, then the bile becomes toxic, and inflammation or heat increases. If the digestive system cannot fully and completely excrete heavier substances, then dampness or mucus begins to accumulate. If the body as a whole or individual cells cannot fully, completely, or properly respire, toxic gases begin to accumulate. It is through the physical manifestation of signs and symptoms that the doctor can identify and correct the cause of the problem.

Tongue Diagnosis

The eyes may be the windows of your soul, but your tongue is the window of your digestive system. When you eat, your teeth decimate food by crunching it like giant hydraulic presses with jagged steel edges, while your tongue darts around and wallows in the food. During its immersion in the food bath, your tongue sends signals to the digestive system about the tastes and other qualities of the food. Think of the whole system, from the tongue to the stomach, as one long, continuous membrane. As the digestive tract undergoes various changes in its state of health, these changes are physically reflected in the tongue.

The following simple observations can help you diagnose conditions that may exist in the digestive tract:

- A **swollen** tongue may indicate dampness.

- A **dry** tongue may indicate inflammation and/or dehydration.

- A **redder-than-normal** tongue may indicate heat and inflammation.

- A **pale** tongue may indicate blood deficiency or anemia.

- A **blue** tongue may indicate thick stagnant blood, insufficient oxygen, or poor circulation.

- A **small, thin** tongue (as if it has shrunk) may indicate Yin (nutrient) deficiency.

- A **thick white coating** on the tongue may indicate mucus.

- A **thin white coating** may indicate cold and dampness.

- A **thick, yellow greasy coating** may indicate heat and dampness.

- A **puffy and swollen** tongue with **visible tooth marks** may indicate weak digestion.

- **Redness around the edges** of the tongue may indicate liver inflammation.

- **Swelling and a bluish tint** of the large veins on the back of the tongue (you can see this when you curl the tongue up) may indicate blood congestion.

- A **withered and quivering** tongue may indicate severe deficiency and nervous exhaustion.

These signs should never be taken alone as definitive diagnoses. They are pieces of information that must be corroborated by other signs and symptoms to form a diagnosis and treatment protocol.

The Pulse

The pulse is another tool herbalists use to diagnose general health conditions. The same cautions I offered about tongue diagnosis apply here as well. TCM pulse diagnosis is a highly specialized skill and takes years to develop. In Ayurveda, doctors use pulse diagnosis to assess the levels of imbalance in Vata, Pitta, and Kapha. Western doctors use pulse diagnosis primarily to determine the condition of the heart.

The following rules may help simplify your understanding of the pulse and its diagnostic value:

- A **fast** pulse may indicate inflammation or fever if bounding (Pitta) or nervousness if weak (Vata).

- A **slow, weak** pulse may indicate Qi deficiency (energy depletion).

- A **slow, strong** pulse may indicate that the person has a strong heart, and possibly is an athlete.

- A **tense or wiry pulse** (like plucking a guitar string) may indicate nervous tension or energy restriction.

- A **pulse floating close to the surface** may indicate the early stages of an infection.

- A **slow, soggy, or slippery pulse** (which tries to slip away from the doctor's touch) may indicate mucus and dampness.

- A **thin pulse** may indicate blood deficiency.

- A **deep pulse** (you need to push down to feel) may indicate weakness and/or deficiency.

- An **intermittent or irregular pulse** may indicate congestion in the heart, as well as potential hormonal or neurological imbalances.

Taste + Temperature = Action

In both TCM and TAM the combination of taste with temperature (warming or cooling) can be used to create a simple basic description of the action of an herb. For example sweet herbs are generally nourishing. A sweet herb with a warming action, such as **bala,** would therefore probably benefit conditions requiring warmth and nourishment, such as illnesses involving nervous system weakness or weight gain and tissue regeneration.

Commonly Used Groups of Herbs

All systems of medicine group together their therapeutic agents with similar actions. In Western medicine, for example, pharmaceuticals are grouped into families, such as blood-pressure-lowering agents or painkillers. More than 2,000 years ago, the ancient *Charaka Samhita* divided herbs into 50 different groups. To avoid repetition, I have placed several very important commonly used herbs into groups based upon commonly needed actions. We will refer to these groups here in Section Three as we explore different body systems and the illnesses that compromise them. Please note that these groups are representative and cannot be wholly complete. Also note that some herbs fall into more than one category.

Heat-reducing group (herbs that reduce heat and inflammation):

Boswellia gum, bromelain, bupleurum root, burdock root, dandelion, flaxseed oil, ginger root, guggul gum, heart-leaved moonseed, holy basil, isatis root and leaves, licorice root, milk thistle seeds, neem leaves, phellodendron root, raw rehmannia root, rhubarb root, sarsaparilla, scute root, turmeric root.

Blood-moving group (herbs that move the blood and remove blood stasis):

Carthamus flower, dang gui root, myrrh gum, prickly ash bark, red clover blossoms, salvia root, millettia stem, carthamus flower, tien chi root.

Digestive-strengthening group (herbs that strengthen weak digestion):

Black pepper, bromelain, garlic bulb, ginger root, ginseng root, trikatu (three peppers), white atractylodes rhizome, cardamom.

Immunity/longevity-boosting group (herbs that increase vital force and strengthen the immune system):

American ginseng root, astragalus root, elderberry fruit, chaga mushroom, cordyceps mushroom, ginseng root, guduchi stem, maitake mushroom, reishi mushroom, shilajatu, Siberian ginseng root, amla fruit, haritaki fruit, ganoderma mushroom, shou wu root.

Blood-nourishing group (herbs that nourish the blood and/or strengthen the tissues):
American ginseng root, alfalfa, dang gui root, deer antler, eclipta, shou wu root, raw rehmannia, shilajatu, amla fruit, white peony root.

Poison-removing group (herbs that remove and/or protect against poisons):
Amla fruit, beet root, burdock root, castor oil, licorice root, triphala, arjuna bark, dandelion root, gotu kola, guduchi stem and berries, schisandra berries, white sandalwood, turmeric root, green tea.

Nervine group (herbs that calm and/or strengthen the nerves):
Ashwagandha root, bala, bupleurum root, ginkgo leaf, gotu kola, kava, muira puama, reishi mushroom, schisandra berry, skullcap, St. John's wort, valerian root, white peony root, wild asparagus root, milky oat seed.

Vessel-strengthening group (herbs that strengthen and detoxify the microvasculature):
Blueberry, gotu kola, hawthorn berry, raspberry, stoneroot, tien chi.

Mucus-reducing group (herbs that remove thick mucus accumulations):
Black pepper, long pepper, bromelain, guggul gum, tangerine peel, turmeric root, fritillaria bulb (chuan bei mu / *F. cirrhosa*), arisaema (tian nan xing /*A.* species), trichosanthes fruit (gou lou / *T. kirilowii*), acorus rhizome.

Diuretic group (herbs that promote urination and eliminate retention of watery fluids):
Dandelion leaf, akebia (mu tong / *A. trifoliata),* plantain leaf (*P. ovata),* capillaris (yin chen hao / *Artemisia capillaris),* punarnava root *(Boerhavia diffusa),* parsley, grifola mushroom (zhu ling / *Polyporus umbellatus),* uva ursi leaf *(Arctostaphylos uva-ursi),* barley water.

Dampness-removing group (herbs that remove thickened fluids from the digestive system and tissues):
Poria mushroom, tangerine peel, pinellia tuber, licorice root, prickly ash bark, oregano leaf.

Warming group (herbs that warm the system):
Aconite, dry ginger, cinnamon bark, black pepper, long pepper, prickly ash bark.

Nutritive group (herbs that promote weight gain):
Ashwagandha root, dates, cashews, bala, cardamom, white atractylodes, ginseng root, dang gui root, cooked rehmannia root.

Wound-healing group (herbs that promote healing of skin, vessels and tissue):
Gotu kola, tien chi root, aloe gel, turmeric root. dang gui root, astragalus root.

Intestinal-healing group (herbs that soothe and heal the intestinal membranes):
Slippery elm bark, marshmallow root, licorice root, chlorophyll juice, wild asparagus root, fennel seed, peppermint leaf, flaxseed oil, kava root.

Formulas: Addition, Subtraction, and Multiplication

Dr. Jim Duke, in his excellent (and free) online Medical Botany course (http://www. arsgrin.gov/duke/syllabus/), says that herbs generally interact in formulas in three ways: (1) antagonism, (2) additivity, and (3) synergy.

Antagonism occurs when herbs or herbal actions work in opposing ways. For example, the coldness of **neem** would be antagonized, or neutralized, by the warmth of **prickly ash bark.** The bitterness of **coptis rhizome** would be antagonized by the sweetness of **licorice root.** Herbalists use this idea to modify the actions of their formulas.

Because individual herbs are complex mixtures of substances, the antagonism that occurs when you combine two herbs is much like the result of mixing two groups of very different people. Imagine, for example, a group of birdwatchers and a group of biologists meeting at a park. Chances are, they would get along quite harmoniously, though individual members of each group might not see eye to eye.

Additivity occurs when herbs simply add to each other. Mixing a group of herbs containing immune-stimulating polysaccharides (like **maitake mushroom** with **ganoderma mushroom**) is additive, as is mixing herbs that contain phytoestrogens. Mixing herbs with similar actions to get additive effects is a common herbal strategy. Most of the herbs in the groups mentioned below have additive effects.

Synergy is a result of the combination of two or more substances that cannot be predicted by simply adding the sum of the parts. Following this phenomenon, individual nutrients must work together for the body to produce its immune response. For example, your body needs less vitamin C if you are getting adequate levels of vitamin E, because these two antioxidants support the regeneration of one another in the body. Herbs like **shilajatu** and **American ginseng root** seem to generally increase and add to the actions of other herbs.

It's All in the Dosage

The same nutrients can affect your body in very different ways, depending on the dose. Individual herbs can act differently, depending on dose. For example, **ginseng extracts** cause blood vessel constriction in small doses and blood vessel dilation in large doses. The same thing is true of individual nutrients, such as vitamin K. While low doses of this vitamin assist blood clotting, high doses (above 1 mg/day) aid calcification of the bone matrix.

Another case in point is vitamin C. At low doses, vitamin C helps generate collagen and elastin, which help keep the body "glued together." At higher doses, however, it becomes a potent antiviral and antioxidant compound.

A final example is niacin, an important B vitamin. At low doses, niacin provides the body with adequate energy metabolism through the action of nicotinamide adenine dinucleotide (NAD). At somewhat higher doses, niacin becomes a valuable vasodilator. When the dosage is increased even more, this vitamin is a potent cholesterol-lowering agent. Niacin was the first drug used in the treatment of high cholesterol.

Most of what we know about how herbs interact with each other is based on empirical knowledge. All mature herbal traditions know how to combine herbs to improve, modify, or amplify their effects. Two examples are Traditional Chinese Medicine's use of **licorice root** to "harmonize" formulas and Ayurveda's combining of three fruits **(triphala)** to create a balanced tonic effect. In fact, because each of the individual tonic fruits in **triphala** work a bit more on Vata, Pitta, and Kapha, this is an excellent example of a well-constructed formula.

A powerful example of drug interaction is the use by South American shamans of the two herbs *Banisteriopsis caapi* vine and the plant *Psychotria viridis*. Scientists discovered that the mixture of an alkaloid (harmine) from one plant and phytochemicals (beta-carbolines) from the other creates a hallucinogenic state resembling schizophrenia.

The areas of antagonism, additivity, synergy, and dosage are exciting ones for the future of herbal medicine. Because this research leads to a different direction than looking for single active ingredients, it is more in harmony with the philosophy of herbal medicine.

Not only can herbs and nutrients work together or in opposition, but all of us can react differently to just about everything. This concept is called **biological** or **biochemical individuality.** Thus, no matter how much we try to standardize treatments (one size fits all), some of us simply will not respond. As a result, I believe we will always need a good doctor-patient relationship with frequent feedback in order to have the best individualized treatments.

I still don't get the big picture.

Are things getting a bit complicated? Let me try to clarify the goal of all herbal medicine.

The central goal of herbal treatment is to restore the body to balance. The nervous system and the mind work together with the digestive, cardiovascular, and circulatory systems to regulate bodily function and health. As I view it, these systems derive from three primary germinal layers, elemental tissues that form in the earliest stages of embryonic development. The tissue layers are called "ectoderm," "mesoderm," and "endoderm," and serve as the precursors to all tissue development (ectoderm–nervous system, mesoderm–blood and heart, endoderm–digestive system).

The large tube that extends from mouth to anus, forming our digestive tract and all its related organs, grows out of the "endoderm" tissue layer. The heart, blood vessels, connective tissue, glandular system, muscles, and bones all derive from the "mesoderm" layer. Finally, the brain and nervous system are composed of "ectoderm" tissue.

These three primary germ layers have evolved together; they are entwined and interdependent, and this complexity reaches all the way down to the cellular level. For example, cell biologists have shown us that each cell in the body has its own musculoskeletal system, consisting of a stiffened skeleton composed of tubules, which are surrounded by a contractile fibrous substance. Each aspect of the living weblike matrix of energies and systems we call the human body is designed to break down and absorb different forms of energy, which it then converts and releases outward in a never-ending flow as we move through the world. For example, the food that we eat contains:

- essential nutrients that we cannot produce in our bodies from smaller building blocks

- energy trapped in chemical bonds in the molecules that make up food

- building blocks (such as amino acids) that our bodies can use

Our digestive systems break down food into component molecules and absorb them. The blood takes these molecules to the cells where they are used as raw materials to produce our own molecules or further broken down to release the energy trapped in the chemical bonds. This energy release occurs only in the presence of oxygen, and our breathing changes to accommodate ever-changing metabolic needs. This process creates waste products that are expelled from the body via exhalation and our eliminative organs. As we move through the world, our nervous system "hears" internal signals (like hunger) and responds, perhaps by looking for food. Likewise, our cells are constantly hearing and responding to messages from the outside as well as sending signals outward. This same process (flow of energy) takes place on many levels.

The goal of this energy flow is a constant movement toward balance among all organs and systems. Health is optimal when the major systems are individually and collectively in balance. When your body is in a state of optimal health, you experience such feelings as love, peace, harmony, and appreciation. Conversely, imbalances in health usually lead to emotional states of pain, fear, depression, and anger. When health breaks down, certain large causative factors can be seen, including inflammation, nutritional deficiencies, and regulatory dysfunction.

This is why I, as an herbalist, am primarily concerned (at the physical level) with a patient's digestive energy, circulatory and metabolic efficiency, and nervous system function. Once these primary regulators are brought back into balance, we can begin to restore a patient to optimal health. One way to do this is to use herbs.

Formula Writing Made Simple

Once you have good diagnostic information and a clear picture of your larger goals, you are ready to choose your herbs according to taste, texture, aroma, nutrition, and so on. Putting together an herbal formula is like writing a recipe.

However, there is an important intermediate step, which is stipulating a strategy. A strategy includes what you want to do to the body, the methods you choose to employ, and the order in which you want to deploy your tools. You have seen in Section Two that herbs are often described by "What they do" to the body, as well as their effects on specific disease processes. This understanding allows us to determine how to employ herbs.

Examples of simple objectives are:

1. To nourish the blood

2. To calm spasms in the legs

3. To reduce inflammation in the liver

4. To improve white blood cell counts

The above were arrived at as a result of diagnostic work. We would choose herbs that nourish the blood, for example, only if the person had anemia or another blood deficiency problem. So, a more complete description of the strategies mentioned above would be:

1. My patient is fatigued and anemic, so I will nourish their blood.

2. My patient is having painful leg spasms, so I will calm the spasms.

3. My patient is fatigued and jaundiced, so I will reduce inflammation in their liver.

4. My patient is undergoing chemotherapy, so I will improve white blood cell counts.

Most patients will have other secondary considerations. They may have blood sugar problems or poor digestion, nervousness, or constipation. In writing the formula, I would want to add some herbs to address these important secondary elements. This would translate the above examples as follows:

1. My patient is fatigued and anemic due to stress and overwork, so I will nourish their blood and add some calming nervine herbs.

2. My patient is having painful leg spasms due to poor absorption and poor diet, so I will calm the spasms, increase their intake of mineral-rich vegetables, and add some digestive herbs.

3. My patient is fatigued and jaundiced due to hepatitis, so I will reduce inflammation in their liver, counsel them on the importance of stopping alcohol abuse, flush the bile out with diuretics and an increase in water intake, and add some antiviral and immune-stimulating herbs.

4. My patient is undergoing chemotherapy, and white blood cell counts have decreased, especially macrophages. The gastrointestinal system is also severely inflamed. Therefore I will nourish the blood with tonics, emphasizing herbs that increase macrophage counts, and I will protect the gastrointestinal system with herbs that coat the intestinal membrane and counteract inflammation.

Don't think this is easy—it isn't—but if you can train your mind to formulate your medical ideas in this manner, you can start to develop your own strategies and begin to think like an herbalist. Once you have identified the appropriate herbs and strategy for treating all aspects of the patient's condition, you can construct your starting formula. Start off simply, working, for example, with a simple formula for mild nausea.

It helps to know that it has been a principle of TCM since its earliest classic text *(Herbal Classic of the Divine Plowman,* first recorded on paper over 2,000 years ago) that most basic prescriptions contain one or two major herbs, along with several supportive ones to improve activity and reduce adverse effects.

Dosage and Process: Healing with Herbs Is Like Playing Football

I heard a group of NFL football players on TV discussing how they sized up an opponent. I was surprised to learn that these professionals did not only look for obvious qualities like strength, size, speed, and agility, but were equally concerned with knee flexibility, grip strength, and peripheral vision. The latter information, I learned, was necessary to determine when an opponent was coming at you from behind. Similiarly, good diagnosis and treatment in herbal medicine involves noticing things that others ignore.

The starting formula (and starting dosage) is like the first play in a football game. The goal is total health. The symptoms and disease states are like the opposing team. After you make your first play (write your starting formula), you will evaluate results, and if necessary restrategize and reformulate your secondary formula and dosages. This is like the football huddle before the second play.

In both China and Nepal, formulas are usually changed every 3 to 5 days. As the problems begin to resolve or stabilize, there are longer periods of time between formula changes. Thus, good herbal medicine is an *ongoing feedback process,* requiring a willingness to continually change tactics. We will discuss this more in the following chapters.

When I was in Nepal, my teacher was making herb doses by scooping up with a spoon (about 2 grams) from his bottles of dried or fresh herbs, and then putting the powders in paper packages. I asked him about the obvious variation in total herb weight, and he told me (this is 10 years ago) something like . . . "Every day the plants change. In the field they get weaker and stronger as the season progresses. In the monsoon season most of the plants get weak, like we do. Each individual plant also has a different strength and weakness. After it is picked, it changes in strength each day. After it is ground up or chopped or boiled it changes in strength each day. After it is mixed with other herbs, this changes its strength also. The patients also are all different. Some of them are weaker and some are stronger. During each day, they change in strength, and they change in strength from morning to evening. If they eat something different, or if they have something to disturb their mind, their digestive strength will be changed. If they don't get enough sleep, they get weaker. So we give the standard dose, and then check in 3 or 5 days. No matter what the result, then we can change the dose to the correct one. We do this each time we see them."

—Vaidya Mana Bajra Bajracharya
(Dr. Mana)
Head of the world's oldest Ayurvedic lineage (700 years)

CHAPTER *10*

Nutrition and Lifestyle

You've got to be careful if you don't know where you're going,
because you might not get there.

—Yogi Berra

Nutrition is the foundation of all herbal medicine treatments. Herbs themselves are simply specialized food sources. Studies of nutrition clearly demonstrate a direct causal relationship between diet and health. Sensible, healthy dietary habits can help prevent disease. By the same token, poor dietary choices can contribute to the deterioration of general health and lead to many diseases. People who take supplements and herbal medicines are healthier than the general population, as are people who follow healthy diets. However, when forced to choose just one practice, those who eat a balanced diet enjoy better health than do those who simply take supplements. Adoption of both practices is ideal for a long and healthy life.

Examining a patient's dietary habits is an integral step in herbal diagnosis and treatment. It is a mistake to treat a nutritional deficiency with herbs. If someone is experiencing frequent coughs and colds due to poor nutrition, giving them **echinacea** is not the answer. Similarly, if someone has constipation because their diet is devoid of fiber, it is a mistake just to give them herbal laxatives. The herbal prescription in such a case should include counseling about the health benefits of a high-fiber diet and suggestions for increasing dietary fiber.

More Than You Can Swallow

The vast field of nutrition encompasses an enormous range of information—more so than even the field of chemistry. Clive McKay, one of the outstanding nutritionists in the early part of the 20th century, estimated that a person would have to read one article every 3 minutes, 8 hours a day, 7 days a week to keep up with the newly published literature on just the *chemical* aspects of nutrition. That estimate was made in the 1930s, and back then they ignored the *medical* aspects of nutrition, as well as any information originating from nations outside of Europe and America. Today, the information load in nutrition has multiplied a hundredfold. A quick search of MEDLINE in October 1999 showed more than 150,000 articles on nutrition.

In 1997, I was one of the speakers at a conference for the Delaware Department of Aging. The keynote speaker, a physician from Hawaii, had everyone stand up. She then challenged us with the following statements, telling those who had to answer no to any of them to sit down.

- Everyone who eats fewer than 5 servings of fresh fruits and vegetables every day, please sit down.
- Everyone who drinks more than 2 ounces of hard liquor or 16 ounces of wine per day, please sit down.
- Everyone who does not get at least 15 minutes of vigorous exercise every day, please sit down.
- Everyone who does not get at least 7 hours of sleep each night, please sit down.
- Everyone who smokes cigarettes, please sit down.

Within one minute, out of an initial 400 people, only 3 remained standing at the end of the exercise (one of them being yours truly). This shows the great gap between public pronouncement and the reality of our lives.

Beyond what is known by food chemists and dietitians, a small sampling of perspectives on nutrition would include psychological, phytomedicinal, energetic, religious, cultural, constitutional, soil chemical, environmental, and ethnobotanical aspects. It is therefore imperative not to hang your flag on a single diet, or on a single aspect of nutrition. I will provide you with functional descriptions here, which will allow you to develop a simplified approach to nutrition based upon the herbal concepts described in this book. This personal approach will allow you to make dietary choices that are complementary to your herbal remedies, enabling you to enjoy a harmonious herbal regimen.

Knowing and Doing

In spite of the modern explosion in health and nutrition books, most people who walk into my clinic don't really have enough practical information to make clear dietary and herbal decisions, and even those who do have information hold numerous misconceptions. For example, many people take over-the-counter or prescription acid-blocking drugs without any understanding of how blocking acid can affect nutrient assimilation, and how this can directly counteract the benefits of even the best diet and supplementation program.

Moreover, even among those who do know the major health protective dos and don'ts, many are still part of the 92% of Americans who fail to consume the necessary 5 servings of fresh fruits and vegetables every day. In theory, people may be aware of the various risks and benefits associated with certain diet and lifestyle choices, but they aren't implementing these healthy practices in their daily lives. Many people resist any new practices that may require them to adapt their lifestyle.

Unfortunately, this usually means that changes designed to support or improve one's health are superseded by other priorities. This unwillingness to adapt or try new things is usually rooted in a patient's psychological or emotional character and may require much persistence to overcome. The patient must come to understand that the road to good health involves a willingness to explore and commit to new directions. It's like the age-old Middle Eastern proverb, "I fear you will never reach Mecca, dear traveler, for you are on the road to Turkestan." Or, in modern parlance, JUST DO IT.

The Benefits of Exercise

The U.S. Department of Health and Human Services issued a report in 1996 on the benefits of regular exercise. Following are several highlights, with my comments:

- Inactive people can improve their health and well-being by becoming even moderately active on a regular basis.

- Physical activity need not be strenuous to achieve health benefits. T'ai Chi and Yoga, for instance, are nonstressful age-old methods of exercise.

- People can achieve greater health benefits by increasing the duration, frequency, or intensity of physical activity.

- Routine physical activity on most days of the week reduces a person's vulnerability to some of the leading causes of illness and death in the United States.

Regular physical activity can improve health in the following ways, according to the World Hypertension League, the American College of Sports Medicine, the report of the U.S. Surgeon General on physical activity and health, and the U.S. National Institutes of Health Consensus Development Panel on Physical Activity and Cardiovascular Health:

- Reduce risk of premature death.

- Reduce risk of death from heart disease.

- Reduce risk of developing diabetes.

- Reduce risk of developing high blood pressure.

- Lower elevated blood pressure.

- Reduce risk of developing colon cancer.

- Relieve feelings of depression and anxiety, similar to the effect of antidepressants.

- Help control weight.

- Help build and maintain healthy bones, muscles, and joints.

- Improve strength and mobility in older adults, decreasing risk of falls and injuries.

- Promote general psychological well-being and improve self-esteem.

The Food Store

The first step in keeping your digestive system healthy occurs when you go shopping at the food store, where you select what will eventually go into your mouth. Thus, if you buy candy, you will eat it. If you buy organic carrots, you will eat them. If you lack will power, keep a list and follow it closely when you shop.

Basic Guidelines for Making Smart Food Choices

- Buy organic products as frequently as possible.
- Drink several glasses of good-quality water every day.
- Buy foods fresh whenever possible.
- Read labels.
- Buy produce with maximum, vivid color.
- Avoid canned/processed foods and foods with too many additives.
- Eat a wide variety of foods.
- Buy produce in season.
- Try something new once in a while.
- Use a variety of herbs and spices.

The regimen you follow for food preparation and consumption is as important as the foods you choose. Following are a few suggestions for balanced, healthy eating, based upon research in the field of nutrition and traditional dietary practices.

Strive to maintain regular mealtimes. Your digestive system adjusts the production of digestive enzymes to coincide with mealtimes. If you eat at the same time every day, you'll be hungrier then, and your digestive power will be stronger. I often see patients who experience ravenous hunger at bedtime, while others have no appetite at breakfast.

Both of these tendencies can add to health problems, so I teach patients how to retrain their appetite and digestion. I tell those who are ravenous at night to avoid eating at that time for 2 weeks. After about 2 weeks, they inevitably find that the hunger has disappeared because the digestive system has adjusted. I tell the people with no appetite in the morning that they must eat a small meal for breakfast every day, and just as with the bedtime eaters, within 2 weeks the problem is resolved. By the way, it is important to rediscover breakfast and to eat that meal every day.

Eat your largest meal at lunchtime. Studies have shown that human metabolism is regulated by pituitary-controlled release of hormones linked to the daily circadian (24-hour) cycle. Ayurvedic doctors hold that digestive energy is highest around noon, and foods eaten at this time are digested more efficiently and are less likely to cause weight gain. Eating late at night can contribute to weight gain.

Eat in a relaxed atmosphere, and allow sufficient time to digest. Sit back and relax after meals for 10 or 15 minutes. Since the practice of relaxing after a meal, although it improves digestion, is unheard of these days, try this little trick to stretch out your mealtime. Get a glass of water or juice and sit back and sip it slowly while you relax after meals.

Learn to cook, and prepare fresh food as frequently as possible. Get a few good cookbooks. When done right, cooking is a form of herbal medicine. For example, I add **Siberian ginseng root bark** to my juice drinks and pick **day lilies** for my salads.

Cook vegetables until the colors jump out at you and bite, but no longer. Once you see this vivid color, it means that cellulose has broken down and the carotenes and bioflavonoids are now easier to see, and thus more available to absorb when you eat. Overcooking degrades these and other nutrients.

Don't stuff yourself. Follow the Yogic rule of eating until your stomach is only three-quarters full. Chronic overeating changes your metabolism and leads to obesity.

Sometimes people don't believe there are benefits to following these rules. If you're skeptical, try doing the opposite. Make sure you stuff yourself whenever you feel tense, try to eat as fast as you can (especially while driving or watching TV), make sure your foods are cooked until they are mush, and pig out right before bed. After a few months of gastric discomfort and weight gain, I think you'll see the light.

Balance the Macronutrients

Macronutrients are fats, carbohydrates, and proteins. Let's consider these components the three legs of a stool. If one leg is longer or shorter, the stool is not balanced. If the quality of wood in any one of the three legs is poor, the stool can break. The quality of each is just as important as the quantity. That's it.

- Too much fat is bad for you, too little fat is bad for you, and the wrong kind of fat is bad for you.

- Too much protein is bad for you, too little protein is bad for you, and the wrong kind of protein is bad for you.

- Too much carbohydrate is bad for you, too little carbohydrate is bad for you, and the wrong kind of carbohydrate is bad for you.

Intake of all three macronutrients should be balanced within each meal to provide the body with the best possible fuel for health maintenance. **Too much or too little of any macronutrient disrupts this balance.** Consider this quote from the Case Western Reserve University School of Medicine:

Adaptation to carbohydrate and fat intake involves changes in a number of biochemical parameters at the cellular level. A change in the concentration of fat or carbohydrate in the blood acts directly to influence metabolic pathways by altering the flux of intermediates into cells. This in turn alters the concentration of hormones and other signaling molecules and changes the rate of expression of genes coding for key regulatory proteins or enzymes in metabolic pathways. These effects occur at different rates and in a tissue-specific manner in response to diet.

In other words, what you eat affects key regulatory processes relating to health. Equally important, each of us has a unique biochemical individuality that affects how we personally react to foods. Some people do better on higher-protein or higher-fat diets, and some don't. There is no way to escape listening to what your own body tells you.

Fats and Oils

Fats and oils break down and supply your body with essential fatty acids (EFAs), which are necessary for normal growth, smooth skin, and healthy membranes. They act as carriers for the fat-soluble vitamins A, D, E, and K. It's true that excess oil (like excess anything else) is bad for health, but the opposite is unhealthy as well. A very low-fat diet can lead to EFA deficiency, which can lead to a host of physical problems including dryness, skin disease, and fatigue.

Illnesses that may respond to EFA balancing and supplementation include acne, AIDS, allergies, Alzheimer's, arthritis, arteriosclerosis, autoimmune disease, breast cysts, cancer, cartilage problems, cystic fibrosis, dermatitis, diabetes, *E. coli* infection, eczema, heart disease, hepatitis, hyperactivity, hypertension, inflammation, neurological disorders, psoriasis, rheumatoid arthritis, skin disorders, stroke, vascular disease, and vision problems.

A sensible course for most of us is to consume moderate amounts of high-quality fats and oils. This is true even for people dieting to lose weight. Intake, of course, should not exceed what is needed to maintain desirable weight. Oils can be divided into two main categories, good and bad, based upon quality and biochemical balance.

Good Fats

Ghee, or clarified butter, is generally good for health and can be used instead of butter. It has a milder taste and does not need to be refrigerated. Some of the best oils are **canola oil, fish oil,** and **olive oil. Borage, evening primrose,** and **flax oils** are most frequently used as nutritional supplements. These oils are balanced in their levels of the two primary EFAs, omega-3 and omega-6, favoring the first. Those who have difficulty processing fats and utilizing these EFAs, can benefit from **borage** or **evening primrose oil** supplementation. Most people do not get enough omega-3 EFAs from the foods they eat. By the way, many people do better with fish oils.

Omega-3 and -6 oils are incorporated into the cell membrane, and cell membranes are responsible for transporting nutrients. When the membranes contain a balance of these oils, they are much more flexible than if formed from animal fatty acids, saturated fats, cholesterol, trans-fatty acids, or excessive omega-6's. For example, omega-3 oils increase insulin transport of sugar into cells. When harmonized with omega-6 oils, they aid in production of healthy prostaglandins. Along with the EFAs, prostaglandins regulate steroid and hormone synthesis, eye pressure, joints and blood vessels, pain and inflammation, immune response, secretions, hormone direction to target cells, fluidity, oxygen transport, platelet stickiness, nerve transmission, energy production for the heart muscle, allergic response, and kidney function.

By the way, don't make the mistake of thinking that only omega-3 oils are good and omega-6's are bad and to be completely eliminated. Although most Americans get too much of the 6's and too little of the 3's, too little omega-6 oil is also bad. Both are essential.

Bad Fats

The worst oil profile comes from excess intake of animal fat in red meats, which are low in omega-3 EFAs, and in trans-fatty acids found in chips, margarine, and processed foods. Other unhealthful oils include overly heated (oxidized) oils such as those found in fried foods, hydrogenated (chemically processed) oils, and oils made rancid through age (commercially sold peanuts are always slightly rancid). Cottonseed oil contains toxic residues, because the plants are sprayed heavily with pesticides during growth.

Lower-quality oils can exacerbate immune and allergy responses. For example, breast milk composition changes according to dietary fat intake, and the milk of mothers whose children have eczema have abnormal or altered fat composition.

Keep Your Oils Healthful

All the oils you purchase should be cold pressed. If they were heated during manufacture, the quality was lowered. A rule of thumb—if oil has been cold pressed, it will be indicated on the label. If you can't find this clearly stated anywhere on the label, don't buy the product.

Always store oil in dark glass bottles to avoid oxidation, and refrigerate them if you're not going to use them up in a reasonable time period. It is wise to buy oils in small bottles and use them within 2 weeks of opening.

Within 5 minutes of cooking, oil changes from its cis (good) structure to the trans (bad) form. However, the addition of antioxidant herbs such as **garlic bulb, ginger root,** or **onion** will delay this degradation for up to 20 minutes, usually long enough to complete the cooking process. Therefore, always add one of these spices as soon as the oil is hot to preserve its freshness during cooking.

Bad fat is usually hidden in store-bought bread products in the form of hydrogenated vegetable oil, so buy bread in the health food store, and be sure to read labels of all other foods to avoid hydrogenated oils. Many environmental chemicals are fat-soluble, another reason to buy organic foods whenever possible.

For the body to properly absorb oils, two things are important to know. First, vitamin E helps to keep the oils from oxidizing, and second, oils absorb more efficiently when emulsified. Oatmeal, corn mush, egg yolks, and tapioca are good emulsifiers.

Throughout this book I will refer to the use of omega-3 fatty acid supplements to reduce inflammation. These oil supplements, found primarily in **flaxseed, borage, evening primrose,** and **fish,** are of great clinical significance. Experienced physicians often use a combination of an EPA and DHA supplement (about 2 1,000-mg capsules three times per day), along with a smaller amount of either **evening primrose oil** or **borage oil** (about 1 500-mg capsule two times a day). Many controlled studies show benefits for a wide range of inflammatory disorders, such as rheumatoid arthritis and inflammatory bowel disorders.

Carbohydrates and Fiber

Carbohydrates are organic compounds composed of carbon, hydrogen, and oxygen. Interestingly, only very small amounts of carbohydrates are found in the human body at any one time, totaling about 1% of body weight. They are found primarily as sugar in the blood, and as glycogen stored in the liver.

Carbohydrates are broken down into two types—simple and complex. Simple carbohydrates are sugars, which are quickly utilized by the body. Complex carbohydrates are starches, formed by the combination of simple sugars into more complex molecules. Your body breaks down starches more slowly than sugars. Fruits, grains, nuts, and vegetables are the primary sources of complex carbohydrates.

The digestion of starches and sugars begins in the mouth and continues down through the small intestine. All carbohydrates are converted, with the help of enzymes, into one of three monosaccharides—galactose, glucose, or fructose. The body uses glucose in three ways: it yields energy directly, it is stored in the liver as glycogen which is released constantly to replenish blood sugar, or it is converted to and stored as fat. Levels of sugar in the blood must be carefully maintained for proper function of your internal organs, and the nervous system is especially sensitive to blood sugar changes. Alterations in blood sugar can affect memory, metabolism, fat deposition, and energy.

Good and Bad Sugars

Natural sugars—found in fruits and vegetables—contain many essential nutrients that aid in their digestion. Refined sugars—found in processed foods such as cakes, pies, and candy—lack these additional nutrients and can therefore potentially disrupt the body's control of blood sugar. Hypoglycemics, diabetics, and people suffering from intestinal infections must be especially careful to moderate their sugar intake. Food labels often mask extra sugars by using names like sucrose, glucose, maltose, lactose, fructose, corn syrup, or natural flavors. They all mean the same thing—sugar, in one form or another.

If carbohydrate intake is very low, the body cannot completely utilize fat. The resulting increase in fat metabolism can produce an undesirable excess of "ketones," acidlike molecules which can damage the body tissues. This process can be avoided by consuming the recommended 50 to 100 grams of carbohydrates per day. Less can be used for weight loss.

I like to distinguish between grain carbohydrates and vegetable carbohydrates. Many people are sensitive to grains (which are relatively new additions to our diet, after the advent of farming). Corn, wheat, rice, and so on can be problematic if you are allergic.

Fiber

Carbohydrates also include cellulose, pectins (gel-like substances that lower cholesterol by binding it to promote excretion and drawing it out of the body), and other substances known as dietary fiber or roughage. Most plant cell walls contain about 35% insoluble fiber, 45% soluble fiber, and various amounts of pectin and other substances. The soluble fibers include mucilages and gums, which mechanically coat and protect the intestinal walls. The fiber substances also absorb water and give bulk to the intestinal contents and stimulate peristaltic movement.

Research has shown that people who consume large amounts of fiber (100–170 grams per day), such as rural Africans, have an average bowel transit time of 30 hours and a fecal weight of 500 grams. Europeans and Americans, who typically eat only 20 grams of fiber per day, have a transit time of 48 hours and a fecal weight of only 100 grams. This allows prolonged exposure to various cancer-causing substances in the bowel.

Insufficient dietary fiber intake has been linked in epidemiological studies to constipation, diverticular disease, irritable bowel disease, bowel cancer, inflammatory bowel diseases, coronary artery disease, and gallstones.

Proteins

Proteins are complex organic compounds made primarily of amino acids. Protein is necessary for growth and develop-

> Because proteins contain a stable amount of nitrogen (about 16%), protein requirements can be determined by a measurement called nitrogen equilibrium. When a healthy adult is in a state of equilibrium, he or she is ingesting and excreting protein in a balanced, desirable way. Scientists have calculated approximately how much protein is needed for this balance as follows:
>
> Infants: 13 grams/day
> Children: 16–28 grams/day
> Adult males: 50–65 grams/day
> Adult females: 45–50 grams/day
>
> In general, intake should not exceed or drop below what is needed to maintain desirable weight. Protein requirements can change with certain disease states. For example, Ayurveda teaches that people with hypoglycemia or nervous dispositions often do better on a higher-protein diet.

ment and for heat and energy production. It also helps us maintain the acid-alkali balance in the body. Using the full set of amino acids, and under the direction of DNA, the body constructs all its proteins, a dazzling array including such essentials as hormones, enzymes, and antibodies.

While we can manufacture certain amino acids ourselves, we need to ingest some (called essential amino acids) from our diet. Without them, our bodies cannot function properly. Inadequate dietary protein intake is perhaps the most frequent cause of immune deficiency in the world. Protein malnutrition results in a reduced number and reduced functions of T-cells, phagocytic cells, and antibody response. Fully one-third of young children in the low-income countries of our world are stunted in growth due to protein-energy malnutrition.

Plants use energy from the sun to synthesize sugar, which they then combine with nutrients from the soil to make amino acids and, finally, proteins. Plants, therefore, are the original source of all the world's protein. In animals, proteins are concentrated in structural and protective tissues, such as bones, tendons, hair, fingernails, and skin, as well as soft tissues such as organs and especially muscles. Animals cannot synthesize their own proteins and must depend on their dietary intake of plants and other animals.

All protein food sources are not equal. Meats, fish, eggs, and milk contain all the essential amino acids, while vegetables are almost always deficient in one or more of the essential amino acids. Fortunately for vegetarians, we can correct amino acid deficiencies by combining foods. For example, we can complement cereals, which are low in the amino acid lysine, with soybeans, lima beans, or kidney beans, which are high in lysine.

Other beneficial combinations include breads with cheese, beans with corn, wheat with beans, nuts with breads, and cereals with milk. Most traditional cultures utilize these particular food combinations extensively. They offer much-needed alternatives for the many people whose protein choices are restricted by health conditions like allergy and inflammation.

The body breaks down protein in the stomach and intestines, and this process leads to the release of energy. Poor protein digestion contributes to many disease processes. If protein digestion is weak, or if there is poor intestinal absorption of amino acids, bacteria can break the protein down into many toxic compounds. Protein digestion can be improved with herbal medicines, hydrochloric acid, or proteolytic enzyme supplementation.

Even though animal products seem ideal as a source of protein, there are some very important considerations. Animal protein sources are more concentrated and contain higher levels of toxins than vegetable proteins, resulting in more work for the liver and kidneys. There is much more protein in a gram of meat than in a gram of vegetable matter, resulting in a higher concentration of nitrogen for the kidneys to process in a typical meal. Excessive consumption of proteins from these sources in lieu of vegetable sources can also lead to relative deficiencies of other necessary plant-based nutritional elements, such as carotenes and bioflavonoids. Therefore, it is usually wise to make sure a good portion of your protein comes from vegetable sources. This important consideration is often overlooked in patients with kidney and liver diseases.

Eat According to the Seasons

Seasonal weather fluctuations affect digestion and the body as a whole. Ayurvedic medicine teaches extensively about this phenomenon, and I have found the following Ayurvedic concepts, taught to me by my teacher Dr. Mana, to be very helpful in understanding how the body reacts to seasonal changes.

When the temperature suddenly drops at the beginning of a cold-weather season, it is very noticeable at first. Everyone finds it difficult to tolerate the cold for a few days until their blood circulation adjusts. In the winter months, the colder weather causes blood circulation to move to the inner parts of the body, away from the extremities. This shift away from the surface creates extra heat in the interior abdominal area, strengthening digestion as well as appetite. During these colder months, the body requires a heavier diet with an increase in caloric intake to maintain heat and warmth. Some people also find that warm drinks such as teas are helpful. Otherwise, a decrease in blood circulation in the extremities can lead to joint pain and may even contribute to arthritis, pain, and slow healing.

I often question people suffering from musculoskeletal pain as to whether they experience cold hands and toes. I remember one particular case of a young man who was always cold. He was also having trouble with his martial arts. He was studying a very acrobatic Japanese style and found that his recovery time and endurance were low. He had strong spiritual beliefs and was following a strict vegetarian diet, eating no meat, fish, or eggs. He was always cold, though he proudly told me his cholesterol level was about 110 (far below normal). I immediately took him out and bought him three fried eggs. Within an hour, he began to warm up.

As spring approaches, blood composition changes as the warmer external air causes the blood to thin. This change causes the body to release accumulated mucus and blood fats into the circulation, resulting in allergies, asthma, loss of appetite, and general sluggishness. Changing to a lighter and drier diet can counteract this.

During the summer, hot air temperatures draw the blood flow toward the extremities and away from the abdominal region. This change can cause weakness, decreased appetite, and digestive disorders in sensitive individuals. A dietary increase in liquids and cooling foods, especially vegetables and

---

Tips for Adjusting to Seasonal Changes

- Increased consumption of meats, fish, and oils can help maintain body temperature during the colder months.
- **Ginger root tea** and **cinnamon bark** are good for warming the system in winter.
- Increased intake of barley, beans, and green leafy vegetables can combat sluggishness as the warmer seasons approach.
- "Spring cleaning" can be done simply by drinking **dandelion tea** or **burdock root tea.**
- Increased intake of sweet fruits and fruit juices, especially watermelon, is good for cooling the system as temperatures rise.
- Increased intake of salads and other fresh vegetables aids the digestion in warm weather.
- **Chrysanthemum flower tea** is an excellent cooling summer beverage. Also useful are **honeysuckle flower tea** and **peppermint leaf tea.**
- **Ginger root tea** and **cinnamon bark tea** are helpful for stimulating digestion in humid weather.

fruits, is usually sufficient to correct these ailments. I recommend staying away from sour, salty, and pungent foods, meats, alcohol, and hot foods during this season, as they simply generate more heat. Instead, make a conscious effort to increase your intake of lighter foods such as fresh salads. A more vegetarian diet in general is better during this time of year. This type of diet naturally cleanses the system and keeps the arteries and other ducts healthy.

Humidity weakens the digestion and the nerves. I follow Ayurvedic principles to aid my digestion when the humidity is high, by changing to a heavier diet with more sour foods. Adding some honey to meal preparations can also help with the digestion of oilier foods.

Special Diets for Illness

In 1978, I helped Dr. Mana to edit a book he wrote called *The Eastern Theory of Diet*. In this book, Dr. Mana shows how diets can be developed based upon body type, seasonal fluctuations of weather, and the taste qualities of different types of foods using the energetic concepts of Vata, Pitta, and Kapha. I was impressed with his ability to offer dietary advice in complete harmony with his understanding of the disease process. Ayurvedic doctors have classified all common foods and spices via the TAM system of energetics. Therefore, if a person had a Pitta (inflammatory) disease and was being given herbs to reduce Pitta, it only made sense to prescribe a diet containing foodstuffs that also reduced Pitta.

Following Dr. Mana's lead, I developed a list of six diets that addressed the most common energetic imbalances seen in the clinic. The diets were based on the common TCM and TAM diagnostic concepts of heat, cold, dampness, dryness, and wind (for a refresher, turn back to the beginning of Chapter 9). If you figure out the major causative factor(s) in an illness, you can easily prescribe a diet that will help overcome the problem.

Here's a simple example. If you had stomach inflammation, you would not eat a chili pepper, and if your digestion were weak and sluggish, you would not want to eat a heavy steak. These suggestions cannot be counteracted by saying, for example, "Steak contains iron, and when you are weak you need iron." That is, the energetics of the food can sometimes take precedence over individual nutrient considerations. If a person has sluggish digestion and needs iron, they should get it from an easy-to-digest source.

General Guidelines for a Healthy Diet and Lifestyle

- Take a high-potency multivitamin and multimineral supplement each day (add extra doses of vitamins C and E when indicated).
- Drink plenty of fresh water.
- Get fresh air and exercise every day.
- Eat meals at a regular time.
- Avoid rushing meals.
- Limit snacks.
- Avoid late-night or bedtime eating.
- Chew food thoroughly.
- Read labels.
- Don't eat anything you can't pronounce.
- Don't smoke.
- Don't drink excess alcohol.

To keep it simple, I have left out cold and dry as separate entities. If there is heat, it drives out cold. If there is dampness, there is no dryness. Also, I use these as a starting point and modify them according to individual needs. Remember, these diets are used during herbal treatments and are not intended to be used all the time.

DIET TO REDUCE WIND (VATA)
Strengthens the Nervous System

I use this diet when a patient experiences any or all of these symptoms: weak digestion, nervousness, fatigue, spasms, dryness, neurasthenia, nerve pain, weight loss, numbness, and tingling.

FAVOR:

General: Foods that are both highly nutritive and easy to digest are key to healing nervous system problems. Favor soups, warm foods, and drinks. Drink spring water, especially with meals. All foods should be fresh, and organic if possible. Try to maintain regular mealtimes and adequate sleep. Use a high-potency multivitamin / multimineral.

Grains: Corn, oatmeal, rice, wheat (unless allergic). Prepare warm cereals or well-cooked whole grains with spices.

Dairy: All dairy products, organic if possible, unless you are allergic or intolerant. If so, use soy or rice milk and other natural substitutes.

Sweeteners: Maple syrup, molasses, Sucanat (natural cane sugar).

Oils: Borage, canola, evening primrose, fish, flax, olive, sunflower. Use healthful quantities unless you have weight problems.

Fruits: Sweet fruits, including berries, grapes, cherries, melon, avocado, coconut, sweet plum, mango, pear, banana, fresh fig. Use freely, including juices.

Vegetables: Well-cooked vegetables, especially asparagus, carrots, celery, cucumber, green beans, green peas, lettuce, okra, potato, pumpkin, squash, sweet potato. Eat freely, especially cooked with spices. Vegetable juices.

Spices: Cardamom, mints, coriander, chamomile, cinnamon, cumin, fennel, ginger (root or tea), mustard, bay leaf, black pepper, salt.

Proteins: Chicken, eggs, duck, fresh seafood, nuts (except peanuts), turkey, pork.

AVOID:

General: Avoid dieting and fasting. Avoid stale foods, ice-cold drinks, canned or prepared foods, chemical additives, processed meats, hydrogenated oils and fats, excess alcohol, candy, cake, sugary sweets.

Sweeteners: Nutrasweet (and other chemical sugar replacers), processed or refined sugars.

Oils and fats: Corn oil, peanut oil, sesame oil. Low-quality or hard-to-digest oils weaken the nervous system.

Grains: Millet (drying).

Vegetables: Cabbage, cauliflower, turnip, zucchini, raw vegetables (except lettuce and carrots) if hard to digest. (All these vegetables should be limited, taken in small quantities, and cooked well to avoid indigestion.)

Spices: Excess amounts of cayenne pepper, chili, cloves, fenugreek, mustard, or hot spices.

Proteins: Beans except lentils (unless taken with spices or "Beano"), peanuts.

DIET TO REDUCE HEAT (PITTA)
Helps Reduce General Inflammation

I use this diet when a patient experiences any or all of these symptoms: inflammation, heat signs, burning pain, acidity, hot flashes, painful joints, skin itching, anger and irritability, tissue destruction, infection, fever.

FAVOR:

General: Two keys to reducing inflammation are increasing intake of fresh fruits and vegetables and avoiding unhealthful fats and oils. All foods should be fresh and organic if possible, and not overly hot in temperature. Drink spring water, at least 6 glasses per day, especially with meals. Stick to regular mealtimes, and avoid snacking.

Grains: Barley, oats, rice, unless allergic. Inflammation caused by grain allergies, especially wheat, is a common problem.

Dairy: Butter, ghee, milk (unless allergic), all in moderate quantities, and organic if possible. If allergic, use soy or rice milk and other natural substitutes.

Sweeteners: Maple syrup, Sucanat (natural cane sugar).

Oils: Borage, canola, evening primrose, fish, flax, olive, sunflower. Use small or moderate quantities.

Fruits: Sweet fruits including avocado, banana, berries, cherries, coconut, grapes, mango, melon, pear, sweet plum, watermelon.

Vegetables: Asparagus, beans, beets, broccoli, carrots, cauliflower, cabbage, celery, cucumber, green beans, green peas, lettuce, okra, potato, pumpkin, squash, zucchini. Eat large quantities of these vegetables (warm, not hot), preferably boiled. Vegetable juices.

Spices: Cardamom, coriander, dill, fennel, fenugreek, ginger, bay leaf, turmeric. Turmeric is strongly anti-inflammatory and may be supplemented at ½ teaspoon two to three times per day.

Proteins: Beans, chicken, eggs, fresh seafood, turkey. Eat moderate amounts, except beans, which can be eaten freely.

AVOID:

General: Avoid spicy, hot, sour, salty, greasy, stale, canned, or prepared foods, hot drinks, chemical additives, hydrogenated oils and fats, alcohol, vinegar, candy, cake, sugary sweets, pickles.

Dairy: Buttermilk, sour cream.

Sweeteners: Molasses.

Oils: Corn, Crisco, peanut, sesame. Low-quality oils are very inflammatory.

Grains: Corn, millet, rye, wheat.

Fruits: Sour fruits.

Vegetables: Hot peppers, nightshade family vegetables (bell peppers, eggplant, tomato).

Spices: Cayenne pepper, chili, cloves, cumin, fenugreek, hot spices, mustard, salt.

Proteins: Beef and other red meats, peanuts.

DIET TO REDUCE DAMPNESS AND MUCUS (KAPHA)
Removes Fluids, Mucus, and Sticky Accumulations

I use this diet when a patient experiences any or all of these symptoms: heaviness, dampness, excess mucus, fluid accumulation, elevated blood fats, nausea.

FAVOR:

General: Light, dry foods work best for reducing dampness and mucus. Favor pungent (spicy), bitter, astringent, and warm or hot foods and drinks. Drink plenty of spring water, especially at meals. All foods should be fresh, and organic if possible.

Grains: Barley, wheat, corn, millet, oats (unless allergic).

Dairy: Small amounts of low-fat milk occasionally (unless allergic), goat's milk.

Sweeteners: Honey.

Oils: Light oils, such as canola, in food preparation. Use very small quantities. Alternatively, use borage, evening primrose, or flax as supplements.

Fruits: Apple, cranberry, guava, pear, persimmon, pomegranate. Eat fruit slightly unripe.

Vegetables: Asparagus, beets, broccoli, cabbage, carrot, cauliflower, celery, eggplant, garlic, green leafy vegetables, onion, potato, pumpkin, radish, sprouts.

Spices: All spices can be eaten freely except salt, which should be avoided.

Proteins: Beans, chicken, fresh seafood (less oily varieties), turkey. Beans can be eaten freely.

AVOID:

General: Do not overeat. Reduce cold foods and drinks, oily or greasy foods, and foods that are excessively sweet, sour, or salty. Reduce or eliminate milk products.

Dairy: All milk products, except small amounts of low-fat milk occasionally.

Sweeteners: All sweeteners except honey.

Oils: All oils, except small quantities of light oils or supplements.

Grains: Excesses of oats, rice, and wheat.

Fruits: Avocado, banana, coconut, dates, figs, and sweet fruits.

Vegetables: Cucumber, okra, sweet potato, tomato, zucchini.

Spices: Salt.

Proteins: Nuts, pork, red meat.

DIET TO REDUCE WIND AND DAMPNESS
Strengthens Nervous System and Reduces Accumulations

FAVOR:

General: Foods that are both highly nutritive and easy to digest are key to healing the nervous system, while avoiding heavy oily and greasy foods to reduce accumulations. Favor soups, warm foods, and drinks. Drink spring water, especially with meals. All foods should be fresh, and organic if possible. Try to maintain regular mealtimes and adequate sleep. Use a high-potency multivitamin / multimineral, as well as a daily 400–800 IU dose of mixed tocopherol vitamin E.

Grains: Barley, corn, oatmeal, rice, or wheat (unless allergic). Prepare warm cereals or well-cooked whole grains with spices. Barley is the best grain to use.

Dairy: Use soy and rice milk and cheeses as substitutes for dairy.

Sweeteners: Honey, molasses, Sucanat (natural cane sugar).

Oils: Moderate use of only high-quality oils and fats is key to reducing dampness and mucus in the body while maintaining adequate EFAs. Borage, canola, evening primrose, fish, flax, olive, and sunflower are best. Use small quantities if you have weight problems.

Fruits: Avocado, banana, berries, cherries, coconut, dark-colored fruits, fresh figs, grapes, mango, melon, pear, sweet plums. Eat freely.

Vegetables: Well-cooked vegetables, including asparagus, beans, broccoli, carrot, celery, cucumber, green beans, green peas, lettuce, onion, potato, pumpkin, squash. Eat vegetables freely, especially cooked with spices.

Spices: Cardamom, chamomile, cinnamon, cumin, fennel, ginger (root or tea), mustard, pepper, salt.

Proteins: Chicken, eggs, fresh seafood, nuts (except peanuts), pork, turkey. Use moderate amounts and cook with garlic, ginger, or onion.

AVOID:

General: Avoid dieting and fasting. Avoid stale foods, ice-cold drinks, canned or prepared foods, chemical additives, hydrogenated oils and fats, excess alcohol, candy, cakes, sugary sweets.

Sweeteners: Nutrasweet and other chemical or processed sugar substitutes.

Oils: Corn, Crisco, peanut, sesame. Low-quality oils contribute to accumulations.

Grains and Vegetables: None necessary to avoid.

Spices: Excess amounts of cayenne pepper, chili, cloves, hot spices, salt.

Proteins: Fatty meats (use lean cuts), peanuts.

DIET TO REDUCE WIND AND HEAT
Strengthens the Nerves and Reduces Inflammation

FAVOR:

General: Foods that are both highly nutritive and easy to digest are key to healing the nervous system, while good-quality oils and adequate fruits and vegetables help fight inflammation. Drink spring water, especially with meals. All foods should be fresh, and organic if possible. Try to maintain regular mealtimes and adequate sleep, and avoid snacking. Use a high-potency multivitamin / multimineral.

Grains: Corn, rice, wheat (unless you are allergic). Favor well-cooked whole grains.

Dairy: All dairy products (unless allergic), especially ghee, organic if possible.

Sweeteners: Maple syrup, molasses, Sucanat (natural cane sugar). Use sparingly.

Oils: Use only high-quality oils and fats to reduce inflammation. Use borage, canola, evening primrose, fish, flax, olive, sunflower in healthful quantities, unless you have weight problems.

Fruits: Adequate intake of fruit is necessary to reduce inflammation. Use sweet fruits, including avocado, banana, berries, cherries, coconut, fresh figs, grapes, mango, melon, pear, sweet plums, watermelon, and so on. Eat freely.

Vegetables: Adequate intake of vegetables is necessary to reduce inflammation. Favor well-cooked vegetables, including asparagus, beans, broccoli, carrots, celery, cucumber, green beans, green peas, lettuce, okra, artichoke, potato, pumpkin, squash, sweet potato, zucchini. Eat freely.

Spices: Cardamom, chamomile, cumin, dill, fennel, ginger (root or tea), salt. Turmeric is also strongly anti-inflammatory and may be supplemented at ½ teaspoon two to three times per day.

Proteins: Chicken, eggs, fresh seafood, nuts (except peanuts), turkey.

AVOID:

General: Avoid stale, canned, or prepared foods, chemical additives, hydrogenated oils and fats, excess alcohol, candy, cakes, sugary sweets.

Sweeteners: Nutrasweet and other chemical or processed sugar substitutes.

Oils: Corn, Crisco, peanut. Low-quality oils are very inflammatory.

Grains and Vegetables: Reduce raw vegetables (except lettuce and carrots) if hard to digest.

Spices: Excess amounts of cayenne pepper, chili, cloves, fenugreek, hot spices, mustard, salt.

Proteins: Beans except lentils (unless taken with spices or "Beano"), peanuts.

DIET TO REDUCE HEAT AND DAMPNESS
Diet for Reducing Inflammation, Fluid, and Mucus

FAVOR:

General: Foods should be very fresh, and organic if possible. Favor light and easy-to-digest foods such as soups, and increase fruits and vegetables. Do not overeat. Reduce oily or greasy foods, sour foods, salt, and hot spices. Avoid prepared foods. Drink spring water, up to 6 glasses per day, especially at meals. Also drink teas. Use foods at moderate temperature, not too hot or cold.

Grains: Use whole grains such as barley, buckwheat, corn, millet, rice, rye (unless allergic). Use breads in moderation.

Dairy: Use soy and rice products as substitutes for milk. Use Spectrum Naturals canola spread as a substitute for butter. Ghee may be used.

Sweeteners: Honey, stevia, Sucanat (natural cane sugar).

Oils: Use only small amounts of cold-pressed canola and olive. Alternatively, use borage, evening primrose, or flax as supplements. Low-quality oils increase inflammation and mucus.

Fruits: Insufficient intake of fruits increases inflammation. Eat several servings of fresh fruit each day, especially those with dark colors, such as blueberries, grapes, strawberries, and watermelon.

Vegetables: Insufficient intake of vegetables increases inflammation. Eat large quantities, preferably cooked or boiled. Use asparagus, beets, broccoli, cabbage, carrots, cauliflower, celery, cucumber, dandelion tea, green leafy vegetables, green tea, lettuce, okra, onion (cooked), parsley, potato, pumpkin, radish, sprouts, zucchini, and every other vegetable you can think of, *except* nightshade family vegetables (bell peppers, eggplant, tomato).

Spices: Basil, dill, garlic, oregano, turmeric.

Proteins: Beans, chicken, eggs, fresh seafood, nuts (except peanuts), seeds, turkey. Beans can be eaten freely.

AVOID:

Grains: Avoid processed or prepared grain and starch products such as snack crackers, unless manufactured by a natural foods company.

Dairy: Avoid all dairy products except ghee.

Sweeteners: Avoid concentrated sweets. Also avoid chemical sugar substitutes.

Oils: Avoid excess intake of oils, especially corn, Crisco, peanut. Low-quality oils increase inflammation and mucus.

Fruits: Reduce intake of light-colored fruits in favor of darker fruits listed above.

Vegetables: Avoid nightshade vegetables, including bell peppers, eggplant, tomato.

Spices: Avoid chilis.

Proteins: Peanuts, red meats.

CHAPTER *11*

The Gastrointestinal Tract: Digestion and Elimination

Wholesome food when devoured is ceaselessly consumed by the digestive fires to produce nutrients which are carried by the winds through the channels to endow the body tissues with happiness, strength, luster, and energy.

—Lord Atreya, 2500 B.C.

The purpose of the gastrointestinal (GI) tract is to digest nutrients from food sources so the body can absorb them to support life. I would estimate that up to half the people who come to my clinic suffer from some sort of digestive problem. In such cases, I must first identify and treat these conditions before I can focus on managing other health concerns. Digestive problems are often directly linked to improper dietary choices, already discussed in the previous chapter on nutrition. Beyond that, a comprehensive understanding of the GI system is your best bet for continued digestive health, so in this chapter we are going to walk through it step by step and learn how to use herbs to repair digestive problems.

Our basic topics of discussion include:

- Understanding the digestive process
- Restoring digestive power
- Coating, soothing, and healing irritated intestinal membranes
- Reducing intestinal acid and inflammation
- Reducing dampness and mucus in the intestinal tract
- Clearing toxic bacteria and fungi from the alimentary system

- Restoring balance to the intestinal flora

- Treating specific gastrointestinal problems

The Food Tube

The digestive tract is a continuous tube, running from the lips to the anus. It is embryologically derived primarily from the primary germ cell layer called the "endoderm" and is supported by a rich network of nerves, lymph tissue, and blood vessels. The tract is lined with soft tissues and membranes that guide food as it passes through, breaking it down and finally absorbing the resultant nutrients into the bloodstream and passing out remaining wastes for elimination. Outpouchings within this tube become the organs we all know, such as the lungs, the liver, and the pancreas, which secrete substances necessary for digestion.

Seen as a whole, the digestive tube is an intelligent nutrient absorption and transport system. As we discussed in Chapter 10, the tongue is the primary digestive sense organ and a very useful tool for diagnosing digestive problems. I always refer to the tongue if I am unsure of an intestinal diagnosis.

The integrity of the membranes lining the GI tract is another determining factor in overall GI health. Insults from dietary errors, diseases, or various chemical or mechanical problems can erode this membrane. It is an unfortunate fact that by the age of 85, two-thirds of the populations in Western countries suffer from diverticulosis. We tend to ignore many digestive problems such as pain, diarrhea, and constipation, or to simply treat them symptomatically instead of resolving them permanently. Prompt identification and correction of GI problems is crucial to maintaining good health throughout life.

Hunger and Appetite

Hunger is a physiological desire for food after a period of fasting, while appetite is the learned or evoked desire awakened by the presence of food. Someone who is extremely hungry may still not have an appetite for disliked foods. As well, someone who is not hungry may still have an appetite for delicious foods. Because hunger is controlled by physiological needs, and appetite is controlled by conditioned or mental factors, it is often important to distinguish these two.

Digestive Power

Most digestive problems are related to imbalances or changes in the digestive power. When the digestive power is strong, your appetite is regular, your system digests food easily and completely, and bowel movements are regular and complete. This combination of factors indicates that the various parts of the digestive system are working together smoothly.

Ayurvedic doctors point out that to maintain digestive power, it is very important to maintain regular mealtimes, choose healthy, well-prepared foods, and exercise portion control. Overeating, not eating enough, skipping meals, eating between meals frequently, or indulging in foods that are overly sweet, greasy, or stale can all stress the digestive function. Emotional stress can also weaken the digestive power, either directly by decreasing hunger or indirectly by affecting appetite.

The Mouth

Digestion begins in the mouth where your teeth break down food and mix it with saliva. Enzymes (amylase and ptyalin) are released which initiate fat and carbohydrate digestion. The saliva is important not only because of enzymes, but also because it contains nutrients and minerals important to remineralize your teeth and to lubricate and protect your mouth membranes. Regular mouth cleaning (brushing and flossing) is important to remove bacteria-encouraging debris and to slow formation of plaque and tartar.

- Ayurveda offers a very useful custom of cleaning the tongue each morning with a metal scraping tool. These tools are available online or in various health food stores.

- **Echinacea tincture** stimulates saliva flow for dry mouth when mixed with water and swished around in the mouth. It is also valuable for stimulating secretory IgA, a protective immune system antibody.

- **Haritaki fruit** is an effective mouthwash, when mixed with cold water, for treating spongy gums and slowing down bacterial growth.

Weak and Irregular Digestion

The stomach produces about 2 liters of digestive secretions per day. Insufficient activity of the nerves that control the stomach can cause a reduction in the production of stomach acid and pepsin (protein-digesting enzyme), which causes a major slowdown of food digestion. Sometimes even the mechanical churning of the stomach is slowed.

Stomach acid and pepsin are strong substances that can turn a piece of meat to liquid and are important to destroy incoming bacteria mixed with foods. When they are reduced in quantity, digestive function is hampered, and hormones and digestive enzymes are incapacitated. When levels are low, patients often report feeling that the food sits in their stomach "like a lump." This reaction causes a loss of appetite, nausea, and distended abdomen. From a diagnostic standpoint, the tongue is often puffy and swollen, and is sometimes pale or has a thick white coating. Weak digestion can sometimes cause paradoxical symptoms of stomach burning, perhaps due to irritation, in which case the standard Western practice of treatment with acid-blocking drugs can be very harmful. Digestion tends to weaken as we age, in part due to reduced hydrochloric acid secretion. For this reason, I always pay special attention to digestion when working with my elderly patients.

Weak digestion is a basic health problem that can become very serious and is often the cause of many seemingly unrelated diseases. According to holistic physician Jonathan Wright, M.D., weak digestion can contribute to arthritis (rheumatoid and degenerative), childhood asthma, acne rosacea, bursitis, chronic fatigue syndrome, depression, diabetes (Types 1 and 2), gallbladder attacks, lupus, macular degeneration, multiple sclerosis, osteoporosis, shingles (herpes zoster), and many cases of cancer. He also warns us that even this list is by no means complete. According to the same report, Japanese researchers found poor digestion to be the reason that some people do not respond to herbal remedies.

Pancreas, Liver, and Lymph

After the digestive process in the stomach is completed, food substances are released into the duodenum, where most digestion and absorption takes place. If (and only if) there is sufficient acid in the duodenum, the body releases two other digestive hormones, secretin and cholecystokinin. These hormones stimulate the gallbladder to secrete bile and the pancreas to release its digestive juices. In other words, poor initial digestion hinders everything further down the line.

Depending on signs and symptoms, it may be important to use herbs that regulate bile flow, such as **dandelion root, bupleurum root, beet root, celandine** *(Chelidonium majus),* **turmeric root, fringe tree bark** *(Chionanthus virginicus),* **rhubarb root,** and **sarsaparilla root.** These herbs are used when there are signs of a sluggish liver, such as poor digestion, fatigue, elevated liver enzymes, nausea, hightened sensitivity to foods or pharmaceutical medications, and poor elimination.

The pancreas produces enzymes that digest protein, fat, and carbohydrate, as well as sodium bicarbonate, an alkalizing agent. These are secreted directly into the small intestine through the pancreatic duct. The alkaline bicarbonate neutralizes the acidic chyme produced in the stomach. When these enzymes are low, they can be supplemented with herbs that have enzymatic action, such as **bromelain** or **papaya.**

Within the membranes of the intestinal tract is a rich network of submucosal lymphoid tissue, called the GALT (gut-associated lymphoid tissue). These compartmentlike tissues behind the intestinal membranes are critically important in immune function, both for the intestinal tract and for the body as a whole.

For example, food particles and immune cells intermingle here, and the GALT maintains a diverse population of mature lymphocytes capable of responding to foreign antigens. Indigestion, malnutrition, or inflammation can adversely affect this tissue (even causing it to atrophy), resulting in a wide variety of immune and inflammatory disorders.

Dietary fat intake is closely associated with the health of both the GALT and the intestinal mucosa, so care in using only high-quality fats in proper quantity can be important in both prevention and treatment of intestinal diseases by maintaining barrier integrity. These facts illuminate why herbalists through the centuries have strongly focused on intestinal health issues when treating problems in other areas of the body.

Strengthening Digestion

Herbs that strengthen digestion include **trikatu,** the famous Ayurvedic combination of **black pepper, long pepper,** and **ginger root.** You can make a variation of this at home by simply combining ground **black pepper** with **ginger powder.** Mix it with honey until a paste is formed, and take ½ teaspoon before meals.

These peppers may be too hot in conditions where the stomach membrane itself is weak or, of course, if acidity is actually too high. You can often determine this in advance by asking the patient about any cravings for warm drinks and spicy foods. In the absence of such cravings, you may want to start with an anti-inflammatory digestive aid like **papaya** or **bromelain** instead of the peppers. Warming, bitter herbs such as **turmeric root** or freshly ground **fenugreek seeds** are also useful in these cases. They stimulate digestion by activating the bitter taste receptors on the tongue, stimulating the nerves to secrete more digestive juices. Sometimes, however, coating therapy is needed (see below).

White atractylodes is perhaps the most commonly prescribed TCM herb for treating poor appetite and digestive weakness with signs of fatigue and diarrhea, a condition called **spleen Qi deficiency.** We often use it in our clinic before resorting to the stronger digestive herbs such as **trikatu** or pancreatic digestive enzymes. It seems to help gently restore digestive energy rather than simply substituting the missing enzymes.

TCM doctors often prescribe **white atractylodes** with **ginseng root, pinellia tuber, tangerine peel, poria mushroom,** and **licorice root** in a classic TCM digestive formula called **Six Gentlemen Decoction.** Elderly patients with weak digestion often benefit dramatically from **ginseng root** or **ginseng-based** digestive formulas.

Some patients do not digest oils properly, and when we use omega-3-rich oils like **flaxseed oil** or **fish oils,** the patients will report that they repeat back. Sometimes there are no obvious signs beyond this, and other times there are problems with dryness, such as dry eyes, or dry skin. In such cases, in addition to the herbs mentioned, pay attention to using foods that emulsify and thus help digest oils, mentioned in the nutrition chapter in the section on oils.

When treated promptly, poor digestion will usually respond very well to herbal treatments. However, when treatment is delayed, or symptoms are masked by the use of acid-blocking drugs or other symptomatic treatments, digestive problems can progress to more serious conditions.

Stomach and Intestine Sensitivity

The stomach churns our food, emulsifies fats, and continues the enzymatic breakdown of foods. In cases of extreme stomach or intestinal sensitivity and inflammation, even simple, gentle herbs can cause a negative reaction. In these cases, before I use the herbs mentioned above, I administer a simple combination of **slippery elm bark** and **licorice root,** about 2 grams two or three times per day. This formula mechanically soothes and coats the intestines. It can be used for several weeks, after which you can safely add other herbs.

Another good choice along with the **slippery elm** and **licorice** is **liquid chlorophyll,** about 1 tablespoon once or twice per day. **These herbs are so safe that they can be used even if you are not sure what your digestive problem is.**

Control of Nausea and Vomiting

Abdominal stimulation by irritants or toxins can activate nausea and vomiting through mechano- or chemoreceptors found in the mucosa of the stomach, jejunum, and ileum. Vomiting and nausea are natural protective responses of your digestive system to prevent intake of noxious substances and should not be inhibited until the cause is removed, if known. However, vomiting can itself be a troublesome symptom as well if prolonged due to irritation rather than an immediate and true toxicity.

- The TCM combination of **ginger root, agastache, pinellia tuber,** and **tangerine peel** offers simple nausea relief. Take 1–2 grams of concentrated extract powders before meals.

- Adding **inula flower** (xuan fu hua or *Inula* species) to the same formula often helps control vomiting. This flower has a strong downward action according to TCM doctors.

Gastric Ulcers

Continued weakness and inflammation of the gastrointestinal membranes can lead to the formation of ulcers. Recent scientific evidence indicates that the *Helicobacter pylori* bacterium plays an influential role in ulcer formation. However, we must remember that pathological organisms flourish only when conditions are favorable. For example, dental plaque can harbor a supply of *H. pylori,* which may allow continual reinfection. In cases of gastric ulcers, we must first address diet, stress, food allergies, liver health, and digestive power.

It is sometimes possible to obtain symptomatic relief with **cooked okra, cabbage juice,** or **bananas.** A few weeks or months of **DGL licorice** therapy can also serve to strengthen the stomach and intestinal membranes. This is very effective, even in some cases of *H. py-*

lori infection. In stubborn cases that do not respond to simple therapy, research indicates that **mastic gum** *(Pistacia lentiscus)* is emerging as a beneficial antiulcer therapy.

Digestive Acid and Heat

When the stomach nerves are overactive, often as a result of tension or stress, the stomach produces more acid. Normally, foods remain in the stomach for 4 or 5 hours and will not pass down through the pylorus (a muscular tissue which controls outlet from the stomach) until they are completely digested. However, in this hyperactive condition, incompletely processed foods pass down through the opening early—one of the physical causes of indigestion and diarrhea.

For example, rapid gastric emptying often occurs from pylorus muscle weakness caused by hypoglycemia. The rapid but incompletely processed and acidic downflow weakens the duodenum, which is alkaline in its function. If it cannot neutralize the acidity, weakening (irritation or erosion) of the duodenal membrane will ensue.

If stress is the cause of the hyperacidity and consequential weakness, dealing with the cause of the stress is the best solution. Herbs that can be useful in this capacity as adjunct therapy are those known to calm agitation, such as **skullcap, kava root,** or **bupleurum root,** along with herbs that reduce acidity like **cardamom seeds** *(Amomum* species) or **dried cuttlefish bone** (used in TAM and TCM, it is a good source of calcium).

General systemic inflammation can also cause stomach acidity because it leads to increased blood circulation and heat in the digestive organs. This heat stimulates the digestive fire. In this condition, there are higher levels of acid in both the stomach and the rest of the intestine, including the duodenum. This causes the general symptoms of gastritis with constipation or duodenitis with diarrhea, usually accompanied by an increase in appetite. The heat in the stomach causes a reduction in the digestive and blood fluids that can lead to excessive thirst and craving for cold liquids. Additionally, heat in the colon causes an increased absorption of fluids out of the colon, leading to constipation.

Laxatives like **rhubarb root** can be useful for initially purging this heat. If the patient is weak, I mix **rhubarb root** with an equal part of **triphala,** which has tonic qualities less likely to further weakness. The herbs are given for 1–2 days at bedtime at dosages enough to cause two to three bowel movements the following day.

Cooling herbs **(heat-reducing group)** can also neutralize these problems, including those that remove heat from the liver. TCM doctors often use **coptis root,** which is very cold in action, to treat heartburn and microbial diarrhea. I use it most frequently in these cases, along with **dandelion root** and **scute root. Boswellia gum** and **phellodendron root** are two other very important herbs for treating intestinal inflammation.

Dampness and Mucus

Eating too many fatty, oily, cold, or difficult-to-digest foods can create conditions of dampness and mucus, which weaken digestion. It is also important to understand that conditions of weak digestion can create dampness and mucus. The increased mucus (sometimes called phlegm) accumulates and inactivates or neutralizes the stomach acidity and the alkaline reaction in the intestines. This results in slowed digestion, which affects all the natural functions of the digestive system. Symptoms of dampness and mucus include a sensation of heaviness, abdominal distention, nausea, and sometimes diarrhea. There will often be a greasy coating or tooth marks on the tongue.

Treatment of these conditions requires herbs that warm and stimulate digestive function along with herbs that break up mucus and/or help to move the stagnant energy. **Poria mushroom, pinellia tuber, black atractylodes, magnolia bark, sausurrea root** (mu xiang or *S. lappa),* and **tangerine peel** are especially effective. Additional useful treatments include **ginger root, black** or **long pepper, coriander seeds,** and **amla fruit.** In cases of extreme nausea, use warming aromatic herbs like **agastache, magnolia bark, and fresh ginger root.** Patience is a true virtue when treating these cases, because conditions of dampness and mucus often take months to completely resolve if they are chronic.

Intestinal Dysbiosis

Intestinal dysbiosis is an emerging medical term for imbalances in the intestinal flora, a concept pioneered by holistic and naturopathic physicians. Think of the membranes lining your small and large intestines as your back yard. In this analogy, the membranes are the soil, and the "good guy" bacteria that inhabit your intestinal tract are the grass. The "bad guys," or inappropriate bacteria, yeasts, worms, or parasites, represent crabgrass that can take over parts of your intestinal lawn.

All in all, scientists have identified more than 400 species of gut microflora, which number in the billions in the average intestinal environment and can be weighed by the pound. The good guys produce beneficial substances including important natural antibiotic and immune-stimulating chemicals, and the bad guys can produce carcinogens, organic amines, and high levels of endotoxin (toxins released into the body when bacteria die). Poor digestion, poor food choices, inflammation, dampness, and stress lead to intestinal flora imbalances.

How the Bad Guys Infest Your Intestinal Lawn

Some of the more common bad guys include yeast *(Candida albicans), Klebsiella, Proteus, H. pylori, Giardia, Pseudomonas, Citrobacter,* and *Cryptosporidia.* Dysbiosis often occurs after long periods of weak or compromised digestion. When digestion is compromised, hydrochloric acid, pepsin, or pancreatic digestive enzymes are low and they fail to sterilize food entering the system. As often occurs in elderly patients, this allows the "bad guy" crabgrass to begin to seed your intestines. Other causes of intestinal dysbiosis include weakened immunity, alterations in intestinal pH, infections, and exposure to chemicals.

"Bad guys" can also colonize the small intestine. As abnormal fermentation increases, symptoms such as gas, bloating, and diarrhea begin to emerge. Over time, as the mucosal barrier erodes, toxins enter the bloodstream and there may be allergy, loss of mental clarity, moderate to severe fatigue, inflammation, and muscle pain. This

> ABC science news writer Nicholas Regush reported the work of parisitologist Dr. Lawrence Kaplow that a type of food-borne roundworm *(Cryptostrongylus pulmoni)* could be a newly discovered hidden causative agent in chronic fatigue syndrome.

is a very real and frustrating problem for patients that conventional physicians often overlook. In severe cases it can even be debilitating. It is one of the hidden causes of chronic fatigue syndrome.

Overuse of antibiotics can kill off the "good guy" bacterial population, resulting in a favorable environment for "bad guy" crabgrass growth. Yeast and similar intestinal infections are often easy to diagnose when patients produce an unusually high level of gas that often distends the stomach dramatically. These infections can also cause patients to wake up during the night during periods when they feel extremely hot, almost as if they are experiencing extended hot flashes. The heat produced by the bad guy organisms can also inflame and dry the intestines, causing constipation.

The Good Guys Fight Back

"Good guy" bacteria, especially *Lactobacillus acidophilus*, *Bifidobacteria,* and *Escherichia coli,* typically inhabit the large intestine. These bacterial species have been used as medicines (in pill form) since the discovery of their beneficial properties in 1908. They are traditionally found in fermented foods such as yogurt and **miso soup,** historically lauded for their many health benefits.

Lactobacillus and *Bifidobacteria* adhere to the cells of the intestinal epithelium and contribute to the equilibrium of gut flora. Because they are positive in action, they are called probiotics (pro-life), as opposed to antibiotics (anti-life). They help conjugate bile acids and antagonize other bacteria, especially the harmful ones that can lead to bowel toxemia, a precursor to skin conditions, cancers, fatigue, and various forms of inflammation. They also reduce incidence of intestinal infections, diarrhea, and urinary tract infections (UTIs).

> Although there has been slow acceptance in the Western world of the importance of yeast in chronic health conditions, Japanese scientists have been aware of this since the late 1960s, when microbiologists discovered that gut fermentation of some species could actually increase blood alcohol levels. The title of one particularly interesting article presented at an international conference in 1972 says it all: "A review of the literature on drunken symptoms due to yeasts in the gastrointestinal tract." In the West, such patients are often put on psychiatric medications.

Recent studies show it to be useful for management of food allergies by improving gut wall integrity, and controlled studies show that consumption of *acidophilus* capsules is beneficial during antibiotic treatment to restore intestinal flora and reduce diarrhea. In an article in the *American Journal of Gastroenterology,* a doctor at Johns Hopkins Medical Center in Baltimore, Maryland stated that "it is clear probiotic agents are becoming an important part of the armamentarium against gastrointestinal problems in infants and children."

I have devised a simple strategy for dealing with this problem, based on Dr. William Crook's pioneering work with *Candida* (yeast) infections. I do not initially differentiate between the different bacteria or yeast species. I simply administer an effective bad guy killer herb such as **grapefruit seed extract** or **neem leaf,** combined with good guy probiotics. The herb **wormwood** *(Artemisia annua)* is also very good for parasites, using 1 500-mg capsule twice a day. These are administered for days, weeks, but seldom for longer than 2 months, unless at reduced dosage.

In addition, I starve the bad guys out by depriving them of their favorite food—sugar—instructing the patient to avoid all cake, pie, candy, fruit, and fruit juice, and to lower dietary intake of complex carbohydrates from grain sources. Regular consumption of vegetables, oils, and proteins of all sorts is still allowed, and this program usually reduces symptoms within a few weeks, if not days.

In the old days, I prescribed this protocol alone, and perhaps six of my initial patients who had suffered for years thought I was a miracle worker. However, my revered status would soon change when the problem recurred several months later. In hindsight, I learned that it is necessary to treat the underlying problems as well. Now I work with patients for a couple of months during or after initial eradication of "bad guy" organisms to strengthen the GI system, following the various protocols outlined in this chapter. This results in long-term benefits for most patients. If symptoms do not clear, there is the possibility that a particularly nasty microbe or parasite is involved, and it then becomes necessary to send the patients for stool tests at a good laboratory (see Resource Guide).

The Large Intestine

The large intestine is wrapped in a layer of fat that acts like a thermal blanket, helping to create heat, absorb fluids, and solidify the stool for elimination. As mentioned earlier, there is a large population of gram-negative bacteria in the intestines, which ferment soluble fibers, starch, and undigested carbohydrates. This fermentation creates short-chain fatty acids, which is the main energy source for the lining epithelial cells. When there are imbalances in this fermentation, caused by problems further up the GI tract leading to increases in bad guy bacteria, putrefactive gases can develop.

These conditions result in serious abnormal fermentation in the intestines, thus producing a large amount of endotoxin, heat, and inflammation. This can cause the fluids to decrease enough to make the stool hard, causing constipation.

Other common causes of constipation include poor digestion, intestinal infections, lack of exercise, not drinking enough water, lack of fiber, sluggish liver, dryness, bowel diseases, and structural or neurological abnormalities.

Whatever the cause, putrefactive gases are harmful. In Ayurveda, they are known to be absorbed into the blood and to trigger inflammation in other areas of the body. To remove putrefactive gases, use the **diet to reduce wind,** along with carminative (gas-expelling) spices, such as **celery seeds, cloves, allspice, dill, fennel, peppermint, sage, cardamom, cumin, caraway,** and **fennel.** These spices work by either inhibiting the offending bacteria or neutralizing the offending gases.

Constipation

After making the appropriate dietary adjustments, I treat constipation with **rhubarb-based** formulas, instructing patients to increase fluid intake. A simple, effective bowel tonic combines **dandelion root, rhubarb root,** and **triphala. Rhubarb root** is, of course, laxative. The **dandelion** stimulates the bile flow while the **triphala** has a general healing effect on the intestinal membranes, combining mild laxative with strong tonic effects. I tell patients to adjust the amount they take each night until they return to proper bowel movements in the morning.

In more serious cases, patients may temporarily require stronger laxatives such as **buckthorn bark, cascara sagrada,** or **senna,** after which they must retrain their bowels to function properly. This is done by increasing water and fiber intake, exercising every day for at least 15 minutes, and attempting to move the bowels at a set time each morning. Drinking some warm **lemon juice** can sometimes serve as an effective intermediate step after a gradual decrease in the use of laxative herbs.

TCM doctors point out that it is sometimes necessary to release tension (Qi restriction) in the intestines. A classic TCM formula for this purpose contains **rhubarb root, immature bitter orange fruit** (zhi shi or *Citrus aurantium),* and **magnolia bark** (hou po or *M. officinalis).*

Diarrhea

Diarrhea, defined as increased volume, fluidity, or frequency of bowel movements, can have many causes. Generally, if the cause originates in the small intestine, the diarrhea is characterized by large quantities of watery and/or fatty stools. If the cause of the diarrhea is a disease in or of the colon, the stools are frequent and often accompanied by blood, mucus, or pus. If the disease is rectal in origin, there are often frequent movements of small amounts of stool.

In cases of acute diarrhea the most important thing to remember is the need to maintain electrolyte balance, especially in children. In emergency cases with signs of dehydration, you can introduce fluids supplemented with table salt. Otherwise, use an electrolyte replace-

---

Recipe for Homemade Electrolyte Replacement Solution

Simmer several of the following chopped vegetables for 2 hours in about 2 quarts of water: green beans, kale, broccoli, cabbage, onion, garlic, parsley, cilantro, celery, baby bok choy, brussels sprouts, asparagus, chard, collard greens, etc. Strain and add:

1 tsp salt (mineral salt is best)

1 cup fresh carrot or tomato juice

1 tsp baking soda

2 tablespoons molasses

1 teaspoon miso

Mix all ingredients together and refrigerate. Drink ½ cup three or four times per day. Take until diarrhea clears up.

---

ment supplement, and always remember to drink plenty of water. There are many acceptable commercial electrolyte supplements on the market, but if you so desire you can make your own version at home. I have my own recipe, provided in the adjacent box for your convenience.

I recommend a short period of water or juice fasting for 1 or 2 days, followed by a gradual reintroduction of mild foods that are very easy to digest. Choose foods such as rice, cooked carrots, miso soup, tapioca, potato broth, potassium broth (made with carrot, spinach, celery, and parsley), applesauce, and **black** or **green tea.** After that, choose formulas as described above based upon the cause, bacterial infection, inflammation, and so on.

Chronic Diarrhea

Bacterial toxins, drugs, liver ailments, various types of inflammation, and poor digestion leading to unabsorbed dietary fat or carbohydrates are the most common causes of chronic diarrhea. To treat chronic diarrhea successfully, you must first identify the underlying causes and treat them with the appropriate herbs as defined earlier.

However, there are several special cases we need to mention because there are times when chronic diarrhea does not respond to direct herbal treatment. Hidden food allergies can often cause chronic diarrhea, as can inflammatory bowel disease, two situations we will explore later in more detail. A severe intestinal infection can also be the culprit, and this will require treatment with strong herbs or antibiotics. A stool test is often necessary to identify the infection causing the condition.

Additionally, some patients may have hydrochloric acid levels that are so low they require direct HCl supplementation. This is especially true with patients over the age of 60. Finally, there are times when none of the usual theories help. In these cases I use **vilwa fruit,** which can sometimes work wonders, very slowly.

In severe cases following a very restricted diet, such as "The Elemental Diet" (very low carbohydrates) can be helpful. Some authorities allow only lamb and pears for a few weeks.

I recommend initiating the following measures immediately to help to control the problem.

- Reduce the size of your meals, and eat 5 or 6 smaller meals throughout the day. Choose from the foods I recommended earlier. The decreased amount of food eases the strain on your digestive system and is less likely to stimulate bowel movements.

- It is important to replace the fluid lost with diarrhea. Drink 6 to 12 cups of fluid per day. Even if you are not thirsty, you must still drink. Try taking it in smaller amounts, about ½ cup of clear fluid every 2 hours.

- Avoid coffee, which can stimulate bowel movements and urination. Sodas also stimulate urination due to their high sugar content. Surprisingly, these fluids can actually lower your total fluid balance by prompting you to excrete more than you take in.

- A temporary low-fiber diet may decrease cramping and gas in severe cases. Choose softer white breads, white rice, and pasta at first. Although you want to limit high-fiber food sources for a period of time, water-soluble fiber supplements such as Metamucil and pectins will help you produce a firmer stool. They can also help absorb irritating excess bile salts.

- Eat foods high in potassium and salt, such as crackers, bananas, baked potatoes, bouillon, potassium broth, chicken soup, and tomato juice. If the diarrhea is severe, use commercial electrolyte replacement solutions, or make your own with the recipe provided earlier.

- Probiotic supplementation is helpful for easing diarrhea. The usual dosage is 2 capsules per day (10 billion organisms) for up to 2 weeks, then 1 capsule per day. The organisms are quickly excreted, so usage should be constant in severe cases.

- Eat fewer fruits, and limit portion sizes. It is probably best to primarily use fruit juices because they provide the nutrients and are easier to assimilate than whole fruits. Unpeeled fruits can be irritating. If you have been told to avoid sugar, you can make **blueberry** or **raspberry** juice in your blender by combining berries, water, and a noncaloric sweetener such as **stevia leaf.**

- For vegetable sources, use well-cooked soups at first, gradually reintroducing cooked and raw vegetables.

- Many people with chronic diarrhea have difficulty digesting milk. Signs of lactose intolerance include gas

---

The following foods get high marks for taste and nutrition and can be used in lieu of milk products:

- Soy milk. Kids especially like the vanilla-flavored forms.
- Rice Sliced Cheese, available in two flavors. Tastes like real cheese.
- Spectrum Naturals Spread, a nonhydrogenated butter substitute.

These and many others are available at most local health food stores.

and cramping after consumption of dairy products in addition to the diarrhea. Some people have to avoid all milk products, while others can use lactase supplements or may be able to tolerate yogurt or cheese. There are several commercially available products that can be used in place of dairy if necessary. See the box on page 293 for a few of my personal favorites.

Hidden Food Allergies

A "food allergy" is an immediate or delayed adverse reaction to the ingestion of a specific food. Common signs and symptoms of such allergies include dark circles and puffiness under the eyes, chronic diarrhea, various inflammations, headaches (including migraine), chronic runny nose, itchy eyes, asthma, hives, poor digestion, mental and physical fatigue, inflammatory diseases, and chronic infections. Food allergy sensitivity usually forms slowly as a result of repetitive consumption of a food.

To test for a hidden food allergy, remove the item completely from your diet for 2 weeks, making sure to read all labels to ensure compliance. After 2 weeks, eat a moderate to large amount of the food in question and see if the reintroduction of the food causes a noticeable adverse reaction over the next 24–48 hours. Common reactions include diarrhea, headache, nausea, hyperactivity, hives or skin itching, fatigue, irritability, bags under the eyes, and insomnia. If any of these symptoms appear, you are most likely allergic to the food and should remove it from your diet permanently. The 2-week abstinence period allows the body to mount a stronger response, allowing for easier identification. If there is no response, you are not allergic to this food and may resume regular consumption. You may want to repeat the test if you are unsure of the result.

Once you have eliminated the offending food from your diet, you may find that after 3–6 months you can eat it occasionally without experiencing an adverse reaction. Eat the food no more than once every 4 or 5 days—several days in a row will probably reactivate the allergy and cause a return of symptoms.

For a list of the most common causes of food allergy, refer to the Appendix. It is also possible to react to an entire class of foods, such as all milk products, citrus fruits, nuts, or chemical preservatives. Remember to check all labels of the foods you eat to make sure none of the foods you are allergic to are hidden in the ingredients.

Irritable Bowel Syndrome

According to a meta-analysis in the *American Journal of Gastroenterology,* **peppermint oil** is an effective treatment for irritable bowel syndrome (IBS), a condition that accounts for 50% of all visits to gastrointestinal doctors! The **peppermint oil** usually relieves intestinal spasms and promotes rhythmic peristaltic movement within a few weeks. Before taking **peppermint,** however, make sure that you are suffering from simple intestinal spasms and not a more serious inflammatory colitis. Of course, you must also identify any food allergies, and correct intestinal membrane health and digestive power. It is never wise to rely on a simple remedy, no matter how effective, without treating the underlying causes of a condition. If patients do not respond to **peppermint,** we use the herbs mentioned next.

Diverticulosis, Diverticulitis, and Intestinal Permeability

Diverticulosis, a condition characterized by sacs or pockets in the colon with no inflammation, is a disease seen most frequently in elderly patients. It affects up to 20% of the population by the age of retirement, and two-thirds by the age of 85.

Researcher A.R.P. Walker pioneered the work linking food, gut function, and disease patterns. He recognized that South African blacks have a very low incidence of colonic problems such as diverticulitis, adenomatous polyps, and carcinoma. Consequently, he postulated that the traditional high-fiber African diet was important for maintaining colonic health. Follow-up studies showed that disease symptoms could be substantially improved with a diet high in fiber-containing whole-wheat bread, cereals with bran, vegetables, and fruits.

While I agree that fiber is of therapeutic importance, we must also consider the other factors discussed throughout this chapter, especially long-term neglected constipation. Also, any of the problems mentioned throughout this chapter can create a condition of increased intestinal permeability, allowing toxins to enter the bloodstream and disturb the immune system.

We can treat diverticulosis and intestinal permeability conservatively but effectively with a high-fiber diet, accompanied by membrane-strengthening herbs like **tien chi root, licorice root, gotu kola,** and **liquid chlorophyll,** or mucilaginous herbs like **slippery elm bark** that coat. Carotene-rich carrot juice is also often helpful. According to tolerance **ginseng root** or **white atractylodes** can be gradually added to strengthen the internal energy. Basic vitamins and minerals are also important.

> I recall one very difficult case. The patient was a woman in her 50s who had been suffering from chronic diverticulitis for two decades, and her diet was severely limited. She could not take even simple Chinese herbs. I began by putting her on a diet of organic baby food, supplemented with 2 grams of **slippery elm/licorice powder** twice per day. After about a month she was able to tolerate Chinese herbs, and Nai-shing brought about a recovery from there, using the herbs mentioned here. In 6 months the patient had gained weight and regained her health.

Diverticulitis is a progression of diverticulosis, caused by inflammation and subsequent perforation of one or more of the sacs in the colon. Milder forms of diverticulitis begin with gradually increasing symptoms emanating from the lower left quadrant of the abdomen. Cases of acute complicated disease present with dramatic onset of abdominal pain, followed by fever. Chronic diverticulitis can be debilitating. The treatment is the same as described but often requires more sophisticated formula changes over a long period of time, along with the addition of anti-inflammatory herbs like **scute root, coptis rhizome, dandelion root, persica seed** (tao ren or *Prunus persica*), **red peony root,** and **boswellia gum.**

Nai-shing has noticed that there is often internal bowel tension contributing to this problem, which accords with both TAM correlation of bowel dysfunction with neurological disturbance (Vata) and the Western clinical observation that antispasmodics are of clinical use with this disease. If there are signs of tension along with the pain, **kava root** or **ashwagandha root** can be added to your formula. **Peppermint oil** or **stoneroot tincture** can be used independently. Use of omega-3 oils like **flaxseed** or **fish oils** are also of benefit to lubricate and reduce inflammation.

Inflammatory Bowel Disease

Inflammatory bowel diseases (IBD) include Crohn's disease and ulcerative colitis. Crohn's disease involves diarrhea, weakness, occasional bleeding, and a diffuse granulomatous inflammation of the entire bowel membrane. In cases of ulcerative colitis the inflammation is limited mostly to the colon. These cases are very difficult to treat with herbs alone. The diseases often progress to the point where patients require surgery to remove inflamed areas of the bowel, and since this does not usually solve the problem, they often experience recurrences.

I usually begin treatment of these conditions with a careful history to identify causative factors. My usual first step is a bland diet, eliminating milk products and other potential food allergens (see Appendix). I then add **slippery elm/licorice powder** to calm things down mechanically, about 6 grams per day in divided doses for up to a month. I sometimes use **liquid chlorophyll** and acidophilus capsules as well. Herbs that can be of great benefit in these conditions when used as simples (single herbs in capsules or tablets) include **tien chi root,** which helps heal the ulcers, and **boswellia gum, turmeric root,** and **licorice root,** which control inflammation. Sometimes plain **green tea** can also be helpful.

Inflammatory prostaglandin levels are almost always highly elevated in these diseases, and studies have shown great benefit in using large amounts of **flaxseed** or **fish oils.** Tinctures can often work at first when patients cannot tolerate powders. For the same reason, I often employ liquid vitamin and mineral combinations to ensure some absorption.

Because IBD patients are invariably deficient in key nutrients, it is necessary to supplement with a liquid multivitamin and liquid multimineral. Studies show that patients are especially prone to elevated homocysteine levels, indicating the need for B_{12} and folic acid supplementation. **Beet root** would also be valuable here.

Vilwa fruit is an important herb for treating colitis. A simple Ayurvedic formula combines **vilwa fruit powder** (60%) with **anise, coriander,** a very small amount of **ginger root,** and an astringent herb such as **black tea.** I recommend using about 2 grams two to three times per day.

It is always best to consult a skilled herbalist when writing formulas for serious diseases like this. The thought processes behind the formulas in this case include assessment of both the digestive power and the inflammation level, as both types of herbs usually are needed. In cases of weak digestion, herbs like **white atractylodes, poria mushroom,** and **ginseng root** should be emphasized.

If the inflammation is more severe, you might emphasize other herbs in the formula, like **scute root, coptis rhizome, boswellia gum,** and **phellodendron root.** When bleeding is present, it is important to add **tien chi root** or another hemostatic. Cases with fixed pain indicate blood congestion, which requires blood-moving herbs like **red peony root** and **salvia root.** If the diarrhea is severe, use astringent herbs such as **vilwa fruit** or **white oak bark.**

CHAPTER 12

Cardiovascular Health and Regulation of Blood

The miracle is not to walk on water. The miracle is to walk on the green earth, dwelling deeply in the present moment and feeling truly alive.

—Thich Nhat Hanh

Cardiovascular disease (CVD) is a serious problem throughout many parts of the world. In the United States, according to the American Heart Association, 58.8 million Americans had one or more types of heart disease in 1998. Since the turn of the 20th century, CVD has been the number one cause of death every year except 1918. The yearly cost associated with these cases is estimated to be in excess of $250 billion, and billions of dollars more have been spent upon research. Yet few people are aware that workable solutions and preventive measures for many heart and circulation problems are available by the intelligent use of a bit of herbal and functional medicine knowledge.

Our purpose here will be to understand how to maintain a strong heart, healthy blood, and good circulation and how to avoid inflammation. We have already discussed the importance of nutrition and how to keep the digestive tract healthy in the chapters on nutrition and the GI tract. Our circulatory system depends upon a good supply of high-quality raw materials. Once food leaves the gastrointestinal tract, it goes to the liver for processing and filtering and then enters the general circulation under the command of the heart muscle. Before we can talk about the blood, we need to understand a little about the liver and the heart.

Understanding the Heart

Imagine a thick tube, about the size of a garden hose and about 2 feet long. Once you have a good mental picture, tie the tube into a knot about the size of your fist. Now picture a hand squeezing the knot, causing water to squirt out of the ends of the tube. When the heart beats, it pumps the blood out into the circulatory system. Imagine also that someone has placed some screens inside the hose to trap and filter particles.

It should now be easy for you to visualize the major components to this system, all of which are important for our ensuing discussion. Your hand represents the electrical impulses that tell the heart to beat. The garden hose represents the tough fibrous muscular outer structures of both the heart and the blood vessels. The screens represent the liver and spleen, filtering out poisons. The inside lining of the hose represents the interior lining of both your heart and its blood vessels. This lining exists in both heart chambers as well as in the vessels that enter and exit the heart. Because these delicate membranes lining the entire cardiovascular system are in direct contact with the blood components and are very susceptible to oxidative damage (deterioration and clogging), we will be spending extra time discussing how to prevent and neutralize this destructive inflammation.

Hearty Considerations

As we breathe, we absorb the Earth's gases. The nose, mouth, trachea, and diaphragm take air into our lungs, bringing life-giving oxygen and gases into our blood when we inhale, and excreting waste gases as we exhale. Moreover, musculoskeletal and myofascial integrity are necessary to prevent blockage of blood and energy flow and to ease the workload of the heart. To stay healthy, the heart of course needs plenty of oxygen, nutrients, exercise, relaxation, pure water, and love, the latter perhaps suffering as the most underappreciated of these necessities.

To understand these issues at a deeper level, it is important to note that the pumping action of the heart is insufficient in itself to propel the blood. It requires the aid of the diaphragm, so good respiration is essential to good blood circulation. Because our degree of muscular tension determines oxygen demand, the more tension we have, the harder our heart and our muscles have to work.

For example, a muscle that has to pull against its chronically tense partner will become overworked, requiring a constant supply of energy (ATP). This will burn up nutrients and increase oxidative stress. By utilizing relaxation tools like T'ai Chi, Yoga, and Qi Gong, we take a big load off the heart. By the same token, periodic regular exercise strengthens our heart. These larger lifestyle issues are important for prevention, always the primary goal of holistic medicine.

Attention to these issues puts us in harmony with the natural cycles of Yin and Yang. We will explore both of these in more depth in Chapter 15 when we discuss musculoskeletal disorders, and in Chapter 17 when we take a look at the respiratory system.

If we fail to heed the aforementioned lessons, our hearts will gradually weaken and fail. Following is a list of the most common heart problems:

1. *Arteriosclerosis.* This term refers to the walls of the arteries becoming thickened, with a resultant loss of elasticity, commonly called "hardening of the arteries."

2. ***Atherosclerosis.*** This is a form of arteriosclerosis in which the cause is the buildup of fatty plaques on the interior lining of the arteries.

3. ***Ischemia.*** This is a lack of oxygen to a tissue usually due to inadequate blood supply.

4. ***Myocardial infarction.*** An infarct is an area of tissue that dies (necrosis) following cessation of blood supply. A myocardial infarction occurs when an infarct forms in your heart muscle. This is commonly called a heart attack and is usually caused by a thrombus (blood clot in the arteries).

5. ***Arrhythmia.*** This is an irregularity or loss of rhythm in the heartbeat. There are several types such as tachycardia, which means faster than normal beating of the heart. These are usually caused by disturbances in the electrical impulses from a special area of the heart called the sinoatrial node.

6. ***Stroke.*** This is a sudden loss of consciousness, followed by paralysis. It is sometimes caused by a hemorrhage in the brain, often due to high blood pressure. The most common cause is a thrombus in a vessel supplying the brain.

7. ***Pericarditis, myocarditis, and endocarditis.*** These are disorders caused by inflammation and swelling in the sheath surrounding the heart, the heart muscle, and the heart muscle lining, respectively.

8. ***Heart failure.*** This is essentially the end stage of failure to nourish, cleanse, and strengthen. Congestive heart failure (CHF) occurs when there is a profound reduction in the ability of the heart to contract and deliver nutrients and oxygen to the tissues. Cardiac output then becomes inadequate to meet the metabolic needs of our many organ systems. Symptoms include shortness of breath upon exertion, fatigue and weakness, and fluid accumulation in the lungs, liver, abdomen, and ankles. This condition is clearly associated with various electrolyte imbalances and nutritional deficiencies, especially magnesium and potassium.

Keeping Your Heart Strong and Healthy

There are many herbal methods for avoiding heart problems. The flavonoid nutrients found in many herbs reduce inflammation and help repair the membranes on the inside of the heart and blood vessels (see **vessel-strengthening group**). Foods that are high in flavonoids include wine that is made from **red grapes,** and **berries** (such as blackberries, blueberries, and raspberries). Both are very good for keeping the heart healthy.

The cholesterol-reducing agents found in herbs in the **mucus-removing group** help prevent vessel clogging. Tonic herbs found in the **immune group** help keep the heart muscle energized. Any of the herbs from the **blood-nourishing group** will strengthen the heart, because the blood nourishes all the muscles, including the heart muscle.

Hawthorn is the preferred heart herb in Western herbal medicine. The leaf and flower of

hawthorn are indicated specifically for treating Stage I and Stage II cardiac insufficiency, as defined by the New York Heart Association. This herb works more on reducing interior lining inflammation.

In Ayurvedic practice, the premier heart tonic is **arjuna bark.** This herb offers a large spectrum of healing benefits that include helping cardiac muscle weakness, easing arterial clogging, and lowering blood pressure. It contains fairly high levels of magnesium and other minerals. **Pomegranate fruit** is also considered a heart tonic in TAM, especially the sweeter varieties, as well as **wild asparagus root.**

For congestive heart failure Chinese doctors often use a compound called "Generate the Pulse," which contains **ginseng root, astragalus root,** and **ophiopogon root** (mai men dong or *O. japonicus).* They also use this formula in cases of heart palpitations and skipped heartbeats, as well as for recovery from severe cardiac trauma.

Another important heart herb is **night-blooming cereus flower** *(Selenicereus grandiflorus).* This herb, used by Eclectic physicians, strengthens the heart action and can correct an irregular pulse due to neurological weakness. It has a strong stimulating action on the sympathetic nerves and may be used for bradycardia. The correct dose for general tonification is 10–20 drops of a 1:5 tincture two times a day. An excessive dose (more than 40 drops) may quicken the pulse. This plant combines well with **hawthorn tincture.**

For detailed descriptions of **ginseng, astragalus, hawthorn, arjuna,** and **wild asparagus,** refer to Section Two.

Research Highlights

- **Bupleurum root, soy products, astragalus root, salvia root,** and **ginseng root** all contain saponins and other phytonutrients that are beneficial to the heart. They reduce lipid peroxide formation in the cardiac muscle and the liver, and they decrease blood coagulation and cholesterol in the blood. Research also indicates that they "act either directly, by blocking the transfer of Ca_2+ ions or modulating the function of Na(+)-K(+)-ATPase, or they help resorb other active principles" (Purmova, 1995).

- Gingerol from **ginger root** mildly increases the heart's force of contraction via beta-adrenergic stimulation in animal models (Antipenko et al, 1999).

- **Gynostemma** *(Gynostemma pentaphyllum* or xian cao), also known as the "herb of immortality," contains triterpenoid saponins called gypenosides. Research has shown that these compounds directly stimulate nitric oxide release, a process that is very beneficial to the heart (Tanner et al., 1999).

- The combination of **ginseng root** and **ginkgo leaf** showed benefit in a placebo-controlled double-blind study on the cognitive function and heart rate at maximum load of 64 healthy volunteers (Wesnes et al., 1997).

- A 10-month clinical study of the heart benefits of **garlic bulb** use showed it to be quite broad, including positive effects on lipids, blood pressure, and platelet stickiness (Steiner and Lin, 1998).

- Fish (and fish oils) are heart tonics. In two studies it was reported, for example, that simply eating fish once per week could reduce the risk of sudden cardiac death by almost 50% (Albert et al., 1998; Kromhout, 1998). Combining fish oils with **garlic bulb** quickens the onset of beneficial effects (Morcos, 1997).

- A controlled multicenter trial in elderly patients showed that the use of high-dose **St. John's wort** is safer with regard to cardiac function than tricyclic antidepressants (Czekalla et al., 1997).

- German researchers working with **hawthorn** report that "rigorous clinical trials show benefit concerning objective signs and subjective symptoms of congestive heart failure" (Weihmayr and Ernst, 1996).

- Other well-researched important heart nutrients include vitamin E, B vitamins, coenzyme Q_{10}, calcium, magnesium, and L-carnitine.

At our clinic, when we see heart patients, we place them on a healthy diet, relaxation, and therapeutic exercise regimen and give them a tonic composed of a selection of the above herbal medicines and nutrients in relatively high doses. If these directions are followed and the herbs taken without fail for months and years, great improvement can often be seen.

One of our patients was a middle-aged medical doctor, whose life and practice were on the skids after he developed early signs of cardiac insufficiency, perhaps related to his disillusionment with his standard medical practice. Now, several years later, he is a much healthier and happier man, with a thriving holistic-oriented practice. His patients love him, because he now loves what he is doing.

Understanding the Liver

The liver is a vascular, secretory, and metabolic organ that resides in the upper abdomen. It receives a dual blood supply from the hepatic artery and the portal vein and is by far our most important metabolic and detoxification organ.

The liver metabolizes (burns) all three macronutrients (fats, carbohydrates, and proteins), providing energy, vitamins, minerals, and other nutrients. Composed of thousands of tiny functional units called lobules, this organ filters over 1,500 mL of blood per minute. If it is not functioning well, toxins spill into the bloodstream or out into the bile causing inflammation and oxidative stress.

The liver is also a major storage organ. Nutrients are extracted, converted, and stored. For example, excess sugars are converted into glycogen and stored for later release. The same is done for fat-soluble vitamins, other essential nutrients (proteins and fats, etc.), and even blood.

Moreover, the liver can also store toxins, hopefully for later elimination. The liver is responsible for the creation and secretion of bile, necessary to emulsify and digest fats and carry away wastes. It also synthesizes various immune and blood proteins necessary for life processes.

Complex chemical substances that enter the liver are neutralized in one of three major ways:

- They are eaten by Kupffer cells.

- They are captured and dissolved into the bile, produced in the gallbladder from components supplied by the liver, and excreted to the intestine.

- They are chemically dismantled, tagged, and sent off by the enzyme systems for elimination.

Kupffer cells are large specialized macrophages (white blood cells) that phagocytize (eat) bacteria, endotoxins, antigen-antibody complexes, and other liver poisons. This makes the liver an important immune system organ. These cells chew up most of the larger particles that enter the liver. However, they produce dangerous oxidative free radicals as a by-product of this process, and the liver requires a sufficient supply of protective antioxidants to neutralize them. We will give a detailed discussion of other immune cells in Chapter 19.

The liver's cytochrome P450 system works on complex chemicals. As substances such as hormones, drugs, alcohol, carcinogens, pesticides, and inflammatory chemicals like histamine enter the system, enzymes oxidize and break down the intruders (a process called phase I detoxification). After that, the liver chemically tags and changes the breakdown products so that they can be excreted (called phase II detoxification). This process also results in the release of free radical poisons, so it is important to supply the body with the protective antioxidant herbs mentioned above.

The liver synthesizes more than a liter of thick, viscous, heavily pigmented, and bitter bile each day to capture, neutralize, and carry away poisons, acids, dying red blood cells, drugs, mucus, cholesterol, lecithin, mucin, chemicals, pigments, salts, and minerals.

Once released by the gallbladder into the intestine, the bile helps emulsify and digest fats. The condition in which the liver is congested or sluggish is known as cholestasis. This often occurs because the bile has become too thick and loaded down with mucus and inflammatory toxins. Of course, evaluation and regulation of dietary habits—especially fat intake—should be the initial and continuing treatment method for permanent resolution of this condition.

By the way, a lot of the mystery concerning how your body reacts to things is eliminated if you realize that sometimes herbs or drugs (and even common foods) help activate individual cytochrome P450 enzymes, which speeds removal of molecules. They can also inhibit the action of these enzymes, which can be useful for keeping certain chemical substances in the general circulation for a longer period of time.

The importance of this acceleration process varies. If we have a "bad guy" chemical in our blood, speeding removal is good. However, if we have a necessary or "good guy" chemical in our blood, speeding removal would be bad.

In the same way, if we have a "bad guy," slowing removal would be bad and if we have a "good guy, " slowing removal would be good. For example, drinking **grapefruit juice** will keep the expensive pharmaceutical drug Viagra in circulation longer, which means you could probably use half as much and save money. Drinking grapefruit juice when taking cardiac glycosides could raise our blood levels and be dangerous.

Individual variations in our cytochrome P40 enzymes help to demystify why there are so many variations in how we respond to drugs and herbs. This is why one man's herbal meat is another man's herbal poison. A well-trained medical practitioner can exploit these facts to your advantage. For more information on this process with common drugs, and a few herbs, look for Dave Flockhart's Drug Table on the web at http://www.dml.georgetown.edu/depts/pharmacology/davetab.html.

Herbs to Help the Liver

When discussing herbs for the liver, it is important to keep in mind that the TCM Liver (with a capital *L*) system differs from the physical liver in several respects, although there is some overlap. We will cover the TCM concepts of **Liver Qi restriction** and **Liver wind** elsewhere. Treating the liver and treating the blood are similar (the filter and the substance being filtered), so some things—such as clearing the blood of fats—will be covered later in this chapter.

The important thing to remember is that the liver is a hot (metabolically active) organ and so tends to get congested and inflamed. Therefore, all the herbs in these categories work to reduce this "heat and damp," but they work in different ways.

Protection

Turmeric root, wheat sprouts, schisandra berries, amla fruit, beet root, and **milk thistle seed** are major sources of protective antioxidants for the liver cells, as are fruits that contain flavonoids, especially citrus fruits. These should be used to prevent development of inflammatory disease, or for damage protection as in the case of persons taking strong chemical drugs or undergoing chemotherapy.

Correcting Deficiency

The liver can become weakened and deficient. If this is not corrected, it can lead to liver atrophy and depletion of glycogen stores, even hepatitis. Signs include fatigue, low blood pressure, hypoglycemia, dry eyes, headache, heat symptoms, and irritability. In such a case, we use **white peony root** and **cooked rehmannia root** to do what is known in TCM terms as nourishing the **Liver blood** and **Liver Yin. Milk thistle seed** also nourishes the liver, stimulating protein synthesis and cellular regeneration. **Shilajatu** and **haritaki fruit** are both very nourishing to the liver. Any of these herbs can also be used to lower elevated liver enzymes.

Heat Removal

To remove excess liver inflammation with heat signs or toxins, you can use **bromelain, bupleurum root, scute root, dandelion root, turmeric root, milk thistle seed, vasaca leaf** *(Adhatoda vasica),* **neem leaf, chrysanthemum flower, salvia root, wild asparagus root,** or **gardenia fruit** (zhi zi or *G. jasminoides).* You can also use any of the herbs from the **poison-removing group** or the **heat-removing group.**

Heat and Dampness Reduction

Heat and dampness are present in the liver with signs of both inflammation and conges- tion or swelling; bile flow is usually slowed. Use cholagogues, herbs that reduce inflamma- tion by moving the bile out more quickly to the intestine. Choose among **bupleurum root, dandelion root, burdock root, eclipta, turmeric root, scute root, capillaris** (yin chen hao or *Artemisia capillaris),* **sarsaparilla root, greater celandine** *(Chelidonium majus),* and **fringe tree bark** *(Chionanthus virginicus).* Laxative herbs like **rhubarb root** can some- times provide even quicker results. **Castor oil packs** over the abdomen are also useful.

Pain Relief

If there is liver inflammation with signs of pain and tension, use herbs that calm the liver and move the blood. Choose from **schisandra berries, white sandalwood, salvia root, wild asparagus root, turmeric root,** and **German chamomile.**

Blood and Blood Circulation

In the same way the blood draws gases from the air, the blood draws its nutrient supply from the Earth. All our important blood nutrients come from the Earth's bounty, as the food we ingest is processed in the intestinal tract. Nutrients are absorbed from the intestines into the portal vein system and then move directly into the liver, which is responsible for clean- ing our blood through filtration and detoxification processes. For this and other reasons al- ready discussed, the quality of the air and food is critical to keeping the blood healthy.

We can compare the blood to a trucking company carrying oxygen and nutrients to the tissues and cells, and carrying away waste products for elimination. To accomplish these parallel tasks, the body uses its many vessels and ducts, an enclosed system that functions like a road system for the serum "nutrient trucks," red blood cell "oxygen trucks," and im- mune system "debris removers." Additionally, the lymph system ducts draw away more fluid wastes. If the blood is pure and full of nutrients and oxygen, and the processes of waste re- moval and circulation are operating efficiently, the cells will remain healthy.

There are tiny grooves inside blood vessels, and as the blood is pumped through the heart (picture the hand squeezing the knot) it swirls outward, creating a centrifugal force that helps propel the blood cells into the tissues. As early as 1932, scientists photographed blood flow in embryos. In the embryonic stages before the heart developed, they demonstrated that the blood circulated in two separate, self-propelled spiral streams.

If the arteries and blood vessels become congested with inflammation and plaque buildup, it creates turbulence that defeats this mechanism leading to selective starvation or overfeeding of tissues. This can lead to critical problems before there is a full blockage leading to a stroke or heart attack.

Blood Circulation—Natural Diagnosis and Treatment

All herbal traditions put a great emphasis on the crucial processes of regulating and improving blood circulation. Many destructive changes to the heart, liver, and all other tissues can be avoided if we keep the blood healthy. Some herbalists have gone so far as to say that if the blood is clean and healthy there will be little or no disease. Several herbal approaches to blood circulation can be applied to treat a large number of health disorders. The protocol you select will depend on your treatment goals.

These basic goals are:

- To nourish the blood

- To improve poor circulation

- To move the blood

- To reduce blood congestion and stasis

- To remove excess blood fats

- To cleanse the blood of inflammation

> I had a case of an 85-year-old woman with a history of congestive heart failure, chronic diarrhea and fluid retention, and persistent anemia requiring blood transfusions every month. To stop the diarrhea and anemia, I added **arjuna bark** for the heart, **bael fruit** for the diarrhea, **ginseng root, schisandra berry, ophiopogon,** and some digestive enzymes to a quart of **alfalfa** tincture. She took it by the teaspoon until it slowed the diarrhea and swelling and restored her appetite. She gained 3 pounds, but her red blood cell numbers continued to drop, so I made her a separate formula of **deer antler, dang gui root, millettia stem, shou wu root, cardamom, amla fruit, ginseng root,** and **shilajatu.** Within a week her blood count numbers stabilized and she was able to avoid further transfusions for several months.

Blood Deficiency—Diagnosis and Treatment

The herbalist's concept of blood deficiency takes on greater significance when you consider how much nutrient deficiency exists in the general population today. According to naturopath and best-selling author Dr. Michael Murray, N.D., more than 80% of certain age groups consume less than the recommended daily allowance (RDA) of select nutrients (reported in Murray, 1996).

The first step in correcting blood deficiency is correcting nutrition and digestion. We can then use herbs to tonify the blood directly, many of which are listed in the **blood-nourishing group.** The Western idea of anemia is similar to, though more limited than, the TCM and TAM concepts of blood deficiency. We can diagnose and treat blood deficiency with herbs even when blood tests indicate sufficient red blood cells or other blood parameters.

The major symptoms of blood deficiency include a pale tongue, weak thin pulse, dryness (especially skin), fatigue, coldness, vertigo, drowsiness, general malaise, heart palpitations, poor digestion, and loss of libido.

I use a variety of herbs from the **blood-nourishing group,** but especially **dang gui root, alfalfa, shou wu root, yellow dock root tincture** *(Rumex crispus),* and **white peony root.** Algae such as **spirulina** *(S. platensis)* or **chlorella** are also valuable. Ayurvedic doctors also extensively use **shilajatu,** as well as **mandura bhasma,** a form of iron ore oxide, which is purified by cooking with various herbs. Herbs that nourish the blood are usually prescribed by traditional doctors along with digestive herbs such as **white atractylodes** or **trikatu** to ensure absorption.

In severe cases of blood deficiency there may be blood loss or bone marrow deficiency (from chemotherapy or advanced age). In these cases I use stronger tonics, concentrating on strengthening the bone marrow with **deer antler.**

When the white blood cells are low, they can be increased by combining herbs from the **blood-nourishing group** and the **immune system group,** such as **ginseng root, dang gui root, maitake mushroom, millettia stem, astragalus root,** and **shou wu root.** We will discuss this more in Chapter 19. There we will break down the effects of herbs on specific white blood cells and immune system chemicals.

Nourishing the Blood to Treat Hair Loss

TCM doctors have a unique application that demonstrates the power of nourishing the blood. They use herbs to nourish the hair roots and treat alopecia (hair loss). At our clinic we have seen several women and a few men restore hair loss using herbs over the course of 6 months to a year or more. TAM doctors differentiate conditions and the appropriate herbal treatment by determining what is causing the hair loss. If the hair is simply falling out it is more of an inflammatory condition and should be treated as such. If the hair is fragile and breaks off, it is more of a deficiency condition that requires nourishment.

Recommended herbal treatments for hair loss:

- I use a base formula of **eclipta, shou wu root, raw rehmannia, cooked rehmannia, salvia root, schisandra fruit, dang gui root, mu gua fruit** *(Chaenomelis lagenaria),*

chiang huo rhizome *(Notopterygium* species), and **dang shen root** *(Codonopsis pilosula),* to nourish the hair roots. The dose is 2 grams of concentrated granules twice per day.

- If the patient is hypothyroid or has a tendency toward coldness (Yang deficiency), I add **deer antler** to the base formula.

- If there are signs that the condition is more inflammatory, I will add herbs to clear liver heat to the base formula, such as **scute root, burdock root,** or **dandelion root.**

- Essential oils can be a good adjunct treatment for alopecia. In a study published in the *Archives of Dermatology,* 44% of patients who massaged essential oils (**thyme, rosemary, lavender,** and **cedarwood**) in a mixture of carrier oils (**jojoba** and **grapeseed**) into their scalp daily had improvement (Hay et al., 1998).

- Herbal treatments for hair loss based upon nourishing blood usually work better for women than men. Herbalist David Winston, A.H.G., and Dr. James Duke, Ph.D., both report theoretical and anecdotal evidence that using **saw palmetto berry** can be of help due to its effect on the inflammatory testosteronelike chemical DHT, which apparently kills off hair follicles (Winston, 1999; Duke, 1997).

Improving Poor Circulation with Herbs

Sometimes just nourishing the blood is not enough. In spite of a good diet and adequate digestion, I often get patients complaining of poor circulation accompanied by symptoms like a weak pulse, cold intolerance, or cold fingers and toes. Again, it is important to first determine underlying medical conditions that may be causing the symptoms, such as iron deficiency anemia, hypothyroidism, cardiac weakness, or vitamin B$_{12}$ deficiency.

Once you have addressed those areas, you can work to directly improve the circulation with herbs. In fact, it is very common for my patients to have circulation or blood problems that are not clearly defined by blood tests.

It is equally common for me to see patients with various forms of fatigue and anemia who do not respond, for example, to simple iron supplements. In such cases, the choice of herbs for treating poor circulation now depends on herbal differential diagnosis. Weakness, coldness, congestion, restriction, and deficiency are among the major contributing factors, and any or all may be present. The patient or doctor must identify which factor is most prominent, which will help in developing the proper treatment protocol, which usually involves mixing herbs from several groups.

TCM analysis tells us that Qi or vital energy deficiency can cause poor circulation because the Qi pushes the blood. If this factor is predominant, the patient will present with weakness, fatigue, a slow, weak pulse, and low digestive energy. I use **astragalus root, ginseng root, salvia root, dang gui root,** and **ginkgo leaves** in these cases. According to TCM theory the **astragalus** and **ginseng** strengthen the vital force (Qi), and the **dang gui** and **ginkgo** nourish and regulate the blood. Scientific studies show that these herbs help dilate and/or regulate peripheral vessels and improve capillary circulation.

If the problem is a consequence of coldness, which slows the blood flow, it is first necessary to differentiate between interior and exterior coldness. In our discussion of diet in Chapter 10 we mentioned that exterior or weather-related cold (low exterior temperatures) moves the blood to the interior areas of the body. Symptoms include cold limbs, cold intolerance, tendency to shiver, joint pain, and sometimes low back and musculoskeletal pain, all related to a Yang deficiency.

I treat this according to the TCM principle "Use heat to treat coldness." Herbs from the warming group like **dry ginger, cinnamon bark,** and **prickly ash bark** are usually very effective.

Do not use these herbs by themselves as long-term treatment. Unless the coldness is very superficial and short-lived, there is usually another causative condition, such as low energy or blood deficiency, which requires treatment to resolve the circulatory problem permanently. In these cases, I use herbs to treat the underlying condition in combination with the warming group herbs.

If the coldness has penetrated to the interior of the body the patient will present with cold hands and feet, combined with symptoms such as poor digestion, abdominal pain, fatigue, nausea, and reduced appetite. In these cases, I use fresh **ginger, black pepper, trikatu, ginseng root, white atractylodes,** and **licorice root.**

A final possible cause of poor circulation is the form of interior tension called Liver Qi restriction in TCM. This common condition is seen in patients presenting with tension, a rapid wiry pulse, cold fingers and toes, and a red tongue. Two major herbs for this condition, often prescribed together, are **bupleurum root** and **scute root.** You can also use **blue citrus peel** (qing pi or *C. reticulata),* **xiang fu rhizome** *(Cyperus rotundus),* and **zhi ke fruit** *(Citrus aurantium).* Calming herbs like **ashwagandha root** and **skullcap tincture** have somewhat similar actions.

Moving the Blood

According to TCM, when the blood flow is impeded the condition is known as "blood congestion." If the blood actually stops moving, the condition is termed "blood stasis." These concepts correspond very closely to the Western medicine stages of blood coagulation, especially platelet stickiness, in which platelets stick together to prevent bleeding. Chinese researchers have investigated this process in detail and have developed commercial herbal formulas to promote blood circulation and inhibit platelet aggregation. These formulas are used in China to treat and prevent strokes and heart attacks.

Because blood stagnation also inhibits tissue repair and removal of waste products, herbs that move the blood can be used to treat a wide variety of health problems, including slow healing, chronic inflammation (discussed in more detail later in this chapter), poor memory, and some forms of headache and vertigo. We have listed some important blood-moving herbs in the **blood-moving group.** Other herbs that have similar properties include **garlic bulb, bilberry, evening primrose oil,** and **turmeric root.**

When blood congestion progresses, it can lead to pain syndromes including menstrual cramps, Reynaud's syndrome, and even life-threatening thrombosis. The same herbs are used to treat these ailments, but using the stronger ones like **persica seed** (tao ren or *Prunus persica),* **carthamus flower, red peony root** (chi shao / *Paeonia rubra),* **prickly ash bark,** and **e zhu root** *(Curcuma zedoaria).* If the congestion progresses to the stage of what TCM doctors call "mass formation," more powerful and potentially toxic "herbs" are used, such as **anteater scales** (chuan shan jia / *Manis pentadactyla)* and/or **dried leech** (shui zhi or *Hirudo nipponia).*

Warning: all blood-moving treatments are contraindicated in pregnancy and patients taking blood-thinning medication. (If there is any uncertainty, adding herbs from the **vessel-strengthening group** to formulas can help prevent chances of bleeding.)

Cleaning the Blood of Fats

Elevated levels of cholesterol and other blood fats contribute to heart disease, arterial clogging, and cardiovascular diseases. The ancient concept of "mucus in the blood," long discounted or ignored, is now an integral concern of modern medicine. The liver is largely responsible for processing and removing fats from the blood. As mentioned earlier, HDL (Happy DL) and LDL (Lousy DL) and other blood fats form your total cholesterol (TC) level. A combined cholesterol level around 180–200 is often cited as the optimal range for the lowest risk of heart attack and stroke. Keeping cholesterol levels low is essential for people who have suffered heart disease and seems to be very important for preventing heart attack and stroke.

Because of this, a huge industry has developed surrounding the Western cholesterol-lowering drugs called statins. However, most people are aware that most of these drugs pose a variety of dangers to the liver. Therefore, many people wisely try to control their cholesterol levels with herbs and lifestyle modifications before resorting to drug therapy. Dr. Mana reminds us that most pungent herbs and foods, such as **ginger root** and **garlic bulb,** will reduce cholesterol, as will many bitter and astringent herbs. In spite of this, I think it is a mistake to simply substitute herbs for drugs. Herbal treatment with accompanying lifestyle changes is the way to go.

Herbs that help reduce and remove blood fats include **guggul gum, arjuna bark, turmeric root, ginger root, black pepper, garlic bulb, hawthorn,** and **shou wu root.** I often mix these herbs together along with some **triphala** to reduce inflammation. I use about 4–5 grams of concentrated powder extracts of these herbs per day. It is often helpful to increase dietary intake of beans as well. If you must use cholesterol-lowering drugs, remember that **milk thistle seed** and **turmeric root** can help keep the liver healthy.

Holistic physician Gerald Lemole, M.D., chief of cardiac surgery at Christiana Care in Wilmington, Delaware, noted that German athletes recovered more quickly during Olympic competition in part due to massage. Dr. Lemole reported that lymphostasis may be a hidden cause of arteriosclerosis, because the more quickly the lipoproteins and cholesterol are cleared from the system, the less time they are in contact with the vessel linings where they can cause damage. Massage, Yoga, T'ai Chi, and just plain old exercise can increase lymphatic flow by as much as 300%. Severe lymphostasis can be treated with **castor oil packs.**

Removing Heat and Inflammation from the Blood

Inflammation is one of the body's primary mechanisms for removing metabolic by-products, debris, and foreign agents. It enables the body to remove damaged cells, neutralize toxins, and fight bacteria, fungi, and viruses. We have already discussed inflammation in the section on the liver, and we will discuss it now from a slightly different angle. In Chapter 19 when we discuss the immune system, we'll examine it again from yet another angle.

The main physiological components of inflammation are pain, heat, and swelling. Pain is the nervous system's response to heat and irritation when the body initiates the inflammation process to burn away offending agents. Swelling and redness appear as fluids leak out of capillaries that have dilated in response to heat. Inflammation goes through several stages before finally allowing the body to heal. Like a prompt, efficient police force, inflammation is usually our friend.

Acute Inflammation

When cells sustain damage or tension from infection, wounds or poisons, allergens or other triggers, they release chemicals that start the inflammation process. The basic process involves first an increased flow of blood to the area, followed by an increase in capillary permeability to allow the immune system access to the area, and finally the arrival of white blood cells (WBCs). The WBCs release various chemicals, a process called chemotaxis, all of which cause the heat, redness, pain, and swelling. The WBCs and their chemical weapons destroy invaders and remove debris. The increased fluids present also contain nutrients to initiate repair processes as the inflammation recedes. Acute inflammation is usually self-limiting.

Chronic Inflammation

Inflammation is always present in our bodies at low, silent levels, and this is buffered by our nutrient and defensive capabilities. When our systems are in balance, destructive and nutritive processes deal with foreign agents efficiently and our tissues are protected. However, moderate or even mild long-term inflammation can be damaging to our health. Chronic inflammation differs from acute inflammation in that there is usually less heat present. Also, there are changes in the balance of immune-messaging molecules toward unhealthy ratios of WBCs and increases of inflammatory chemicals.

The more obvious signs of long-term inflammation can include fluid retention, musculoskeletal pain and stiffness, allergies, intestinal pain, chronic red eyes, chronic postnasal drip, burning sensations, poor concentration, and poor digestion. Modern biomedical analysis shows us how long-term mild inflammation (at levels just slightly above normal) can contribute to the development of arteriosclerosis, arthritis, calcium deposits, chronic fatigue, skin diseases, cancer, and numerous other conditions.

Our cells have their own signaling systems designed for self-protection during acute inflammation, but they can be overwhelmed if the battle goes on too long. This is why severe or long-term inflammation can be damaging to the body.

For example, we now know that various inflammatory triggers in the blood cause the release of damaging chemicals, including vascular adhesion molecules (VCAMs) or intracellular adhesion molecules (ICAMs), both of which help initiate common forms of heart disease, such as arterial clogging and heart attacks.

Review of Common Sources of Chronic Inflammation

Herbalists offer several explanations for the preponderance of chronic inflammatory conditions in our modern society, noting that in traditional societies we see much less of it. Following is a list of common causes of inflammation.

- Incomplete diet, which leads to basic nutrient deficiencies and eventually immune system weakness or poor repair processes.

- Dietary intake of low-quality fats and oils, which leads to increased production of inflammatory chemicals.

- Insufficient dietary intake of fresh fruits and vegetables, which leads to deficiencies in carotenes, flavonoids, and other anti-inflammatory plant nutrients.

- Digestive imbalances in the intestines, which lead to intestinal dysbiosis and production of toxic gases and inflammatory compounds that enter the blood.

- Exposure to environmental toxins, chemicals, or prescription pharmaceuticals.

- Genetic errors of metabolism that alter body chemistry toward inflammation.

- Lack of exercise, which leads to cardiac weakness and eventually to poor supply of oxygen and nutrients to tissues and failure to neutralize and carry away wastes.

- Weakness or failure in one of the detoxification organs or systems, such as the liver, lungs, kidneys, skin, urinary system, lymphatic system, venous system, or bowels.

- Congestion or blockage in the vessels or organs, which leads to the accumulation of waste materials.

I could cite numerous examples to support all of the above causative factors. Instead, I offer a single chilling example. Scientists have been reporting the presence of pesticides in the amniotic fluids of pregnant women since the early 1980s. In 1996, one group reported: "We analyzed polychlorinated biphenyl (PCB), DDT, hexachlorocyclohexane (HCH), and heptachlor in subcutaneous fat tissue and other tissues (placenta, liver, kidney, lung, brain, thymus, muscle, heart) of 34 fetuses and dead children. These substances were found regularly in placenta, in fetal subcutaneous fat tissue and in fetal organs. They therefore can influence possibly early and sensitive stages of intrauterine development."

Herbal medicines can, of course, be of great benefit in reducing inflammation, as long as you realize that using herbs to block inflammation without dealing with its cause will not work very well. Since these causes range from the subtle (genetic imbalances) to the gross (poor nutrition), we must examine different methods. Our solutions must proceed from understanding both the causal process and the symptoms. Traditional herbal systems compare this to treating the root and the branches of an ailing tree.

Detoxification First

To quickly remove toxins from the blood, we can use detoxification methods. It is interesting to note that, in nature, animals fast when they are ill and sometimes eat grass to induce vomiting. Detoxification has long been a part of all the major herbal healing systems. In Ayurveda, it was elevated to the status of one of the original eight branches of medicine. Even today, the use of emetics to cleanse the stomach of poisons is a standard ER treatment.

All of us recognize the importance of cleansing our skin by bathing, cleansing our food by washing it before use, and so forth. In herbal medicine this concept can be expanded to encompass ideas such as cleansing the colon with laxatives or washing the sinuses to treat chronic sinusitis. Sweating therapy is used to stimulate removal of oils and fluids. Fasting is used to change metabolism at first toward a catabolic phase, where chemicals and toxins are released from storage and broken down, eventually leading to an anabolic phase where rebuilding of healthy new tissue occurs. I should mention that in Ayurvedic medicine, there are strict rules about who should and should not undertake cleansing therapy. The very weak or very ill are told to avoid fasting and strong purgatives or laxatives.

Detoxification can be accomplished by short-term use of any herbs that stimulate one of the eliminative organs, including skin (sweating agents), lungs (expectorants), kidneys (diuretics), intestines (laxatives), lymphatic system (oils), or liver (cholagogues and choleretics).

Fasting involves abstinence from all food and drink for a specific period of time. This practice has proven beneficial for many conditions, including heart disease, pancreatitis,

PCB and DDT contamination, autoimmune diseases, arthritis, food allergy, psoriasis, eczema, IBS, asthma, and depression. Immune function is stimulated in the days and weeks following a fast, as well as a general sense of well-being.

A short fast (3–5 days) can be implemented on a Wednesday or Friday to allow for rest on the weekend. Many people like to do this at the end of winter, calling it "spring cleaning." To do so, make the last meal one of only fresh fruits and vegetables, or vegetable soup. Drink only spring or distilled water during the fast. Rest as much as possible, doing only light tasks such as walking and bathing. Bathe frequently, but only using warm water, not hot water. Break the fast with only fruit on the first meal, followed by vegetable soups the rest of the day. Return to normal foods the following day.

Laxatives such as **rhubarb root** or **castor oil** are easy to use to cleanse the colon. You can also use any commercial herbal laxative pill, though I prefer balanced herbal laxative formulas. Laxatives flush out stores of endotoxins from the bowel, speeding recovery from both chronic degenerative and acute febrile diseases. One reason this is helpful in detoxification may be that endotoxins increase free radical production in the liver.

Traditional Analysis of Inflammation

Ayurvedic doctors focus not on the innumerable specific toxins but on restoration of balance to the carrier mechanisms. They call these mechanisms toxic bile **(Pitta dosha)**, salty mucus **(Kapha dosha),** and putrefactive gases **(Vata dosha),** all identified by direct observation and by inference.

If there is inflammation with toxic gases, the affected tissue or organ will exhibit more pain, stiffness, and gradual degeneration. If there is inflammation with toxic bile, there will be relatively more heat and rapid tissue destruction. If there is more toxic mucus there will be more heavy sensation, swelling, and blockage.

By looking for the relative preponderance of these symptoms in addition to the usual signs of pain, heat, redness, and swelling, it is possible to fine-tune herbal choices. If the inflammation has more swelling, for example, herbs from the **heat-removing group** would be chosen along with a small amount of herbs from the **diuretic group.** If there is more pain and dryness, herbs from the **heat-removing group** would be given along with a small amount of herbs from the **nervine group.**

TCM doctors observe that chronic inflammation often involves blood stagnation or a heat and dampness condition. In cases of blood stagnation you would mainly use herbs from the **blood-moving group** along with herbs from the **heat-removing group.**

Analyzing still further, if the blood stagnation is caused by Qi restriction, herbs that release the restriction, such as **bupleurum root,** would be most useful. If the blood stagnation is caused by deficiency of Qi (because Qi moves the blood), add **ginseng root** or **astragalus root** to the **heat-removing** and **blood-moving** herbs. In the presence of heat and dampness, choose herbs from the **heat-removing group** along with a small amount of herbs from the

diuretic group or **dampness-removing group.** There are many more possibilities, but this should give you a general idea. Obviously, it takes a trained herbalist to make the best herb choices in each condition.

Removing Blood Inflammation

It is not enough to know the causes and type of inflammation to formulate the proper treatment protocol. You also have to understand where you are in the process.

For example, if the inflammation results from external trauma, the initial treatment should include herbs that focus on the immediate problem, followed by wound-healing herbs such as **tien chi root.** If the inflammation results from an infection, the focus treatment should involve cooling herbs with antimicrobial properties, such as **isatis root.** If the inflammation results from weakness and deficiency, you would use nutrient herbs like **flaxseed oil** or **maitake mushroom** or tonic antioxidant herbs like **amla fruit.**

I recall a conversation I had with a medical doctor after returning from Nepal many decades ago. He was also a Ph.D. and professor of biochemistry. Initially open-minded, he wanted to know about my experiences, so I told him I had witnessed Dr. Mana treat many cases of acute and infectious hepatitis successfully and quickly. I explained that part of Dr. Mana's treatment included herbs that reduced inflammation in the liver and bile duct. My curious friend was skeptical, saying that it was not possible that the action of an herbal anti-inflammatory could be specific to a particular organ. He used the *V* word that some M.D.'s and scientists like to use to intimidate herbalists—voodoo.

Naturopaths and holistic M.D.'s rely on scientific research and specialized tests to identify the inflammatory chemicals that are out of balance in different types of disease, and explain why. For example, it is important to know that cases of eczema can involve weak action of the delta-6-desaturase enzyme, which can affect the body's levels of prostaglandins. Knowledge of this problem allows the naturopath to choose **evening primrose oil** as a remedy, because it bypasses the missing chemical link, neutralizing the inflammatory process. Similarly, knowing that the inflammation of multiple sclerosis relates to problems digesting dietary fats gives us a clinical treatment advantage.

It is also very important to identify the location of the inflammation. This knowledge enables TCM doctors to use specific plants for specific organs. Originally believed to be something of a "voodoo" custom (see the story in the adjacent box), this is now a widely accepted herbal practice. The breakthrough in understanding lies in the concept of tissue-specific antioxidant activity. It turns out that many plant chemicals such as carotenoids and flavonoids have affinities for specific tissues. Part of this can be explained by whether the plant nutrients are fat or water soluble, but there is more to it than that. For example, **milk thistle seed** phytochemicals go to the liver, **ginkgo leaf** chemicals increase glucose and oxygen transport across nerve cell membranes, and lycopene from **tomatoes** goes to the macula. Since my earliest days as an herbalist, I have trusted the observations of traditional doctors regarding the use of specific herbs to treat tissue- or organ-specific inflammation or deficiency. It's nice to know my faith in herbs has a scientific basis.

Common Herbal Treatments for Inflammation

Anti-inflammatory herbs can be grouped according to the specific organs and tissues they treat most effectively. Following are some common classifications.

- **Intestinal Inflammation:** Choose from **beet root, bromelain, scute root, coptis rhizome, boswellia gum, licorice root, dandelion root, phellodendron bark, sarsaparilla root, triphala,** and **turmeric root.** To coat and soothe irritation, use **slippery elm bark.** To flush out inflammation, use **rhubarb root** for 1 or 2 days.

- **Joint inflammation:** Choose from **boswellia gum, bromelain, scute root, flaxseed oil, guggul gum, myrrh gum, phellodendron bark,** and **turmeric root.** If there is deficiency, choose from **deer antler, amla fruit, alfalfa leaf, dry ginger, raw rehmannia root,** or **wheat sprouts**. The nutritional supplement **glucosamine sulfate** is also useful for deficiency joint inflammation as is the traditional Ayurvedic tonic **Yogarajaguggulu.** For topical treatment apply **castor oil packs.**

- **Kidney inflammation:** Choose from **scute root, alisma rhizome** (ze xie or *A. plantago-aquatica),* **capillaris** (yin chen hao or *Artemisia capillaris),* **phellodendron bark,** and **stinging nettle leaf.** If there is deficiency, choose from **astragalus root, cordyceps mushroom, rehmannia root** (cooked and raw), **shilajatu,** and **stinging nettle seed.** For topical treatment apply **castor oil packs.**

- **Lung inflammation:** Choose from **beet root, boswellia gum, scute root, chrysanthemum flower, garlic bulb, tulsi, peppermint leaf,** and **turmeric root.** If there is deficiency, choose from **American ginseng root, cordyceps mushroom, reishi mushroom, schisandra berries,** and **wild asparagus root.**

- **Sinus inflammation:** Choose from **scute root, echinacea, forsythia flower, honeysuckle flower** (jin yin hua or *Lonicera japonica),* and **wild chrysanthemum flower.** To soothe the sinuses, put a few drops of **flaxseed** or **sesame oil** mixed with **white sandalwood** in each nostril.

- **Skin inflammation:** Choose from **burdock root, dandelion root** or **leaf, moutan, neem, red clover blossom, red peony root, sarsaparilla,** and **turmeric root.** If there is deficiency, use **dang gui root, gotu kola, raw rehmannia root, shilajatu,** or **shou wu root.** Skin inflammation sometimes yields to 1 or 2 days of bowel flushing with laxatives like **rhubarb root** or **castor oil.** For topical treatment, apply fresh **aloe vera gel** or **aloe** preparations with **olive oil, black tea bags,** or **castor oil.** For itching, use tinctures with menthol crystals derived from **mint oils.**

- **Stomach inflammation:** Choose from **scute root, coptis rhizome, fresh ginger root, peppermint leaf, burdock root, boswellia gum, fennel seed, licorice root, kudzu, triphala,** and **turmeric root.** To coat and soothe irritation, use **flaxseed oil** (long term) or **slippery elm bark** (short term).

- **Thyroid inflammation:** Choose from **bugleweed** *(Lycopus virginicus),* **capillaris** (yin chen hao or *Artemisia capillaris),* **scute root, gardenia fruit** (zhi zi or *Gardenia jasminoides),* and **prunella** (xie ku cao or *P. vulgaris).*

- **Pancreas inflammation:** Choose from **moudan bark** (mu dan pi or *Paeonia suffruticosa),* **persica seed** (tao ren or *Prunus persica),* **carthamus flower, benincasa fruit** (dong gua ren or *B. hispida),* **guggul gum, rhubarb root, bromelain,** and **shilajatu.**

Treating Serious Inflammation

The general list of herbs offered above provides a starting point. There are many inflammation-related diseases, and we will be going into greater detail in the next chapters. Here I will discuss two special forms of inflammatory disease in greater detail to make it clear how herbs are applied in real-life clinical situations. The detail presented here is indicative of how trained professional herbalists think.

Venous Insufficiency

After the arteries and capillaries deliver nutrients to the cells, the veins return the blood to the heart and lungs for "recharging." Veins are larger than arteries and can easily suffer from inflammatory damage, especially in cases of poor circulation or blood stagnation. Varicose or abnormally dilated tortuous veins are usually found in the legs, resulting from the high venous pressure and relatively poor tissue support for the superficial veins.

> A diet high in dark-colored fruits, especially citrus varieties and berries, is a very important step in preventing venous problems.

Dr. Mana points out that the elasticity of the vein depends on a normal expansion-contraction cycle controlled by the nerves. If there is a constant dilation from pressure or neurological incompetence, the failure to expand and contract causes the tissue to dry out and lose elasticity. The resulting lack of motion allows the blood to stagnate. Histological studies show that chronic venous insufficiency and varicose vein formation are characterized by a loss of contractile strength in the tissues and by an increase in secretion and collagen deposits. **Consequently, the treatment goals for venous insufficiency are threefold:**

- To restore the elasticity and tone of the venous walls

- To remove blood congestion and exudate sludge

- To restore neurological competence

To treat simple spider veins, I use a tincture of **stoneroot, butcher's broom rhizome** *(Ruscus aculeatus),* **horse chestnut seed** *(Aesculus hippocastanum),* and **gotu kola.** These herbs seem to directly heal and restore elasticity to the venous walls and remove inflamma-tion. Apply the tincture directly to the af-fected area twice per day, and the veins will usually begin to disappear in a month or so. The same compound can be taken internally. I recommend about 35–45 drops three times per day. To remove blood congestion, I recommend the **blood-moving herbs** mentioned in our earlier discussion about moving the blood. To strengthen neurologi-cal force, I usually add **astragalus root** to these formulas.

> Oil massage can also be very useful. Soak a thick cloth with warm salt water and apply it to the veins. This is even more powerful if the salt water is made with a decoction of bael fruit.

Jaundice and Hepatitis

The term *hepatitis* is actually a catchall for inflammation of the liver. About 90% of pa-tients with serious liver disease develop jaundice and/or acute liver cell injury. The most common causes of liver disease are viral hepatitis and alcohol-, chemical-, or toxin-caused liver disease.

Modern medical science divides viral hepatitis into four strains, based upon the type of virus (A, B, C, or E). Hepatitis with jaundice is usually found in types A and E, both of which are classified as contagious. Modern society has experienced a major increase in the incidence of certain viral strains of the disease, particularly hepatitis B and C. In fact, hep-atitis C is now being referred to as a "silent epidemic." Herbal medicine has much to offer in the way of treatment for these difficult diseases.

TCM and Jaundice

In TCM, jaundice is divided into two basic groups, called **Yin** yellow disease and **Yang** yellow disease. **Yang** yellow disease is actually acute jaundice or acute hepatitis. **Yin** yellow disease is chronic jaundice caused either by external toxins and dampness or by excesses of alcohol and greasy food. These factors weaken the digestive system and eventually block the liver. The blocked liver backs up, causing jaundice.

TCM doctors formulate based upon whether there is more heat or more dampness. **Capillaris** (yin chen hao or *Artemisia capillaris*) is used as the main herbal treatment, adding other herbs as needed. **Capillaris** is bitter and pungent in taste and cool in property. It removes heat and dampness from the liver and gallbladder, increases bile secretion, and is diuretic. It is used for symptoms such as intermittent fever and chills, bitter taste in the mouth, nausea, and loss of appetite. It is the number one herb for treating jaundice, gallbladder disorders, and hepatitis.

For chronic hepatitis TCM doctors use **capillaris** in high doses, along with many other adjunct herbs, including **dandelion root, isatis root and leaf, bupleurum root, scute root, turmeric root, white peony root, salvia root,** and **licorice root.**

Ayurveda and Jaundice

In general, Ayurvedic texts divide hepatitis into four main conditions: anemic hepatitis (pandu kamala), contagious hepatitis (aupadravika kamala), acute hepatitis (kumbha kamala), and chronic hepatitis (halimaka). The early Ayurvedic texts include hepatitis as a subset within their chapters on anemia. As they described it, in an anemic condition the liver becomes overactive as it filters the by-products of the dead red blood cells, leading to liver weakness.

With chronic hepatitis, there is no obvious swelling and blockage in the liver. Only the symptoms of anemia and pallor can be identified. This condition can stay in the body for many years, with periods of remission and exacerbation of liver inflammation.

Ayurveda diagnoses this condition as a disease of Vata and Pitta, as it involves mild chronic inflammation (Pitta dosha) coupled with "reversed liver nerve function" (yakrit udavarta). In reversed function of the hepatic nerves, the upper function of the liver becomes more active, while the lower function is relatively inactive or sluggish. Ayurveda points out that this sort of neurological overactivity usually causes mild pain.

According to Ayurveda, the main causes of hepatitis can be classified into three groups as follows:

1. Overuse of heat-generating foods and behaviors. In general, heat-generating foods are sour, pungent, or salty in taste and have the physical effect of capillary dilation. Causative factors thus include excessive or daily use of high-fat foods, roasted or fried foods, butter, ghee, alcohol, milk products, coffee, vinegar, pickles, chili, and other hot spices. All of these aggravate Pitta.

   Heat-generating behaviors include heavy physical labor, summer heat, working or living in indoor environments which are excessively hot (such as working over a stove), emotional upset (especially anger), and excessive daytime sleeping.

2. Improper medical treatment. Treatment with or exposure to strong chemical agents, such as astringent drugs to stop diarrhea, exposure to pesticides, and antibiotics can all weaken the liver.

3. Direct contact with an infected person's bodily fluids, stool, or food. Transmission rates are much higher at times of epidemic outbreaks. Control extends to obvious pre-

cautions with sexual contact, using the same eating utensils, food, plates, cups, or water, and poor hygiene.

Hepatitis B and C have a relatively low rate of cure with Western medicines at the time of this writing, and the available treatments are very expensive and have strong side effects. The drug cocktails (combinations), which seemed to offer hope in 1998 in spite of sometimes horrific side effects, are now showing signs of viral recurrence after drug discontinuation. Furthermore, I am not convinced that the drugs themselves do not damage the liver. There is even some controversy whether or not hepatitis C is truly a virus. It may simply be a sign of chronic liver damage, possibly with multiple causes, leaking RNA particles picked up by the currently inaccurate testing methods.

A science editor of ABC News stated, "No one's been able to come up with a hepatitis C virus, purify it, inject it into an animal and cause hepatitis."

Ayurvedic physicians were unaware of the seriousness of the complications of these new forms of chronic hepatitis until this was made clear with the emergence of new diagnostic tests around 1989 and the reports in the literature and press. Until that time, patients with hepatitis B and C symptoms were treated with basic hepatitis herbs, liver tonics, and rasayana (longevity tonics). Hepatitis B responded well to Ayurvedic treatments, but hepatitis C (originally called non A/non B) responded much more slowly.

When blood tests finally became available around 1991, Dr. Mana began to keep records at his Kathmandu clinic of patients with B and C strains after utilizing his Ayurvedic treatments. Dr. Mana also noted and spoke out about the emotional shock that awaited patients when told that the diseases were not curable and could cause liver cancer and cirrhosis. In

> Dr. Mana is known throughout Nepal for his effective treatments for all forms of hepatitis. I imported his medicines for several of my patients, and they all responded very well, as indicated by a drop in the total viral load, some as much as 90%. One even went into complete remission.

Ayurvedic thinking, this type of fear progressively weakens the entire nervous system (Vata). The fear adds to the burden of the illness, and can speed up progression.

Dr. Mana has developed several complex herbal tonics (containing up to 40 herbs each) for all forms of chronic hepatitis, and has treated literally thousands of patients during his four decades of active practice since 1955. Some important known herbs include **shilajatu, guduchi stem, turmeric root,** and **triphala.** However, many herbs he uses in his formulas are unavailable outside Nepal. Patients visit him from all over the world to be treated for chronic hepatitis, with many patients now importing herbs from Nepal utilizing FDA allowances for personal importation (see Resource Guide). The treatment takes from 6 months to 2 years. His success is so high that cab drivers in Nepal will recommend foreigners see him if they look yellow.

Western Herbalists Treating Chronic Hepatitis

At the 1999 American Herbalists Guild Annual Symposium, I talked with several prominent herbalists, including Michael and Lesley Tierra and David Winston. All of them reported cases with similar results to those I had experienced in the clinic, dropping liver enzymes into the normal range, and viral loads by as much as 50–90%. Dr. Terry Willard reported a high level of complete extinction of hepatitis C at his clinic in Canada. To my knowledge, only Dr Mana and Dr. Willard have reported multiple cases of hepatitis C clearance.

After reviewing TAM, TCM, and Western medicine approaches to this disease, I developed a series of treatment protocols with herbalist Kirk Moulton of Chicago that also achieved good results (lowering of liver enzymes to normal). We decided that we would use the Internet, not to "promise a cure," but to share our understanding, experiences, and treatments with the public at large. People who work with us on the web site share their histories and results, both positive and negative, and we post these contributions anonymously. The protocols and medicine choices change as we learn from many sources, including the patients themselves. We hope patients find this useful and will help us identify the most effective means for solving this problem. If you'd like to take a closer look, the web site address is: **http://hepatitis-alternatives.com/** You may also contact my clinic directly (see Resource Guide).

Because I learned about some of the herbs we used for these protocols from Dr. Mana, I send a large portion of any resulting income back to his clinic in Kathmandu.

Gallstones

Gallstone formation *(cholelithiasis)* is another disease with a very low incidence in primitive societies, yet in modern society it affects more than 20% of women and 8% of men over the age of 40. Each year hundreds of thousands of gallbladders are surgically removed, at great cost.

Seventy-five percent of all gallstones consist primarily of cholesterol, while the rest are formed from pigments (calcium bilirubinate), bile salts, bile pigments, inorganic calcium salts, and other minerals. It is important to know the composition of the stone because pure cholesterol stones are far easier to dissolve with prescription medicines. Therefore, it is necessary to see your doctor for the appropriate tests to determine the size and type of stone before trying herbal therapy. Herbal and chemical medicines do not always work or may work only temporarily, so as with most diseases, prevention is the best strategy. In traditional terms, gallstones are a result of heat and dampness leading to blockage.

The symptoms of gallbladder disease are often silent. The most common warning signs are dyspepsia, nausea, belching, and vomiting. Patients may also experience episodic pain in the upper right quadrant of the abdomen, jaundice, or infection. Some cases also present cystic or common bile duct obstruction. Cases of blockage or severe pain require emergency medical attention.

Prevention and Treatment of Gallstones

- Obesity causes more cholesterol to be secreted in the bile, so preventive measures include exercise and weight control. Obese individuals are far more likely to develop gallstones than individuals at a healthy weight.

- Dietary fiber inhibits cholesterol stone formation by reducing the biliary cholesterol saturation.

- My recommended **diet for heat and damp** (refer to Chapter 10 on nutrition) as well as moderate use of healthy fats and oils can help improve liver and bile function, clear blood fats, and aid in keeping the intestinal flora healthy.

- Diets that promote quick weight loss with drastic caloric restrictions can promote gallstone formation.

- Exercise can prevent gallstone formation. The Harvard School of Public Health reported in 1999 that women who exercise regularly (2–3 hours per week) cut their risk of gallstones by as much as one-third.

- Drinking several cups of **dandelion tea** each day can prevent gallbladder attacks.

- Volatile oils, such as the limolene found in **lemons,** can help dissolve gallstones. The European prescription herbal medicine Rowachol, made primarily from mint oils, has also demonstrated effectiveness.

- At our clinic we use a product called **Mentharil,** made by Phyto-pharmica, to treat gallstones. This sort of therapy takes many months to work and exhibits better results when combined with pharmaceutical bile acid therapy.

- **Milk thistle seed** and **turmeric root** both increase the solubility of bile, which helps prevent stone formation, and can aid in elimination of small stones. I recommend about 2 grams of **turmeric** and 600 mg of **milk thistle extract** per day.

- The standard TCM prescription called **Jin shi san** (JSS) or **San jin tang** has been shown in clinical trials to dissolve gallstones in a large percentage of patients. Analysis of bile showed that JSS increased the amount of bile acid and decreased the bilirubin and mucus. A form of this formula, **Lysmachia 3,** is available from ITM.

- The Chinese name **jin qian cao** applies to several different herbs capable of dissolving gallstones. The most popular of these herbs are **jin qian cao herb** *(Lysimachia christinae)* and **guang jin qian herb** *(Desmodium styracifolium).*

According to TCM theory, if stones are small enough you can treat them by removing heat and dampness from the gallbladder. One basic Chinese formula contains **jin qian cao**

herb, capillaris *(Artemisia capillaris),* **bupleurum root, scute root, dandelion root,** and the **inner lining of chicken gizzard** (ji nei jin or *Gallus domesticus).*

TCM doctors also use **rhubarb root** that has been soaked in wine and fried (to reduce the laxative effect). With signs of more severe heat and inflammation you might include **turmeric root** and extra **dandelion.** In cases with more pain accompanied by spasms, **cordyalis tuber** (yan hu suo or *Corydalis yanhusuo)* and **white peony root** would be helpful.

CHAPTER 13

The Nervous System:
Brain, Nerves, and Mind

If you gaze long into an abyss, the abyss will gaze back into you.
—Friedrich Nietzsche

The close link between the mind and the brain took a long time for us humans to discover. The ancient Chinese believed the heart was the true seat of the mind, while the brain was just excess bone marrow. The Greeks thought the brain worked like a radiator, cooling the blood. I remember talking to an old naturopath, Dr. Marsteller, who had participated in some early experiments in brain surgery at Hahnemann College in Philadelphia in the 1920s. He told me they knew so little back then he thought the practice fell just short of legal murder.

Today, many of us think of the brain as a complex computer that processes information at lightning speed. Others say the best analogy is that of a hologram, reflecting throughout our physical being any and all changes in nervous system energy or function. But whatever we think today, tomorrow it will be different. Although they have progressed rapidly in the past decades, both neurobiology, the science of the brain and how it functions, and psychology are still in their infancy. Nervous system diseases, including mental disorders and neurodegenerative conditions, remain among the most difficult to understand and to treat.

Nonetheless, I believe there are miracles awaiting us in the near future. Herbal medicine will be part of this. As always, I like to look into the past, as well as the future.

The Ayurvedic Qualities of Mind

According to Ayurvedic medicine, the mind has three primary qualities. The first is called *suddha sattva*, and it refers to a pure mind, with clarity of perception and filled with peace and love. The second is called *rajasa sattva*, denoting an aggressive mind, filled with anger and desire. The third is called *tamasa sattva*, a mind filled with inertia and sloth. The condition of pure mind promotes health, while the aggressive and slothful mind-sets promote disease.

Functionally, there are three things I suggest you keep in mind if you want mental peace. First, your mental state largely depends on the usual suspects—lifestyle, sleep, good nutrition, exercise, and so on. Second, there is a well-developed system of traditional psychology which I judge to be of immense depth and benefit. See the offerings of the Institute for the Study of Human Knowledge mentioned in the Resource Guide. Third, practicing T'ai Chi, Yoga, deep relaxation, prayer, or meditation enables us to reprogram and gain some voluntary control of our nervous system, so we can turn off stress and enter into a blissful mental state.

What It Takes to Relax the Mind

If you think you understand this already, take note of this lecture given by martial arts master Kuo Feng-chih to his students, described by Robert Smith in the book *Pa-Kua*. The last sentence gives one of the keys to health benefits. I will simplify for brevity:

> Several months have passed since I began teaching you. Although we have practiced many hours, your progress is slow because you have failed to grasp the concept of the internal (nei chia). You must learn to quiet the mind and soften the muscles, an almost spiritual feat which depends upon the revolutionary idea that the mind can "will" relaxation. You must practice this "willing" of a tranquil flow from your eyebrows to the soles of your feet. Your mind must travel this imagined route until all distracting thoughts are shut out, your nerve-endings sharpened, but your mind at ease, completely free of all impatience and anxiety. Your whole being must enter a state of bliss, and your mind will thus become liberated. When this happens, your body and limbs will attain a happy unencumbered circulation of oxygen and blood.

The Nervous System, Simplified

As we have discussed, the nervous system and its related systems are one of the three large primary systems controlling our bodies. Nerve cells themselves are biological miracles. The DNA in individual nerve cells is extraordinarily active, doing things scientists can only guess at. Nerve cells process information in milliseconds with electrical and chemical pulses that travel along their length, feeding information into a geometrically expanding circuitous web.

The brain and spinal cord make up the **central nervous system** or **CNS,** while the peripheral nerves and ganglia comprise the **peripheral nervous system** or **PNS.** The PNS is further divided into two subsystems, **autonomic** and **somatic.** The autonomic division of the PNS controls involuntary bodily functions, including glands, smooth muscle, and the heart. The somatic nervous system controls voluntary bodily functions.

The autonomic system comprises two subsystems, known as the **sympathetic** and **parasympathetic** systems. The sympathetic nervous system is generally stimulatory in nature and is known as the "fight-or-flight" system. The parasympathetic nervous system is generally calming in nature. Most organs in our bodies receive stimulation from both sympathetic and parasympathetic nerves, controlling the excitability or lack thereof of the organ in question.

Brain Chemistry, Simplified to the Point of Absurdity

The body has many ways of signaling, necessary for coordination and control. For example, when the glands of the body release chemical messengers called hormones into the bloodstream, these act on receptor molecules anywhere in the body. These "messages" can stimulate a cell to do many things, including manufacture chemicals like estrogen, or even cause changes in the operation of the genetic material—DNA. The chemicals from a particular part of the body fit into locations on receptor molecules as a key fits into a lock. Local messaging (paracrine signaling) works in a similar way, when neighboring cells communicate with chemical secretion "messages," as happens at sites of infection.

The nervous system has a special form of communication called neuronal signaling. It differs from hormonal signaling in that the "messages" travel over private lines, your nerve cells with their enlongated shape. The brain and nerve cells talk with each other via **neurotransmitters,** chemical messaging molecules that send information across the synapse (junction) connecting one nerve cell to another nerve cell or a muscle. When an electrical impulse traveling along the nerve reaches the axon, this biochemical neurotransmitter is released and crosses the synapse to a synaptic receptor, where it stimulates or inhibits the receiving neuron.

There are more than 300 known neurotransmitters, including the endorphins and acetylcholine. A class of neurotransmitters called "neuropeptides" can also deliver complex messages to other parts of the body, even to receptors on single immune system cells.

We can look at neurotransmitters as fingers on a hand, and the receptor sites as keys on a piano. Each finger has its place on a particular key, and the resulting pressure produces an expected "note" or reaction. Thus, the modern explanation of how the body accomplishes certain tasks is linked to its quite elaborate chemical messaging systems.

> It is interesting to note that herbs are not single molecules. Rather, they are composed of complex groups of chemicals. Unlike the single-molecule "finger" that plays a chemical message "note," herbs are capable of playing chords, and when combined properly, herbal formulas can play symphonies.

Signals received by cells regulate basic life processes:

1. If the cell receives adequate signal stimulation, it survives. Otherwise, it dies.

2. Additional signals beyond survival can stimulate division (growth).

3. Other additional signals promote specialized changes known as cell differentiation.

Herbal medicines can act on the nervous or hormonal systems (or any cell), partly because they contain molecules with pieces that resemble the "keys" found in the chemical messaging systems. These pieces fit into the receptor sites. Herbs can thus regulate life processes.

Phytoestrogens, for example, are plant chemicals that gently mimic the action of the body's natural estrogens and can help alleviate the postmenopausal symptoms of estrogen deficiency women experience. This is a case of an herb attaching to and stimulating a receptor site chemical reaction.

These herbs and other substances that stimulate receptor sites are called "agonists." Other herbs have the ability to attach to receptor sites and block the chemical reaction. These agents are called "antagonists." Biochemists classify synapses into different groups according to the type of neurotransmitters they utilize.

Brain Chemicals, Simplified

Specific nutrients are required for your nervous system to function properly. For example, choline is a nutrient found within the B complex that is essential for manufacturing the excitatory neurotransmitter acetylcholine. Choline is found in grains, legumes, and egg yolks and especially in lecithin. A superior form of lecithin made with high levels of phosphatidylcholine is used in Germany for many liver disorders, including chronic hepatitis and cirrhosis.

The brain uses acetylcholine for many processes. This neurotransmitter is very important for memory as well as movement, coordination, and stamina via action on the skeletal muscles and the heart.

"Cholinergic nerve synapses" are those that release and respond to the acetylcholine. "Cholinergic chemicals" are those that increase the production or release of acetylcholine, or prevent its degradation. Because of this, researchers have been looking for ways to boost acetylcholine to improve memory in Alzheimer's patients and decrease the depression caused by bipolar disorder.

Theoretically, safe forms of plants or plant extracts might be beneficial to improve memory, strengthen muscles, promote peristaltic movement, and decrease eye pressure via this mechanism. This is a fertile area for herbal research.

- **Ginseng root extracts** (ginsenosides) have been shown in animal experiments to directly increase production of acetylcholine.

- Both **shilajatu** and **ashwagandha root** are used as brain and memory tonics in Ayurvedic medicine. In one rat study, Indian researchers found that several groups of extracts from these two herbs preferentially stimulated cholinergic cascades in the cortical and basal forebrain areas, increasing receptor capacity. They concluded that this could help "explain the cognition-enhancing and memory-improving effects of extracts from **ashwagandha** observed in animals and humans."

- In one screening, the Chinese herb **evodia fruit** (wu zhu yu / *Evodia rutaecarpa*) strongly inhibited an acetylcholine-destroying enzyme. In live animal studies it was shown to have strong antiamnesia action, and a fraction was found to be more potent than Tacrine, the only drug for Alzheimer's disease approved by the FDA (Park et al., 1996). In TCM this strong-smelling herb is considered to be very hot and is used to warm the liver with signs of coldness, headache, and stomach pain. Therefore, I would consider using it only as part of a balanced formula in patients with both symptoms (amnesia and internal coldness).

Conversely, anticholinergic chemicals inhibit acetylcholine release and/or response. Curare is a strong anticholinergic, which explains why it paralyzes muscles.

- The anticholinergic action of the herb *Swertia japonica* is effectively used in Japan to calm intestinal muscle spasms.

- Ayurvedic doctors use **suchi** *(Atropa acuminata),* a relative of **belladonna,** as a sedative, narcotic, and antispasmodic. Both **belladonna** and **suchi** contain the anticholinergic alkaloid atropine, long considered to be the "active ingredient." However, in an interesting demonstration of whole-plant action, Italian researchers found in animal experiments they could produce "significant biological activity" using whole-plant extracts which contained low levels of atropine.

Adrenaline and Noradrenaline

"Adrenaline" and "noradrenaline" are neurotransmitters stored in the adrenal glands that control the adrenergic nerve synapses. Adrenaline is released in emergency response to physical stress and tends to stimulate the heart and relax the muscles in the GI tract. This helps explain the well-known "fight-or-flight" response, in which muscles must be stimulated to fight, while the bowels must be relaxed to remove waste quickly for rapid flight.

We know that the body manufactures monoamines from dietary amino acids. Based on this knowledge, scientists were able to understand the mechanism that makes dietary supplementation with the amino acid **tryptophan** an effective sleep aid and antidepressant. This discovery was hailed as a breakthrough in nutritional neuroscience until the FDA outlawed the sale of tryptophan after a poisoning incident caused by faulty manufacture.

"Noradrenaline" (also called "norepinephrine") is similar in nature, but it does not relax the muscles of the lungs or increase heart output. Instead, it strongly constricts blood vessels to raise blood pressure.

We have different types of adrenergic receptors that take up the adrenaline and noradrenaline released into our system. The physical result of adrenaline or noradrenaline uptake depends on the type of receptor involved. For example, **beta-adrenergic** receptors stimulate the heart, which is why "beta-blocker" chemicals are used to calm the heart and lower blood pressure. The endorphins we produce in our bodies bind to **opiate receptors** and act as natural painkillers.

- Herbs such as **opium poppy** and **corydalis rhizome** *(Corydalis yanhusuo)* reduce pain by binding to opiate receptors.

- The alkaloid ephedrine, found in the TCM herb **ephedra** (ma huang), stimulates these receptors. This explains why **ephedra** is known to relax and open the muscles surrounding the lungs in asthma, but too much will overstimulate the heart and raise blood pressure.

- **Red pepper** was examined in a controlled clinical study for its effects on dietary energy production. Subjects received either 10 grams of **red pepper** or a placebo with their meals. The herb recipients experienced increased energy (heat) production for 30 minutes and carbohydrate metabolism for a period of 150 minutes, after which metabolism returned to normal. The effect was a result of a short-term beta-adrenergic stimulation. This could prove useful for some patients who have difficulty digesting carbohydrates.

  It also means patients with hypertension taking beta-blockers might not want to eat large amounts of **red peppers.** However, considering the short period of time and large amount of herb involved in the study, it is not cause for major concern. I wouldn't suggest eating 10 grams (5 teaspoons) of **red pepper.** Traditional usage dictates mild dosage.

- The powder of **puskaramula root** *(Inula racemosa),* traditionally used for asthma and allergies due to a potent bronchodilating effect, was investigated in animal studies and found to have beta-adrenergic activity. TCM doctors use a related species, **inula flower** *(Inula chinesis* / xuan fu hua), for wheezing excessive sputum and to "direct the Qi downward." It is a very useful plant to stop vomiting and hiccups.

Mood-Managing Neurochemicals

We achieve chemical management of mood through modern drug therapy by focusing on imbalances in a group of neurotransmitters called "monoamines," which include **sero-**

tonin, melatonin, dopamine, epinephrine, and **norepinephrine.** The body manufactures all of these neurotransmitters from dietary amino acids. As with the other brain chemicals mentioned, mood-altering drugs either increase the production or inhibit the breakdown of these neurotransmitters, altering nerve cell stimulation. Within the cerebral cortex, **glutamate** acts as the primary stimulatory neurotransmitter, and **GABA (gamma-aminobutyric acid)** acts as the primary inhibitory neurotransmitter. **Serotonin** is also of particular importance, because it is a natural antidepressant and tranquilizer.

It is important to maintain good levels of important brain chemicals. However, you must remember that mental and emotional symptoms are signs that something needs to be corrected. Numerous foods and herbs act on the receptor sites that control mood, and your body can't efficiently manufacture these neurochemicals without proper nutrition. Taking a multivitamin and watching your diet is a good start, and should always be tried as a first step before using herbs. **Ginseng root** has been shown to raise brain levels of numerous monoamines.

According to a report in the journal *Lancet,* melatonin is one of the natural ingredients of the commonly used antimigraine herb **feverfew.** I'm not sure what this might mean in a clinical application, but it is a surprising reminder that plants can contain very specific hormones that are known to influence human brain chemistry. Melatonin, produced in the pineal gland, is related to circadian (day-night) cycles. **Feverfew** is used to treat migraine headaches.

People taking monoamine-oxidase-inhibiting drugs (MAO inhibitors) must avoid fermented cheeses, yeast-containing products, alcohol of any type, and pickled herring due to a chemical interaction with tyramine, an **ephedra**-like chemical. For the same reason, the herb **ephedra** should never be taken with these drugs.

Certain fractions of **ginkgo leaf** have shown strong MAO-inhibiting action, which may partially account for its neuroprotective and neurorestorative effects (Wu et al., 1999). There is some theoretical concern that additive effects indicate it should not be taken with MAO-inhibiting drugs. The same concerns have been raised for **St. John's wort,** but so far there is no direct evidence of any problems in this regard. Rather, it now seems that this herb exhibits broad-based neurotransmitter uptake inhibition of serotonin, dopamine, noradrenaline, GABA, and L-glutamate. This action is strong, but because it is well distributed across many chemical pathways, strong interaction with other drugs in this class has not so far been problematic, although it does speed clearance of other drugs. A similar argument can be made for **kava root.**

Nitric Oxide

The remarkable tiny gas molecule nitric oxide (NO) functions as a signaling molecule that works in response to nerve cell stimulation. It penetrates directly into cells and sets off reactions. It sends signals between nerve cells and also to endothelial tissues (vessel linings), where it acts as a potent vasodilator. When NO is released from nerves in the penis, it causes the blood vessel dilation required for erection, which is how the drug Viagra works. NO also doubles as a destroyer molecule in activated immune cells. Numerous herbs have shown the ability to modulate nitric oxide activity in test tube and animal studies. These studies have not reached the level of clinical significance yet, but they point to another area of research.

Research Highlights

- Both **ginkgo leaf** and **ginseng root extracts** were able to induce cerebral blood vessel relaxation via NO pathways (Chen et al., 1997). This, of course, leads to increased blood and oxygen flow to brain tissues.

- Many plant flavonoids, including those found in **green tea leaves,** have shown anti-cancer effects in a variety of test tube and animal models. One mechanism of action is through modulation of nitric oxide–related inflammation (Liang et al., 1999).

- **Garlic bulb** activates NO release, and in a controlled experiment, garlic-fed animals were able to neutralize a chemical that inhibited NO, preventing them from developing high blood pressure (Pedraza-Chaverri et al., 1998).

- **American ginseng root** has shown the ability in animal studies to increase NO release in blood vessels, indicating a potential role in cardiovascular disease treatment (Yuan et al., 1999). **Chinese ginseng root extracts** have shown similar actions in heart tissue (Varga et al., 1999).

- Other herbs that have shown effects on NO in test tube and animal studies include **dandelion root** (Kim et al., 1999), **aged garlic** (Ide and Lau, 1999), **schisandra berries** (Panossian et al., 1999), **licorice root** (Nose et al., 1998), and **aloe vera leaf** (Izzo et al., 1999).

Is That All There Is?

As I mentioned earlier, herbalists believe it is important to discuss not only the "hardware" of the brain and nervous system but also its "software," the mind and emotions. All of these chemical reactions and responses are essential to our understanding of the nervous system, and focusing on hormones and neurotransmitters can certainly offer us insight into mental processes. But we all know that they are only part of the answer. Psychological factors obviously are involved in nervous system health. I don't believe we can improve our lives by simply taking "happy pills," whether pharmaceutical or herbal.

One of the greatest difficulties the healer faces is a decision between the two basic thought trends that color most of what we do in this field. The **causal-mechanistic mode,** which focuses on physical aspects of health, is common among scientists but also appeals to many practitioners of natural medicine. I certainly do this myself, as I love scientific discussions about signaling molecules and receptor sites. There is nothing wrong, and a lot right, about this method.

However, we must not forget the equally important **teleological approach,** which focuses on the emotional and spiritual aspects of health. This mode involves the influence and consequences of the intertwined components we call thoughts, principles, personality traits, moods, or even soul and spirit. There is no doubt that each individual is composed of different physical and nonphysical aspects, and the goal of healing is to bring about an effective and balanced integration of these aspects. To live one's life in conflict, without tasting an integrative path with heart, is to live in sorrow.

I have a story I'd like to share with you, about a breast cancer patient I treated. She came to me, as so many others do, looking for herbs and vitamins to help her fight this disease. During our initial conversations, I found out she was unhappy at her job as a schoolteacher but found real happiness when singing for her church. As I listened to her, an idea popped into my mind. I wondered if she had ever thought of pursuing a gospel singing career. She had thought about it, she said, and told me of her idea to create "teaching plays." She would go to local schools, wearing the clothes of her great-grandmother who was born in 1863, and teach the students the history of American slavery through song. I thought this was a wonderful idea and encouraged her strongly.

To make a long story short, she went ahead with her plan, and now she makes a living doing what she loves. She is a minor "star" of sorts in our area, and schools from neighboring states are now booking her appearances years in advance. By the way, her cancer disappeared after her first surgery, she breezed through chemotherapy using herbs, she discontinued tamoxifen and all further treatment with Western medicines by choice after 1 year, and she has been cancer-free since 1997.

The Mind Controls the Body

The *Mind/Body Health Newsletter* regularly publishes research examining the ways that the mind can directly affect health. The following findings are some of my favorites:

- Hostility toward one's spouse elevates blood pressure and lowers immune response.

- People who regularly contribute their time and energy to help others are far less likely to die from all causes of disease than noninvolved persons.

- Having a window in one's office that affords a view of trees and flowers increases job satisfaction.

- People who experience stress are six times as likely to become infected by a cold virus.

- Having a pet decreases one's chance of getting heart disease.

Oriental Neurology

To increase our understanding of how the nervous system operates, and to give us some additional insights into how to use herbs for mental and nervous system complaints, it is important to explore and incorporate traditional ideas. Both TCM and TAM use similar concepts to emphasize the belief that nervous function (sensation, thought, and movement) depends upon a subtle supply of energy flowing throughout the body.

> To understand why it is important to look at the large picture before examining the small, imagine you came from Mars and were given a bear's tooth to study. Although the tooth contains a very few cells with the DNA code for the whole bear, it takes a lot of work to get this information out. If you were able to see the whole bear first, it would become much easier to know where the tooth fit in and what it probably did.

In TCM this energy is the Qi (chi), while in TAM it is called **Prana** (first energy), the life force derived from breath which, in conjunction with **Oja,** a "vital water," nourishes Vata and activates the nerves.

In TCM, a similar concept to Oja is **Jing** (the essence of **Kidney Yin),** equated with male and female sexual energy (sperm and egg). Both systems caution that poor breathing habits or wastage of Oja or Jing lead to nervous system weakness.

Conversely, conservation of sexual energy and skillful breathing practices can dramatically increase one's supply of Qi, with a corresponding increase in intelligence, neural sensitivity, balance, regenerative power, coordination, and memory.

> As a T'ai Chi instructor for 20 years, I have taught the following types of people to feel Qi energy flow through their body:
>
> Secretaries
> Medical doctors
> Ph.D.-educated scientists
> Schoolteachers
> Biochemistry professors
> CEOs
> Athletes
> Senior citizens
> Kids
> Hippies

This energy described in the traditional systems is not simply a theoretical concept. It is a palpable entity, something that can be felt and experienced. This is common knowledge among natural medicine therapists, energy healers, martial artists, and people who meditate. Herbal medicines can also increase Qi or Oja, changing our innate feelings of energy and well-being. Martial artists and people who meditate use **ginseng** root to increase their Qi.

According to Nai-shing's reading of the ancient Chinese writings, Qi was originally defined as a nutrient steam that was absorbed from the digestion of foods (like the steam from a cooking pot) and distributed to organs and nerves through invisible tubes called acupuncture channels. Far from being a purely "made-up" philosophy, it was based upon the fact that people who practice meditation and breathing arts can feel the flow of this energy.

Because most physiologists study only neural pathways and hormone receptor reactions, and most do not meditate, little attention has been paid to the difficult-to-measure or subtle energy flow systems in the human body. However, modern researchers have demonstrated that the perineural cells that form the sheaths around bundles of nerves are involved in a number of important nervous system phenomena, including reaction time, control of growth and regeneration of nerves, navigational control, and wound healing.

These functions closely resemble the heightened physical skills that develop over time in skilled T'ai Chi practitioners and Yogis. To the advanced practitioner, this energy takes on a life of its own and resembles pulses of blissful energy that courses through the whole body in waves. Over time, it sharpens and perhaps even heals the nervous system. Maybe we should broaden our investigations of these phenomena in our search for new neurological remedies.

No matter how much I talk about it, no one will be convinced Qi exists until they experience it themselves. It's simple. Stretch your arms out really long in front of your body, lock your elbows, and pull your fingers back toward your nose. Stretch until it hurts a bit for 5 or 10 seconds. Then, relax your arms and shake your hands out for a few seconds. Immediately calm your mind, and place your open palms facing each other with about 2 inches of air between. Close your eyes and move your hands very slowly (as if you were squeezing the Charmin), not going closer together than 1 inch or further apart than 2 inches, until you feel a magnetic-like force field between the open palms. Once the 85% of you who are capable of feeling this force do so, rotate your hands out of alignment and back again, maintaining the same space, and you will feel the strength of the field change. The ability to feel this energy is greatly expanded by practicing Yoga or T'ai Chi, or by practicing the breathing exercises mentioned in Chapter 17.

Nerve Tonics—Don't Worry, Be Happy

In TAM and TCM medical theory, the Qi (or Prana) increases when there is mind-body harmony. Conversely, signs of Qi deficiency include muscle weakness, slow pulse, mental confusion, digestive disturbances, immune system weakness, and mood disorders. Properly prescribed tonic herbs such as **astragalus root, ginseng root, gotu kola, shilajatu, Siberian ginseng root bark,** and **white atractylodes** can increase the vital force and help alleviate these conditions.

The ideal nerve tonic is one that would make us smarter, happier, and more physically and biochemically efficient. The search for such medicines began in ancient times. In the Himalayan Mountains, sages, wealthy merchants, and kings coveted medicinal plants believed to bestow happiness, intelligence, and even enlightenment. They were called "Soma" plants, but they reportedly died out thanks to greed, secretiveness, and hoarding.

Today we do not have any plants that possess this level of power, but we do have some excellent herbal nerve tonics. Of course, any of these herbs can be used in combination.

- My favorite calming nerve tonics from our nervine group are **ashwagandha root** (both forms), **milky oat seed, skullcap, kava root,** and **American ginseng root.**

- My favorite stimulating nerve tonics are **ginseng root, shilajatu, bacopa, gotu kola, St. John's wort,** and **ginkgo leaf.**

Following are my personal recommendations for treating specific conditions with nerve tonics:

- If a patient tends toward moderate to severe nervousness or nerve exhaustion, I choose **skullcap** and **milky oat seed,** both of which seem to cause an immediate calmness. This sometimes occurs within 30 minutes, partially because I use both herbs in the easily assimilated tincture form.

- If a patient needs nourishment and calm strength, I choose **American ginseng, ashwagandha root,** or **bala,** all of which fortify nerve strength over time. **Cordyceps mushroom, schisandra berries, wild asparagus root,** and **shilajatu** are also useful for strengthening the nervous system.

- I make a simple and convenient Ayurvedic nerve tonic (used since ancient times) by combining **wild asparagus root** or **fresh asparagus root** with eggs. We now know that eggs contain lecithin, a convenient source of choline, as well as easy-to-assimilate protein. To increase general mental and physical energy I frequently use **Siberian ginseng root bark,** at a dosage of 2 2,500-mg pills three times per day, or in tincture form 35–45 drops three or more times per day.

A Note of Caution

The complexity of psychological problems often dictates the need for professional help, particularly in moderate to severe cases. **If you are taking a prescription medication for depression or anxiety, you must consult with your physician before discontinuing it. Discontinuation without medical supervision may be life threatening.**

Rules for Good Mental Health

In Ayurvedic thought, strong mental health is synonymous with virtue. The ancient texts made frequent and eloquent reference to religious virtues. Honesty, courtesy, and respect for others are the basic ingredients for mental well-being. Almost as important is the belief that the sense organs must be trained and used carefully. It is imperative that we avoid overstimulation of the senses, which can lead to damage. This dangerous stimulation includes but is not limited to loud noise, bright light, and excessive vibration. TAM doctors recommend a peaceful atmosphere for most of life's activities. One can only wonder what the ancient writers would think of today's world.

Ancient cultures engaged in physical and spiritual practices such as breath control, mental focusing exercises, memory practice, visualization, and meditation to train the sense organs. One goal of these training exercises is to reach a quiescent (tranquil or serene) spiritual place where the deepest muscle tissues relax and blood flow equalizes. This stimulates the release of healing energy (and probably some neuropeptides as well) and has an extraordinarily beneficial effect on health.

Anxiety, Depression, and Anger

Love is our primary positive emotion, and anxiety, depression, and anger are our primary negative emotions. To understand the distinction between them, let's recall the two branches of the autonomic nervous system.

The sympathetic system is the fight-or-flight system, and it kicks in during emergency situations. Symptoms include rapid heartbeat or heart palpitations, muscle tension, constriction of the throat, cold hands, and rapid shifting of thoughts and emotions. This nervous defense system correlates closely with either functional anger (fight) or fear (flight). When these physical manifestations appear in response to real danger or a bona fide emergency, we classify them as the fight-or-flight response, an intelligent short-term response.

However, in cases of long-term anxiety, fear is excessive or amplified in relation to the actual situation. The anxiety response often results from fear of future events rather than the current reality. The same is true of prolonged or easily triggered anger. Anxiety is usually a Vata imbalance, and anger is a Pitta imbalance.

While useful in the short term, the following herbs are not substitutes for underlying causes of anxiety or anger, which can range from hypoglycemia to family problems and job dissatisfaction. Since both anger and anxiety stem from sympathetic nervous system activity, the same herbs can be used for both. However, in anxiety states, it is often necessary to add warming and nourishing herbs, and with anger states it is often helpful to add some cooling herbs.

- Calming nervine tonics such as **milky oat seed tincture, ashwagandha root, skullcap tincture,** and **valerian root** can often manage simple anxiety states.

- **Kava root** has proven useful for treating anxiety.

- **Scute root** and **bupleurum root** can be added to reduce internal heat and restriction (more for anger), and **white atractylodes** can be added to warm digestion and increase nourishment (more for the poor digestion associated with anxiety).

Good nutrition, exercise, and study are all essential for relaxation. As a T'ai Chi teacher, I know that learning to relax deeply takes some time and effort. Therefore I think of herbs as immediate and short-term solutions, while the lifestyle methods are essential for long-term solutions.

Note: Stimulating herbs like **St. John's wort** and **ginseng root** should not be used for anxiety unless combined with calming herbs.

Depression

The symptoms of clinical depression include loss of interest in or pleasure from normal activities, a desire to sleep all the time, recurrent thoughts of death or suicide, fatigue, and feelings of worthlessness and guilt. Depression is more **Kaphaja** (caused by Kapha) in nature. Before using herbs to treat depression, it is important to look at the whole physiology to rule out physical causes like hormone imbalances and dietary problems. Here are some suggested herbal treatments for depression.

- **St. John's wort** has been shown to inhibit the breakdown of several neurotransmitters including serotonin. This action makes it a useful treatment for depression.

- **Ginkgo leaf** also acts on serotonin and has been shown to relieve depression in the elderly.

- **Bacopa, gotu kola,** and **white peony root** can increase cognitive function.

- **Siberian ginseng root bark** can improve mood and general physical energy.

- The combination of **shilajatu** and **ashwagandha root,** mentioned earlier, can be useful for depression.

- I often find that depression relates to dampness and/or mucus accumulation. Look for a greasy coating on the tongue and a slippery pulse. In these cases I use herbs such as **pinellia tuber** and **tangerine peel.** When there is added Qi deficiency, I add **ginseng root.**

- **Muira puama** is particularly useful in cases where there is lack of interest in sex.

- Don't forget the benefits of **cocoa bean** or **chocolate** as mild mood-altering herbs.

- **Valerian** and **kava roots** are sedating and should not be used in depressive states unless combined with stimulating herbs.

Insomnia

Insomnia is extraordinarily common in Western society, affecting as much as 30% of the population, with 12% having moderate to severe sleep disturbance. Sleep disturbances are linked with heart disease and can predict heart events. Psychological problems account for a large amount of sleep disturbances, and vice versa. Insomnia and sleep disturbance is pervasive among the elderly and, though I disagree, is considered to be normal. The total direct cost for insomnia in the United States in 1995 was estimated to be $13.9 billion.

Prescription medications account for a large amount of sleep disturbances, as insomnia is a side effect of many drugs. I have met many patients whose sleep has improved dramatically as a result of simply weaning off unnecessary medications and replacing them with healthy diet and lifestyle changes. A woman called me once and told me that she had stopped taking five prescription medications and replaced them with a multivitamin and vitamin E. Most of her symptoms disappeared, and her sleep returned to normal.

It is very difficult for patients to recover from illness unless they get enough good-quality sleep. Insomnia can be caused by many factors, and you must dig deeper to identify the underlying causes if the methods outlined here do not produce results within a few days. Sleep apnea, for example, should also be ruled out as a cause. I have seen many patients recover from insomnia after they cleaned up their diet and lifestyle.

- Any of the herbs found in the nervine group can be of use. For simple insomnia, I often mix tinctures of **valerian root, passionflower,** and **skullcap.** Dr. Duke points out that it is not single elements like valepotriates that cause the effect of **valerian,** but the synergy of the different parts working together.

- Simple **chamomile tea** may prove sufficient in mild cases.

- **Kava root** is a simple traditional remedy for insomnia, as is **lemon balm tea** *(Melissa officinalis).*

- Regular exercise can improve sleep, as can liver detoxification routines.

- Nai-shing says that the premier TCM herb for insomnia is **sour date seed** *(Ziziphus spinosa* / suan zao ren). Second is **schisandra berries.**

> ### A Case of Age Reversal
>
> In 1977 I met my first T'ai Chi teacher, Master Dee Chao. Master Chao proved to be an amazing example of age reversal. At age 61 he was overweight and suffered from stomach ulcers, chronic fatigue, and irregular heartbeat, and arthritis so bad he could not even dress himself. His doctors in Taiwan told him he had only a year or so to live. He began to study T'ai Chi even though his teacher told him it was hopeless, that it was too late. He persisted, practicing daily, until his body gradually improved. He ultimately achieved Qi control, and it took him only 7 years to totally rejuvenate his body. When I met him he was in his early 70s, strong as an ox, and moving with the fluidity of a professional dancer. His diet consisted of typical Chinese home-cooked food, and I noticed he ingested quite a few herbal tablets along with his wines. That was it—daily T'ai Chi practice, good food, and TCM tonic herbs.

- Hypoglycemia is often a hidden cause of insomnia. Treatment of blood sugar imbalances, described later in this chapter, can solve this problem.

- Insomnia is often caused by circadian cycle disturbances. In this case, exposure to bright light at appropriate times can help realign the circadian rhythm.

- Restless-leg syndrome can be a cause of insomnia. TCM doctors see this as wind resulting from a failure of the blood to nourish the muscles. They treat it with a combination of **dang gui, chaenomelis fruit, white peony root, millettia root, tortoiseshell** (gui ban), and **siler root** (fang feng / *Ledebouriella* species). Folic acid (35–60 mg per day) has also been found useful for this condition. Lentils contain high levels of this nutrient.

- **Rauwolfia root** can be used under the supervision of a qualified herbalist for short-term relief of insomnia as long as you follow appropriate cautions. I have often added it to tinctures to increase the effects of other calming herbs.

- In patients with depression and insomnia, the blood-brain barrier (BBB), which filters molecules coming into cerebral circulation, seems to block uptake of 5-HTP (5-hydroxy L-tryptophan), the precursor chemical for the natural relaxant serotonin. The seed of the African plant *Griffonia simplicifolia,* now found in health food stores, can be used to correct this and induce sleep because it contains high amounts of 5-HTP in a lipid-soluble form that is better able to cross the BBB.

- As always, Yoga, T'ai Chi, and meditation are recommended.

Alzheimer's and Dementia

Currently, more than 4 million people in the United States suffer from Alzheimer's disease (AD) or other dementias. AD affects 47% of people over the age of 85. In AD, in addition to degenerative changes and atrophy, individual brain cells begin to produce a sticky proteinous substance that swells the interior of the cell (neurofibrillary tangles) and "gums up" the exterior (amyloid plaques). In essence, the brain petrifies.

One of our patients was a retired judge who has been eating a healthy diet and taking numerous vitamin and herbal supplements since the 1960s. His vitamin supplements include vitamins B and C, both of which have now been shown important in dementia prevention, as well as **Siberian ginseng root bark.** Up to the age of 94, he maintained a full schedule of board meetings and charitable functions, and his mind remained as clear as a bell until an unfortunate fall took his life.

Causes of dementias include hardening of the arteries and ministrokes. Inflammation is a major contributor to neuronal damage in neurodegenerative disorders such as AD, Parkinson's disease, multiple sclerosis (MS), and amyotrophic lateral sclerosis (ALS). Nitric oxide inflammation has been shown to play a specific role in neurodegeneration. Blood flow to neural tissue is another important consideration.

The historical use of herbal medicines to treat dementia diseases like Alzheimer's varies according to the different traditions.

According to TAM and TCM theories, dementias result from multisystemic decline and brain destruction due to aging, and thus can be prevented or slowed by maintaining overall health and using tonics. Consequently, our preventive and treatment goals are the reduction of oxidative damage, reduction of cellular toxins and inflammation, and improvement of cerebral circulation and oxygen and glucose transport.

- Neural circulation can be improved with blood-moving herbs, especially **corydalis rhizome** (yan hu suo), which slows the breakdown of choline.

- According to studies of the pharmacological properties of **gingko leaf,** gingkolides exhibit antioxidant, neuroprotective, and cholinergic activities relevant to Alzheimer's disease mechanisms.

- In numerous well-controlled clinical studies in Europe and the United States, extracts of **ginkgo leaf** have proven "effective therapy for a wide variety of disturbances of cerebral function, including multi-infarct dementia, early cognitive decline, and mild-to-moderate cases of the more severe types of senile dementia including Alzheimer's disease."

- Tonics that can prevent mental and neurological decline include **flaxseed oil,** DHA (docosahexaenoic acid from fish oils), **guggul gum, rehmannia root, amla fruit, American ginseng root, ginseng root, ashwagandha root, dang gui root, garlic bulb, gotu kola, guduchi stem, shou wu root, maitake mushroom, milk thistle seed, ganoderma mushroom, shilajatu,** and **Siberian ginseng root bark.**

- Antioxidant protection comes from eating lots of fresh fruits and vegetables and using herbs like **amla fruit, triphala,** and **wheat sprouts.**

- Because neurotransmitters and other brain chemicals are formed from amino acids, and digestion declines with age, digestion-strengthening herbs like **bromelain** or **trikatu** can be used to ensure proper protein and nutrient assimilation.

Attention Deficit Disorder

Attention deficit disorder (ADD) and attention deficit hyperactivity disorder (ADHD) are clinical names for symptoms typically related to problems with attention. These conditions appear most frequently in school-age children, although they can affect people at any age. People suffering from these disorders seem incapable of coping with school, work, or life in general and they are constantly distracted, moody, and sometimes aggressive. The most common psychiatric children's disorders are ADHD, anxiety disorders, depression, substance-use disorders, and conduct disorder.

Parents often come to our clinic hoping to wean their children off drug therapy. Immediately we note that ADD is a Vata disorder, disordered nervous energy. Second, we notice that ADHD is a Vata-Pitta disorder, attention dysfunction with the additional problem of excess/disordered energy or inflammation. Sometimes we see poor mental performance in school related to Kapha, with signs of poor digestion (dampness), sluggishness, and perhaps a greasy coating on the tongue. This differential diagnosis allows us to pinpoint and work on the underlying causes of these disorders.

Vata disorders are caused by excess nervous system stimulation, including bright lights, loud sounds, a complex rapidly changing environment, and stressful situations—a snapshot of today's world. Therefore, all children with ADD or ADHD would theoretically benefit from quiet meditative time, or time with nature.

In fact, it is my clinical experience that exercise and/or stress reduction practices can be extremely useful in managing ADD or ADHD symptoms. Many adults with ADHD have reported vigorous daily exercise to be their most important management tool, and parents of children have reported similar results. However, this approach seems to work slowly over time, and although there is a biological basis, no well-designed studies have been done. Studies done in other stressed patient populations, such as airline crews, make it very likely, in my opinion, that reports of benefits are real.

For example, college students using Yoga to control the stress of exams reported "improved concentration, self-confidence, improved efficiency, good interpersonal relationship, increased attentiveness, lowered irritability levels, and an optimistic outlook in life."

- One condition that can cause, or at least exacerbate, ADD is hypoglycemia. Refer to the section below for treatment options.

- A review of the ridiculously sparse literature on diet related to this problem shows that dietary changes definitely have positive benefits on some children. A controlled clinical study of a nutritional supplement showed some benefit. Dr. William Mitchell, one of the founders of the John Bastyr Naturopathic University in Seattle, suggests daily dietary intake of foods rich in aromatic polyphenols, such as **apricots, russet potatoes, yellow onions,** and **broccoli.** These would reduce inflammation and oxidative stress.

After correcting any underlying problems, we have found it helpful in our clinic to employ one or two of the following four strategies.

- If the child is aggressive and agitated, they can often be calmed with **kava root, valerian root,** or **milky oat seed** and **skullcap** tincture. Numerous commercial tinctures and capsules contain one or more of these herbs. Unlike many pharmaceutical calmatives, the calming action of these herbs is not associated with decline in reaction time, alertness, or concentration. **Ashwagandha root** is also quite calming, reducing Vata and Kapha.

- To improve memory and concentration, I use **bacopa, gotu kola, guduchi stem, shilajatu,** and **valerian root.** Maharishi Ayurved manufactures a syrup called MA 674 that contains many of these herbs. Some children respond to **St. John's wort.**

- To "calm the spirit" and reduce mucus and inflammation according to TCM theory, we use **Acorus tablets,** available from ITM. The tablets contain 12 herbs tested in China for the treatment of ADD and ADHD. They are made in small (300-mg) size, easy for children to swallow.

- If the child requires increased nutrients, Nai-shing will often make a formula using herbs designed to nourish the Yin energy, considered useful for the brain. Such herbs include **rehmannia root, tortoiseshell,** and **lycium fruit** (gou qi zi). She may also include herbs to "open the heart orifices," such as **polygala root** (yuan zhi) and **acorus rhizome** (shi chang pu). **Polygala root** is considered good for releasing pent-up emotions, and Ayurvedic doctors also use **acorus rhizome** as a brain tonic and for memory problems.

Most ADD children require at least two of the above strategies. In addition, I have heard many personal reports of the value of **grapeseed extract** and **evening primrose oil** supplementation in this condition, both of which would reduce inflammation and oxidative stress.

Hypoglycemia

Poor carbohydrate metabolism or poor glycogen storage in the liver often causes hypoglycemia, because both make it difficult for the body to control blood sugar levels. Symptoms of hypoglycemia include nervousness, the need to eat frequently, craving for sugar, shakiness, and the inability to concentrate or think properly. The diagnostic standard is blood sugar levels below 50 mg/dL, and abnormal response to a sugar challenge given in a test called the glucose tolerance test.

In TAM, this problem is linked to low blood pressure and is considered to be the result of weak digestion and blood deficiency (rasaksaya). The problem is often found in nerve-natured (Vata prakriti) patients. It is treated by combining digestive herbs and general rasayana tonics.

I normally treat hypoglycemia with a product called **Hyporil,** manufactured by Phytopharmica. It helps the body with carbohydrate metabolism and contains several B vitamins and digestive enzymes.

- Eating frequent meals, up to six per day, and increasing protein intake will often alleviate this problem. I have people follow the **diet for reducing wind,** which strengthens the nervous system (refer to Chapter 10 for the complete diet). Some people also find it useful to balance their dietary intake of carbohydrates, proteins, and fats according to the principles outlined in the "Zone Diet" by biochemist Barry Sears.

- Especially important is to avoid simple sugars. Complex carbohydrates are more slowly absorbed carbohydrates and reduce the glycemic index (a measure of how fast sugars enter the blood) and therefore lower insulin production.

- For more serious cases I sometimes construct an herbal formula using a tonic called **shilajatu rasayana.** This medicine, which contains both **shilajatu** and **triphala,** tonifies the blood and aids the liver in storing sugars.

- Because the liver is the major storehouse for sugars, liver tonics such as **dandelion root, milk thistle seed, bupleurum root,** and **white peony root** may also help with hypoglycemia. Look for signs of restricted energy (Liver Qi restriction), with a tense wiry pulse.

- Digestive aids like **ginger root, black pepper,** or **trikatu** are always useful and should be combined with general tonics like **shilajatu, dang gui root, ashwagandha root, cooked rehmannia root, shou wu root,** and so on. The standard tonic **chyvanaprash** is also useful.

- Hypoglycemia may be a symptom of more serious underlying diseases, such as chronic hepatitis, diarrhea or chronic diarrhea, anemia, and urinary diseases. These should be investigated and ruled out.

Neuropathy and Neuritis

The term *neuropathy* (also called *neuritis)* is defined by symptoms and location. Although neuropathy can affect any nerve, the term usually is used for the cranial nerves, the peripheral nerves (in your extremities), and the autonomic nerves. Symptoms are either numbness to pain, temperature, and pressure or painful burning sensations.

Neuoropathies include diabetic neuropathy, Guillain-Barré syndrome, post-herpetic neuralgia, and other forms of neuropathic pain/damage. Diabetic neuropathy is a common long-term complication that causes persistent painful sensation or loss of sensation, most commonly in the hands, feet, and legs. It affects an estimated 1.3 million diabetic patients in the United States and, if severe, can lead to amputation of affected limbs. About 50% of diabetics develop neuropathy after 25 years, and approximately 56,000 amputations in the United States each year are due to diabetic neuropathy.

Nerves get the same types of problems as other tissues—inflammation, toxicity, swelling, permeability, and so on, yet patients are often very frustrated by the inability of physicians to stop neuropathy using anti-inflammatories or painkillers. It is important to know that neuropathies are resistant to treatment partially due to special protective structures which exist around the nerves.

For example, peripheral nerves are protected in many ways. Each nerve cell has a long axon along which electrical impulses travel. Larger axons are wrapped by a protective myelin sheath coating (not all axons are myelinated). The axons are additionally protected by several sheaths of connective tissue. When these barriers are penetrated or otherwise dysfunctional, inflammatory cells can infiltrate, causing neuropathies with demyelination, inflammation, pain, and atrophy. Because it's as though each nerve cell is wearing several pairs of thick gloves, it takes longer for these nerves to get sick, and longer to get better. Therefore, herbal and nutritional treatments must be given for long periods of time, months and years.

Antioxidant therapy can often help with diabetic neuropathy. In a double-blind study of 21 patients, 900 mg of vitamin E for 6 months showed significant results.

However, of all the antioxidants, alpha-lipoic acid (ALA) seems to be the strongest. ALA is an approved medicine in Germany, where it has been used to treat diabetic neuropathy for over three decades. Studies have repeatedly shown that a 200-mg dose of ALA three times per day shows significant results within 6 months for most diabetics. ALA has the ability to restore missing electrons and extend the life of other antioxidants, such as vitamins C and E. This activity is crucial in neuropathy because it is difficult to remove inflammation from the affected nerve tissue due to its complex barriers. The concentration of antioxidants that ALA supports seems to slowly build up in the tissue, removing inflammation and allowing repair to occur over several months.

To reduce the general inflammation, I use **evening primrose oil.** The Ayurvedic herb **bala** can be useful. Acupuncture often benefits neuropathy. **Periwinkle extract** or my own Myelin Sheath Support formula can be used (see Resource Guide).

Research Highlights

- To help speed and improve this antioxidant healing process I use the mentioned vitamins along with herbs from the blood-moving group, including **salvia root, red peony root,** and **carthamus flower** (Qian et al., 1987).

- **Licorice root,** which has been shown to reduce diabetic cataract formation in rat studies, may help reduce the inflammation of neuropathy by reducing a chemical called aldose reductase (Aida et al., 1990).

- **Ginkgo leaf** has shown specific benefit for optic neuropathy in a placebo-controlled human study (Chung et al., 1999).

- Commercially available preparations of capsaicin, the strongly pungent ingredient in **red peppers,** can be applied externally to block the pain of neuropathy (Fusco et al., 1997).

Multiple Sclerosis

In 1976, I met one of Dr. Mana's patients, a person with multiple sclerosis who had regained the ability to walk. Dr. Mana's success with this disease is such that for many years he has had patients flying in to Kathmandu from America, Europe, and Japan for treatment.

Multiple sclerosis (MS) is a difficult disease to treat. It is characterized by recurrent patches of inflammation on the brain, spinal cord, and optic nerves caused by immune system attacks. MS remains one of the most frustrating diseases for patients and physicians because there is no cure or agreed-upon therapy. Fifty percent of patients are unable to work or perform household duties 10 years after the onset of the disease, 50% are unable to walk unassisted after 15 years, and 50% are unable to walk at all after 25 years.

The main Western therapeutic strategy is to use a form of interferon (INF-beta) to turn down the immune attack in the central nervous system. Although this approach slows progression, it is associated with flulike symptoms, headaches, edema, and other side effects. In my opinion, this approach, when used alone, is like stopping a brawl by sending in the cops, but leaving the door open so more bad guys can come in. By itself it is not enough.

Several years ago, I noticed a correlation between Dr. Mana's Ayurvedic approach and the work of MS researcher Roy Swank, M.D., Ph.D. Both of them paid particular attention to the use of fats and oils in the diet. In one study of 144 MS patients who followed a low-fat diet for 36 years, Swank demonstrated that at each level of severity of disability, the patients who followed the diet showed less deterioration than those who consumed more fat. Defaulting from the diet reactivated the disease. In other words, reducing fats has a similar effect to the interferon therapy, slowing or stalling of progression, but without reported side effects.

In 1996, I began to formulate an herbal medicine complex using herbs from Nepal, China, and the West, based on my analysis of various herbal and nutritional approaches. The main strategies were to:

- Decrease intake of low-quality fats and oils and any other offending foods that increase inflammation-causing lipid peroxides. Use the **diet for wind and heat,** but with only low levels of high-quality fats.

- Increase elimination of immune-caused inflammation via antioxidant mechanisms.

- Improve digestion and processing of fats.

- Stimulate repair of the blood-brain barrier to slow immune migration.

- Down-regulate central nervous system inflammation.

- Strengthen overall nervous and metabolic energy.

Some of the herbs I have found useful for accomplishing these treatment goals include **bacopa, boswellia gum, bromelain, salvia root, hawthorn, turmeric root, amla fruit, licorice root, ginseng root,** and **ashwagandha root.** I also have patients take lipoic acid (250 mg twice a day) and DHA (also 250 mg twice per day), two nutrients which have independently shown promise in MS.

With the small number of patients I have treated, it is impossible to prove in a scientific sense that my treatment works. Almost without exception, the patients who have continued report increases in energy and strength. In addition, Dr. Abel and I have had some partial success in reversing some cases of the related disease optic neuritis. However, with the relapsing-remitting form of MS, though the average time between attacks is about 1 year, some people can have periods where it seems to disappear for years. Nonetheless, it is difficult to explain the results of the two patients mentioned below in terms of placebo. I have been in communication with several neurobiologists and hope to obtain funding for a clinical trial.

In 1999 Dr. Michael Tierra, founder of Planetary Formulas, offered to produce my formula. It will be called **Myelin Sheath Support** and should be available from Source Naturals (distributors of Planetary formulas). I realize that it is possible that others will pirate my formula, but I hope that does not happen. I could not have done this without the inspiration of Dr. Mana. Therefore, a solid percentage of all commissions we make in selling this formula will go back to my teacher in Nepal to help him to build his dream of an Ayurvedic Research Center to restore the precious yet threatened Ayurvedic traditions and plants of Nepal.

Here are two reports from users of this formula.

From Ivy Creighton, a mother in New York whose daughter, Donna Waldren, had lost most sensation and motor control in her legs, feet, arms and hands, and was unable to sit up or feed herself.

Dear Dr. Tillotson,

I am writing to tell you how impressed I am with the early results of your MS treatment. Donna is feeling burning sensations in her toes and feet and legs. Not to mention the energy she's feeling. I am so excited that I will be ordering your formula every month from now on.

Thank you, I am very happy.
(signed) Ivy Creighton

Note: In March 2000, Donna regained the ability to sit up and feed herself, and motor control of her legs began to return. Barbara can now ascend two flights of stairs with her cane.

Progress Report from the St. Francis Rehabilitation Center in Wilmington, Delaware (released with the consent of the patient) from Kenneth Dill, P.T., ordered by David Jezyk, M.D.

Re: Barbara Starling
Diagnosis: Multiple Sclerosis

Barbara Starling is a 51-year-old female who was first diagnosed with MS in 1990, though she reports noticing symptoms many years prior to that time. She reports that since 1990 her primary form of transportation has been a wheelchair due to decreased strength and balance. She states that her symptoms and function continue to decline until she was at her worst in 1997. Since the middle of 1997 (18 months) she has been using herbal treatments with surprising results. She has progressed so well she was sent to our facility to begin physical therapy to regain strength, balance and begin gait training . . . muscular endurance has doubled . . . This is uncommon with Multiple Sclerosis patients this far advanced . . . She reports 50% decreased pain so far stating, "It doesn't feel like I'm walking on hot stones anymore." She now ambulates with a straight cane as her primary locomotion. She can usually walk up to two hundred feet before needing to rest. She can also walk without assistive devices 25-30 feet . . .

Both Ivy and Barbara have given permission to be called or interviewed about their experiences. Barbara can be reached at (302) 235-0769, and Ivy at (212) 877-1570. For access to the **Myelin Sheath Support** formula, refer to the Resource Guide.

CHAPTER 14

Endocrine and Metabolic Disorders

Freedom from the desire for an answer is essential to the understanding of a problem.

—Jiddu Krishnamurti

The endocrine system consists of the glands and other structures that produce and release hormones. These include the thyroid, pancreas, pituitary, adrenal glands, and gonads. Hormones are chemical substances formed in one organ or part of the body and carried in the blood to another organ or part. Generally, because hormones strongly influence metabolism, they are grouped as metabolic disorders, including problems with bone (such as osteoporosis) and lipid metabolism (cholesterol problems), which are covered in other chapters.

Most endocrine gland problems are caused by a deficiency of hormone production, excessive hormone production, or abnormal glandular growth (neoplasm). In addition, glandular function must be seen in relationship to other systemic processes.

Hormone resistance, for example, occurs when there are adequate blood levels of a given hormone, but not enough of the hormone enters the cells. Also, inflammatory processes or infection can injure the secreting tissues.

All of these issues must be carefully analyzed to pinpoint the underlying causes. Often, when we treat and remove the cause, we can favorably affect future glandular function. If the gland has been too severely injured, we can work on neutralizing resulting problems.

Diabetes

Diabetes is a disorder of carbohydrate metabolism caused by inadequate production or use of insulin, the hormone secreted by beta cells in the pancreas. Type 1 diabetes (insulin-dependent diabetes mellitus or IDDM) is also called "juvenile diabetes," as it appears most often in children under the age of 15. This autoimmune disease affects about 10% of the diabetic population.

The more prevalent Type 2 diabetes (non-insulin-dependent diabetes mellitus or NIDDM), is also called "adult-onset diabetes," as it appears most frequently in adults over the age of 20. The age-related terms are becoming outdated, however, because NIDDM is now showing up in increasing numbers in children, and IDDM is appearing more frequently in adults. It is very important to differentiate between the two types, partly because the dietary and nutrient requirements vary in some important ways.

Major symptoms of diabetes include excessive thirst, fatigue, and frequent urination. The long-term health problems that can result from diabetes are mostly vascular. Fluctuations in blood sugar shock the mural cells in tiny capillaries, gradually weakening and narrowing them. Most diabetic problems result from this breakdown in the vascular system. The resultant damage is usually much more severe in patients with poor blood sugar control and/or poor nutritional status.

Through a process called "glycosylation," excess sugar attaches to the hemoglobin in the red blood cells and makes it more difficult for them to deliver necessary oxygen to your tissues. When there is a lack of insulin, the body burns fat instead of sugar, causing an increase in toxic acids called "ketones."

Diabetics who do not have the necessary discipline to take proper care of their health risk blindness, kidney failure, burning nerve pain, and early death. Because of the horrific cost of poorly managed diabetes, and because it is so easy to avoid or slow the onset of problems with simple lifestyle and diet changes, specific programs designed to increase patient awareness and compliance are now rapidly being developed by the health care insurance industry.

It is possible to live a long and healthy life with diabetes. As I mentioned in the Introduction, I was diagnosed with Type 1 diabetes (IDDM) in 1961 at the age of 11. Now, almost 40 years later, I have not suffered any major diabetes-related health problems. I have been able to accomplish this through strict discipline, by adhering pretty much to every guideline explained in the following chapters. The herbs I take vary according to signs and symptoms.

I would like to emphasize here the importance of listening to your body. As a child, when I found out I was diabetic I went to the library and read everything I could on the subject. The books available at that time told me I had no options and that gradual deterioration would inevitably lead to severe complications. I was terrified, and I decided to do everything I could to stay healthy.

I began by cutting out all dietary sugars except fruit. I spent the next 10 years learning, through trial and error, how to manage my disease. For example, I figured out by 1965 that eating blueberries made me feel good, as did exercising daily.

When my early doctors gave me insulin, I followed their instructions to the letter and assumed I couldn't change the dose. I remember one particular day when my sugar level was very high. I called my doctor, who told me I could change my dose by two units. I did just that and immediately felt better. From that moment on, I took on the responsibility of adjusting my own insulin as needed.

Back when the early blood sugar monitors first came out, before they were available in drug stores, I stood in line to get one at a medical supply outlet. I began to adjust my medicines and foods to keep my sugars on an even keel. Remember, this all occurred decades before researchers demonstrated the importance of exercise and good blood sugar control, and the benefits of flavonoids in blueberries. I did these things because, instinctively, I "knew" they made me feel better. I listened to my body. You can do the same.

In spite of my efforts, by the time I reached my early 20s, I began to exhibit early signs of diabetic problems. My skin tone was pale and I had some stiffness in my joints. My sugar levels would sometimes fluctuate way too much. When I was 26 I met Dr. Mana, my Ayurvedic teacher, in Kathmandu, Nepal. He started me on herbal medications, and this put me on the road to true control of my disease.

The following steps are crucial to gaining complete control of your disease:

- Thoroughly understand the disease and its relationship to your whole person.

- Learn how to manage the disease properly, which will help you detect and treat any problems that may arise while they are still small.

- Adopt the necessary nutrition and lifestyle habits, and incorporate herbal supplements that can prevent or repair problems.

Understanding Your Type of Diabetes

Type 1

The pancreas contains groups of beta cells called "islets" that secrete insulin. Type 1 diabetes (IDDM) mellitus results from a progressive destruction of these insulin-secreting beta cells by "T-lymphocytes," a type of white blood cell. This destruction may be triggered by errors in the production of the insulin molecule, or perhaps by viral invasion. These errors stimulate the white blood cells (T-cells and macrophages) to attack and destroy the beta cells producing the insulin. Type 1 diabetics always need insulin and must maintain excellent control of their insulin levels to avoid serious health problems.

Type 1 diabetics often require a diet higher in protein, vegetables, and healthy fats, with restrictions on sugars and grain carbohydrates such as wheat and corn. This type of diet alone will lower blood sugar, reduce craving for sweets, and lower levels of glycosylated hemoglobin. However, each patient's nutritional requirements are unique. Some do better on the HCF (high carbohydrate and fiber) diet usually recommended for Type 2 diabetics. The HCF diet is high in cereal grains, legumes, and root vegetables and restricts intake of fats and simple sugars. Because many studies do not distinguish between high- and low-quality fats, it is difficult to interpret the scientific data. This diet will not work if the fats consumed are of low quality or excessive in amount.

Type 2

Type 2 diabetes, the more common form, is characterized by onset at a later age and is often associated with obesity and poor diet. The average American consumes 9% of his or her daily diet in the form of simple sugars, resulting in a significant reduction in nutrient and mineral intake. This nutritional decline is increased by a modern trend of decreased nutritional value in ordinary foods. The high levels of dietary sugar stress the pancreas and the liver and overall sugar regulation. This may result in depletion of insulin supplies, or cells may become resistant to the insulin. The incidence of Type 2 diabetes is much higher in countries where the general population follows the standard American diet (the "SAD diet"). Native populations such as American Indians and aborigines who abandon their traditional diets develop the disease much more frequently than populations that maintain their native diets.

Insulin resistance is a major concern for Type 2 diabetics. Although the body produces enough insulin, for some reason the cells resist using it. Blood sugar control worsens as abnormal fat stores increase and obesity increases insulin resistance. Therefore, weight loss is often all that is needed for Type 2 diabetics to reduce their medicine requirements. Some successful patients can even come off their prescription medications altogether.

Prescriptions are not a substitute for healthy living. Various prescription pills for NIDDM can "wear off" and stop working after a few years as the body builds a tolerance to them. This phenomenon has been known to occur in up to 40% of patients. You must learn to identify and utilize lifestyle alternatives. For example, it appears that a **garlic bulb** (two cloves per day) and **onion** (one medium bulb per day) can lower blood sugar by about the same amount as prescription medicines in some patients.

Type 2 diabetics sometimes do well on the HCF diet, which is high in cereal grains, legumes, and root vegetables, with restrictions on fats and simple sugars. Conversely, some patients do better on the higher-protein diet usually recommended for Type 1 diabetics. As I stated earlier, each person's nutritional requirements are unique, so it is necessary to listen to your body to manage your diet and your disease successfully.

Ayurvedic Understanding of Diabetes

Traditional Ayurvedic Medicine (TAM) doctors were perhaps the first to classify diabetes as a separate disease, calling it "madhumeha," which means "honeylike urine." They noticed that patients with this malady had ants attracted to their urine. Ayurveda identified two distinct types of diabetes since ancient times. Earlier, we discussed the Ayurvedic body types, and in this disease, the Vata or nerve-natured person is more likely to get Type 1 diabetes. The obese person with strong appetite (Pitta-Kapha type) is more likely to get Type 2 diabetes.

Although Ayurveda had no idea of insulin, it is certainly clear they understood long ago that the thin and wasting physical condition typical of young diabetics was related to digestive problems and presence of sugar in the urine. As they described it, the nerve-natured person was by nature thinner and restless and had a weaker digestive system, which accounted for their generally low weight. At the same time, the highly restless nature often displayed a craving for sweets. Putting high levels of sugars into a weak digestive system created dryness and heat, and favored promotion of toxic gases (Vata dosha). This in turn weakened the major digestive organ called agnyasaya, Sanskrit for pancreas. As Ayurvedic physicians began to have access to modern physiological teachings, they began to relate these ideas to Type 1 diabetes and hypoglycemia.

They described another scenario with regard to Type 2 diabetes. When someone is obese, constantly eating heavy and/or sugary foods, and has strong digestive energy (Pitta-Kapha personality), the pancreas can become overactive. There is an increase in bile flow to the intestine to digest the fats, and weight gain ensues. In this condition, secretions are increased, and the mucous membranes and arteries are "working overtime." These increased secretions cause blockages in the vessels and ducts, as well as obesity. The secretions and blockages irritate the nervous system and change the physical properties of the blood. The altered sugars (called "greaseless sugar") cannot be absorbed, so they exit through the urinary system as "honey-urine." Although Ayurveda has no concept of "insulin resistance," it is obvious they were describing Type 2 diabetes in another way. Because we now know the duct and membrane blockages tend to slow blood flow and metabolism, that excess fats change cell receptor sites, and high levels of sugars stimulate insulin release, it is easy to speculate that the physical conditions described in the traditional literature could be causative of insulin resistance.

This would also make it more clear why Type 2 diabetes often recedes or disappears when patients lose weight. Adding their understanding to modern understanding, we see that Type 2 diabetes is a disease of obesity and insulin resistance (Western understanding) and poor fat digestion and resultant excess mucus exudation and duct blockage (Eastern understanding). This broadens our therapeutic options.

Management: Lifestyle Rules for Both Diabetic Types

- **Regular *daily* exercise is essential for diabetics.** A sedentary period will elevate your blood sugars within half a day. A few hours of exercise will bring sugars down. Regular (and frequent) exercise is helpful for burning fat and improving cardiovascular health. This consequently improves circulation and metabolism, which will help your body fight off other diabetes-related symptoms. In one study that followed a group of nurses for 8 years, the ones who exercised the most had a 54% lower incidence of diabetes than the sedentary subjects. Diabetics must keep moving. One of the Ayurvedic treatments for diabetes is to walk 2–3 hours per day while taking **shilajatu** and **garlic pills,** and following a careful diet.

- **The appropriate amount of insulin is the one that causes the least fluctuation in your blood sugar levels and keeps you at a healthy weight.** You may have to experiment under a doctor's supervision to find your proper insulin dosage and the best times of day for you to take insulin. Some patients also need to use more than one type of insulin. There are both long- and short-acting forms.

- **Check your blood sugars several times per day, and act accordingly.** If your sugars are above 150, it is a good idea to delay meals. Otherwise, food will cause them to rise above 200, leading to the production of toxic ketones. You might want to consider using Humalog, the fast-acting insulin, to bring down levels quickly. Check your levels 2 hours after eating, when sugars are usually highest, and take a few units of Humalog right then and there (I learned this trick from another diabetic). Other strategies that will help stabilize sugar levels include increasing exercise on the spot, or reducing food intake on your next meal. Consciously figure out how to keep your levels from getting too high.

- **Relaxation and stress reduction techniques have also been shown to reduce insulin needs in some patients.** Learn T'ai Chi, meditation, or Yoga. Studies have shown that such stress reduction tactics can reduce medication need and reduce sugar levels.

- **Check your glycosylated hemoglobin (HgbA1c) every 3–4 months, to find out how well you are controlling your blood sugars.** This test requires a doctor's prescription.

- **Get a yearly eye examination by a good ophthalmologist**. Diabetics are more prone to retinopathy, glaucoma, and cataracts. The earlier treatment is initiated, the greater the success. If you develop retinopathy, there are herbs that can resolve the problem even in cases where bleeding has started (refer to our discussion of all three diseases in Chapter 16 for more information).

- **Avoid artificial sweeteners.** There is concern they are toxic to nerves, and diabetics are more susceptible to this reaction. Try **stevia leaf** or d-xylose, available in most health food stores. These natural sweeteners will not increase your blood sugar.

- **Eat more beans.** Your body metabolizes beans slowly, which slows down the absorption of sugars from the intestinal tract, aiding your body's regulation of sugar levels. A diet high in fiber is very helpful for diabetics due to this beneficial action.

- **Eat lots of berries, especially blueberries. Blueberries** (or **bilberries**) contain anthocyanins, plant chemicals that help repair tiny blood vessels especially in the eyes. Consume about 1 quart of fresh or one bag of frozen **blueberries** per week. **Blueberries, blackberries,** and **raspberries** are also low in sugar.

- **Take your vitamins.** Diabetics can benefit greatly from vitamin supplements. I recommend taking a multivitamin twice each day, as well as the following:

- Vitamin C (2,000 mg), which makes collagen and keeps capillaries strong.

- The B vitamins, including niacin, zinc, and other minerals, which are important for sugar metabolism.

- Vitamin E and essential fatty acids (EFAs), which are important for cell membrane stability.

- Alpha-lipoic acid, which protects nerves, decreases insulin resistance, and can reverse neuropathy.

- Quercetin (1,000 mg per day), one of the most powerful bioflavonoids, which prevents capillary leakage.

- Always take a multimineral if you have diabetes. Three minerals that are known to lower blood sugars are GTF chromium (200 mcg per day), manganese (5–15 mg per day), and vanadium (20 mg per day for 2 weeks, and then 2 mg per day). Interestingly, one study showed that herbs traditionally used to treat diabetes contained higher-than-normal levels of chromium. Barley also contains high levels of chromium.

Herbal Treatments for Both Diabetic Types

Numerous herbs can affect blood sugar levels and overall diabetic status. For a complete list of the herbs that can affect blood sugar, refer to the Appendix. However, be aware that there have been reports of other herbs in many parts of the world that act on blood sugar levels, so this is a fertile field for continued research.

- **Turmeric root, black atractylodes rhizome, fenugreek seeds, bitter melon** (which contains an insulinlike molecule), **prickly pear cactus** *(Opuntia fuliginosa,* used by Native Americans), **ganoderma mushroom, gymnema, Malabar kino** *(Pterocarpus marsupium),* **green tea, maitake mushroom, devil's club root bark** *(Oplopanax horridum),* **jambul seed** *(Syzygium jambolanum),* **fig leaf** *(Ficus carica),* **Siberian ginseng root bark,** and **bay leaves** can help regulate and lower elevated blood sugars.

- Ayurvedic doctors use a complex mineral formula called **trivanga bhasma** to lower blood sugars, not available in the Western world due to its heavy metal content, albeit purified. This is prescribed side by side with digestive medicines such as **garlic** and

trikatu for both by types of diabetes until the urine is free of sugar, and then discontinued in favor of the medicines listed below.

- Long-term use of **shilajatu** and **triphala** is excellent for improving energy in Type 1 diabetics and reducing long-term complications. This is the combination Dr. Mana gave me in 1976, and I still take these herbs frequently. Herbs that promote digestion such as **garlic** or **trikatu** are also important, as well as high-quality oils to maintain membrane moisture and health. If the patient is emaciated, **ashwagandha root** is used. For Type 2 diabetes, in addition to **trivanga bhasma** and digestive medicine, weight-loss medicines and those that open blockage are useful, especially **shilajatu** mixed with **agnimantha root** and **bark** *(Premna integrifolia)*.

Research Highlights

- Some studies indicate that the use of niacinamide (a form of niacin, also called nicotinamide) very early in the disease process can sometimes prevent the destruction of beta cells. Some patients have had complete reversal (Cleary, 1990). The reason it works is that it inhibits monocyte/macrophage function in the peripheral blood, preventing production of the beta-cell-destructive cytokines interleukin-12 and tumor necrosis factor-alpha (Kretowski et al., 2000).

- Herbs from the **vessel-strengthening group,** especially **tien chi root,** act directly on capillary vessel weakness, thus preventing diabetic complications. **Tien chi root** is one of my herbal mainstays. I take it several months each year to prevent vessel and eye damage.

- Diabetics suffering from neuropathy may benefit from acupuncture, alpha-lipoic acid supplements, and **ginkgo leaf** (Reljanovic et al., 1999; Chung et al., 1999).

- Coenzyme Q_{10} (CoQ_{10}) can help with heart problems and blood sugar control in diabetics. In one study as many as 59% of patients responded to supplementation (reported in Murray, 1996).

- **Evening primrose oil** was shown in a double-blind clinical trial of 22 diabetics with neuropathy to reduce pain and improve motor function after 6 months of supplementation (Jamal, 1987).

- Chinese research shows that herbs from the **blood-moving group** help prevent diabetic complications (Huang et al., 1997). I use herbs from this group several months per year for preventive purposes—I recommend you do the same.

Thyroid Disease

The thyroid is a two-lobed gland usually situated in the front of the lower neck. It stores and secretes thyroid hormones that play a major role in regulating various metabolic rates throughout the entire body. Any abnormality in thyroid function can affect every cell in the body.

Hypothyroidism

Hypothyroidism, or a slowing of thyroid function, can range from subclinical deficiency, with only subtle symptoms, to severe life-threatening myxoedema. Major symptoms of underactive thyroid include unusually slow pulse; cold intolerance; fatigue; depression; dry and coarse skin; lethargy; tingling and/or numbness in the hands and feet; dry hair; hair loss (particularly the outer third of the eyebrows); high cholesterol; muscle cramps; heavier and more frequent menstrual periods; digestive changes such as constipation, bloating, heartburn, and loss of appetite; and unexplained weight gain.

Hypothyroidism is often caused by Hashimoto's disease, an inflammation of the thyroid that can occur alone or may appear in conjunction with Graves' disease. Hypothyroidism can also result from iodine deficiency or damage to the pituitary gland. Subclinical thyroid dysfunction, which does not usually present any symptoms, may occur in as many as 10% of women over the age of 60 and is often mistaken for other diseases. It has been linked to many problems including heart disease, depression, elevated cholesterol, bone loss, and poor circulation. Returning your thyroid to normal function can decrease blood levels of homocysteine, thereby reducing your chances of developing coronary and cerebrovascular diseases.

It is a mistake to assume that clinical blood tests for thyroid function are infallible. In fact, it is my clinical experience (shared by other holistic doctors) that persons whose blood tests do not show problems often continue to have symptoms. When treated with either thyroid hormone or herbal alternatives, many of these patients improve dramatically. The simple tried and true method of taking the basal body temperature with a thermometer is often a more accurate way to assess thyroid status, and is certainly less expensive than laboratory evaluations. Blood tests measure the amount of thyroid hormone that is produced by the body and circulated in the blood, but they cannot tell if the body is utilizing the hormone properly at the cellular level.

Interpreting Your Blood Tests

Patients are often confused by their blood tests, so here is a simple summary of the most common ones:

1. **TSH.** Thyroid-stimulating hormone, or thyrotropin, stimulates the thyroid to release more thyroid hormone. If it is high, it means your thyroid is underactive, and TSH is

trying to stimulate it. If the TSH is low, it means the thyroid is overactive. Because TSH is high before other tests show problems, it is used to detect hypothyroidism. It is not as sensitive for hyperthyroidism.

2. **Total serum T$_4$.** Thyroid hormone (thyroxine or T$_4$) is the iodine-based compound that is released by your thyroid gland to stimulate metabolism. This number is high if you have hyperthyroidism, with a greater than 90% accuracy. Other more complex tests are used if this test is uncertain, such as serum T$_3$, a precursor.

3. **Serum thyroid antibodies.** This test measures if your immune system is attacking your thyroid. High levels indicate Hashimoto's thyroiditis.

Herbal Treatment of Hypothyroidism

Treatment of thyroid problems with natural means can take a long time. It is important to continue to take your thyroid medication and work with your doctor. If these herbal methods are successful you may be able to decrease your medicines, but this is by no means certain.

To measure your basal temperature, keep a thermometer by your bed at night. Upon waking (don't leave the bed at all), shake it down below 95 degrees, and place it in your armpit for a full 10 minutes. Move as little as possible. Record the temperature for 3 days. Menstruating women need to do this on the 2nd, 3rd, and 4th day of menstruation. **Normal basal temperature should be between 97.6° F and 98.2° F.** Low temperatures may indicate hypothyroidism, and high temperatures may indicate hyperthyroidism.

Herbs That May Alter Thyroid Function

Betel leaf *(Areca catechu):* dual role, inhibits or stimulates thyroid function depending on dosage

Bugleweed leaf *(Lycopus* species): inhibits thyroid function

Coleus root *(Coleus forskohlii):* may stimulate thyroid function

Guggul gum *(Commiphora mukul / Balsamodendron mukul):* may stimulate thyroid function

Holy basil leaf *(Ocimum sanctum):* may inhibit thyroid function

Lemon balm leaf *(Melissa officinalis):* may inhibit thyroid function

Lithospermum root *(Lithospermum* species): inhibits thyroid function, may reduce thyroid swelling

Mother of thyme plant *(Thymus serpyllum):* inhibits thyroid function

Stoneseed plant *(Lithospermum* species): inhibits thyroid function, may reduce thyroid swelling

Xing ren seed *(Prunus armeniaca):* inhibits thyroid function, may reduce thyroid swelling

Zi cao root *(Lithospermum* species): inhibits thyroid function, may reduce thyroid swelling

Deficiency of any one of many basic nutrients, especially iodine, can slow thyroid hormone production and utilization. Daily intake of a multivitamin and multimineral can help solve this problem (see Resource Section). Thyrosine Complex by Phyto-Pharmica works well (see Resource Section).

Goitrogens are naturally occurring substances that block the body's utilization of thyroid hormone. These substances can range from chemicals in the water supply to common foods such as cabbage, mustard, cassava root, soybeans, peanuts, pine nuts, and millet. The cooking process can inactivate goitrogens, so be sure to avoid raw forms of these foods. Authorities such as Dr. Jim Duke believe that cruciferous vegetables (such as cabbage) exert a deleterious effect only when there is iodine deficiency and may be beneficial in the presence of sufficient iodine.

Kelp fronds *(Fucus versicolor)* are a very rich source of micronutrition, minerals and trace minerals. They are especially high in iodine and potassium, useful for increasing underactive thyroid function and for alkalizing blood chemistry. Experienced clinician Dr. William Mitchell, N.D., has observed that low T_4 levels often increase slightly with 6 **kelp tablets** once a day at lunch. Other varieties of **seaweed** are also natural sources of iodine and can serve as beneficial dietary additions in cases of hypothyroidism. It is important to moderate your dietary intake of iodine-rich foods, especially when taking prescription thyroid medications. An overdose of iodine can interfere with thyroid tests and can even lead to hyperthyroidism or a goiter.

TCM doctors believe hypothyroidism is a Yang deficiency disease (see research note below), and they prescribe combinations of **purified aconite, deer antler, astragalus root, ba ji tian root** *(Morinda officinalis),* **epimedium herb, dry ginger root,** and **cinnamon bark.** The dosage is usually about 6 to 9 grams per day of the 4:1 concentrated powders. These herbs are very strong and need to be prescribed by a qualified TCM practitioner.

The unique herb **coleus** *(C. forskohlii)* can be used to strengthen thyroid function by increasing intracellular cAMP levels.

In addition to prescription medications and herbal remedies, regular exercise also helps stimulate healthy thyroid activity.

Hyperthyroidism

Hyperthyroidism is the primary manifestation of a group of diseases characterized by an overactive thyroid gland and increased production of thyroid hormone. Major symptoms of hyperthyroidism include rapid heartbeat resulting in palpitations; heat intolerance or sweating; emotional symptoms including but not limited to irritability, anxiety, and insomnia; tremors; exhaustion; softer, finer hair; hair loss; easy bruising; lighter and more infrequent menstrual periods; muscle weakness; eye problems such as itching, watering, bulging, and double vision; and weight loss.

Graves' disease, an autoimmune disorder, accounts for more than 80% of all cases of hyperthyroidism. An overactive thyroid can also result from a toxic goiter condition seen most frequently in women over 60, or from taking too much synthetic thyroid hormone.

Western treatments include irradiation of the thyroid, surgical removal of the thyroid, and pharmaceutical preparations. Due to the danger of vision loss, Graves' disease should always be managed and monitored by a licensed physician.

Herbal Treatment of Hyperthyroidism

Herbalists use **bugleweed** and other *Lycopus* species plants in tincture form to treat hyperthyroid symptoms (tincture form, 30 drops twice a day). Animal research supports its effect on reducing blood levels of thyroid hormones.

According to Dr. Jim Duke, many studies suggest that herbs rich in rosmarinic acid, such as **bugleweed, lemon balm** *(Melissa officinalis),* and **verbena** *(V.* species), may possess "amphithyroid" qualities. This means they are capable of acting on the thyroid in either direction, exciting hypoactive and depressing hyperactive thyroids. This suggests that these herbs may be used to treat both conditions—a fascinating but unproven possibility. There is no historical record of using these herbs in this fashion, so I am taking a wait-and-see attitude. Dr. Duke also tells us that broccoli contains phytochemicals that are capable of reducing thyroid hormone production.

Chinese doctors believe that hyperthyroidism is a Yin deficiency syndrome with deficiency heat signs, and they primarily use **self-heal** *(Prunella vulgaris* or xie ku cao). Use this in a high dose—it should constitute about 20% of your total formula. Interestingly, this herb also contains rosmarinic acid. A typical TCM hyperthyroid formula might include **self-heal, raw** and **cooked rehmannia, fritillaria bulb** (chuan bei mu or *F. cirrhosa),* **scrophularia root** (xuan shen or *S. ningpoensis),* **glehnia root** (sha shen or *Adenophora tetraphylla),* **scute root, coptis rhizome,** and **phellodendron root.**

On a personal note, we have treated three patients in our clinic with a combination of these herbs and nutrients. All three patients have experienced a gradual cessation of symptoms and improvement in blood test results, and they have been able to avoid surgery thus far. Two cases seem to have stabilized on a maintenance dosage of herbs. It is difficult to express how grateful patients in danger of losing their thyroid glands are when they discover herbs can prevent this.

Research Highlights

- A study of 89 cases of hyperthyroidism and 20 cases of hypothyroidism caused by Hashimoto's thyroiditis were analyzed via blood tests to check for correlation with TCM differentiations. In patients with Yin deficiency, the T_3 and T_4 hormone levels were higher than normal, and the TSH lower than normal. In patients with Yang deficiency, the T_3 and T_4 hormone levels were lower than normal, and the TSH higher than normal. This study showed that the TCM differentiations were almost exactly correlated with Western diagnosis (Chen et al., 1990).

Adrenal Glands and Function

The adrenal glands, situated over the kidneys, are generally most responsible for the body's response to stress. Their regulatory function involves the release of a number of important hormones. The inner part of the adrenal gland secretes adrenaline (epinephrine) and noradrenaline (norepinephrine)—hormones that help regulate our "fight-or-flight" response and also exert some control over digestion, heart rate, and respiration. The outer part of the adrenal gland secretes a different set of hormones called corticosteroids, all of which are manufactured in your body from cholesterol.

Corticosteroids have three basic functions:

- Cortisol, corticosterone, and cortisone regulate blood sugar and help "turn off" the immune system when activated by a stressor.

- Mineralcorticoids regulate mineral and salt balance in the body.

- 17-ketosteroids, including DHEA, are sex hormones. DHEA may also be an antiaging hormone.

All of these hormones allow us to meet challenges by regulating our mental and muscle energy and nutrient stores to allow the body to deal effectively with crisis situations. However, they work very hard to do this. Severe exhaustion after acute or chronic illness can lead to a state of adrenal gland deficiency and, in some cases, to atrophy of the adrenal cortex. This atrophy is also common in aging.

This syndrome should be addressed any time a patient has endured severe stress, such as the death of a loved one, or has fought a long-term illness. Patients report an extreme fatigue, the key factor being no reserve energy at all to deal with problems, or "spells" of weakness and dizziness. Low blood pressure is common.

Herbal Treatment for Weak Adrenal Function

- Dietary regulation combined with a good multivitamin/mineral combination is a very effective way to strengthen the adrenal system. For a detailed list of recommendations, refer to the treatment diets in Chapter 10 based upon signs and symptoms. It is important to keep potassium stores high and sodium levels low to restore adrenal function, so be sure to eat a variety of potassium-rich foods like carrots, potatoes, bananas, tomatoes, apples, peaches, oranges, flounder, and salmon.

- I consider **Siberian ginseng root bark, American ginseng root, shilajatu,** and **licorice root** to be the major herbs for strengthening the adrenals, but all other adaptogenic and tonic herbs from the **immunity/longevity group** are useful. Moderate doses should be used over a long period of time.

- T'ai Chi, meditation, Qi Gong, or Yoga practice is essential to restore weak adrenals.

- Serum cortisol tests can sometimes detect weak adrenals, but holistic doctors prefer to do more complete testing of all major adrenal hormones.

CHAPTER 15

The Musculoskeletal System

I have never let my schooling interfere with my education.
—Mark Twain

The musculoskeletal system is composed of muscles, connective tissue, bones, and joints. The tough, dense, and protective character of these tissues contrasts sharply with the softness of our internal organs. The bulk of the musculoskeletal system develops during the third trimester of pregnancy, forming a coating the shape and strength of which is intimately connected to our sense of self, as well as to our mobility, physical power, vital force, and general well-being.

TCM doctors note that there are two basic types of health problems with musculoskeletal tissues—degeneration and pain or blockage. They generally treat degenerative changes in bones or tissues with nourishing and digestive herbs, and pain or blockage with herbs that open blockages, improve circulation, and reduce inflammation. Diseases of this system can be divided into categories depending on which of the four components they affect.

The Importance of Collateral Bodywork in Treatment

Manual healers from all schools point out that proper alignment and balance are necessary for energy and fluids to flow freely throughout the body and to relieve pain and blockage. It is my personal clinical observation that when treating most diseases of the musculoskeletal system, we must use herbal and nutritional approaches hand in hand with skillful bodywork such as physical therapy, chiropractic, rolfing, or osteopathy.

Mechanical misalignments and tensions both contribute to and prevent healing of these problems. I believe that combination therapy can often dramatically improve results in these areas.

Diseases of the Joints

Osteoarthritis

Osteoarthritis is a degenerative disease of the joints associated with aging. The disease mostly affects the spine and large weight-bearing joints and is often characterized more by degeneration of the articular cartilage than by inflammation. The first thing to do is to make sure the digestive system is working properly, especially in the elderly. Look for signs like poor digestion and low appetite (See Chapter 11).

I have found the herb **devil's claw root** *(Harpagophytum procumbens)* helpful in many cases of arthritis with inflammation and pain, taken either by itself or as part of a combination formula, about 2 grams twice a day as a crude powder, or 60 drops of tincture three times per day.

Herbs from the **blood-nourishing group** are also essential to slow, and hopefully reverse, joint degeneration. They act on the structural components of ligament and bone. TCM doctors frequently use **raw rehmannia root, dang gui root, shou wu root, millettia stem, eucommia bark** (du zhong or *E. ulmoides),* **drynaria rhizome** (gu sui bu or *D. fortunei),* **psoralea seed** (bu gu zhi or *P. corylifolia),* and **deer antler.**

Glucosamine sulfate is extraordinarily effective, so I always use it to treat this disease. This substance is an amino-sugar extract derived from the exoskeletons of shrimp, lobsters, and crabs. As people age, they lose the ability to manufacture their own supply of glucosamine sulfate. More than 300 scientific investigations and 20 double-blind studies have shown that patients treated with this nutrient experience an improvement rate between 72% and 95% in various forms of osteoarthritis. The recommended dosage is 750 mg twice per day. It is important to use the sulfate form because, according to the studies I've seen, it is the most effective. It takes up to 6 weeks to see results, at which point patients often experience pain relief that exceeds the results from aspirin treatment.

Glucosamine sulfate is not a painkiller—it literally repairs the joint tissue. This translates into dramatic and long-lasting results. However, in spite of the treatment's effectiveness, we must remember that it does not reverse or cure the underlying degenerative process that causes the disease.

Traditional Ayurvedic medicine (TAM) doctors consider osteoarthritis (sandhigatavata) to be a degenerative process caused by any food, behavior, or condition that results in poor blood circulation, dryness (Vata), or low nutrient supply to the joint. Their treatments emphasize use of the following strategies:

- Try a gentle and slow oil massage (do not disturb the joint), using the standard tonic oil **narayana taila,** which contains **wild asparagus root** as a main component.

- The oil massage should be followed by application of a warm compress soaked in a warm decoction made from **bala,** using gentle range-of-motion manipulation.

- The well-known tonic **yogarajaguggulu,** which contains **guggul gum,** is a standard Ayurvedic medicine for osteoarthritis, used for several months.

- A second general tonic should also be prescribed to supply nutrition, such as the ones mentioned in the **immune/longevity group.**

- Use the **diet to reduce wind,** along with carminative (gas-expelling) spices, especially **celery seeds.** Other carminatives include **cloves, caraway,** and **fennel.**

To control arthritic inflammation (as opposed to degeneration), it is often important to use herbs from the **heat-reducing group.** TCM doctors use **phellodendron bark** and **scute root** to control inflammation, in combination with other herbs like **myrrh gum, fang feng root** *(Ledebouriella* species), and **qin jiao root** *(Gentiana macrophylla).* They also use a relative to **boswellia gum** called **ru xiang gum** *(B. carterii).*

Beware of NSAIDs—aspirins and aspirinlike compounds, including acetaminophen. Unlike many natural anti-inflammatory herbs, these pharmaceutical products cause damage to mucosa, cartilage, and joints. One would therefore expect that herbs containing salycilate compounds would cause the same problems. Interestingly, I have used the European prescription herbal tincture **Phytodolor,** which contains three such herbs, **common ash bark** *(Fraxinus excelsior),* **aspen leaf/bark** *(Populus tremula),* and **goldenrod aerial portions** *(Solidago virgaurea),* and it does not seem to cause stomach upset or bleeding, as correctly stated in the promotional literature. This may be because the slow onset of action (several days) creates less concentrated action on the stomach mucosa. Another trick is to use **DGL licorice** to protect the mucosa.

Most herbal anti-inflammatories do not cause stomach problems. **Turmeric root,** for example, works partly via cyclooxygenase inhibition (COX-2) activity, similar to the prescription drug Celebrex. Such medicines do not damage the mucosa because they work in a different biochemical way.

A good base herbal formula might start with **boswellia gum, myrrh gum, scute root,** and **turmeric root.** Add other herbs as discussed, and adjust as follows:

- If the patient tends toward coldness, try adding **ginger root** or **prickly ash bark.**

- If heat and inflammation are severe, add **phellodendron bark.**

Thus our typical osteoarthritis treatment program consists of:

1. Glucosamine sulfate supplements: 750 mg twice per day

2. An herbal formula for inflammation

3. Additional nourishing tonic herbs and basic vitamins to slow degeneration

4. A healthy diet, bodywork, oil/herb massage, exercise, and vitamin supplements

The relative proportion of the formula that tonifies and the formula that reduces inflammation depends on signs and symptoms. In elderly patients, for example, tonification and digestion are usually emphasized.

The following therapies can also be useful additions to your treatment protocol.

- Some patients, especially those over the age of 60, require digestive aids to ensure proper absorption of nutrients. Digestive herbs like **bromelain, white atractylodes, and ginseng root** can be added to the formula in these cases.

- Essential fatty acids (EFAs) are essential to control deficiency-based inflammation, so I use **fish oils** along with **borage oil** or **evening primrose oil.**

- Acupuncture can help alleviate pain and stimulate natural healing powers.

- Women must remain aware of hormonal changes that can affect arthritis and bone loss. In cases of hormone involvement, collateral treatment may be necessary (for further detail see Chapter 18).

You can also treat bursitis and Sjögren's syndrome with these methods (refer to the dry eye discussion in Chapter 16). Naturopaths also recommend vitamin B_{12} injections as a useful addition.

Gout

Gout is a form of arthritis caused by an increase in the production of uric acid and its deposition in the joints, kidneys, and other tissues. It is often characterized by acute onset with severe pain. It frequently affects the big toe (up to 90% of all cases), especially in the first attack. The concentration of uric acid in the body is a compound total determined by the amount eaten (in foods), how much the body produces, and how much is excreted in the urine. Excessive dietary intake of fatty foods or ingestion of alcohol or drugs often precedes gout attacks. However, 85% of cases are caused by failure to excrete sufficient urea via the urine.

Standard allopathic treatment involves inflammation control with NSAIDs and uric acid control with Allopurinol or other drugs, along with avoidance of alcohol, fats, refined carbohydrates, and foods high in purine, such as organ meats (liver, kidney) and sardines.

All three systems of medicine suggest dietary restrictions. The importance of reducing purine-rich foods is clear. TAM doctors suggest dietary limitation of vinegar and burnt or fried foods, as well as avoidance of damp environmental conditions and overeating. TCM doctors pretty much agree, calling this a disease of heat and damp, so the **heat and damp-ness diet** can be followed. It is also important to drink plenty of pure water, which has a natural diuretic effect.

An important clinical differentiation is whether the patient is an underexcreter of uric acid (85%) or an overproducer (15%). This is determined by testing the urine for uric acid levels. Underexcreters are treated with the drug Allopurinol, which works by blocking xanthine oxidase, the liver enzyme that produces uric acid while breaking down purines. Overproducers are treated with agents that stimulate urinary excretion of uric acid. With that in mind, we can examine herbal alternatives.

Because it is necessary to stop the severe pain, acute gout attacks should be treated with strong anti-inflammatories whether herbal or pharmaceutical. In most cases it is best to use Western medicines to get through a crisis. Steroid injections are commonly used. Mild anti-inflammatories may be used for long-term management, but not as the sole treatment. Any of the herbs from the **heat-removing group** or **poison-removing group** may be used for this purpose. One anti-inflammatory that is potentially very useful is **bromelain,** the anti-inflammatory and digestive herb.

Herbal Strategies to Inhibit Production of Uric Acid

Anecdotal reports indicate that eating large amounts of flavonoid-rich **cherries** (up to ½ pound per day) can be beneficial for gout. Several patients in the past have come in and told me this works for them. This makes sense, because numerous naturally occurring flavonoids have been tested that inhibit the effects of xanthine oxidase. These include those found in **bupleurum root, green tea, capillaris root, tangerine peel, perilla leaf** (zi su ye or *P. frutescens),* and **kudzu.** Quercetin has also been shown to do this. The easiest herbal way to control uric acid production may be to eat **cherries,** drink **green tea,** and watch your diet.

Herbal Strategies to Enhance Excretion of Uric Acid

Promoting excretion of uric acid through urination is a bit more problematic. You cannot simply use any diuretic—you would have to use one that expels the uric acid. Thiazide diuretics, for example, commonly used to control high blood pressure, can increase gout risk and uric acid blood levels if prescribed in high doses. The minidoses of aspirin used to prevent heart attacks can slow uric acid excretion by 15%.

I was unable to locate studies measuring the effect of different herbs on uric acid excretion, with the exception of some studies reported by Dr. Duke in his superb book *The Green Pharmacy*. He reports that **devil's claw** *(Harpagophytum procumbens),* **olive leaf tea** *(Olea europaea),* and **stinging nettles** *(Urtica dioica)* have some weak historical use data and pharmacological evidence showing they can increase urinary output of uric acid. However, there are numerous diuretic herbs traditionally found useful for removing gouty accumulations. For this reason we can predict they would stimulate removal of uric acid. (Some simple urine testing could easily determine the truth of this.)

- One of the best simple herbal treatments for gout is daily ingestion of **celery seeds** *(Apium graveolens)*. TAM doctors also use these seeds to treat other forms of pain and swelling.

- Ayurvedic doctors use the protocol mentioned for osteoarthritis for gout, along with a standard TAM tonic called **kaisaraguggulu,** which contains **guggul gum, guduchi stem,** and **triphala.** (The full formula is given in Chapter 19.) This tonic has traditionally been used to increase uric acid excretion, and Dr. Mana has told me he has successfully used it on many patients.

- Western herbs reputed to remove uric acid accumulations include **cleavers** *(Galium aparine),* **hydrangea root** *(Hydrangea arborescens),* **buchu leaf** *(Barosma betulina),* **parsley root** *(Petroselinum crispum),* **parsley piert** *(Aphanes arvensis),* and **gravel root** *(Eupatorium purpureum).*

Sciatica

The sciatic nerve is the largest nerve in the body, running from the lumbar and sacral plexuses down the back all the way to the buttocks and thigh. Compression or inflammation at the base of the sciatic nerve is typically the primary cause of sciatica. Characteristic symptoms include a sharp electrical shooting pain down the leg, accompanied by numbness, tingling, and sensitivity to touch.

The primary therapeutic goal is relief of the compression on the nerve. You can relax the muscles and ligaments in the lower back directly with acupuncture or other forms of physical therapy. Chiropractic manipulation of the spine is also useful for restoring proper function to "locked-up" joints.

To construct a formula for treating sciatica, always use herbs that help relieve external spasm, such as **kava root, valerian root,** and **millettia stem.** Western-trained herbalists and TAM doctors both use **lobelia** *(L. pyramidalis)* to treat sciatica, and this is the strongest treatment in my experience. TCM doctors note that the combination of **white peony root** and **licorice root** in high doses for a short period of time is also useful for relieving the associated spasms.

In cases with more congestion, cold, and restricted circulation, add herbs that open blockage like **salvia root, prickly ash bark, tien chi root, liquidambar fruit** (lu lu tong or *L. taiwaniana),* **turmeric root, dang gui root, myrrh gum, cinnamon twig,** and **ginger root.** You can also make this formula as a tincture and apply it topically to the site of pain. A simple tincture combination of **cayenne pepper** and **lobelia** can be useful for both internal and external use, often affording quick relief. (See Resource Section.) All of these herbs can also be made into a tea and soaked into a cotton cloth for direct warm application. In cases with more inflammation and heat, add herbs like **bromelain, boswellia gum, phellodendron root,** and **scute root.** It may be better to use cold applications here. You will find that some of the TCM blood-moving herbs mentioned are the basic ingredients in "secret" commercial applications sold at martial arts stores for treating athletic injury (see Nai-shing's "Secret Joint and Muscle Healing Elixir" below).

Carpal Tunnel Syndrome

The median nerve passes through the space formed by the arch of the wrist bones and surrounding ligament (the flexor retinaculum), forming the carpal tunnel. Carpal tunnel syndrome is a painful condition caused by compression of the median nerve. Common symptoms include weakness, tingling, and aching pain. The condition occurs most frequently in people who perform repetitive work with their hands, such as typists and carpenters.

Dr. Jeff West, D.C., one of the chiropractors I have worked with, often gets dramatic results by simply restoring movement to the wrist bones with specialized adjustments. Many of his very grateful patients have been able to avoid surgery this way. The operation not only is very expensive but involves cutting the ligament to relieve the pressure, which further destabilizes the joint and can lead to more serious dysfunction later on. Naturopaths and M.D.'s cite scientific studies that have shown the benefits of high doses of vitamin B_6 to treat carpal tunnel syndrome.

At our clinic, in addition to the above treatments, we use herbs from the **blood-moving group** along with acupuncture.

Diseases of the Bones

Osteoporosis and Osteomalacia

Osteoporosis refers to a gradual and generalized loss of numerous components of bone substance that results in decreased bone mass. It is often associated with aging, as more than 50% of Americans show signs of osteoporosis after the age of 50. Bone loss is typically greatest in the spine, hips, and ribs. In its advanced stages it leads to pain and tendency toward bone fractures. Coffee, alcohol, and smoking are known contributors to calcium loss, but soft drinks are the worst offenders thanks to their phosphoric acid content. Phosphoric acid leaches calcium out of bones. Osteomalacia is a softening of the bones caused by calcium loss (the adult equivalent of rickets) and can be treated with the same herbs and nutrients as osteoporosis.

As with osteoarthritis, the first step in treating these problems is to ensure that all digestive processes are working properly. As people pass the age of 60, the digestive system weakens, resulting in reduced absorption of nutrients. Herbs from the digestive group can help combat this problem. In addition to improving absorption, it is also necessary to supplement the diet directly with easy-to-absorb nutrients. I use a formula called "Osteoprime," developed by well-known holistic Drs. Alan Gaby and Jonathan Wright. Research has shown that it contains all necessary bone-strengthening minerals and nutrients in proper proportions, including easy-to-absorb forms of calcium and magnesium. Exercise is also an essential component of any osteoarthritis treatment regimen, as is exposure to sunlight to get your daily dose of vitamin D.

Micronutrients are also important. Boron, for example, is a mineral necessary for vitamin D metabolism, which in turn stimulates calcium absorption. Foods that contain high levels of boron include asparagus, cabbage, dandelion, peach, plum, quince, and strawberry. A healthy, proportional diet is the best way to keep sufficient concentrations of micro- and macronutrients. It can be a delicate balance, as in the case of protein. Excess protein can leach calcium out of your system, while protein deficiency can lead to metabolic weakness.

In China, most families eat "bone soup" once or twice a week. They make it by cooking animal bones, seaweed, and vegetables for a few hours, often adding **astragalus root, dang gui root,** and **dioscorea root** (shan yao or *D. opposita).*

According to Nai-shing, the best TCM herbs for osteoporosis are **bu gu zhi seed** *(Psoralea corylifolia),* **deer antler, drynaria rhizome** (gu sui bu or *D. fortunei),* and **eucommia bark** (du zhong or *E. ulmoides).* To these, you can add herbs from the blood-nourishing group, such as **dang gui root, millettia stem, cooked rehmannia root,** and **shou wu root.** ITM makes a pill called "Drynaria 12" that contains many of these herbs.

Osteoporosis is clearly associated with the reduction in hormones that occurs after menopause. Dr. Duke tells me that according to his database, **bu gu zhi seed** *(Psoralea corylifolia)* is currently one of the world's richest sources of the phytoestrogens daidzein and genistein. Part of its reputation in China as a useful treatment for osteoporosis may be due to its hormonal effects. Similar herbs from the West include **alfalfa, black cohosh,** and **red clover blossoms.**

The piezoelectric shock that occurs during exercise (as a result of compression) has long been thought to stimulate bone growth. It is a well-known fact that athletes and martial artists have stronger bones than less active people. Research has shown up to 20% more bone mineral content in the dominant arm of tennis players. We also know that long periods of bed rest will result in a loss of bone mass. Researchers are developing vibrating devices that will stimulate and help strengthen bones.

Advanced Qi Gong ("skillful energy breathing," also spelled **Chi Kung)** and T'ai Chi practitioners often have bones much stronger than normal. It is a well-known aphorism that "a real T'ai Chi master has arms like iron bars wrapped in cotton." I have felt the extraordinary bone heaviness of a few 80- and 90-year-old masters. My own bones are also heavier than normal due to my 20+ years of practice. The bone strengthening seems to occur around 1 or 2 years after the T'ai Chi player succeeds in "sinking the Qi," a specific skill that takes a few years of ardent practice under correct guidance to develop.

At our clinic we treat osteoporosis with a combination of hormone balancing, dietary measures, regular exercise, Chinese herbs, and Osteoprime. We have seen several cases of stabilization and reversal of osteoporosis in postmenopausal women using this strategy.

Diseases of the Muscles

Muscle Spasms and Cramps

Spasms and cramps affect both the smooth and the skeletal muscles. Small vessels that enter the muscles and subdivide into permeating capillaries deliver nutrition to the tissues. Muscle contraction depends upon the conduction of electrical impulses via minerals called electrolytes (potassium, sodium, and chloride). Other minerals including calcium also play very important roles. If nutrient supply declines in a local area of tissue, or if free calcium is not removed, the affected muscles can go into spasm. Magnesium helps to maintain the intracellular homeostasis of potassium and calcium, so in natural medicine circles it is said, "If it spasms, give magnesium." Nutrient supply can also decline as a result of poor circulation, poor nutrition, inflammation, mechanical trauma, and overuse of pharmaceutical medications. We must address each of these problems individually.

A major and often overlooked cause of back pain and stress is simple muscle tension, which often precedes and sets the stage for nutrient problems by restricting circulation. One common cause is the postural stress that results from sitting at a desk at work for hours at a time. Simply stretching out periodically, or getting regular manual therapy, can provide considerable relief.

To calm muscle spasms with herbs and nutrients, patients should use daily mineral supplements, especially full-spectrum products that contain all 13 essential minerals and vitamin D. Manual therapy or local applications of heat can be helpful, and a tincture of **lobelia** and **cayenne pepper** can often provide quick relief. TCM doctors recommend long-term use of **siler root** (fang feng or *Ledebouriella divaricata)* and **dang gui root** to treat muscle spasms. **Kudzu root** taken internally is very useful for tension and spasm, especially in the neck and shoulders.

> When I was young, I used to get leg cramps and severe muscle spasms several times a year. After I began to watch my diet and emphasize nutrition in my late teens, I never had this problem again.

Backache and Lower Back Pain

Low back pain occurs when the connective tissues and discs go into spasm or become damaged and/or inflamed. A complex muscle called the *quadratus lumborum* is the one most commonly involved in low back pain. Visualize a web of muscle fibers attached to the bottom of the lower ribs that extends down to the hipbone on both sides of the spine. Since humans are "upright animals," the low back is subject to numerous forces that can weaken or destabilize this muscle. Functionally, this muscle serves to stabilize the lumbar spine and acts as a "brake" when bending to the side. It is so important that complete paralysis of the quadratus lumborum makes walking impossible. Therefore, strengthening and restoring mobility to this muscle is a main object of therapy.

The most useful method is to combine herbs that relieve spasm, restore flexibility, increase circulation, and reduce inflammation. A good combination might include **carthamus flower, myrrh gum, prickly ash bark, turmeric root, boswellia gum,** and **lobelia herb.** TCM doctors also use **tu huo root** *(Angelica pubescens),* **lu lu tong fruit** *(Liquidambar taiwaniana),* **eucommia bark** (du zhong or *E. ulmoides),* and **loranthus branches** (sang ji sheng or *Viscum album).* When a patient with low back pain experiences degenerative changes due to osteoarthritis, treat according to the guidelines provided in our discussion of osteoarthritis.

Tension Headache

You can treat tension headaches with the same herbs used for muscle spasms, especially **kudzu root.** However, in many cases this may not be sufficient. The tension is often internal, so successful treatment requires herbs that relax us internally. Use herbs from the nervine group, like **kava root, milky oat seed, skullcap,** and **white peony root.** Chinese doctors also like to use **chrysanthemum flower,** which combined with **peppermint leaves** and **ginger root** makes an excellent tea for tension headaches. You can get **dried chrysanthemum flower** at your local oriental grocery store or health food store.

Nai-shing's "Secret Joint and Muscle Healing Elixir"

Tien chi root
Dang gui root
Carthamus flower
Persica seed (tao ren or *Prunus persica)*
Cnidium rhizome (chuan xiong or *Ligusticum wallichii)*
Millettia stem
Myrrh gum
Corydalis rhizome (yan hu suo or *Corydalis yanhusuo)*

Take about 2 ounces of each of these crude herbs (powdered) and mix into a bottle of high-proof wine or gin, enough to cover it completely. Shake it a few times a day for about 2 weeks. Strain and rub over joints several times per day to speed healing.

Postural imbalances in the spine and lower parts of the body are often neglected or overlooked causes of tension headaches. Misalignment prompts the upper neck and shoulders to increase tension to improve stability. Such external tensions can be treated with the same herbs and external methods mentioned earlier.

Healing Wounds and Traumatic Injuries

Chinese martial artists have known for centuries that herbs can help speed recovery from athletic or traumatic injury. Such herbs were often coveted and sometimes kept secret. Today, most "wounds" I see result from either surgery or motor vehicle accidents.

Bromelain can speed wound healing dramatically, and I often prescribe 2 tablets three times per day (2,000 mg strength) on an empty stomach for a few weeks. Perhaps even more effective is **tien chi root,** at a dose of 2 500-mg tablets two or three times per day. For healing the skin and superficial fascia, I use **gotu kola tincture,** about 25 drops three times per day for a while, usually about 3 weeks. More complex TCM formulas include **tien chi root** with herbs from the **blood-moving group** and a few anti-inflammatory and pain-relieving herbs (see box).

I can't tell you how many surgical patients have returned to tell me that they healed much more quickly than their physicians expected. Rapid wound healing is important because it results in the formation of less scar tissue and therefore fewer related problems down the line.

Fractures

Treat fractures by taking high doses of bone-strengthening herbs including **tien chi root, drynaria rhizome** (gu sui bu or *D. fortunei)*, **deer antler,** and **eucommia bark** (du zhong or *E. ulmoides)* for about a month. If you have an opportunity, ask your doctor about bone growth stimulation to heal fractures. This practice involves exposing the cells at the site of fracture to a pulsed electromagnetic field. The recommendations in our osteoporosis discussion can also be helpful when treating fractures.

Muscle Atrophy

Digestive weakness is the most common cause of muscle atrophy. Most cases occur in the elderly and in young children, and it can be an especially devastating condition for both patients and family in cases where there is thought to be no known cause. According to TCM, since

> My own father began to lose weight and his appetite when he passed the age of 80. Nai-shing wrote him a tonic formula, and he soon gained his energy and weight back. He still requires this medicine.

the blood nourishes the muscles, simply combining herbs from the **digestive group** and the **blood-nourishing group** can help heal this problem. Be sure to add strong pure tonics like **dang gui root, astragalus root, Siberian ginseng root bark,** and **ginseng root.** In severe cases, I also recommend stronger pancreatic digestive enzyme pills.

Diseases of the Connective Tissue

The connective tissues are fabriclike substances that form a matrix that wraps and fills all the spaces in the body, even extending into the innermost parts of cells. All the major bodily systems—the circulatory system, the nervous system, the digestive tract, the musculoskeletal system, and each individual organ—are surrounded and supported by the connective tissue.

With the exception of cartilage, all the connective tissues are highly vascular. Collagen is a fibrous, insoluble protein in connective tissue. It represents about 30% of the total body protein. The diseases that affect this tissue are collectively known as connective tissue disease (CTD), or sometimes collagen vascular diseases. These include systemic lupus erythematosus (SLE), scleroderma, rheumatoid arthritis, and combinations of these three diseases, called mixed connective tissue diseases or MCTDs. They share many characteristics, so the herbal treatments discussed here can be used for all these problems.

Rheumatoid Arthritis, Lupus, and Scleroderma

Rheumatoid arthritis is characterized by fatigue, weakness, and gradually intensifying joint pain. The pain usually begins in the small joints, eventually affecting all the joints in the body. It is an extremely painful and disfiguring condition.

Lupus (SLE) is an inflammatory CTD that occurs predominantly in young women—90% of all cases are diagnosed in this portion of the population. Although it can develop slowly over time, lupus often starts with a fever or acute infection. Most patients complain of arthritislike pain, swelling, and skin inflammation, and there is often a characteristic butterfly-shaped reddening on the cheeks. Lupus can spread to the brain, kidneys, lymph glands, lungs, and other tissues. There is a strong suspicion that part of the cause involves hormonal abnormality. For example, there is a higher incidence of the disease in women taking synthetic estrogen supplements. Patients should avoid prolonged sun exposure as it often exacerbates the disease.

Scleroderma is a CTD characterized by progressive thickening and stiffening of the skin, followed by atrophy and changes in pigmentation. It can progress to the internal organs, eventually leading to death.

Treatment of CTDs

The high level of inflammation and tissue destruction that occurs with CTDs points clearly to a weakness in the body's detoxification systems. Alteration in blood chemistry parameters indicates a need for immune and general tonification, as well as additional support of the digestive system. The seriousness of these diseases often necessitates concomitant use of strong Western anti-inflammatories such as prednisone when a patient is in crisis. The swelling and pain dictate a need to remove dampness and blockage.

To understand the connective tissue you must realize that it is elastic. Moreover, it is not found just in our fibrous well-known "gristle." Connective tissue proteins are also found within cells in the contractile filaments, stiff tubes, and connecting trabeculae, and some even surround the genetic material.

Just as the discovery of the virus erased the supposed dividing line between "life" and "nonlife," scientists are now moving away from the traditional rigid view of the body as a collection of separate cell units with distinctly different functions. As they delve deeper into the physical tissue, it is possible to find the same or similar patterns, tissue types, and functions repeating themselves at all levels.

It is essential to seek professional help in serious or advanced cases. Nutritional experts emphasize the need to check for food allergies. Many patients benefit from dietary elimination of cow's milk products, wheat, oats, barley, rye, and grains containing the proteins gluten and gliadin. As in most inflammatory diseases, **fish** and **flaxseed oils** are often used to treat CTDs. Long-term use of **borage oil** has also been shown to benefit rheumatoid arthritis patients. The combination of both oils together has been reported effective by numerous practitioners.

According to Jonathan Wright, M.D., author of the *Nutrition & Healing Newsletter,* digestive weakness is very common. He says, "I can't remember the last time I saw someone with lupus who had a normal stomach test; usually there is no stomach acid and pepsin at all, or very little. Replacement hydrochloric acid and pepsin capsules are almost always necessary."

Hollywood news media reports in 1999 claimed that actor James Coburn recovered from a severe case of RA using a nutritional supplement called methylsulfonylmethane (MSM). MSM is an easily assimilated food source of nutritional sulfur that helps strengthen connective tissue. MSM has captured interest among the nutritional science community because of its ability to strengthen and maintain joints and collagen structures. It is also a scavenger for free radicals and foreign proteins. Patients usually use 1,500 mg of MSM twice a day. Initial onset of action is typically 3 to 6 weeks, with maximum benefits seen at 3 months. I have used it with moderate success. It sometimes works very well, and sometimes does not work at all.

TAM doctors suggest using anti-inflammatory herbs, along with laxative, diuretic and, digestive herbs, for 6 months or longer. Effective anti-inflammatory herbs include **triphala, guggul gum,** and **guduchi stem.** Interestingly, they also use plasters that contain sulfur—MSM cream would perhaps be the modern equivalent. One unique medicine that may be of benefit is **narayana taila,** a complex medicated oil also used to treat osteoarthritis.

Antibiotic treatment with minocycline has been shown effective in rheumatoid arthritis, lending credence to the idea that there may be an unknown infectious component to CTDs. In fact, allopathic doctors are increasingly using two antibiotics, sul-

Dr. Jezyk and I once saw a very serious case of scleroderma. This young woman was basically turning to stone. A friend of mine brought her to us after she had been to a specialist at a famous hospital. She was on an experimental drug protocol, but there had been no results in close to a year. Nonetheless, she kept a positive attitude, always trying to smile, which really impressed me. I spent some time with her and told her all the facts. I was concerned when she did not come back for her second visit, and upon inquiry I discovered that she was afraid. After I called her and calmed her fears she agreed to give it a try, and after 2 months on the herbs, she returned with a written report from her specialist. He said that she was improving greatly. She could now move her elbows and arms. She could walk better. There was "impressive softening" of the skin. I was elated, thinking the herbs were working really well. The patient promptly corrected me, stating that she thought it was the combination therapy. The specialist thought that his experimental medicine was finally beginning to work. What do you think?

fasalazine and minocycline, that have been shown effective in treating rheumatoid arthritis. I have seen Dr. David Jezyk, a holistic M.D., put rheumatoid arthritis patients into temporary remission using these medicines. This treatment can serve as a good beginning for a holistic program.

Along similar lines, and as a result of my own experiences in developing protocols for MS (another autoimmune disease), I have concluded that immune system tonification is an important component of treatment. I often use herbs like **ginseng root** and **astragalus root.**

Dietary counseling is essential. I often find that the **diet for heat and dampness** is the best choice, along with the appropriate herbal treatments mentioned in Chapter 11. The exercises of T'ai Chi and Yoga, combined with "breathwork" such as Qi Gong and Pranayama, work to restore energy and elasticity directly to this tissue and are therefore fundamental to the treatment of CTDs.

I treat CTD patients by first helping them to understand the importance of strict dietary control as outlined above. I think it is important for patients to accept the fact that CTDs do not respond to "quick fix" methods. I then formulate at least two long-term herbal combinations, choosing herbs primarily from the following lists, emphasizing different herbs depending on the patient's signs and symptoms. My choices are highly individualized.

Herbs for treating CTDs:

- To strengthen the body's own antioxidant status and liver removal of toxins, choose from **amla fruit, dandelion root, milk thistle seed, wheat sprouts,** and **white peony root.** I often use 2 or 3 grams of concentrated **wheat sprouts** for a minimum of 6 weeks early in the therapy.

- To directly remove inflammation and swelling, make a combination of herbs that reduce heat or heat and dampness such as **ashwagandha root, boswellia gum, honeysuckle flower, licorice root, raw rehmannia root, rhubarb root, willow bark, guduchi stem,** and **turmeric root** (concentrated). I also use **flaxseed** or **fish oil.** The combination called **Phytodolor,** discussed earlier, is also a good choice.

- For digestive support, refer to Chapter 11.

- To strengthen the immune system and fight toxic microorganisms, choose from the **immune/longevity group.**

- To remove blockage, choose herbs from the **blood-moving group.**

- To remove dampness and swelling, choose from **black atractylodes, coix, dandelion leaf,** and **phellodendron bark. Phytodolor** is also useful for this.

- To strengthen the connective tissue itself, choose from herbs and nutrients like **glucosamine sulfate, gotu kola leaf, bamboo sap** (*Bambusa* species), flavonoid-rich fruits, multimineral combinations, **hawthorn, stone root,** and MSM. In scleroderma cases, MSM is also useful topically, as a cream.

Combinations of these herbs must be used in moderate to high doses for a long period of time and chosen and adjusted according to patient response. Although we have not succeeded in completely reversing CTDs, many of our patients have experienced slowed progression and a noticeable reduction in symptoms. We have put some patients into remission, but it is too early to know if these will last. You can add breathing and stretching exercises to the regimen once the patient has progressed enough to do them comfortably. This usually occurs a few months into treatment. Moderation is the key.

CHAPTER 16

Herbal Ophthalmology

Discovery consists in seeing what everyone else has seen and thinking what no one else has thought.
—Albert Szent-Györgyi

The sense organs are our windows into the world. Few of us truly realize how precious sight and hearing and our other senses are until we are threatened with their loss. For example, vision loss is one of the greatest fears of our aging population, equal only to fear of cancer. The sound of a bird's chatter, the rustling of the leaves in the wind, and the glint of the last ray of sunlight over a still lake have become sought-after luxuries in this chaotic modern world, when long before they were a daily blessing.

According to the ancient Ayurvedic doctor-sages, the five senses are gifts from the Gods of the Five Elements. The God of Fire draws the light of vision into our eyes, the God of Earth brings smells to our nose, the Sky God carries sounds to our ears, the Water God carries tastes to our tongue, and the Air God imbues our skin with feeling. Echoing this ancient insight, I believe it is essential to our health and happiness that we learn to protect, nurture, and sharpen our senses. In this chapter we will discuss how to optimize eye health and how to preserve our precious vision.

A Simplified Description of the Eye

The eye uses light to create vision. The skull contains two eye sockets made of bone and layered with fat. The eyeball itself, which rests in the fat of the socket, is a Ping-Pong ball-like structure that consists of three layers, or coats. The tough outer coat is made of collagen, and the circular fingernail-sized area of collagen at the front, which is transparent to let in light, is called the "cornea." The rest of the outer coat is white and is called the "sclera." This

Note: Parts of this chapter were excerpted from Dr. Abel's book *The Eye Care Revolution* (New York: Kensington Books, 1999).

coating continues all the way around the eye to the back, where it becomes the outer coating of the optic nerve, which enters the eye from the back. The inside of the eyeball contains the iris, the lens, and two fluids called "aqueous humor" and "vitreous humor."

The middle layer of the eyeball (covered by the sclera) is musclelike and embedded with a weblike supply of small nutrition-bringing arteries and waste-removing veins. It is called the "uvea," or uveal tract. The front part of the uvea forms the "iris," the colored portion of the eye which opens and closes to control light intake, the middle is the "circular ciliary muscle," and the back is the "choroid." The "pupil" is the opening in the iris.

Behind the iris is the "lens," which is suspended from the ciliary body. The ciliary body can focus the lens and secretes the thinner fluid (aqueous humor) which fills the small space behind between the cornea and the lens. If this fluid gets congested or obstructed, it contributes to elevated eye pressure, or glaucoma.

The cornea and the lens focus light onto the rod- and cone-shaped cells of the retina, which catch the light focused by the cornea and the lens. These photoreceptor cells send nerve fibers to the optic nerve, which forms a cable leaving the back of the eyeball. Thus, focused light is converted to electrical impulses that go back to the brain for interpretation.

Attached to the eyeball are six muscles that control the movements of the eyes so they move together harmoniously. The eyelids, lashes, and overhanging brow protect the eye from harmful external elements, such as dust and overly intense light. The thickly fat-layered orbit protects the eyeball against external blows and trauma.

Ancient Ophthalmology

It seems certain that organized ophthalmology started with Ayurveda. One of the original eight branches of Ayurvedic medical study is the Shalakya Tantra (Mouth, Eyes, Ears, Nose, and Throat). The fascinating story of the genesis of this early medical division is recorded in the *Charaka Samhita,* the earliest classic of Ayurvedic medicine (c. 2500 B.C.) and the most detailed of all ancient medical texts. This book records the story of how specialists in each of the eight branches were chosen during a years-long ancient world medical gathering in the Himalayas. Patriarchal eye specialist Videhadhipati Janaka, the king of Videha, championed the ancient school of Shalakya Tantra. Videha was located within what is now known as the district of Janakapura in Nepal. According to Dr. Mana, Dr. Janaka, like the scholars heading each of the other schools, was charged with compiling the practical knowledge gained by different physicians of his era in his field. He wrote the first authentic textbook in the field, the *Videha Tantra,* and the comprehensive practical knowledge of Ayurvedic ophthalmology was a major chapter of this work. This text was lost. However, Dr. Susruta, a well-known contemporary of Dr. Janaka and the head of the surgical school, quoted sections of the *Videha Tantra* in detail in his *Susruta Samhita,* devoting an entire section to the Shalakya Tantra. Dr. Susruta performed the first cataract operation.

In the years following the origin of the school of Videhadhipati, numerous scholars—Drs. Janaka, Nimi, Katyayana, Gargya, Shataki, Saunaka, and Chakshusa, among others—

contributed their unique knowledge to the field of eye disease. Their original commentaries and books have also been lost, so our knowledge of them comes from existing references to their books. One of the most important sources is the *Madhava Nidana*, written by Dr. Madhavarara in the 13th century. *Atankadarpana* by Sri Kanthadatta in the 15th century also contains many commentaries on ophthalmic diseases.

TCM scholars also report that the earliest books mentioning eye diseases were lost. During the Sui dynasty (A.D. 581–618), a book by Dr. Tsao Yuan-fang called *Physiology of Diseases* (Zhu bin yuan ho nen), discussed various eye diseases in its Chapter 26. During the magnificent T'ang dynasty (A.D. 618–906), there was a rapid integration of foreign and domestic influences from Confucianism, Taoism, and Buddhism. Dr. Sun Si-miao's classic book *One Thousand Golden Formulas* (Qian jin yao fang) introduced over 80 eye formulas. Dr. Wang Tao's *Secret Medical Book* (Wai t'ai pi yao, c. 725) mentioned numerous eye treatments that were specifically ascribed to Ayurvedic influences brought in by traveling monks. Newly introduced medical procedures included surgery for cataracts using the Ayurvedic techniques mentioned earlier (albeit with golden needles) and the use of artificial eyes made from beads. The almost identical classification of glaucoma and cataracts by color (white cataracts, blue cataracts, etc.) is a starkly clear confirmation of the Ayurvedic influence. The T'ang dynasty set up programs to promote medical education, and from that time forward ophthalmology was separated as a distinct medical discipline.

In 1996, Dr. Abel and I traveled to Nepal to meet with Dr. Mana, and we prevailed upon him to formulate a concise compilation of the Ayurvedic knowledge of eye diseases. We compiled Dr. Mana's information into an unpublished manuscript entitled *Ayurvedic Ophthalmology*. This book contains Dr. Mana's detailed translation of the first recorded cataract operation from *Susruta Samhita*, about 2,500 years ago. For a description of the procedure, refer to the end of this chapter. Please note that in order for this to make sense in English, it was necessary to draw some information from other contemporary surgical descriptions.

The Cherokee also have a tradition of cataract surgery over a thousand years old. They did "couching," or pushing the cataract down through a small incision, which has the advantage of preserving the lens. According to David Winston, A.H.G., Dean of the Herbal Therapeutics School of Botanical Medicine, eyedrops such as **bull-nettle** *(Solanum carolinense)* and **hoary-pea** *(Tephrosia virginiana)* were used to great effect to desensitize the eye. The same herbs would be used internally for pain, along with **Indian pipe** *(Monotropa uniflora)* and **turkey corn** *(Dicentra canadensis)*. One person would hold the eyelid, and another would perform the surgery with a sharp blade of thick wild grass.

Ophthalmology and Herbs in the West

Although reports of many remedies for various eye conditions exist in the Western herbal and Eclectic traditions, they have been minor parts of these traditions. Dr. Rudolph Weiss, in his textbook *Herbal Medicine,* states: "Generally speaking, not much can be achieved with herbal drugs for eye diseases." However, certain medicines have always stood out, such as **jaborandi** *(Pilocarpus* species), which was widely used in folk medicine for dry mouth and eye diseases.

By 1648, Spanish botanical writers seemed aware of its use, and in 1875 the alkaloid pilocarpine was isolated. It is used in the form of eyedrops to treat glaucoma. Drs. Ellingwood and Lloyd, in their 1919 classic *American Materia Medica, Therapeutics and Pharmacognosy,* mention that "ophthalmologists claim excellent results from its use **[jaborandi]** in a number of diseases of the eye."

An ophthalmic textbook by Kent Foltz, M.D., published in 1900, details the homeopathic and herbal treatments used by Eclectic physicians for various eye diseases. In his preface, Dr. Foltz states, "That drug action is the same in ocular lesions as in other organs is unquestionable, but this fact is ignored as a general rule, and the local application of remedies alone is usually dwelt upon to the exclusion of other equally important measures. . . . The generally accepted plan of treating the eye as an independent and isolated organ should be abandoned . . . on account of the influence exerted by remote structures."

It is clear that Dr. Janaka, Dr. Tsao, and Dr. Foltz and their colleagues laid the philosophical and practical groundwork for holistic ophthalmology in the past, stressing whole-body interactions. Now, with modern breakthroughs in nutritional biochemistry and with more attention to clues from our herbal ancestors, we are in a position to find effective new solutions for serious chronic eye diseases.

Ayurvedic Health Care of the Eye

Hygiene and health care strategies for preserving the senses are a part of the Ayurvedic traditions. This section, excerpted from the unpublished manuscript *Ayurvedic Ophthalmology,* contains many lessons of importance.

According to the Ayurveda, the eye is one of the five sense organs and is connected directly with the brain. It is a highly sensitive organ, very closely related to the functioning of the mind. The mind is not visible, but its activity can be partially monitored by observing the eyes. Fear, grief, lust, anger, peace, happiness, and suffering reveal the state of the mind as they alter the facial muscles around the eyes. Observation of the patient's eyes is very important for the Vaidya (Ayurvedic doctor) to understand physiological problems.

The eye was created by the Fire Element. The eye captures within itself the fire of the universe, allowing perception of the constant and ever-changing flux of colors and shapes of objects. Any radiation of heat or light, whether originating from the sun or from an electric filament, belongs to the Fire Element. Because it captures fire and heat, the physical structure of the eye requires immersing the cornea, lens, and retina in the cooling aqueous and vitreous humors. This is the Ayurvedic explanation as to why the eye is so adversely affected by excess heat.

Again, the eyes prefer cooling sensations, and they reject excess heat in any form. This is the central idea Ayurvedic Vaidyas emphasize in caring for the eyes. Hygienic measures such as washing the face three to four times each day and taking regular baths, as well as living and working in areas with adequate ventilation or outside in the fresh air, the ancient practice of peering at the moon to benefit from looking into the distance at its cooling rays, and a healthy diet are all ways of promoting the cooling sensations.

Similarly, practical methods of avoiding excess heat include protection from the sun's heating radiation, staying cool in the summer, and avoiding excess amounts of foods that have heating or inflammatory effects. Ayurvedic doctors routinely recommend protecting the eyes from the heat of a sauna, for instance, by holding a cloth soaked with cold water over them.

To maintain the natural power of vision, a *collyrium* (external application) made of a microfine powder of purified antimony can be painted across the entire bottom eyelid each night, making a line about ½ inch in width directly under the lash. This may prevent cataract formation. Eyedrops made by dissolving a condensed paste extract of **darvi root** *(Berberis asiatica)* in water can be used to wash the eyes every fifth day or once a week. These eyedrops clean the eyes and help keep the duct system open. They can also prevent and cure chronic conjunctivitis (see below).

Reading, writing, and working with concentrated vision under poor or tense conditions is not good for the eyes. Examples are poor lighting, viewing minute objects, or prolonged eye work at either near or distance. The negative effect of keen concentrated vision can be the cause of refractive error, especially nearsightedness.

All foreign objects, including dirty water, sweat, dust, pollution, and smoke, are harmful to the eye. They can damage the conjunctiva, cornea, lacrimal duct system, and blood circulatory functions, potentially causing corneal ulcer, pterygium (a membranous film that forms over the eye) and epiphora (excessive tearing).

Sudden changes in temperature are not good for the eye. Examples are sudden immersion in cold water after exercise, hard labor, working near a fire, or being outside in the sun. This type of excessive practice can harm the natural function and elasticity of the optic nerve, veins, and arteries.

Awakening frequently at night or sleeping during the day is not good for the eye. Night work, excess napping, and insomnia are common contributing problems. Waking at night can cause dryness of the eye, while sleeping during the day can cause excess exudation. Dryness and exudation are systemic problems that may contribute to many eye diseases.

A diet high in liquids, and/or excess liquids at night such as milk, tea, coffee, is not good for the eye. This can cause abnormal pressure in the eyeball, which is full of water. In another way, the lacrimal glands, which are usually less active at night, can secrete excessively and disturb sleep.

The bad habit of withholding the natural urges to defecate, urinate, or expel gas is detrimental to health in general and also is not good for the eye. It can be the cause of Vata dosha, which is related to refractive errors.

The eye reflects the negative (and positive) states of the mind; emotions, such as anger, grief, unbearable suffering, mental weakness or tension, an angry or aggressive temperament, deep grief, and so on are not good for the eye. The tension created by these emotions can harm the natural function of the optic nerve, vascular, or lacrimal systems.

Withholding the emotional urge to cry is not good for the eye. This can impair the natural function of the lacrimal glands, causing either dryness or epiphora (tearing).

Any traumatic injury to the head can damage the brain. In this condition, the eye, being directly attached to the brain and the brain being a source of vital energy of the eye, can have functional disorders affecting the optic nerve, vein, and artery. Functional defects include paralysis of the eye, visual field loss, optic nerve ischemia, and hemorrhage. Excess use of alcohol is also bad for the eye. Alcohol can weaken the overall health of the liver, blood and circulation, which is related to some eye diseases.

Prolonged poor weather, including abnormal levels of heat, cold, or rain, weakens the general health of all living beings. The outbreak of epidemic eye diseases like conjunctivitis is related to such weather problems or problems of indoor ventilation. The physical and emotional stress of poverty, poor diet, chronic progressive diseases, and emotional difficulties can impair the natural function of the nervous and vascular systems. Cataract and refractive error are very commonly related to these circumstances.

Overindulgence in sex is not good for the eye. This can impair the natural functioning of the optic nerve. It is considered a well-investigated fact in Ayurveda that preservation of semen plays a major role in strengthening the function of the nervous system. Overindulgence in concentrated sweet foods also is not good for the eye and can cause eye disease, especially diabetic eye problems.

Any eye disease that is not properly treated can be the direct cause of another eye problem. Neglect of conjunctivitis especially can weaken the natural functions of the eye and cause other eye diseases. This factor is very important for the doctor to understand when managing the health care of the eye.

Diseases of the Eye

In order to diagnose and treat chronic diseases with herbs, both the specific understandings of eye anatomy and biochemistry, and systemic, nutritional and energetic considerations are necessary. Developing formulas emphasizes the use of very specific herbs that remove inflammation and blood congestion from the eye. This is because from the traditional (and now modern) point of view certain herbs (as well as foods) have an affinity for ocular tissues.

The correlation between vitamin A intake and vision has been known for a long time, and we now know that specific carotenoids are equally beneficial to the eye. **Lutein, zeaxanthin, and lycopene** should be included in everyone's diet for prevention. To get **lutein** and **zeaxanthin,** eat lots of spinach, collard greens, kale, and mustard greens. The red carotenoid **lycopene** is found in watermelon, guava, and pink grapefruit, though tomatoes are by far the best source. **Lycopene** is made more bioavailable by cooking in oil, so using tomato sauce with some olive oil is probably best. To get high enough levels of lutein to treat eye diseases, supplementation is necessary, and many companies are now providing this nutrient in pill form.

There are many herbs used traditionally for eye problems. In our clinic we commonly use **buddleia flower** (me meng hua or *B. officinalis),* **chrysanthemum flower, lycium fruit** (gou qi zi or *L. chinense),* **cooked** and **raw rehmannia root, elderberry, celosia seed** (qing xiang zi or *C. argentea),* **boswellia gum, turmeric root, wild asparagus root, blueberry or bilberry fruit, tien chi root,** and **triphala. Conch shell** (shi jue ming or *Haliotidis diversicolor)* and **tortoise shell** (gui ban) are also used, the former to "drain fire downward," and the latter to nourish the blood and "suppress Liver wind" (for deficiency and mild sedation). We will refer to these herbs often as we discuss formulas for eye conditions.

Cataracts

The crystalline lens of the eye is a specialized epithelial structure developed from the ectoderm embryonic layer, enveloped in a surrounding capsule developed from the mesoderm. The lens is sufficiently elastic to be acted upon by muscles of accommodation, which then allows light from objects to be focused onto the retina. Because the lens has neither nerves nor blood vessels, it depends on the internal flow of fluid inside the eye (aqueous humor) to provide oxygen and nutrients, especially scavenger and chaperone molecules, and to remove toxic products. Over time, the older focusing fibers are pushed into the center, oxidative stress from sunlight causes haziness (alteration in light transmission) or a film to develop. Any clouding of the lens is called a cataract.

The lens focuses light constantly, from distant objects to near objects. Short light wavelengths such as ultraviolet light are especially toxic. UV light creates more free radicals, which can accelerate the clouding of the lens over the years. A cataract may be central (called nuclear), peripheral (in younger fibers near the outer edge of the lens), or subcapsular (at the very front or very back of the lens). Cataracts are the number one cause of blindness in the world. It is a preventable and treatable condition.

Symptoms of cataracts include hazy vision, glare, difficulty focusing at distance or on the printed page, rapid eye fatigue, and even double vision. Some people will develop second sight. This means that as they grow older, they may see better without their glasses because the cataract actually changes the prescription of the eye. Always have your vision checked to see if your glasses can be improved.

Studies in the United States are gradually accumulating evidence that antioxidant nutrients can help prevent cataract formation. Epidemiological studies clearly show that high dietary consumption of fruits and vegetables is an important preventive measure to reduce the risk of cancer, coronary heart disease, and cataracts.

Among the dietary antioxidant nutrients shown to be important in cataract prevention (from epidemiological and controlled studies) are vitamin E, vitamin C, glutathione, curcumin, and the carotenes lutein, zeaxanthin and vitamin A. You can augment the action of glutathione by consuming foods containing high levels of sulfur such as onions, avocados, eggs, asparagus, and garlic. Dietary sources of carotenes include carrots, pumpkins, spinach, collard greens, kale, squash, watermelon, asparagus, broccoli, and cantaloupe.

There are many common risk factors associated with cataract development, and most are avoidable.

- Sunlight, because of UV light, is a major cause, especially if your body has a low antioxidant bank account. Ask for UV blockers not only in your sunglasses but also as a coating for your regular glasses.

- Dehydration can hasten the development of cataracts. Drink 6 to 8 glasses of water per day to avoid dehydration. Sodas, iced tea, coffee, and other caffeinated beverages do not fulfill this requirement.

- Drink alcohol sparingly—moderate amounts of red or white wine may be beneficial.

- Smoking and secondhand smoke are known causative factors in many ailments. Don't even try to argue this one. STOP smoking, and avoid smoky environments.

- Recent studies have identified obesity as a factor in the development of cataracts. Follow a diet and exercise program to combat obesity. Limit sugar intake, eat lots of raw vegetables and salads, and drink plenty of water.

- Diabetes, heart disease, hypertension, and arthritis (and the medications that treat them) can contribute to the formation of cataracts. For example, cholesterol-lowering drugs frequently speed up the formation of cataracts by virtue of their effect on the liver. Ask your doctor if you can decrease your dose, or if there are any other natural means of controlling or treating these conditions.

- There are more than 300 commonly prescribed medications that speed up cataract formation when coupled with sunlight exposure. Ask your pharmacist about your medication. Wear your UV-protective sunglasses to eliminate this possibility so you don't have to discontinue necessary medications.

- Lack of exercise is a causative factor in all age-related disorders. Cortisone also accelerates cataracts.

- Estrogen apparently has a protective effect against cataracts. Studies show women are almost twice as likely as men to develop cataracts after the age of 50, so it makes sense to use herbs and natural estrogen and progesterone that aid with menopausal symptoms (refer to Chapter 18 for our discussion on menopausal treatment).

- Get plenty of sleep, because night (darkness) is when your eyes get a chance to rest and to heal. They are bombarded by light and the formation of free radicals all day, and this is the opportunity for the liver and other parts of the body to send the necessary antioxidants and minerals to replenish the tissues of the eyes.

The goal of herbal therapy for cataract prevention is to keep the lens sufficiently bathed in solutions rich in antioxidant nutrients. To do this, your body needs to keep high levels in your system at all times. If the levels are high enough, those in your aqueous humor will also be high. As in life, you should strive to save more in your bank account than you spend.

Various free radicals participate in cataract formation. The reduced form of the molecule called glutathione is a key cellular antioxidant that has been shown to reduce oxidative stress and eliminate poisons in both test tube and animal studies.

The body's production of glutathione in the liver is dependent upon a diet high in fruits and vegetables (providing precursors), membrane transport activities of the three sulfur amino acids (cysteine, cystine, and methionine), and adequate conversion of methionine to cysteine via the trans-sulfuration pathway. Therefore, any of the many herbs and nutrients that aid this biochemical process are valuable in cataract prevention. Nutrients include NAC (N-acetyl-cysteine), MSM (methylsulfonylmethane), alpha-lipoic acid and SAMe (s-adenosylmethionine).

Many herbs affect glutathione status because they contain glutathione (or members of the glutathione family) or otherwise boost its action. Some of these are **elderberry, blueberry, astragalus root, milk thistle seed, turmeric root, garlic bulb** and **oil,** and especially **wheat sprouts.**

Additionally, imaging studies using magnetic resonance microscopy have been done on eye lenses to clarify how water transport takes place. Results show that as lenses age, there is a reduction in the rate at which water can enter the lens cells. This of necessity also causes a decrease in the rate of transport of nutrients and antioxidants. This shows why prevention is best, when the lens can still absorb the nutrients, and also why it is so difficult to reverse the damage. Here are some strategies to protect your vision.

- Two equally important factors in healthy eye care are quenching free radicals and reducing whole body inflammation. Use antioxidant vitamins, make sure you avoid unhealthy fats and oils, and use a supplement supplying omega-3 fatty acids. Currently, several companies make nutritional supplements that are designed for the eyes. Martek makes Neuromins brand of DHA and Carlson produces Super DHA. These are a good way to start. Check for one with lutein, such as Ocuvite with lutein.

- **Turmeric root** has been shown to prevent cataract formation in animal studies. I estimate you would need about 2 500-mg capsules twice per day to get enough for this protective effect. Less is necessary when taking other vitamins.

- **Triphala,** the Ayurvedic "three-fruits" compound, is extremely high in antioxidants and has been used for centuries to treat a wide variety of eye problems including cataracts. Use 1–2 grams per day.

- Eclectic physicians stress the importance of digestive and liver health in avoiding cataracts. Two herbs recommended for "hepatic torpor" are **celandine** *(Chelidonium majus)* and **fringe tree bark** *(Chionanthus virginicus).*

- Dr. Abel has been using **MSM eyedrops** and monitoring their effects on cataract progression. MSM (methylsulfonylmethane) is a natural, biologically active, and easily absorbed (due to low molecular weight) form of sulfur. Preliminary results indicate a slowdown of cataract progression, but drinking water and practicing good nutrition and exercise can do that too.

Complex Formulations

TCM herbs traditionally used to prevent cataracts include **celosia seed** (qing xiang zi or *C. argentea),* **plantago seed** (che quian zi or *P. ovata),* **chien li flower** (qian li guang or *Senecia scandens),* **lycium fruit** (gou qi zi or *L. chinense),* and **buddleia flower** (me meng hua or *B. officinalis).* These would be used in formulas along with herbs for systemic imbalances, based upon signs and symptoms.

The most common imbalances are:

- **Spleen Qi deficiency** (digestive insufficiency). Use **ginseng root, white atractylodes, poria mushroom, dang gui root, white peony root, cimicifuga rhizome** (sheng ma or *C. foetida),* **kudzu, siler root** (fang feng or *Ledebouriella* species), **schisandra berry, tangerine peel,** and **licorice root.** Other herbs from the **digestive group** may be used.

- **Kidney deficiency** (degenerative changes associated with aging). Use raw and cooked **rehmannia root, dioscorea root** (shan yao or *D. opposita),* **cornus fruit** (shan zhu yu or *C. officinalis),* **poria mushroom, moudan bark** (mu dan pi or *Paeonia suffruticosa),* **dang gui root, kudzu,** and **schisandra berry.**

- **Liver heat/wind clouding the vision** (inflammation). Use **white** and **red peony root, chrysanthemum flower, gentiana root** (long dan cao or *G. scabra),* **bupleurum root, cnidium rhizome** (chuan xiong or *Ligusticum wallichii),* **conch shell** (shi jue ming or *Haliotidis diversicolor),* and **scute root.**

For maintenance treatment (prevention of cataract progression), Ayurvedic doctors use **Sukhavata Varti,** a tablet made from equal parts of **kataka fruit** *(Strychnos potatorum),* **conch shell** *(Haliotidis diversicolor),* **trikatu,** mineral salt, sugar, **seafoam** (cuttlefish bone), **darvi extract** *(Berberis nepalensis),* honey, **vidanga seeds** *(Emblica ribes),* **purified realgar** (manashila bhasma), and chicken eggshell. It is very effective, used not only for cataract, but also pterygium, corneal ulcer, conjunctivitis, itchy eyes, and skin lesions.

This formula, currently illegal to import because it contains **realgar** (arsenic), must be prepared by an experienced Ayurvedic doctor and made into a tablet (see section on heavy metals in the safety chapter). Arsenic is now being investigated for its effect on leukemia. "Seafoam" is the common name for **cuttlefish bone** *(Sepia* species), which is found floating on seawater, then collected and dried into a layered natural product.

To prepare **Sukhavata Varti,** make a fresh paste each day by rubbing the tablet into a small amount of water on a flat, clean plate made of unpolished marble or stone. A small amount of paste is then carefully and fully diluted in pure water, strained, and a few drops placed into the eye several times per day. Dr. Abel has never used this.

Glaucoma

Glaucoma is another leading cause of blindness in the elderly. There are several types of this disease, all of which could cause damage to the optic nerve in the back of the eye. Peripheral vision examinations can detect glaucoma, even in cases where eye pressure is not necessarily elevated. Age and smoking are major causative factors in this disease, as is stress, because excess adrenaline (the fight-or-flight stress chemical) elevates eye pressure. Poor circulation can also contribute to glaucoma. High blood pressure medications can actually cause blood pressure to drop too low at night, with a negative effect.

Most people develop the open-angle variety of glaucoma, also called primary open-angle, or chronic simple glaucoma. Other types of glaucoma are congenital, narrow-angle, secondary, and low-tension. Many people with higher pressures or enlarged optic cups are put into the category of glaucoma suspect. The disease is characterized by either damage to the optic nerve through a mechanism of elevated pressure in the eye, poor blood supply in the optic nerve, or both.

Conventional treatment options include eyedrops, laser therapy (especially for the narrow-angle variety), and surgery and are required if the patient continues to lose peripheral vision (tested by visual field exams).

The fluid pressure between the iris and the cornea builds up because the trabecular meshwork (the filter on the eye's drainpipe) becomes unable to do its job properly. This is a bit more complex than it sounds. Recent evidence shows that there is a functional relationship between the ciliary body, which pulls, and the trabecular meshwork, which then distends and blocks fluid outflow. Originally thought to be a passive participant, the trabecular meshwork, it now seems, has the ability to contract and open itself for fluid drainage.

The goal of internal herbal therapy is to preserve visual function and maintain the health of the optic nerve. The ideal medicine for glaucoma should improve microcirculation to the back of the eye, nourish photoreceptors and nerve fibers, reduce IOP (intraocular pressure), calm stress, and improve fluid drainage. Elevated eye pressures and regular eye examinations to check results should, of course, be handled by an ophthalmologist during herbal therapy.

Certain chemicals found in foods have been shown to relax the trabecular meshwork without tightening the ciliary muscle. Two of these chemicals are called "tyrosine kinase inhibitors" (TKI) and "protein kinase C inhibitors" (PKCI). According to Dr. Duke's database, these substances are found in high amounts in beans, including yellow split pea, black turtle beans, baby lima beans, large lima beans, anasazi beans, red kidney beans, red lentils, soybeans, black-eyed peas, pinto beans, mung beans, and azuki beans. Quercetin is also a TKI, so eat lots of **yellow-skinned onions,** drink some **green tea,** and eat **garlic** and **broccoli.** The levels of specific chemicals gained by eating these foods are not extremely high, but given the multiple benefits with regard to cancer prevention and cardiovascular disease, it makes good sense to include them in the diet.

With all of this in mind, we can begin to formulate. A good formula would include herbs from the following groups, along with herbs for specific whole-body problems, such as poor digestion and essential fatty acid deficiency.

- To directly reduce IOP (intraocular pressure) with internal medicines, use **coleus** *(Coleus forskohlii),* **jaborandi** *(Pilocarpus jaborandi),* **gou teng twigs** *(Uncaria sinensis),* **abalone shell** (shi jue ming or *Haliotidis diversicolor),* **oyster shell** (mu li or *Ostrea gigas),* or **xie ku cao spike** *(Prunella vulgaris).* Caution: a trained herbal practitioner or holistic physician must administer these. They can be especially useful if eyedrops fail to control pressures.

- To improve blood flow to the eye and prevent destruction of the retinal neurons and ganglion cells, choose herbs from the **blood-moving group,** especially **ginkgo leaf** and **bala.**

- To improve fluid drainage choose from **punarnava root** *(Boerhavia diffusa),* **water plantain rhizome** (ze xie or *Alisma plantago-aquatica),* or **cinnamon twig** (as diuretics; this method makes sense in TCM and TAM but does not have a strong basis in Western understanding).

- To nourish and moisturize the intraeye membranes choose from DHA, **flaxseed oil, evening primrose oil, cooked rehmannia root,** and **triphala.**

- To reduce nervous tension and calm the sympathetic nervous system, choose from the **nervine group.**

- The phytochemical apigenin competes with chemicals that overstimulate PKC (protein kinase C) activity, and so we find potential glaucoma benefit with apigenin-rich **parsley, chamomile flower, feverfew,** and **chrysanthemum flower,** the last of which has long been used by TCM doctors for eye inflammation. In a similar fashion, curcumin from **turmeric root** is also able to reduce PKC activity. Both apigenin and curcumin also have anticancer activity.

- Pharmacological studies have shown that certain **ginseng root glycosides** reduce activation of PKC.

Complex Formulations

The Shanghai research hospital reported an effective rate of 96.6% using the following formula based upon the TCM treatment principles of moving the blood to remove stagnation and warming the Yang to reduce fluids: **raw rehmannia root,** 12 (parts), **red peony root** 9, **dang gui** 12, **achyranthes root** (huan niu xi or *A. bidentata)* 15, **poria mushroom** 12, **grifola mushroom** (zhu ling or *G. umbellata)* 12, **water plantain rhizome** 12, **cinnamon twig** 6. The dose would translate into about 9–12 grams per day of concentrated 4:1 granulated Chinese herbs.

Using complex formulations of herbs based upon signs and symptoms, including a **triphala-**based tonic formula from Nepal (called **trifola**), we have worked with Dr. Abel's group to successfully reduce eye pressures and preserve visual field in numerous patients since 1998, including patients sensitive to steroid eyedrops.

Lifestyle and other adjunct treatment options that may aid in the management or prevention of glaucoma include:

- Good nutrition, especially reduced consumption of alcohol and caffeine and increased intake of foods high in vitamin C such as bell peppers, broccoli, citrus fruit, brussels sprouts, guava, kale, parsley, and strawberries.

- The elimination of artificial sweetners.

- Daily exercise for 30 to 40 minutes

- Smoking cessation. Reduction of caffeine.

- Deep breathing exercises to reduce stress

- Increased intake of spring water, up to 6 glasses per day

- Bowel regulation if the patient is constipated (both Eclectic and Ayurvedic physicians reported this)

- Massage of the eyeball, which appears to have a beneficial influence in some cases

- Acupuncture for eye pressure headaches

Macular Degeneration

Age-related macular degeneration (AMD) is the leading cause of blindness in Americans over the age of 65. The disease results from damage to the center part of the light-sensitive retina, the place where light rays come to a focus in the eye. This yellow-colored center is called the "macula" or "macula lutea." Here our most detailed vision occurs. It is an extremely metabolically active area. The cone cells are packed tightly together in the macula, and each cone cell has a nerve fiber that communicates with the visual areas of the brain. Destruction of the macula imperils central vision, and once it has deteriorated sufficiently, there is no known treatment that can restore vision.

There are two forms of macular degeneration. The common "dry" form occurs in 90% of cases. It develops slowly, and while it does not cause complete blindness, patients experience a significant loss of vision.

About 10% of patients develop the "wet" form of macular degeneration. Blood vessels under the retina begin to grow offshoots that exude and bleed into the retina, causing scarring and blockage. These new blood vessel offshoots are abnormal, and they easily become leaky. The resultant blinding can be rapid and severe. Only regular eye examinations can detect these problems before there is vision loss.

To understand cause and treatment, it is important to know that the macula has a very high concentration of yellow pigments, derived primarily from two carotenoids, lutein and zeaxanthin. This pigment layer under the retina, the RPE or retinal pigment epithelium, nourishes the macula and removes waste from the photoreceptor cells (the cones). Lack of proper nutrition can thus hasten macular destruction. Good oxygen supply has a preventive effect by stimulating RPE cells, but poor blood flow diminishes this effect.

Important causative factors of macular degeneration include:

- Free radical damage that occurs when and ultraviolet and blue light from the sun passes through the eye lens. Smoking, poor nutrition, and weakened immunity all increase free radical activity.

- Deficient supply of nutrients including lutein, zeaxanthin, zinc, taurine, B vitamins, and essential fatty acids. This can be attributed to either insufficient intake or poor digestion. Multiple studies indicate the protective effect of spinach and lutein. Zeaxanthin can be made from lutein.

- Oxidized fatty waste products have also been implicated as causal factors. Tiny waste products called drusen accumulate in and behind the retina and may stimulate macrophages to produce damaging inflammation. Moreover, a large epidemiological study (Beaver Dam Eye Study and Nutritional Factors in Eye Disease Study) showed that a high intake of saturated fat and cholesterol was associated with increased risk for early age-related macular disease.

- Oxygen or nutrient starvation, which triggers chemical signals that initiate abnormal blood vessel growth. Examinations show that elderly patients often have less than two-thirds the blood flow to the back of the eye that occurs in younger people.

Natural medicine treatment centers on improving both blood flow and macular nutrition. Patients should examine digestion and general health and should take an eye vitamin rich in basic nutrients, as well as a tonic herbal supplement of sufficient potency. Important herbs include **tien chi root** (high doses in wet form), **dang gui root, triphala, salvia root, blueberry, bilberry, hawthorn, lycium fruit, ginkgo leaf, tortoise shell, American ginseng root, cooked** and **raw rehmannia, ginseng root, wild asparagus root, shilajatu,** and **elderberry.**

Dry Eye Syndrome

Many people experience inadequate tear supply or eye discomfort sometime in their lives, perhaps on an airplane, in a dry, overheated room or in a dusty workplace. But upwards of 10 million Americans suffer from a significant dry eye condition that may be related to other symptoms.

The classic "Sjögren's-associated" dry eye affects up to 2% of the population and presents with a characteristic triad of symptoms—dry eye, dry mouth, and arthritis. Other causes of dry eyes include medication, dehydration, inflammation of the eyelids or skin, previous eye surgery, systemic diseases such as rheumatoid arthritis, thyroid disease, lupus, sarcoidosis, and even poor blinking habits (such as staring at a computer). Your doctor can tell you if you are suffering from Sjögren's syndrome or other specific diseases.

Tears are not just made up of water. They have three separate components:

1. Oil (from the Meibomian oil glands in the eyelids)

2. Mucous secretions (from the goblet cells deep inside the eyelid)

3. Watery tears (the "aqueous" tears from the lachrymal gland and accessory lachrymal glands located in the conjunctiva of the eyelids)

The innermost layer of tears in direct contact with the eye is the mucous layer, which is also called "mucin." The mucin coats the surface of the cornea. The watery tears comprise the middle layer, sticking to the mucin and keeping the eye moist. The outer tear layer is composed of oil from the Meibomian glands; it is deposited like an oil slick on the outside of the watery tears to slow their evaporation from the surface of the eye. Every time you blink you sweep the tears across the cornea and into the drainage ducts, called "puncta."

Symptoms of dry eye syndrome include irritation, burning, redness, mucus accumulations, itching, light sensitivity, and even tearing. In fact, when cells fall off the cornea it can be downright painful. Mild eye muscle problems or inadequate reading glasses may make the symptoms worse. A routine eye examination can exclude other causes of irritation such as conjunctivitis, faulty glasses, or contact lens trouble.

Caffery notes: "The effect of diet on tear function is illustrated clearly by malnutrition-induced xerophthalmia. Dietary habits in well-nourished North American society have been implicated as a cause of some tear dysfunction. A review of the ocular literature suggests that sufficient dietary protein, vitamins A, B$_6$, and C, potassium, zinc and taurine may be necessary for normal tear function. Excesses of dietary fats, salt, cholesterol, alcohol, protein, and sucrose have been associated with or suggested as causes of tear dysfunction." The essential fatty acid gamma-linolenic acid (GLA) has been shown beneficial in Sjögren's-associated dry eye.

Standard allopathic treatment consists of wetting drops and plugging therapy. This is valuable but ultimately is symptomatic and does not address the deeper issues. Natural medicine therapy is directed at reducing inflammation, improving your environment, evaluating your drugs and diet, and using herbs and nutrients that directly or indirectly nourish and moisten. As you read the following suggestions, remember the three components of tears, and that:

- Vitamin A and carotenoids aid epithelial tissue and goblet cells in production of mucin.

- The watery component of tears requires that you drink lots of water.

- The oily component of tears is dependent upon adequate essential fatty acids.

- Treating *all* of the above three represents holistic nourishment therapy, but removal of causes is equally important.

Recommendations

Use artificial tears. These are available in nonpreserved (sometimes expensive and inconvenient), minimally preserved, or fully preserved varieties. There are some new types of artificial tears that offer patients more options. Ointments at bedtime are often helpful in reducing morning symptoms. Refer to the "Dry Eye" chapter in *The Eye Care Revolution* for more details.

Try punctal plugs. These reduce tear loss. Every time you blink, tears exit through the little holes (puncta) in the inner corner of your eyelids. If the exit route is plugged, the tears you make or supply with eyedrops will remain in place longer. Several companies make removable plugs that can be tried for either short or long periods.

Modify your environment. Is your home, bedroom, or workplace too dry? Is there sufficient humidity? If you suffer from dry eye symptoms especially in the winter, place a humidifier in your bedroom, or put a pie pan with some water in it over the heating ducts. Houseplants can also help regulate humidity.

Remember to blink. Many of us stare at computers and get lost in our work and simply forget to blink. Other people have weak lower lids, which do not contribute the necessary 20% involved in completing a blink. You or your eye doctor may notice that the lower lid doesn't move with a routine blink. Fortunately, with a forced or voluntary blink, you can close the eye. Inadequate eye closure while sleeping may also contribute to dry eye symptoms.

Take a look at your current medications. Common drugs for intestinal problems, depression, allergy, and colds may dehydrate sensitive tissues in your body. If they are necessary, you may have to compensate for this dehydration by drinking more water. Ask your pharmacist or doctor if any of your current medications may cause dry eye.

Take a break from your computer. Look away and every 20 minutes exercise your eyes.

Evaluate your diet. Drink at least 6 glasses of water per day, and limit sodas, caffeine, and alcohol. Include fish, soy and other legumes, and seeds in your diet. These provide essential fatty acids to protect cells and stabilize the tear film. Omega-3 and -6 fatty acids from plant sources (such as **flaxseed, evening primrose,** or **borage oils**) or from cold-water fish (such as salmon, mackerel, sardines, halibut, and cod) are loaded with these good fats. A good supplement is a gelcap containing about 200–500 mg of DHA (docosahexaenoic acid), and perhaps an additional 500-mg gelcap of **evening primrose oil.** Take one gelcap of each twice daily with meals. Double or triple the dose if your have significant inflammation.

Two thousand years ago TAM (Traditional Ayurvedic Medicine) doctors made a wash of **licorice root, turmeric root, haritaki fruit** *(Terminalia chebula),* and **Himalayan cedarwood** *(Cedrus deodara)* ground with goat's milk to treat dry eyes. For children, the treatment was mother's milk applied as drops in the eyes.

You can sometimes get moisture into the eyes simply by squeezing the eyelid with your fingers to milk out fluids. Another simple method is the eyedrops made by rubbing the fingers in water, mentioned above.

Vitamin A eyedrops or vitamin A + E liposomal spray can be of important use. (See Resource Guide.) Alan may suggest a few drops of an herbal ophthalmic solution called **rue-fennel tincture,** made by Herb Pharm. **Rue-fennel tincture** is also good for conjunctivitis (see below). By the way, the correct way to use eyedrops is not to pull the bottom lid open looking in the mirror. Lie down on your back and place the dispenser near the inner depression of each eye (closest to the nose), being careful not to touch the skin or eye. Let one or two drops fall in, and then blink several times to spread the solution over the ocular surface.

Complex Treatments

Complete treatment of dry eyes at our clinic almost always involves systemic herbal medicine formulas. Some patients, especially those over the age of 60, need digestive aids to ensure proper absorption of nutrients. Beneficial herbs from the digestive group like **bromelain, white atractylodes,** and **ginseng root** can be of help. Dry eyes are often associated with menopause and Reynaud's syndrome. The same herbs and supplements we use to treat osteoarthritis appear to help strengthen membranes such as the conjunctiva, as well as the mouth, nose and ears (refer to Chapter 17 for details). In addition to EFAs, we often use glucosamine sulfate 750 mg twice per day in our clinic to treat dry eyes.

We then make a tonic formula of blood- and/or Yin-nourishing herbs that moisten, choosing from herbs like **alfalfa root, American ginseng root, cooked rehmannia root, dang gui root, shou wu root, shilajatu, white peony root, lycium fruit, wild asparagus root,** and **triphala.** I recommend about 2 grams twice per day of the concentrated extracts for long-term use. If successful, there will be a gradual improvement in general health over several months time and a slow return of moisture to the eyes. See Resource Section to order from Chrysalis pharmacy.

Pink Eye

Conjunctivitis, caused by the common adenovirus, is a common plague of the schoolyard and office. It is also known as "pinkeye." Some varieties of this highly contagious virus can be transmitted by infected pools of water and are usually short-lived (3 to 4 days). However, other strains occur often in wintertime and spread because people are clustered together. This can actually set off epidemics.

Children are more likely to develop an associated cold from the virus than are adults. The eye can become red (from pink to blood red), with swollen lids, tearing, and discharge. In some cases, the other eye will become involved shortly after the first. Rubbing increases the chance of spreading the virus to the second eye and to family and friends.

Dr. Abel published an article in the *Annals of Ophthalmology* about using iodine as a treatment for conjunctivitis. Subsequently, Dr. Thomas Neuhann, a German ophthalmologist, informed Dr. Abel that he had been using this treatment since experimenting on himself in the 1980s. As it turns out, a Czechoslovakian researcher who used more frequent doses in treating an epidemic in his town has published a paper as well. Dr. Abel's "new" treatment will soon be available to ophthalmologists in a single-dose pack.

If the eyes are stuck together upon waking or you have a small, tender lump in front of your ear (the site of a related lymph node), it's probably pinkeye.

Doctors used to just treat this condition with antibiotic eyedrops, which, however, have no effect on virus multiplication. Occasionally, eye doctors will treat with a steroid eyedrop, which will help quiet the eye (reduce the swelling) two-thirds of the time, but also may inhibit your white blood cell defenses. In some patients, this treatment can actually prolong the condition.

Good hygiene is always important and is an effective way to avoid this infection. Avoid rubbing your eyes after touching other areas of your body (e.g., nose) or foreign objects (e.g., currency). Wash your hands frequently. Use paper towels and tissues instead of cloth towels and handkerchiefs, and avoid using eye makeup or wearing contact lenses until the infection has healed. If a person with pinkeye uses cloth towels, keep the towels in an area where no one else will use them, and wash all linens in hot water.

One hundred fifty years ago, an Ohio doctor used iodine as a matter of course to treat eye infections. For some reason, this effective treatment got lost along the way, as do many simple and effective herbal treatments.

Dr. Abel has rediscovered this treatment for conjunctivitis. A 5% povidone iodine solution, commonly used to prepare all patients for eye surgery, is an inexpensive, simple, and rapidly effective cure for viral eye infections. You can either swab it on the inside of the eyelids or use it as a drop. This treatment will resolve the infection completely for many people within 24 hours. This is the treatment of choice if it is available. Always treat both eyes to prevent spread of the infection.

For home treatment, the alkaloid berberine has well-documented antibacterial effects. It is used in Germany as a treatment for hypersensitive eyes, inflamed lids, and chronic and allergic conjunctivitis. TAM doctors make eyedrops by dissolving a condensed paste extract of **darvi** *(Berberis asiatica,* which contains berberine) in water. Native Americans and Eclectic physicians used **goldenseal root** *(Hydrastis canadensis),* which also contains appreciable levels of berberine, for the same reason.

Preparations of either of these plants can be used to wash the eyes every few hours in acute cases, and every fifth day or once a week to clean the eyes, help keep the tear ducts open, and prevent infection. They can also prevent and cure chronic conjunctivitis, but it takes a few days. Be sure to filter herbal eye solutions made from teas carefully before use with a coffee filter to remove any particulate matter. Use an eyecup, and wash with this mixture (approximately 1 or 2 minutes for each eye) several times per day.

> **Blast from the Past**
>
> In the 11th century A.D., Dr. Chakrapani administered a treatment for trachoma, viral follicular conjunctivitis, and swelling of the eyelids. "Take the powders of mineral salt, *Piper longum, Saussurea lappa, Uraria lagopoides,* and *Desmodium gangeticum,* and boil in a decoction of **triphala.** This medicament is made into tablets which are used to make eyedrops freshly prepared and placed in the eye each day."

Felter noted that the addition of boric acid to **goldenseal root** extract added greatly to its antibiotic and anti-inflammatory action. At our clinic, I use a sterile commercial eyewash compound for conjunctivitis called **rue-fennel compound** (made by Herb Pharm) which contains boric acid, **goldenseal,** and some other mildly astringent herbs. I sometimes combine it with **Viva-drops** (from Vision Pharmaceuticals), which contain vitamin A. Five to 10 drops of **rue-fennel compound** carefully added to 1 ounce of **Viva-drops** makes an eyedrop which is very effective and easy to use.

Remember, however, that if conjunctivitis worsens, you should see a doctor immediately, because it can infect the cornea and cause clouding.

Chronic or Recurring Conjunctivitis

If conjunctivitis is chronic or frequently recurring, internal treatments may be indicated. TCM doctors usually divide these into four basic categories, based upon signs and symptoms, and treat with formulas for several months. This level of differentiation usually requires a professional TCM doctor.

Start with a base formula of **celosia seed** (qing xiang zi or *C. argentea),* **chrysanthemum flower,** and **buddleia flower** (me meng hua or *B. officinalis).* This should comprise about 35–50% of your formula. Then add additional herbs as follows:

- **Heat related.** Add **dandelion root, forsythia fruit** (lian qiao or *F. suspensa),* **honeysuckle flower** (jin yin hua or *Lonicera japonica),* **scute root, cassia seed** (jue ming zi or *Cassia tora),* and **siler root** (fang feng or *Ledebouriella* species). During an acute episode the same formula can be used to speed results by simply adding **isatis root.**

- **Heat and damp.** Add **scute root, gentian root** (long dan cao or *G. scabra),* **plantago seed** (che quian zi or *P. ovata),* **coptis rhizome** (huang lian or *C. chinensis),* **poria mushroom,** and **phellodendron root.**

- **Wind and heat.** Add **schizonepeta herb** and **flower** (jing jie or *S. tenuifolia),* **siler root, honeysuckle flower, bupleurum root,** and **mentha** (bo he or *M. haplocalyx).*

- **Dryness from deficiency.** Add **raw rehmannia root, glehnia root** (sha shen or *Adenophora tetraphylla),* **scrophularia root** (xuan shen or *S. ningpoensis),* **ophiopogon root** (mai men dong or *O. japonicus),* **white peony root, wild asparagus root,** and **lycium fruit** (gou qi zi or *L. chinense).*

Chronic Eye Inflammation (Uveitis)

Any inflammation inside the eye is called "uveitis." Depending on where the inflammation predominates, it is termed "iritis" (iris), "pars planitis" (ciliary body), or "choroiditis" (choroid). Because these areas are linked together and fed by the same vessels, they can be treated as a group. Patients often report seeing floaters and complain of blurred vision as well as light sensitivity and redness, usually in only one eye. The eye doctor sees redness just outside the cornea and detects cells floating in the anterior chamber. These are either white cells (inflammatory cells) that have leaked out of blood vessels or pigment from the iris.

The most frequent known cause is trauma to the eye, including surgical trauma. Other causes include connective tissue disorders (CTDs), such as lupus and rheumatoid arthritis, and sarcoidosis. Uveitis can also occur as a complication of AIDS. Many uveitis patients also complain of dry eyes. As in CTDs, conventional use of steroids is important during flare-ups to prevent vision loss. For a review of the basic CTD treatment protocols, refer to our discussion in Chapter 15.

Ophthalmologists are seeing more and more cases of uveitis with no apparent origin, which currently is stumping Western physicians. This is why Dr. Abel moved into the fields of nutritional biochemistry and herbal medicine. He and I feel strongly that there are answers to be found. For one thing, we have both found that there are almost always systemic problems associated with uveitis and iritis. We look for signs and symptoms—especially dry skin, digestive disturbance, nervousness, constipation, coated tongue, fatigue—and treat accordingly. Using these strategies we have put many patients into prolonged remissions.

A basic formula for chronic uveitis consists of two parts, which should be 70–80% of the formula:

1. For reducing the inflammation choose from **chrysanthemum flower, turmeric root, buddleia flower, gentian root, elderberry, cclipta, dandelion root, conch shell,** and **triphala.**

2. There is always some blood congestion in chronic uveitis. For this, use **tien chi root** (high doses), **red peony root, bromelain, salvia root** (high doses), **persica seed** (tao ren or *Prunus persica),* and other herbs from the **blood-moving group.**

Modifications

- If there are signs of Yin deficiency or weakness, add **tortoise shell, cooked** and **raw rehmannia, wild asparagus root,** and **dang gui.**

- If there is an excess of sticky mucus exudation, add **pinellia tuber** and **tangerine peel.**

- If there is edema and swelling around the eye socket and eyelid, add **poria mushroom, coix** (yi yi ren or *Coix lachryma),* and **honeysuckle flower.**

- If the inflammation is severe, add **coptis rhizome, boswellia gum, scute root, forsythia fruit** (lian qiao or *F. suspensa),* and **gardenia fruit** (zhi zi or *G. jasminoides).*

Adjunct Therapies

- **Beneficial oils** found in fish (EPA and DHA) reduce inflammation. This can be duplicated in the diet by eating fish—3 or 4 servings per week of mackerel, salmon, tuna (especially albacore), cod, or halibut. To help assimilate the oils, make sure you take at least 100 IU of vitamin E each day.

- **Blueberries** (and **bilberries**) contain anti-inflammatory plant pigments that are good for the eye. Eat about ½ cup of blueberries per day on average, or about 1 bag of frozen blueberries per week. You can use other berries as well, but 75% should be blueberries. These can be fresh, cooked, or frozen, as the pigments are relatively heat and cold resistant. Freezing actually makes them somewhat more bioavailable.

- Use one of the eye vitamins found in health food stores to provide antioxidant support. Typically these contain antioxidant vitamins A, C, and E, as well as riboflavin, zinc, lutein, selenium, rutin, **bilberry extract,** and NAC (N-acetyl-cysteine).

Research Highlights

- The book *Chinese Medicine Secret Recipes* reported on a clinical trial at one of the TCM hospitals in Shangha that claimed a success rate greater than 99% using the following formula for uveitis: **tien chi root** 100 grams, **dang gui root** 15, **red peony root** 12, **cnidium rhizome** (chuan xiong or *Ligusticum wallichii)* 10, **persica seed** 6, **carthamus flower** 8, **salvia root** 20, **conch shell** 30, and **tortoise shell** 15 (Hu et al., 1991). The equivalent dose to that used in the study, if you use commercially available dried decoction powders, would be about 9–12 grams per day.

- In a study of 32 patients with chronic eye inflammation (anterior chamber uveitis), a 375-mg dose of curcumin (**turmeric root** extract) three times per day for 3 months showed improvement comparable to the effects seen with a similar cortisone dose (Lal et al., 1999).

- Vitamin E has been shown beneficial to prevent trauma-initiated uveitis in animal models. Because trauma often initiates uveitis, it makes good preventative sense to use this antioxidant vitamin to protect yourself in case of accidental eye injury. (Pararajasegaram et al., 1991).

- A controlled animal trial showed marked reduction in uveal and retinal inflammation and swelling in experimentally induced uveitis by interperitoneal injection with quercetin (Romero et al., 1989). Quercetin is available in pill form.

Optic Neuritis and Optic Atrophy

"Optic neuritis" is an acute or chronic inflammation of the optic nerve. Often a nerve demyelination (destruction of the protective myelin sheath around the nerve fibers) takes place, similar to multiple sclerosis. Multiple sclerosis, diabetes, poor circulation, trauma, chemical poisoning, and other less common eye insults can cause it. There is often a sudden loss of visual acuity and pain with movement of the eye. The eye doctor can diagnose optic neuritis by examining the back of the eye. There is venous engorgement around the optic nerve head and arterial contraction. There are often small hemorrhages near the swollen optic nerve.

Optic neuropathy is often the first sign of multiple sclerosis (MS). Two follow-up studies showed a greater than 40% development of MS after 8 years. There is also a strong nutritional correlation. An epidemic of neuropathy broke out in Cuba in 1991, and an analysis showed that those affected had a broad range of specific dietary deficiencies, including a sugar intake exceeding 15% of total caloric intake, alcohol consumption and low intake of protein, fats, and micronutrients especially B vitamins.

As far back as 1976, it was noted that "an enriched feed, specially prepared to affect reproduction of mice, significantly suppressed the onset of disease in subacute myelo-optico-neuropathy virus-infected mice, whereas low-calorie feed enhanced the incidence of disease." One researcher noted that "since sunlight influences the metabolism of fatty acids in the retina, it may also influence the development of retrobulbar optic neuritis—a common antecedent of multiple sclerosis."

Ocular toxicity has resulted from many prescription medicines, including isoniazid, thioridazine, steroids, and amiodarone therapy. Therefore, it can safely be assumed that a good diet with nutrient enrichment, attention to digestion of fats, and avoidance of toxins will be protective.

The goal of herbal therapy at the time of onset is to quickly remove blood congestion and restore arterial circulation. Immediately give 2 grams of concentrated **tien chi root** three times per day for up to a week, then reduce the dosage to twice a day for several months. This can be done in conjunction with standard Western use of steroid therapies to reduce swelling. In addition, I use high doses of antioxidants, DHA (an important end-stage fatty acid), lipoic acid, and blood-moving herbs that cool, such as **salvia root** and **red peony root.**

In one case Dr. Abel referred a patient from Philadelphia who had lost vision in one eye down to 20/400, and three ophthalmologists told him that there would be no return of vision. Although I did not see him until 6 weeks afterwards, we were able to restore vision to 20/80 in a month or so. I think that ideally patients should be given this herbal therapy within 1 week of onset. Another patient returned from count fingers vision to 20/20.

When prevention and emergency treatment fail, there is a role for long-term herbal treatment. Although it is widely believed that neurological regeneration is not possible, this is changing, and there are some encouraging signs in the research field. The goal of long-term herbal therapy is to reduce residual optic nerve inflammation, improve microcirculation, nourish the optic nerve, and stimulate nerve repair as much as possible. This strategy is also useful for optic neuropathy. Optic atrophy and optic neuritis share many characteristics, but with atrophy the shrinkage of the arteries and resulting pallor are more pronounced. Although progress is very, very slow, I have seen some mild to moderate improvements in vision. We use a complex protocol similar to the one described in the section on multiple sclerosis. Important herbs in addition to the ones mentioned include **ginkgo leaf** and **bala.**

I remember one very interesting case in which a Southern lady had completely lost both vision and sense of smell for close to a decade. After about 6 months on the protocol, she began to report flashes of light. Such subjective observations are difficult to assess and often are attributed to wishful thinking. However, one day she suddenly regained the ability to smell vanilla, and a few months later coffee. Although there was no further improvement over the next 6 months, I think that we may have a partial answer.

If MS is diagnosed, use Myelin Sheath Support (see Resource Guide).

Diabetic Retinopathy

Almost half of the estimated 16 million people in the United States who have diabetes will develop some degree of diabetic retinopathy, by far the most common form of diabetic eye disease. The retina weakens and bleeds, endangering vision. Good blood sugar control and blood pressure management, as well as yearly examinations and treatment, are the best methods of preventing eye complications due to diabetes. This is discussed in detail in Chapter 14. However, even with good control, I have seen patients develop retinopathy after having diabetes for more than 20 or 30 years. I believe this is preventable with herbal supplementation.

Ophthalmologists have a special advantage in identifying and treating retinopathy because they can directly see the blood vessels and the tiny capillaries in the eye. Therefore every diabetic needs an annual dilated eye exam. Eye doctors know that these oxygen-sensitive blood vessels can become abnormal and exhibit ballooning (microaneurism), fat leakage (exudate), and blood leakage (hemorrhage). Scattered capillary leakage throughout the eye causes a condition known as background diabetic retinopathy, while leakage in the central retina causes macular edema. Oxygen starvation can also cause a third and more severe form of the disease called proliferative diabetic retinopathy, in which new blood vessels grow uncontrollably on the surface of the retina and may even bleed into the eye (vitreous hemorrhage).

To quickly stop retinal bleeding, I recommend **tien chi root,** 1,500 mg twice per day. Continue this essential herb long term (up to several years) to prevent further bleeding episodes. **Yunnan Paiyao capsules,** commonly found in Chinese grocery stores, can also be used. After 2 weeks, add herbs to improve blood flow to the eye from the **blood-moving group** (see page 253), taking about 2 grams of concentrated powders per day. I use the **tien chi root** by itself for 2 weeks because its antihemorrhagic action ensures that the mild blood-thinning actions of the blood-moving herbs do not affect the delicate recently hemorrhaged vessels. If **tien chi root** or **Yunnan Paiyao capsules** are not available, you can substitute **bilberry extracts** containing about 180 mg anthocyanosides per day.

To improve general blood vessel health once you have had retinopathy, I recommend continued regular use of herbs from the **vessel-protective group** forever. **Bilberry** and **blueberries** are especially important, and I recommend using ½ cup per day, or approximately 1 bag of frozen blueberries (available year-round) per week. Use organic **blueberries** if you can get them; also Quercetin, 1500 mg daily.

Research Highlights

- A clinical study on 48 eyes was done to measure the ability of the Ayurvedic preparation called **saptamrita lauha** in absorption of retinal hemorrhages. Rapid absorption of hemorrhage was observed in both diabetic and hypersensitive subjects. Mean duration for absorption was about 17 days, with complete clearance in 3 eyes, and partial clearance in the rest. Follow-up studies showed a 25% recurrence in treated eyes, compared to greater than 50% recurrence in control eyes (Sharma et al., 1992).

- Making this medicine requires a starting drug called **lauha** (iron) **bhasma,** considered to be a powerful astringent tonic. One method of making **lauha bhasma** is to soak iron for 7 days in **pomegranate juice,** then roast it seven successive times to create a purified iron oxide powder. You can then make **saptamrita lauha** by mixing two parts of **lauha bhasma** with one part each of **licorice root, haritaki fruit, vibhitaki fruit, amla fruit,** ghee, and honey. The standard dose is 250 mg twice a day (Namjoshi, 1978; Nadkarni, 1954).

- Bensky and Gamble report that two cases of retinal hemorrhage were treated with decoction of **forsythia fruit** (lian qiao or *Forsythia suspensa).* At 4 weeks there was good resorption of leakage and some visual acuity improvement (reported in Bensky and Gamble, 1993).

Retinitis Pigmentosa

Retinitis pigmentosa (RP) is a slow, progressive deterioration of the retina that results in diminished vision as it progresses. It is often hereditary. The rods that govern peripheral vision are first affected, and peripheral vision gradually deteriorates as time passes and the condition worsens. Night vision also worsens. The pigment degenerates in a way that can be seen by ophthalmologists, until gradually the optic nerve disc changes appearance, and finally central vision is affected. Cataracts may also develop.

Another contributing factor seems to be excessive production of cortisol in response to extreme stress. Immunologist Alfred Sapse, M.D., announced in March 1988 that not only does elevated cortisol contribute to this disease, but treating people with anticortisol drugs improves the condition. Dr Sapse believes that there are two separate components to this disease, one hereditary and the other autoimmune, related to stress and cortisol levels. He also points out that failure to notice connections between cortisol and chronic disease is due to the fact that cortisol levels often swing dramatically due to 24-hour (circadian) rhythms.

Research seems to indicate that patients with this disease have numerous nutritional and metabolic abnormalities. Microscopic examination shows major problems in (1) the daily renewal and shedding of the photoreceptor outer segments, (2) light energy transmission, and (3) vitamin A metabolism.

There is also the presence of deposits in the retinal pigment epithelium. Though not deficient in the amino acid taurine, RP patients appear to have faulty cellular uptake of it. Both the red blood cells and the sperm of RP patients are deficient in the important fatty acid DHA. The cause of this is the inability to biosynthesize DHA even if dietary levels are adequate, so it must be given directly. The problems with DHA and vitamin A metabolism no doubt extend to several other nutrients. The cellular antioxidant methionine is a major source of both taurine and cysteine and can be supplied directly by taking **wheat sprouts.** Large doses of vitamin A (up to 30,000 IU per day) and lutein 20 mg daily can help hereditary retinitis pigmentosa.

Given this backdrop, there are three ways to deal with this: directly add the needed nutrients, add precursors to drive cellular uptake, and stimulate general metabolic energy through a variety of mechanisms. I hypothesize that all three need to be done simultaneously to maximally overcome the metabolic barriers, and with the third component herbal medicine has much to offer.

To summarize, elevated stress levels weaken general energy and, combined with genetic metabolic weakness, cause a gradual atrophy of the retina. From a TCM perspective this is definitely a deficiency condition (Yin, Yang, Essence, Liver blood, etc.). There is also blood congestion. Therefore, in addition to the specific nutrients mentioned, we would want to write a formula that calms stress, strengthens the Qi, nourishes the blood, Yin, and Essence, and strongly breaks down blood congestion to get fresh blood into the atrophied tissue. We also want to repair tissue as much as possible. This requires a complex formulation, choosing herbs from each of the following groups:

- To strengthen the Qi, use **white atractylodes, astragalus root, huang jing rhizome** *(Polygonatum sibiricum),* and **ginseng root**.

- To break down blood congestion, choose from **persica seed** (tao ren or *Prunus persica),* **salvia root, red peony root, tien chi root, ginkgo leaf, prickly ash bark,** and **zedoary root** (e zhu or *Curcuma zedoaria).*

- To nourish the tissue, choose from **dang gui root, shou wu root, elderberry, triphala** or **amla fruit, blueberry** or **bilberry, white peony root, eclipta, lycium fruit, cuscuta seed** (tu si zi or *C. chinensis),* **wheat sprouts,** and **gotu kola.**

Variations

If there is more Yin deficiency, add **cooked** and **raw rehmannia root.** If there is more Yang deficiency, add **deer antler** or **astragalus seed** (sha yuan ji li or *A. complanatus).* If there are signs of tension or Liver Qi restriction, add **bupleurum root** and **ashwagandha root.**

Nutrients

Taurine, CoQ_{10}, Vitamins A and D, lutein, L-carnitine, DHA, vitamin E.

Research Highlights

- 54 patients (106 eyes) with hereditary RP were treated for 3 months with TCM herbal therapies. Computer-averaged oscillatory potentials (OPs) of electroretinograms (ERG) were recorded to measure changes in the physiological functioning of the retina. The results showed that cone activity could be moderately improved even in advanced patients, while rod potentials could be improved only in patients with less-advanced retinal degeneration (Wu, 1995).

- A follow-up study confirmed earlier results and found that "TCM treatment could also enhance the bioactivity of nerve network and therefore have a definite significance in retarding the progression of disease and keeping the central vision." (Wu and Tang, 1996).

Refraction Problems: Near- and Farsightedness

Myopia or nearsightedness is defined as seeing better at close ranges than at a distance. This is because the eye is longer than normal, or the cornea is more curved than normal. This causes light coming from distant images to focus in front of the retina instead of on it.

Hyperopia, or farsightedness, is when vision is better at a distance than close up. Farsighted individuals have a short eye or a flatter cornea that doesn't bend light enough, so the image focuses behind the retina. Glasses, contact lenses, and now refractive surgery can correct these problems. However, there still may be a role for natural medicine. Review the "gazing at the moon" exercise mentioned earlier in this chapter, then consider this information:

- Even simple changes like taking frequent breaks while doing close work can reduce eyestrain and stop your vision from changing.

- In 1996, H. S. Seung, M.D., published his finding in the *Proceedings of the National Academy of Sciences* that the brain is able to hold the eye in one position because it stores a memory of the eye position in the visual cortex.

- A clinical trial of adults in good health, aged 62 to 75 years, showed they could be trained to read more efficiently after training that consisted of rapid visual processing, oculomotor, and guided reading training.

- A double-blind controlled clinical trial done in India using an Ayurvedic eyedrop was shown in early myopic patients to correct refractive errors while in advanced myopic conditions it slowed the progressive deteriorations.

- An examination was done of the nutritional status of 24 children who developed myopia between the ages of 7 and 10 years as compared to the status of 68 subjects who were not myopic at the age of 10 years. Researchers reported that "children who developed myopia had a generally lower intake of many of the food components than children who did not become myopic. The differences were statistically significant for energy intake, protein, fat, vitamins B_1, B_2 and C, phosphorus, iron, and cholesterol."

- High levels of myopia among Chinese students are now being addressed through herbal treatment, acupuncture-point eyeball massage, improved architectural design of school buildings, and (most happily for the kids) lessening of homework assignments.

- A study done in Russia using infrasound pneumomassage for 10 days stabilized the course of progressive myopia, shown by examinations done 3 years after the treatments.

- Height, weight, and vision of 3,884 students were measured in China, revealing that vision and weight were positively interrelated whereas there was no correlation found between vision and height. Researchers pointed out that poor nutrition and poor food choices can explain the correlation between vision and weight.

- Animal studies have revealed that "the quality of the retinal image may be an important regulator of the matching of refractive state to growth of the ocular globe." In other words, as you grow your eyeball also grows and must maintain a precise relationship between size and focus. In young, rapidly growing birds, fitting them with optical devices that degraded the quality of their retinal images interfered with the normal eye growth and resulting in severe myopia. Researchers have also found correlations between eye growth and deficiencies in calcium, vitamin D, and ocular temperature. This lends credence to the idea that the "lights, sounds, and colors" of today's world may cause changes in eyeball growth.

- A series of Scandinavian studies of the biomechanics of the developing sclera were done on rabbits and humans. Initially, they gave injections to rabbits, which stabilized the connective tissue on the surface of the eyes, consequently stabilizing refractive errors. A controlled follow-up study done on 240 human eyes also showed improved stabilization. A third study was done on 612 children and adolescents with high myopia (a yearly progression of over 1.0 D) using a scleroplastic operation. The myopia "remained stable in 95.7% cases 1 year after the operation, and in 71.9%, 7 years after the operation." Researchers stated, "It can be concluded that non-surgical and surgical techniques of correcting the biomechanical properties of sclera for the treatment of progressive myopia as well as discriminative methods of determining the indications to these procedures have proven to be effective."

Taken collectively, these studies show that refractive errors are most probably the result of a complex interaction between environmental conditions (the images we see as we grow up), nutritional factors, and biomechanics. Dr. Abel and I are intensively investigating these factors in an attempt to determine methods that parents can implement to prevent their children from developing refractive errors.

Summary

Herbal and nutritional therapy have a clear role to play in the treatment of both common and unusual or difficult-to-treat ocular disorders, especially where Western medicine does not have causative understanding or effective treatments. The many studies showing the benefits of various nutrients and a few herbs for eye problems should be impetus to explore further the reports coming from China and India with regard to the benefits of their traditional eye herbs. Adopting a healthy lifestyle will reduce the three major stressors that negatively affect eye health: UV light, inadequate nutrition, and stress.

Keep in mind Dr. Abel's four pillars of eye health:

1. Wear sunglasses.

2. Eat and supplement well.

3. Make wise lifestyle choices.

4. Incorporate natural options into the preventive and therapeutic regimens.

Cataract Surgery 2,500 Years Ago*

To have a successful white cataract operation, wait until the lens is completely opacified. Otherwise relapse may occur. After the operation, problems such as brain injury, overexertion, overindulgence in sex, vomiting, or fainting can be the cause of relapsing cataract. Also, postoperative infection can occur.

Before operating, the condition of the cataract has to be checked very well. There are several contraindications. If the opacity of cataract has the shape of a half moon, or a water bubble, or a pearl, there should be no operation. The same is true if the cataract is not movable, or irregular, or thin at the center, or painful, or red.

The operating room must be neat and clean. Cataract operations are best done during the seasons with moderate temperature, and there should be minimal interference from wind or sun. Before the operation, the patient should imbibe a greasy meal and rest to ensure strength. When he arrives for surgery, a warm moist compress should be placed over

*Translated from ancient Ayurvedic text, including Suruta Samhita, by Dr. Mana.

the eye as a preparation. The patient should then be placed in a sitting position. This is better because the patient has to lock their vision inwardly onto the nose to hold the eyes steady.

An instrument called Yavavakra is used for the operation. It is very important to handle the instrument in the proper way, requiring that the surgeon have full confidence. The eye has to be properly opened surgically. Remember that the piercing should be at the center of the conjunctiva, thus avoiding veins. The incision should start laterally and move medially. Piercing upward or downward or in the opposite direction is prohibited.

While piercing, when the instrument enters toward the pupil, some water bubbles will come out making a sound. At that time, place drops of woman's breast milk into the eye to control the pain and irritation. A warm compress made of sedative herbs should be applied around the eyes.

After that, the white coating of the mucus of the lens has to be pushed or scratched out. Any part of it left inside the lens area has to be dislodged by having the patient blow hard with their nose closed. When the operation is completed, the eye becomes clear just like the sky without clouds, and the patient feels better with no pain. This is the sign of a properly done operation. He can see!

After removing the instrument, apply a medicinal ghee ointment over the operated area, and place a proper bandage. After that, the patient should have complete bed rest, lying on the back. During the recovery time, the patient should have no burping, coughing, shaking of the body, and so on. He should stay motionless in a disciplined way.

Then, every 3 days the bandage should be changed, and the eye washed out with a decoction of plants that control the irritation and pain (Vata). A new compress should be applied around the eye. This treatment should be continued for at least 10 days. After that, the patient can have normal activity, but still taking a light diet. It is not advised to operate on a patient if they are suffering from old age, asthma, bronchitis, pulmonary tuberculosis, or any other serious disease.

CHAPTER 17

The Lungs, Nose, Throat, Skin, and Ears

The phenomenon of Tao is elusive, but there is substance to it.
Vacant and dark, it yet contains a vital essence.
This vital essence is very real. It is verifiable.
From past to present its name has not been obliterated,
Because it is ever-present at the center of all things.

—Lao Tsu

The Respiratory System

The respiratory system consists of the lungs and the associated organs and tissues that surround them. The lungs themselves are tender and spongy, divided into five lobes. They rest on the diaphragm, the thick musclclikc organ that divides the upper chest from the lower digestive organs. Air travels from the mouth and nose into the pharynx and trachea, then down into the bronchial tubes into the lungs. TCM doctors believe that the lungs also absorb Qi (vital force) from the air. This Qi rides into the body on the air as wetness rides on water.

According to the Western point of view, the main actions of the lungs are exchange of oxygen and carbon dioxide and maintenance of systemic acid-base balance. Scientific investigations have confirmed the holistic theory that a weblike interconnectedness exists between all human body structures. With the lungs, it is clear that problems arising in many other tissues and organs directly affect lung growth, structure, and function. For example, the lungs can be affected by nutritional factors, obesity, blood factors, stress, and problems in the pancreas, liver, and kidneys. In the same way, anything that supports the lungs and proper breathing will benefit the rest of the body.

For example, a recent discovery that illustrates the medical importance of oxygen intake is that giving a patient extra oxygen during and after surgery reduces by half the occurrence of postsurgical infections. Therefore, in this section we will explore many different ways to support and strengthen the lungs.

Purify Your Home Air Environment

Since ancient times, the lungs have been recognized as tender organs, very susceptible to external influences like heat, dust, chemicals, particulate matter, and various other irritants. This is an important issue to approach in today's environment, as home air pollution is often 10 times as great as outdoor pollution. In this respect, our young children are like the canaries in the coal mine, revealing to us the cost of poor air quality. C. Arden Pope of Brigham Young University, who studies the economic costs and health effects of air pollution, reported findings that linked infant deaths to high air pollution, including a survey of 4 million infants reported by the U.S. Environmental Protection Agency. Infants living in cities with high levels of "particulate pollution" are 46% more likely to die of respiratory ailments and 26% more likely to die from sudden infant death syndrome (SIDS). Common pollutants include household molds, bacteria, dust, and tobacco.

Therefore, the first step in maintaining respiratory health is to keep your home air as healthy as possible. This is especially important for allergic conditions like asthma or sinusitis. I suggest the following:

- Purchase a HEPA air filter. These air filters are used in hospital operating rooms to filter out minute particles. They are now sold at department stores.

- Wash your bedsheets and pillowcases in *hot* water. This will kill dust mites, which can make allergies and asthma worse.

- Get a dehumidifier if your basement or home is damp. Dampness encourages mold, fungus and bacteria to grow. Kill fungus directly by spraying it with antifungal sprays available in the grocery or hardware store.

- Place some healthy houseplants in strategic places. Dr. Wolverton of NASA recommends devil's ivy *(Epipremum aureum),* the Boston fern *(Nephrolepis exalta),* and the lush and leafy dwarf date palm as plants to keep in the home to reduce air pollution and toxins, including fungal toxins.

- Purchase nontoxic household cleaning material. Go to a local health food store and see what they have to offer as replacements. Also avoid perfumes and other chemicals. Also avoid polyester and try to wear clothes with natural fibers.

- Get a new vacuum cleaner with a *good* filter on it so you are not inhaling atomized poisons when you clean.

- Thoroughly vacuum the whole house the first time, and then wash your pets three times per month thereafter with water and shampoo. This will reduce animal dander by 90%.

- Get an electrostatic air filter (sold by Sears and other companies) to eliminate household dust in addition to the HEPA filter mentioned above.

- Get an ozone generator if you really want to destroy poisons, including carpet chemicals and toxic gases. These little machines produce ozone, which breaks down fungi, toxins, and numerous small molecules. Contrary to some instructions, they should be run when no one is in the rooms being treated, to avoid irritating the lungs.

Strengthen the Lungs

To strengthen your lungs, practice breathing exercises such as those taught in Yoga and Qi Gong. These help with blood oxygenation, increase hydrochloric acid production, improve blood circulation, improve peristaltic movement, encourage lymph movement, slow the brain waves, and massage the lower abdominal organs. It is impossible to overstress the importance of improving blood oxygen levels and breath control as a component of vibrant health.

Here is a simple breathing exercise I teach my patients, a variation of the ones taught to me by Master Wang Yen-nien, former chairman of the World T'ai Chi Association. I give it to all my patients with lung problems:

Begin by lying on your back with knees elevated and feet on the ground. Place a paperback book on your navel. Learn to breathe diaphragmatically, through the nose, pushing down with the diaphragm on the inhale while relaxing the perineum muscle, the belly, and the kidneys. This will cause the book to rise as you inhale if you do it properly. Breathe out through the nose in the same way, pulling the diaphragm up, causing the same body parts to gently contract, causing the book to go back down.

Breathe as slowly and deeply as possible, but without tension or discomfort of any kind. The tongue should rest lightly on the roof of the mouth. Time yourself for 10 breaths. This is your basic rate, usually about 5–15 breaths per minute. Go as slowly as you comfortably can, but if you feel the need to breathe in faster the next time after a breath, it means you are going too slowly. No oxygen deprivation is allowed. Feel completely comfortable as you practice. Keep this practice up every day until you can breathe 20 breaths in 5 minutes (inout, in-out, in-out, in-out each minute), 4 breaths per minute. When you accomplish this, your oxygen capacity should be better upon testing.

Herbs for Treating Lung Conditions

Patricia A. Cassano of Cornell University reported that "The difference in lung function between people who consumed above-average amounts of four major antioxidants and those who consumed lower-than-average amounts "was approximately equivalent to the difference between nonsmokers and people who have smoked a pack [of cigarettes] a day for 10 years."

Therefore, take antioxidants and eat plenty of carotenoid-rich carrots, tomatoes, winter squash, apricots, red peppers, and so on. To deal with lung conditions, make a formula from one or more of these categories, based, of course, upon signs and symptoms.

When the lungs are too dry, there will be symptoms of dry mouth and tongue and perhaps dry cough. Construct a formula by choosing from lung-nourishing herbs that soothe, such as **wild cherry bark** *(Prunus* species), **raw rehmannia root, glehnia root** (sha shen or *Adenophora tetraphylla),* **ophiopogon root** (mai men dong or *O. japonicus),* **apricot seed** (xing ren or *Prunus armeniaca),* **licorice root, wild asparagus root, Irish moss** *(Chondrus crispus),* **slippery elm bark,** and **marshmallow root** *(Althaea officinalis).*

If the lungs are very weak, there will be symptoms of shortness of breath, fatigue, weakness, inability to inhale and exhale fully, and an increased susceptibility to upper respiratory infections. Here it is important to strengthen the lung energy with herbs from both the **blood-nourishing** and **immune groups.** Use herbs such as **astragalus root, cordyceps mushroom, schisandra berries, amla fruit, ginseng root,** and **American ginseng root.** The standard Ayurvedic tonic **chyavanaprasha** is also very useful.

For simple mild lung inflammation, use the herbs mentioned in Chapter 12. If there is hotter inflammation or infection in the lungs, there will be symptoms like fever, sore throat, red tongue with a yellow greasy coating, sticky sputum, and difficulty in breathing. Choose from herbs that reduce inflammation and/or fight infection like **scute root, turmeric root, boswellia gum, chrysanthemum flower, echinacea, tulsi, forsythia fruit, isatis root** or **leaves, vasaca leaves** *(Adhatoda vasica),* **oregano leaf, honeysuckle flower** (jin yin hua or *Lonicera japonica),* **morus bark** (sang bai pi or *M. alba),* and **coptis rhizome** (huang lian or *C. chinensis).*

If there is dampness and mucus in the lungs, there will be congestion, wheezing, a heavy sensation, cough, craving for hot drinks, and a thick greasy coating on the tongue. Herbs that reduce mucus in the lungs include **pinellia tuber, garlic bulb, tangerine peel, bromelain, trichosanthes fruit** (gou lou or *T. kirilowii),* **osha root** *(Ligusticum porteri),* **vibhitaki fruit, yerba santa leaf** *(Eriodictyon californicum),* **she gan rhizome** *(Belamcanda chinensis),* and **fritillaria bulb** (chuan bei mu or *F. cirrhosa).*

If there is tension or spasm in the lungs, it needs to be relaxed. The premier TCM herb for this is **ephedra** (see cautions), in TAM it is **vasaca leaf** *(Adhatoda vasica),* and in Western herbology it is **lobelia. Licorice root, apricot seed, aguru wood, fritillaria bulb, khella seed** *(Ammi visnaga),* and **fresh skunk cabbage root tincture** *(Dracontium foetida)* are also of great use. All of these must be prescribed by a qualified medical herbalist.

Upper Respiratory Infections

There are more than 200 different rhinoviruses that cause upper respiratory infections and many more microorganisms that can infect the lungs. The usual symptoms of such infections are sore itchy throat, watery eyes, fatigue, nasal congestion, mucus, and sometimes fever and cough.

At the beginning stages, quick use of heat-clearing herbs can be of great benefit. Many people are aware that use of **echinacea tincture,** 1 teaspoon every 2 to 3 hours, can often stop a cold in its tracks. **Ginger tea** and honey can also be useful.

TCM doctors use the traditional formula **"Honeysuckle and Forsythia powder"** commonly known as **Yin Chiao** or **yin qiao san** pills. These are usually available over the counter at Chinese herb shops and grocery stores. (Remember, these pills, though primarily made of herbs, often contain small amounts of aspirin and occasionally antibiotics.) These work very fast and effectively in the first 24–48 hours of a viral or bacterial infection. Use 3 of the 500-mg tablets three or four times per day. If the infection is very strong, we also give **isatis root** and **leaves** as well.

A simple Ayurvedic home remedy for colds is just to drink plain **ginger tea** with honey every 2 to 3 hours. Pour boiling water over a teaspoon or 2 of freshly ground **ginger** and steep for 10 minutes.

To stop infectious coughs, combine **ephedra, apricot seed, isatis root, isatis leaves, licorice root, trichosanthes fruit,** and **vasaca leaf** as 60–70% of a basic formula, then add herbs from above categories depending on the different symptoms.

These herbs relax and open the lungs, slow the coughing, and fight infection. Because the lungs are so delicate, the secondary choices and proportions of each herb are very important. If you use too many very hot herbs when the lungs are inflamed, you can worsen the condition. If you use too many cold herbs when the lungs are cold and damp, you will worsen the condition.

Research Highlights

- A randomized, double-blind, placebo-controlled, multicenter study using 3 tablets three times per day of a combination of **echinacea root, wild indigo root** *(Baptisia tinctoria),* and **thuja leaf** *(Thuja occidentalis)* followed 263 patients. Results showed a rapid onset of improvement of cold symptoms (Henneicke-von Zepelin et al., 1999).

- In a randomized double-blind study using an extract of **chuan xin lian** *(Andrographis paniculata)* on 158 patients, researchers concluded, *"Andrographis paniculata* had a high degree of effectiveness in reducing the prevalence and intensity of the symptoms in uncomplicated common cold beginning at day two of treatment. No adverse effects were observed or reported" (Caceres et al., 1999). This herb is very clinically effective for viral infections.

Asthma

Asthma is a chronic lung condition characterized by airway obstruction, spasm and hyperresponsiveness in the bronchial tubes, or inflammation and swelling in the lining tissue. It is often an advanced stage of allergies and currently is increasing in prevalence and severity. This disease can be life threatening and must be managed by an allergist to avoid crisis and to handle emergencies. During asthma attacks, patients have severe dyspnea due to bronchial spasms and hypersecretion of mucus, leading to air passageway obstruction. These attacks can be true emergencies leading to death.

The first step in treating asthma is to remove systemic inflammation and reduce allergy by detoxifying the liver and blood, as mentioned in Chapter 12. After that, construct a base formula using **ephedra, apricot seed, boswellia gum,** and **licorice root,** about 10 grams of each herb (concentrated powder granules). This relaxes the lung tissue and reduces cough and inflammation. If the patient has elevated blood pressure, delete **ephedra** and substitute **aguru wood, khella seed,** or **coltsfoot flower** (kuan dong hua or *Tussilago farfara)*. This should comprise about 50% of your formula.

Choose secondary herbs for the rest of your formula from the groups mentioned above, and always add a few herbs for weakness and deficiency. Use about 2 or 3 grams three times per day for several months. Nourishing lung syrups can also be made using honey mixed with tinctured herbs taken from the above lists. A commercial formulation of use is **honey-loquat-flavored oral demulcent syrup** (nin jiom pei pa koa), available from TCM herbalists. Although categorized as a sore throat remedy, the syrup nonetheless contains several lung-nourishing herbs.

TAM doctors point out that weakness of the inhaling and exhaling functions points to a hidden neurasthenia which can benefit from use of tonics at low dosage over a sufficiently long period of time. They also warn that asthma can be related to digestive problems, constipation, and kidney problems, as well as cardiac dysfunction, obesity, and edema. All of these must be treated separately.

They recommend a strict regulation of the external environment and diet. Asthma patients with a cold lung condition are told to avoid excess cold, as might occur during swimming or when drinking icy cold drinks. Those with inflammation have to be careful with overexertion (especially leading to breathing through the mouth), summer heat, and working near stoves. The bedroom and workspace must be well ventilated and properly heated and cooled.

You should notice that the herbs we use for asthma are almost the same as the herbs used for upper respiratory infections, except that we do not use strongly antibacterial herbs like **isatis root** and **leaves, forsythia fruit,** and **honeysuckle flowers.** Instead, we use a higher proportion of tonic and nourishing herbs, because chronic lung illness always weakens the tissues. Also, don't forget to choose the appropriate diet from Chapter 10. The methods mentioned here for treating asthma can also be used for chronic bronchitis or chronic cough after the severely inflamed state has passed.

Research Highlights

- A randomized controlled trial using **boswellia gum** involved 40 patients who had suffered from bronchial asthma for 3 to 15 years. They received 300 mg three times per day for 6 weeks. Researchers reported that "70% of patients showed improvement of disease as evident by disappearance of physical symptoms and signs such as dyspnea, rhonchi, number of attacks . . . as well as decrease in eosinophilic count. . . . Only 27% of patients in the control group showed improvement" (Gupta et al., 1998).

- A study of the clinical properties and mechanisms of action of **coltsfoot flower** showed benefit in bronchial asthma and chronic obstructive bronchitis (Ziolo and Samochowiec, 1998).

- Although **tea leaves** and **coffee** can offer symptomatic relief from asthma, they deal with only a small part of the problem. Therefore it is no surprise that a study of adults who used this strategy showed an increased hospitalization rate, probably due to a delay in using more efficacious methods (Blanc et al., 1997).

- A review of evidence suggests that dietary salt reduction, magnesium supplementation, and use of EFAs all have value in reducing asthmatic symptoms (Ziment, 1997).

- Early British researchers were so impressed by the antiasthma effects of the Ayurvedic herb **anthrapachaka leaf** *(Tylophora indica)* that it was officially admitted into the Bengal pharmacopoeia in 1844 (Nadkarni, 1954). It produces uniform and certain results, stimulating phagocytic function while inhibiting the humoral component of the immune system. Researchers at Johns Hopkins concluded that an extract from this herb constituted a new class of antiallergy agent (Gnabre et al., 1994). In asthma patients, use a 1:5 tincture, giving only 15–30 drops once per day for no more than 7–10 days per month. The results are long lasting and will continue for up to a month after stopping. Excess dosage may create nausea and vomiting, so this herb should be prescribed only by a qualified herbal practitioner. Medi-herb, distributed by Standard Process Company, sells this tincture.

- **Ginkgo leaf oral liquor** was shown to significantly reduce clinical symptoms and pulmonary function of asthmatic patients (Li et al., 1997). It has also shown benefit in children's asthma (Keville, 1996).

Smoking

My clinical experience with patients who are attempting to stop smoking indicated that most are unable to succeed for whatever reasons. My personal feeling is that it simply requires sheer will power for the first month, forcing yourself not to smoke as though your life depended upon it—which it does. After that, the physical addiction symptoms will be gone, and the rest is largely psychological. People tend to revert to smoking after quitting when facing stressful situations, and it is impossible to avoid stress forever. Herbs can help, but they cannot solve the problem.

To reduce craving during withdrawal, and to handle situations of postsmoking stress, use calming nervines like **milky oat seed, kava root,** and **skullcap tincture. Lobelia herb** *(Lobelia inflata)* contains an alkaloid called lobeline, which has a chemical structure similar to nicotine, and has been reported by some practitioners to mask the withdrawal symptoms of nicotine addiction. Consult a professional before using this herb.

To repair damage to the lungs from smoking, if it is not too late, use the same herbs and methods of differentiation mentioned for chronic respiratory problems. Emphasize herbs that reduce lung inflammation combined with herbs that soothe and nourish.

Diseases of the Ears

Tinnitus

Tinnitus is the condition where the patient hears noise such as ringing, buzzing, hissing, whistling, or roaring in the absence of an acoustic stimulus. It is usually associated with a loss of hearing. There is no easy treatment for this condition, because it is a symptom with multiple causes. It can be caused by obstruction of the ear canal, infections, inflammation, eustachian tube obstruction, otosclerosis, Miniere's disease, toxic reactions to chemicals or pharmaceuticals, heavy metals, hypertension, arteriosclerosis, acoustic blast injury, and so on. Hearing and imaging tests can differentiate between sensory and neural hearing losses, arterial obstruction, and other causes. Periwinkle products may also help.

Since several of these causative factors are related to effects on blood flow and on the transport of oxygen and glucose across nerve cell membranes, **ginkgo leaf** has proven effective in some cases.

I recommend using 60 mg of **gingko** twice per day for a few months, at which point you can assess its effectiveness. I now ask our patients to go in for auditory testing if they want a defined herbal treatment. When hardening of the arteries is known to be the culprit, for example, the methods outlined in Chapter 12 can be of benefit, especially herbs from the **blood-moving group.** Also read the section on Neuropathy.

Research Highlights

- One examination of a small group of patients with chronic tinnitus or noise-induced hearing loss showed that 47% had a vitamin B_{12} deficiency. Doctors observed some improvements in 12 patients taking B_{12} supplementation (Shemesh et al., 1993).

- A controlled clinical trial of patients with persistent tinnitus compared Western medicine (WM) with traditional Chinese medicine (TCM). Control subjects received a prescribed oral WM (Valium, nicotinic acid, vitamin B, Lidocaine, etc.), and WM-TCM patients received the same medication along with TCM herbs. The effectiveness of the WM treatments significantly increased with concomitant TCM treatment (Yang DJ, 1989).

- A multicenter double-blind clinical study of 103 patients with tinnitus concluded, **"Ginkgo biloba extract** treatment improved the condition of all the tinnitus patients, irrespective of the prognostic factor" (Meyer, 1986).

Ear Infection (Otitis Media)

The *Journal of Otolaryngology* reported in 1998 that we spend over $3 billion per year to treat acute otitis media (AOM) with drugs and surgery. Some of the organisms that commonly cause AOM *include Streptococcus pneumoniae, Haemophilus influenzae, Aspergillus* species, and *Moraxella catarrhalis.*

Problems with eustachian tube drainage are an important causative factor in these infections. The eustachian tube helps drain exudates and mucus from the middle ear. In young children, this tube is not fully formed, so chiropractic adjustments are reputed valuable in some cases to help with drainage, though no long-term studies have been done. In cases where dietary errors, allergy, or other factors cause abnormal exudation, bacteria can easily multiply, leading to infection.

To treat the immediate problem, we make herbal ear drops with **mullein flower** *(Verbascum thapsus)* and **garlic bulb** in an olive oil base. These are now commercially available, which is the recommended form to ensure sterility. To make them stronger, I add one or two drops of **grapefruit seed extract** or **oregano oil** per ounce. This usually does the trick, and part of the secret may be the penetrating quality of the **garlic** and **oregano,** which allows it to pass through the surface into the interior.

Echinacea tincture in high doses can also add to the effectiveness of the treatments. Some children have lowered immunity, so immune tonic formulas using herbs from the **immune-enhancing group** can be of value. In chronic cases it is necessary to check for food allergy, especially to milk products.

Research Highlights

- In test tube studies against *Aspergillus,* an aqueous **garlic extract** and concentrated **garlic oil** showed similar or better inhibitory effects than several pharmaceutical preparations, while demonstrating lower toxicity and similar minimum inhibitory concentrations (Pai and Platt, 1995).

- In a review of numerous studies concerning breastfeeding, doctors concluded, "Convincing studies demonstrate significant protection during breastfeeding against diarrhoea, respiratory tract infections, otitis media, bacteraemia, bacterial meningitis, botulism, urinary tract infections and necrotizing enterocolitis. There is also good evidence for enhanced protection for years after the termination of breastfeeding against *Haemophilus influenzae* type b infections, otitis media, diarrhea, respiratory tract infections and wheezing bronchitis.

"In some reports breastfeeding has also improved vaccine responses. Several studies show that milk may actively stimulate the immune system of the offspring via transfer of anti-idiotypic antibodies and lymphocytes. This may explain why breastfeeding diminishes the risk of developing coeliac disease. Some investigations suggest that there may also be a similar effect on allergic diseases and autoimmune diseases, as well as inflammatory bowel diseases and certain tumours" (Hanson, 1999).

- Another study of 200 children indicated that "the risk of developing otitis media in an infant is two times greater if a pacifier is used and five times greater if bottle fed or attending a day care facility (Jackson and Mourino, 1999).

Progressive Hearing Loss

Progressive hearing loss is one of the four most prevalent chronic conditions in the elderly. Until the last decade little attention was paid to studying causative factors related to nutrition and blood parameters. An analysis done by Department of Ophthalmology at Harvard Medical School of malnourished Allied prisoners of the Japanese during World War II and among Cubans malnourished during the recent economic embargo showed a rapid onset of visual loss and a high incidence of hearing loss.

In 1999, the *American Journal of Nutrition* reported a clinical study showing that women aged 60–71 with hearing impairment had 48% lower serum vitamin B_{12} and 43% lower red cell folate than women with normal hearing. A Spanish study of cochlear microcirculation in patients with sudden-onset hearing loss showed high blood viscosity (stickiness) and "a notorious increase in aggregability." Moreover, use of high-dose vitamin therapy and hyperbaric oxygen therapy was able to improve recovery rates in cases of sudden sensory neural hearing loss.

As early as 1984 Chinese researchers were able to improve sudden hearing loss using injections of **salvia root,** and in 1986 a French controlled clinical trial using **ginkgo leaf extract** was able to do the same thing.

It seems that both sudden and age-related hearing loss can be prevented by dealing with the causative factors. Good nutrition and attention to factors affecting blood flow and blood viscosity, both of which are also vital for cardiac health, are discussed in further detail in Chapter 12. Herbs from the **blood-moving group** are key factors.

Vertigo

I remember one particularly instructive case early in my apprenticeship with Nai-shing. We saw a gentleman who had suffered from vertigo for more than a decade and gotten no relief from Western medicine. Nai-shing diagnosed him with the Chinese syndrome called **Liver Wind.** She explained that long-standing hyperactivity of Liver Yang with signs of heat stirs up wind in the liver, leading to symptoms of trembling and vertigo. She treated him with two basic TCM herbs to quell this problem, **gou teng twigs** *(Uncaria sinensis)* and **tian ma rhizome** *(Gastrodia elata)*. Within a month his symptoms had subsided, and they were completely gone in less than 6 months. Nai-shing then said to me, "See, Liver Wind really exists, and now it is gone."

Since that time I have seen her treat several other cases, and I have never found another herb combination that works as well. If the vertigo patient has more heat symptoms, simply add cooling herbs that work on the liver, such as **scute root** and **chrysanthemum flower,** to the basic two herbs. If there are signs of deficiency, add liver-nourishing herbs like **white peony root, eclipta,** and **cornus fruit** (shan zhu yu or *Cornus officinalis)*.

Diseases of the Nose

Chronic Sinusitis

Sinusitis is a general term for inflammation of the sinus, commonly caused by bacterial or viral infection or allergy. Other causes include blockage from polyps, enlarged turbinates, scar tissue, dental infections, and a deviated septum, all of which require surgical intervention. In cases of infection, there may be symptoms of pain in the forehead, upper jaw, and face, as well as increased discharge of mucus. This condition is often far more complex than it appears. The first step is to reduce as much as possible allergy triggers, such as pets, molds, fungus, and poor indoor air.

Chinese doctors routinely use **Pe Min Kan Wan** ("Stop the allergic sinus") pills, over-the-counter pills that decrease sinusitis symptoms and fight sinus infections. They can be used to fight infections already in progress, on an as-needed basis for control of occasional symptoms, or continuously during a course of 6 to 12 weeks for a generalized anti-inflammatory and membrane-healing effect. After two courses, it is advised to stop use of the pills to determine whether the symptoms will return. Many patients report that the relief lasts for up to half a year before they need to use the pills again.

These world-famous pills, formulated at factories in mainland China, contain **chrysanthemum flower, honeysuckle flower, scute root,** and about 10 other herbal medicines. They exert antiallergy and anti-inflammatory actions and help reduce postnasal drip. Authentic **Pe Min Kan Wan** includes small amounts of an alkaline extract of animal bile, famed for its strong anti-inflammatory action. Exercise caution when purchasing these products, because low-cost brands sometimes substitute less expensive ingredients and chemical drugs such as Tylenol and antihistamines for the high-quality herbal ingredients (see safety chapter). To be sure you are getting a good-quality product, you may want to see a TCM doctor who has a trusted source.

In our clinic we also use the Neti Pot, a small teapot-shaped vessel that can be filled with salt water. Originally used by Indian Yogis to clean the nostrils, the design of the pot allows control of the water flow to help break loose and remove all foreign matter, opening sinus blockage. It is a superior treatment to salt nasal sprays because it allows greater control of water pressure and deeper penetration into the sinus cavities. After a few weeks of practice, many patients find they can pour a thin stream of salt water into one nostril until the stream comes out the other nostril into the sink. Removing mucus and opening clogged sinus cavities during the off-seasons can calm immune response and aid in reduced allergies the following year. Use the Neti Pot once each week during that time for a preventive effect.

You can also use **grapefruit seed extract** and **oregano oil** nose drops to kill sinus infections in the early stages. Put 2 or 3 drops of each into a 1-ounce dropper bottle and snort 2 or 3 drops every 2 to 3 hours. Gel Masks, available at drug stores, are used for warm heat application and can often open sinuses, especially during early stages of infection.

TAM doctors make nose drops by adding small amounts of herbs to pure sesame oil. For general inflammation, add 5 or 10 drops **white sandalwood oil** to a 1-ounce dropper bottle. Drop 2 or 3 drops into each nostril two to five times per day, or as needed.

Use of **eyebright tincture** *(Euphrasia officinalis)* is very effective for short-term symptomatic relief of allergy-related persistent burning, itching eyes with copious discharge of watery mucus.

Disease of the Mouth, Throat, and Lungs

Laryngitis / Pharyngitis

Laryngitis is an inflammation of the laryngeal mucous membrane and vocal cords, and pharyngitis is an inflammation of the pharyngeal mucous membranes. These diseases cause a dry sore throat, hoarseness, and loss of voice. They can be very serious and require immediate medical attention if they occur in infants. Before diagnosing laryngitis or pharyngitis it is important to rule out strep throat.

To treat simple cases, you can find **slippery elm bark** or **horehound** *(Marrubium vulgare)* lozenges at your health food store. Herbal teas can often be useful treatments even for serious cases. Make a tea from herbs that fight heat and inflammation, like **honeysuckle flower, tulsi, forsythia fruit, peppermint leaf, ginger root, echinacea, mullein flower,**

licorice root, scute root, and **isatis root** or **leaves.** Add 20–40 drops of the very effective tincture of **white sage** *(Salvia apiana)* and drink a cup every 2 to 3 hours, making sure to gargle a bit.

Periodontal Gum Disease / Gingivitis

Gingivitis describes an inflammatory condition of the gums, wherein the gums become swollen, spongy, and prone to bleeding. Eventually pockets form in the gums, where bacteria can live in peace and exude acids that eat away at the bone, ultimately causing the teeth to loosen. The best way to avoid this problem is with regular dental care and careful flossing and brushing. It is very helpful to drink tea, which contains high levels of tannins. Various dental cleaning devices can also be of great benefit.

It is common knowledge among herbalists that the toothpaste called Viadent contains **bloodroot** *(Sanguinaria canadensis),* which has been shown to prevent the formation of plaque from bacteria. East Indians use toothpaste made from **neem leaf,** which is also quite antiseptic. In advanced cases of gum disease, in addition to

> Dr. John Christopher, an early-20th-century herbalist, used to have his patients put pure oak bark powder on their gums at night. Oak bark is very high in tannins and will really tighten up your gums. I've tried it, but I prefer Viadent, commonly sold in pharmacies.

dental work we advise patients to use a commercial product called **Ipsab** (see the Resource Section), which contains **prickly ash bark** and a small amount of iodine. This medicine really works to kill infection and strengthen the gums.

Diseases of the Skin

The skin is our largest sense organ. The outer layer, the "epidermis," covers our skeleton and protects us against injuries and invasion by pathogens. It also regulates body temperature, aids in elimination of toxins, and prevents dehydration. The "corium," or inner layer, is composed of connective tissue and filled with nerves and nerve endings, lymphatics, blood vessels, sebaceous and sweat glands, and elastic fibers. The health of the skin is intimately related to the health of the blood, and many skin conditions can be related to internal factors.

Dryness

Dryness is often the first sign of a skin disorder. The softness and luster of the skin depends upon the proper function and health of the outermost layer, the epidermis. Drinking enough water is a given, of course. Beyond this, regular oil massage helps maintain this layer of the skin. In India, I met an 85-year-old Ayurvedic doctor whose skin was like a child's, thanks to daily oil massage. TAM doctors use numerous medicated herbal oils, especially **Narayana Taila,** extensively and very effectively to treat skin diseases. **Narayana Taila** is a well-known Ayurvedic oil containing over 40 herbs.

The two classes of nutrients useful for combating skin dryness are EFAs (essential fatty acids), found in **flaxseed oil** or **fish oils,** and carotenes, found in carrots, apricots, and other sources. Dryness of skin is sometimes a sign of deficiency, as in postmenopausal women. In these cases, herbs used to treat that particular condition will alleviate the associated dryness. Herbs that are effective for treating skin conditions from nutrient or blood deficiency include **gotu kola, raw rehmannia root, dang gui root, shilajatu,** and **shou wu root.** External application of fresh **aloe vera gel** or **aloe** preparations with **olive oil** can also be very effective.

Skin dryness may also be caused by a generalized inflammation. In these cases, anti-inflammatory and liver herbs such as **boswellia gum, burdock root, sarsaparilla root, moutan bark** (mu dan pi or *Paeonia suffruticosa),* **red peony root, dandelion root** or **leaf, turmeric root, neem leaf,** and **red clover blossoms** can be helpful. Treat itchy skin with tinctures containing menthol crystals derived from **mint oils.** An excellent product for skin itchiness is called **grindelia-sassafras compound** by Herb Pharm (see Resource Guide).

Eczema /Atopic Dermatitis

Data from worldwide epidemiological studies have shown that the prevalence of many allergic conditions has steadily increased in every decade since the 1940s, especially allergic rhinitis, asthma, and eczema. The skin of eczema patients is dry, thickened, and itchy. Lesions may occur, sometimes worsened by scratching, with papules, red patches, weeping fluid, and, in advanced cases, hyperpigmented plaques with a ridged appearance. Eczema patients often develop asthma.

Allergy- and eczema-prone children and adults often are severely deficient in omega-3 fatty acids and have digestive problems. A food allergy connection to eczema is clear, especially in infants and younger children.

For example, there is often marked intestinal inflammation and food allergy. Beginning solid foods too early (before the age of 4 months) may cause more than double the incidence of eczema, and this can be explained by the passage of the new foods into the immature GALT (gut-associated lymphoid tissue), causing immune reactions.

The severity of inflammation caused by food allergy is often underestimated. Among the problems associated with milk allergy, for example, are allergic shock in the newborn, skin and respiratory airway inflammation, acute and chronic gastroenteritis, and atrophy of the intestinal villi. As we learned in our discussion of digestion, dietary improvements and testing for food reactions can quickly and directly reduce the activation of inflammatory mediators in the gut, so attention to diet and food allergy is the obvious first step in these cases. Simple use of acidophilus, for example, can significantly improve the clinical scores of infants with allergic skin conditions.

In infants, many experts promote breastfeeding as a primary mechanism of preventing atopic dermatitis, but in breastfed babies who have the condition, cessation of breast-feeding may eliminate the problem. This would logically point to the health of the mother's breast milk, and at our clinic I have seen various children's ailments cleared up by directly treating the breastfeeding mother.

For example, Ayurvedic doctors use **turmeric root** to purify breast milk. They use a simple test of letting a drop of breast milk fall into a glass of water and watching it dissolve. The more uniformly it disperses into the water, the healthier the milk.

There are many abnormalities in the microcirculation of the skin in eczema patients. There is a visible blanching and a measurable reduction of the radiating skin temperature. The effects are often baffling, as the blanching worsens with the application of nicotinic acid, which normally acts as a vasodilator. These reactions could be explained by the presence of potent and long-acting immune mediators of vasoconstriction and inflammation such as endothelins, which are associated with allergic inflammation and asthma.

Collectively, these findings point to the importance of an integrated approach to eczema, starting with treatment of food allergies and digestive abnormalities. Lowered levels of stomach acid must be treated. While many patients will benefit from the use of healthy oils, a subset of patients (especially children or people whose problems started in childhood) may have difficulty in properly or fully metabolizing fatty acids. The body must first transform linolenic acid to gamma-linoleic acid (GLA) using an enzyme called delta-6-desaturase. If this chemical process is impaired for any reason, the use of "ready-made" **evening primrose oil** or **DHA** may then become very effective.

During the course of treatment, local attention to the skin inflammation itself is necessary to reduce itching and prevent tissue damage. This is especially important to help prevent the problems that result from topical steroid use. Emollient substances can be useful, and I prefer using **olive oil** with **aloe vera gel.** Topical application of **witch hazel** *(Hamamelis virginiana)* or **castor oil** can also be useful, as can soaps or oils containing **white sandalwood** (chandanam or *Santalum album).* Many uncomplicated eczema cases respond to such simple strategies.

Once all these causative factors have been examined and cared for, it is then possible to treat the problem directly with herbs based upon signs and symptoms:

- In cases where there are signs of increased coldness and deficiency, emphasize blood-nourishing and blood-moving formulas that contain herbs like **dang gui root, shou wu root, red peony root, red clover blossom tincture, stinging nettle tincture,** and **shilajatu.**

- In cases of increased heat and inflammation, use formulas with herbs that reduce inflammation in the liver and blood, such as **burdock root, Oregon grape root** *(Berberis aquifolium),* **neem leaf, bromelain, quercetin, turmeric root, raw rehmannia root, licorice root,** and **gotu kola.** Other appropriate Chinese herbs include **moutan**

bark, scrophularia root (xuan shen or *S. ningpoensis)* and **kochia fruit** (di fu zi or *K. scoparia).* It is interesting to note that both TCM doctors and Western herbalists use **scrophularia root** and **burdock root** to treat eczema. **Gotu kola** is especially important, due to its skin-healing effects and ability to improve cutaneous microcirculation.

Fungal Infections

Dr. Duke points out quite correctly that mixtures of antifungal herbs work better than single herbs, and he cites research to back this up in his book *The Green Pharmacy.* He states: "After all, essential oils are complex combinations of chemicals that evolved to protect plants against fungi and other diseases and pests."

"Synergy is the rule in nature, so it makes sense that combinations would work better than a single, isolated essential oil constituent." To treat simple external fungal infections, I mix some **thyme** or **oregano oil,** about 10–20%, into **tea tree oil.** Apply this twice daily to the affected area, for months if necessary. For persistent toenail fungus, put the herbal oils on some cotton and tape it right onto the toenail. Other potent antifungal herbal oils include **garlic, turmeric, cinnamon bark, tulsi, clove** *(Syzygium aromaticum),* and **neem.** Combination treatments of topical Western antifungals with herbals have also been shown to be effective. See the safety sections for cautions when dealing with these volatile oils.

Internally, we often find that patients with persistent fungal infections are suffering from an internal condition of dampness, or heat and dampness. Appropriate systemic treatment is thus indicated, primarily choosing herbs from the **heat-removing** and **dampness-removing groups.**

Bruises, Cuts, and Scrapes

To heal bruises quickly, use 1–2 grams of **tien chi root** twice per day. This even helps speed up healing from surgical wounds or traumatic injury. If you tend to bruise easily, increase your intake of fruits rich in bioflavonoids and vitamin C. With cuts and scrapes, **gotu kola tincture** can also help heal the skin. Use 35–45 drops twice per day for as long as needed. Other useful topical treatments include **plantain leaf** (from your yard), **comfrey ointment, aloe vera gel** and **Triphala Powder.** These herbs can also help relieve sunburn.

Psoriasis

Psoriasis is a chronic skin disease characterized by dry, scaly, and inflamed elevated areas (papules and plaques) of various sizes. It affects up to 2% of all people in the United States. Psoriasis often follows a pattern of relapse and remission. It can vary from a few small patches to an almost complete covering of the skin. Naturopathic physicians suspect incomplete protein digestion, poor liver function, bowel toxemia, and increased blood endotoxin levels in the development of psoriasis. TAM doctors make psoriasis causation more clear, postulating that there is a slow-acting poison trapped in the inner layers of the skin, and that the causative factors are arteriole overexudation and failure of venous drainage due to venous stasis. TCM doctors attribute it to blood stasis, dryness, or heat and dampness.

The process of psoriasis is revealed in the dynamic interaction between the top layer of the skin (epidermis) and the dermal layer it contacts. Blood vessels embedded in the underlying dermal layer transport in blood cells that communicate with keratinocytes (cells) in the surface epidermis. Under ordinary circumstances, healthy blood would support healthy skin. In psoriasis, microscopic examination of the lesions shows dilated tortured vessels, and the lesions contain elevated levels of mast cells and histamine. The presence of these inflammatory toxins and exudates apparently alters the skin cells, and, as a result, they divide rapidly, causing the thick, scaly lesions to form. Ayurvedic literature also notes that insect bites can be triggers for psoriasis.

Upon closer examination, we find that the lesion formation is indirect in nature, caused by epidermal cell stimulation driven primarily by altered immune cells. Researchers at Loyola University were able to induce full-fledged psoriasis in normal skin by injecting it with lymphocytes from psoriasis patients.

In other words, altered (sick) immune cells signal the epidermal cells to multiply. This may also explain why sunlight temporarily helps psoriasis, because UV light can alter the abnormal epidermal cells back toward normal, but as long as the immune cells remain sick, the psoriasis will return in the absence of UV stimulation.

This research seems to support the Ayurvedic explanation that toxins trapped in the dermis are causative and must be cleaned out. Such toxins could cause the immune cell changes and inflammation noted by researchers. In any case, I have personally seen Ayurvedic treatments given in Nepal reduce severe psoriatic lesions in less than 2 weeks.

Utilizing the beneficial effects of sunlight, modern allopathic treatment uses UV light along with chemicals called psoralens (called PUVA treatment). These chemicals can be found in herbs like **bishop's weed** *(Ammi visnaga)* and **vakuchi seeds** *(Psoralea corylifolia),* herbs used historically by both TCM and TAM doctors for psoriasis.

In one Chinese study, intramuscular injections of a **psoralea extract** resulted in a 24% cure rate. Dr. Duke points out that ancient Egyptians and Indians rubbed their skin with plants containing psoralens and then sat in the sunlight to treat psoriasis.

Addition of the herb **katuki** *(Picrorhiza kurroa)* was reported to strengthen the activity and speed the effects of allopathic psoralens and sunlight treatment. Taking advantage of this, I have been able to duplicate this by mixing **katuki** and **psoralea** into a powder (4:1 concentrate) and giving 2 grams twice per day to patients with both psoriasis and vitilago, a skin disease characterized by spreading patches of discoloration. This treatment must be combined with at least 20 minutes of daily exposure to sunlight or UV radiation. Several times I have seen dramatic results within a few weeks. This is the first step in treatment, and it must be followed by blood cleansing to prevent recurrence.

- Many of our long-term patients have benefited from detoxification, fasting, food allergy control, and improvement of liver function with herbs like **milk thistle seeds, burdock root, dandelion root,** and **turmeric root.**

- In 1974, an Indian Central Drug Research Institute screening of Indian medicinal plants identified a plant chemical called forskolin found in *Coleus forskohlii*. **Coleus extract** (available in pills standardized for forskolin content) has the ability to help activate the cell-regulating chemical cAMP, beneficial for psoriasis patients.

- Ayurvedic doctors use blood-cleansing formulas, along with the standard formula called **kaisara guggulu.** Its main ingredients are **guggul gum, guduchi stem, triphala,** and **black pepper.** The full formula is given in Chapter 19.

- In cases of increased inflammation, with itching and angry red patches, I recommend **sarsaparilla, honeysuckle flower, boswellia gum, raw rehmannia root, neem leaf, red peony root,** and **salvia root.**

- In cases with signs of blood stasis, thick scales that do not subside, and mild itching, I recommend **red peony root, salvia root, carthamus flower,** and **turmeric root.** Topical application of **tea tree oil** can also be helpful.

- In cases of increased dryness, the lesions appear browner in color, with fur, itching, and scaling. I recommend **raw rehmannia root, white peony root, dang gui root, tribulus fruit** (bai ji li fruit or *T. terrestris),* **astragalus root,** and **licorice root.**

Hives and Angioedema

Hives (urticaria) are raised red skin weals caused by allergy (mast cell degranulation). They usually appear suddenly and disappear rapidly, only to return again. If they last for more than 5 or 6 weeks, hives are considered to have become chronic. Any number of antigens can cause hives, including antibiotics, aspirin, curare, and various chemicals or foods. These antigens can remain dormant until stimulated by pressure, heat, cold, or other stimuli. Angioedema is a more severe condition with diffuse swelling of the lips, hands and feet, respiratory tract, and so on.

TAM doctors call the condition of hives "cold bile disease" (sitapitta), and TCM doctors call it "wandering wind evil." I actually developed this problem several years ago, and it took me a while to figure out the best way to treat it. I did not respond to any of the normal herbal therapies for removing inflammation from the liver and blood. The condition persisted for more than a full year.

As it turns out, a stool test revealed that I had a hidden and symptomless intestinal infection. Once I treated the infection, the problems decreased by about 50%. Unfortunately, the food allergies I had developed during the time my intestine was secretly infected were still active. I worked on clearing up intestinal inflammation and eliminating offending foods from my diet, and I got 75% better. I returned to health only when Dr. Mana gave me a formula containing condensed **neem leaf powder** (which is very cold and stops skin itching), mixed with hot and spicy **yavani seeds** *(Trachyspermum ammi),* which have an action similar to **thyme.** Both **neem** and **yavani** are potent anti-inflammatories and antifungals, and the treatment worked. I used standard intestinal-healing herbs for several months, and the hives have never returned.

The first step in treating hives is to resolve digestive problems, hidden intestinal infections (intestinal dysbiosis), and liver problems. It is also often necessary to identify and remove hidden food allergies. After that, you can use herbal formulas to treat the prominent signs and symptoms. In addition to the **neem**-and-**yavani** combination, try the following:

- If there are signs of severe heat and itching, use blood-cooling herbs such as **raw rehmannia root, red peony root, honeysuckle flower, chrysanthemum flower, peppermint leaf, licorice root,** and **boswellia gum.**

- If there are signs of deficiency, and the patient has an aversion to wind and perhaps a pale tongue, use **salvia root, cinnamon twig, dandelion root, dang gui root, astragalus root, white peony root,** and **licorice root.**

Research Highlights

- One controlled clinical trial tested for hypersensitivity reactions in children with chronic urticaria. According to the results, 75% of the subjects had clear reactions to one or more foods or food additives, especially coloring agents and preservatives (Ehlers et al., 1998).

- According to a review of Chinese research published in the *Archives of Dermatology,* acute urticaria can be treated effectively with acupuncture. L-111 (Quchi), Sp-10 (Xuehai), Sp-6 (Sanyinjiao), and S-36 (Zusanli) were the four most commonly prescribed acupuncture points. Injecting the acupuncture points with vitamin B_1 was also reported effective (Chen and Yu, 1998). These clinical trials were not placebo-controlled.

- In a series of rigorous studies, researchers found convincing evidence that certain food ingredients provoke urticaria symptoms and sustain the disease in a majority of patients. In one trial, by following a diet avoiding preservatives, dyes, and other natural pseudoallergens, 73% of patients experienced remission of more than 6 months' duration, as compared to 24% of controls. Remission started within the first 3 weeks of following the diet (Henz and Zuberbier, 1998).

- Researchers have also identified a potential link between *Helicobacter pylori* infection and chronic hives, though the data are still conflicting (Wedi and Kapp, 1999). Make sure to have your doctor test for this possibility.

- One very interesting study attempted to determine the most frequent food allergy skin reactions in children, and to find the most frequently involved foods. Researchers reported that certain food allergens are frequently responsible for specific skin manifestations. The foods that most commonly cause allergic skin reactions are fish, eggs, and milk. About half of the children who developed atopic dermatitis were sensitive to fish, half of the children with angioedema were sensitive to eggs, and half of the children with hives were sensitive to milk (Oehling et al., 1997).

- In a 3-year trial, researchers gave 279 infants an allergy-prevention regimen and compared them to a control group of 80 infants. The regimen included prolonged breast milk feeding, hypoantigenic weaning, and protection against adult smoking. Researchers reported that "the incidence of allergic manifestations was much lower in the intervention group than in the non-intervention group at 1 year (11.5 versus 54.4%, respectively) and at 2 years (14.9 versus 65.6%) and 3 years (20.6 versus 74.1%)" (Marini et al., 1996).

CHAPTER 18

Kidney, Urinary, Genital, and Gynecologic Disorders

Basically, I no longer work for anything but the sensation I have while working.

—sculptor Alberto Giacometti

The Kidneys

Our kidneys, the pair of organs located in the lumbar (lower back) region, are involved in functions of filtration, regulation, and excretion. They share the stage with intestinal and liver filtration to keep the blood healthy and clean. They excrete various end products of body metabolism in the form of urine and regulate the concentrations of various ions in the extracellular fluid, including hydrogen, sodium, and potassium.

Nephritis and Nephrosis

Inside each kidney is a network of tiny blood vessels that filter the blood, removing waste products. In a typical human lifetime, enough fluid passes through the delicate tubules to fill a railroad boxcar. The delicate nature of the kidney vessels renders them vulnerable to weakness, especially in the presence of aggravating conditions like diabetes and hypertension.

Nephritis is a general term for inflammation of the kidneys, which causes the filtration system to break down. There are many types. Nephrosis refers to degenerative changes in the kidneys and renal tubules that result from disease. When the kidney's filtering vessels are damaged, proteins can leak out into the urine, and waste products accumulate in the blood.

Nephritis and nephrosis are often secondary problems that result from other diseases. Early signs of kidney problems include edema, anemia, and various salt imbalances. These symptoms can result from various conditions including nutritional imbalances, hepatitis, urinary diseases, liver and spleen problems, heart disease, abdominal tumors, connective tissue diseases, and diabetes. Any causative conditions must be treated individually. As a kidney problem becomes more serious, urine concentrations of albumin and creatinine increase. A simple urine "dip stick" test can detect these substances. Your doctor can also perform a more sensitive microalbumin test for tiny amounts of albumin.

Herbal Treatment of Nephritis and Nephrosis

- **Nettle seed tincture** has emerged as a useful treatment for nephritis.

- Low-protein diets are always prescribed for severe kidney disorders because they lessen the metabolic strain on the kidneys. However, the prescriptions rarely specify the types of protein that should remain in the diet. As a rule, vegetable protein is much easier on the kidneys.

- Avoidance of low-quality fats and oils helps reduce kidney inflammation.

- Vitamin E supplementation has been shown to slow the progression of nephropathy.

- A traditional TAM formula for treating progressive kidney disorders combines **shilajatu** and **triphala.** Dose: 2 grams twice a day.

- The well-known TCM formula called **Rehmannia six** is an effective kidney treatment. It contains cooked **rehmannia root, astragalus root, cornus fruit** (shan zhu yu or *C. officinalis),* **moutan bark** (mu dan pi or *Paeonia suffruticosa),* **water plantain rhizome** (ze xie or *Alisma plantago-aquatica),* and **wild yam root** (han yao or *Dioscorea opposita).* Other useful TCM herbs include **cordyceps mushroom** and **perilla seed** (su zi or *P. frutescens).*

- Animal studies have shown the simple combination of **astragalus root** and **cooked rehmannia root** to be a markedly effective treatment for protein and blood in the urine, causing improvement and recovery of renal functions and reduction of edema, anemia, and anorexia. The combination had no adverse effects on functions of the liver, kidney, heart, and GI tract.

- According to Japanese researchers, combining a TCM formula with low-dose prednisone treatment in autoimmune nephritis is a superior protocol to using either treatment alone. The tested formula contained **white peony root, dang gui root, tangerine peel, astragalus root, cinnamon bark, ginseng root, white atractylodes, cooked rehmannia root, schisandra berry, poria mushroom,** and **poygala root** (yuan zhi or *P. tenuifolia).*

- The Heibei Provincial Hospital reported their findings in a study of 89 cases of chronic nephritis divided into five TCM diagnostic categories and treated accordingly. Researchers found that the curative effect of the treatments was closely related to control of blood in the urine and improvement of microcirculation. This suggests, first, that herbs like **salvia root** and **tien chi root,** as well as herbs from the **vessel-**

strengthening group, would provide positive results, and second, that professional TCM diagnosis may be critical.

Benign Prostatic Hyperplasia

Benign prostatic hyperplasia (BPH, also known as benign prostatic hypertrophy), or swelling of the prostate, is characterized by symptoms of bladder outlet obstruction, progressive urinary urgency and frequency, increased nightly urination, and urination with reduced force and caliber of urine. Patients with BPH typically present with an enlarged, inflamed, and swollen prostate smooth muscle, glandular epithelium, and stromal tissue in the periurethral region of the prostate.

Experts estimate that BPH affects 50–60% of men between 40 and 59 years of age in the United States, resulting in a projected annual overall cost of hospital care and surgery of over $1 billion per year. Neglect of prostate inflammation and swelling can lead to a rise in prostate-specific antigen (PSA), which in turn may indicate an early stage of prostate cancer. Prolonged obstruction can also result in uremia, also known as chronic renal failure.

Analysis of BPH biochemistry shows that it is an androgen-dependent disorder of metabolism primarily reflecting changes in steroid levels in aging men. Testosterone and other hormone levels decrease with age after the age of about 40. This causes an increased concentration in the prostate of dihydrotestosterone (DHT), an inflammatory androgen derived from testosterone. The accumulation of inflammatory DHT results in congestion and swelling of the prostate. In TCM terms, patients with this disease have heat and dampness in the lower abdomen.

Some BPH patients have shown benefit from the following lifestyle changes:

- Be sure to drink 6 to 8 glasses of pure spring water each day for a harmless diuretic effect. This can aid the kidney in removing metabolic wastes. Insufficient water intake is a general causative factor in most inflammatory diseases.

- Engage in regular exercise, which is necessary for maintaining muscle and cardiac tone and good blood circulation. Due to its anatomical location the prostate is especially subject to venous congestion. A sedentary lifestyle may exacerbate this congestion.

- Follow a diet tailored to reducing inflammation and swelling in the prostate. This is generally accomplished by eating plenty of fresh fruits and vegetables and limiting poor-quality fats and oils. The diet should also be as free as possible from pesticides and other contaminants, since many of these compounds, such as dioxin, increase DHT. Also avoid diethylstilbestrol (DES) because it produces changes in rat prostates that are histologically similar to those caused by BPH.

- Increase your dietary intake of soy. Soybeans and soy foods can decrease circulating levels of endogenous estrogens, replacing them with less inflammatory phytoestrogens. Estrogen levels in men increase with age, which facilitates the activity of DHT by enhancing the amount of androgen receptor protein present in the tissue. This may explain the lower incidence of BPH in Chinese males, who consume soy products at least two times per week.

- Follow a higher-protein and lower-fat diet to reduce the very inflammatory chemical 5-HETE.

- Increase your zinc intake. Zinc has been shown to reduce the size of the prostate—as determined by rectal palpation, X-ray, and endoscopy—and to reduce symptomatology in the majority of patients. The clinical efficacy is probably due to its critical involvement in many aspects of androgen metabolism. Intestinal uptake of zinc is impaired by estrogens but enhanced by androgens. Since men with BPH have elevated estrogen levels, zinc uptake may be low.

Herbal Treatment of BPH

Saw palmetto berry *(Serenoa repens)* is the best-known herb for BPH. David Winston, AHG, reviews in great detail the scientific and traditional literature supporting its use for BPH in his book *Saw Palmetto for Men and Women.* He explains how combining it with other herbs into an integrated formula based upon signs and symptoms yields superior clinical results. He also argues against the pigeonholing of this herb as useful only for BPH, mentioning benefits for cystic acne, stimulation of sexual maturation in delayed puberty, and male infertility.

An important **saw palmetto** mechanism of action is inhibition of the inflammation-promoting enzyme 5-alpha-reductase, an action which it shares with **stinging nettle root** *(Urtica dioica),* another herb useful for BPH. However, these actions are not strong enough to account for the reported results. A closer look at the research shows that the positive actions are due to a number of related mechanisms, such as inhibition of inflammatory arachidonic acid metabolites and inhibition of epithelial growth factors.

Saw palmetto basically acts as a nutritive tonic, strengthener, and normalizer (amphoteric) of the male reproductive system. It is of course specifically helpful in improving the symptoms associated with an enlarged prostate gland. It is also useful for genitourinary tract infections. Numerous open and placebo-controlled studies in large populations have also demonstrated the efficacy of African **pygeum bark** *(Pygeum africanum)* in the treatment of BPH and prostate inflammation. However, the effectiveness is less than **saw palmetto,** and there are some minor side effects.

To remove venous congestion in the prostate area, I recommend a tincture of **saw palmetto, stinging nettle, stone root, gotu kola, white sage** *(Salvia apiana),* and **horse chestnut,** about 45–60 drops three to four times per day. A commercial formulation containing a similar constellation of herbs is available from Herbalist & Alchemist (see Resource Guide).

Europeans have used a particular form of **flower pollen** to treat prostatitis and BPH for more than 25 years. Produced by A. B. Cerncile of Sweden, the product is marketed under the name **Cernilton.** Although its mechanism of action is not yet completely understood, it has been shown quite effective in several double-blind studies without any reported side effects. It seems to be effective in both BPH and chronic prostatitis.

Traditional Chinese Medicine offers some insights into the treatment of prostate problems. In simple terms, a TCM doctor would write a prescription based on the concept that there is both heat (inflammation) and dampness (swelling) in the prostate, restricting the flow of urine. There may also be a deficiency condition weakening the kidneys. A BPH formula can be constructed from the following lists of herbs. With 4:1 concentrated granules, the dose would be 6 to 9 grams per day. After 1 or 2 weeks, the doctor would reassess the patient and adjust the relative proportions of individual herbs according to signs and symptoms, perhaps deleting certain herbs and adding others.

The following herbs could be included in a basic BPH formula:

- **Phellodendron bark** to remove heat and dampness

- **Rhubarb root** to soften the swollen gland and purge heat and dampness

- **Black atractylodes rhizome** to dry out the dampness

- **Coix seed** (yi yi ren or *Coix lachryma)* to aid removal of dampness

- **Persica seed** (tao ren or *Prunus persica)* to break up blood congestion

- **Talcum** (hua shi or calcium carbonate) to reduce heat, soothe the urinary tract, and open obstruction

- **Licorice root** to reduce heat and nourish

- **Shi wei leaf** *(Pyrrosia lingua)* to promote urination and reduce heat

- **Dandelion root** to detoxify and remove heat and dampness

- **Anteater scales** (chuan shan jia or *Manis pentadactyla)* to reduce swelling and promote the discharge of pus

- **Lu lu tong fruit** *(Liquidambar taiwaniana)* to promote urination, soften the swollen organ, reduce pain, and unblock the tubes and channels

Based on the following characterizations and symptoms, you can personalize the formula for each patient by adding the appropriate herbs.

With predominant inflammation:

- **Scute root** to drain heat

- **Coptis rhizome** (huang lian or *C. chinensis)* to drain fire (strongly anti-inflammatory)

With a predominance of swelling:

- **Water plantain** (ze xie or *Alisma plantago)* to promote the flow of urine and leach out dampness when there is stagnation and urinary difficulty

With signs of coldness (cold limbs, aversion to cold):

- **Purified aconite** (fu zi or *Aconitum palmatum)* to alleviate pain and warm (professional use only)

- **Cinnamon twig** (gui zhi or *Cinnamomum cassia)* to promote blood circulation and warm

In patients suffering from deficiency or elderly patients, consider adding:

- **Sang ji sheng twigs** *(Viscum album)* to tonify the kidney and remove dampness

- **Eucommia bark** (du zhong or *E. ulmoides)* to strengthen weakness in the organ

- **Scrophularia root** (xuan shen or *S. ningpoensis)* to relieve toxicity and inflammation, soften nodular swelling, and nourish in the later stages of inflammatory diseases

With severe blood and venous congestion, common in the later stages of BPH:

- **Red peony root** to promote blood circulation and remove swelling and pain

- **Zedoary root** (e zhu or *Curcuma zedoaria)* to remove blood stasis, promote the movement of Qi, alleviate pain, and dissolve accumulations

With general fatigue and weakness:

- **Ginseng root** to strengthen vital force and decrease fatigue

Adding to the traditional understanding, **ginseng root** possesses a variety of well-studied pharmacological properties. Animal studies show that **ginseng root** increases testosterone levels while decreasing prostate weight, as well as stimulating corticosterone secretions. This would seem favorable to BPH patients, since increased testosterone could mean decreased DHT and improved intestinal zinc absorption, and decreased prostate size would help alleviate the symptoms. At our clinic we have seen many patients relieved of BPH symptoms using herbal strategies from the Western, Ayurvedic, and TCM systems. We usually start with Western herbs, due to their ease of procurement, and utilize more complex formulations from the other systems if these are not sufficiently successful.

Urinary Tract Infections

The urinary tract includes the kidneys, bladder, ureters (the tubes that connect the kidney to the bladder), and urethra (the tube that leads from the bladder to the outside). Urinary tract infections (UTIs) are caused by bacteria which usually originate in the urethra before moving backward into the bladder where they can then grow and flourish. The main symptoms of UTIs are urinary urgings, frequent urination, pain or burning during urination, and cloudiness or blood in the urine. Some patients may experience low back pain (often radiating upward), dizziness, and nausea. Acute cases require antibiotics.

Urinary tract infections occur more frequently in women than in men. The infections can be divided into three categories.

1. *Urethritis* is an infection of the urethra. This is a viral infection usually transmitted during intercourse.

2. *Cystitis* is infection of the urinary bladder.

3. *Pyelonephritis,* or kidney infection, occurs when the bacteria in the bladder migrate to the kidneys and is much more serious than the other two types of UTI. In these cases it is important to see a doctor or medically trained herbalist immediately.

To prevent UTIs, women should wash the perineal area daily with a mild unscented soap, and change tampons and sanitary napkins frequently. After using the toilet, wipe from front to back to keep bacteria away from the urethra. In addition, wash the hands and genitals before and after sexual intercourse, and use lubricants to avoid bruising the urethra. Avoid wearing tight clothing, which can increase heat. Drink plenty of pure water each day.

I also advise patients who suffer from frequent UTIs to make a solution of 5 drops of **grapefruit seed extract** in 4 to 6 ounces of water, with which both partners should wash their genitals before and after sexual intercourse. Regular use of probiotics containing *Lactobacillus acidophilus* may also be a valuable preventive measure. With any infections that occur from the mouth all the way down to the colon and urinary system, it is important to reduce intake of sugars so the bacteria don't decide to have a party and invite their friends.

As far back as the early 1800s, Europeans noticed that drinking **cranberry juice** was beneficial for preventing and treating UTIs. Scientists have recently identified the source of this benefit. **Cranberries** contain a natural chemical that weakens the ability of the bacteria to attach to the urinary tract. However, it requires a very high level of this chemical to obtain a strong beneficial effect, so it is usually best to buy the concentrated pills now available in health food stores. Interestingly, TCM doctors often add **talcum** to their formulas as well because it is slippery and reduces heat. One might wonder if the heat is reduced because the infectious organisms also find it slippery.

We treat UTIs in our clinic with a combination of the following two strategies. (We always administer the herbal treatments as teas or tinctures.)

- Choose three or four strong anti-inflammatory and antiseptic herbs to reduce heat and infection, especially those with diuretic properties, such as **guduchi stem, phellodendron root, dandelion leaf, yin chen hao** *(Artemisia capillaris),* **varuna** *(Crataeva* species), **buchu leaf** *(Barosma betulina),* **uva ursi leaf** *(Arctostaphylos uva-ursi),* and **cleavers herb** *(Galium aparine).* This should comprise about 70% of your formula.

- Use herbs that soothe and coat the urinary tract, such as **talcum, slippery elm bark,** and **marshmallow root.** This should comprise the remaining 30% of your formula, or can be administered separately as powders or cold water infusions.

Research Highlights

A clinical trial in India looked at the Ayurvedic herb **varuna** as a UTI treatment. Of the 84 cases studied, patients with urinary tract infections accompanied by painful, burning urination experienced a cure rate of 55%, along with 40% improvement and 5% failure rates (Pramod, 1982). An additional study resulted in an 85% improvement rate (Deshpande et al., 1982). This herb also increases bladder tone (reported by Bone, 1996).

Kidney Stones

Formation of stones in the kidney or the urinary tract is a frequent problem, affecting 5–10% of Americans in their lifetimes. They develop when substances like calcium oxalate or phosphate, uric acid, or magnesium phosphate are too concentrated in the urine. Eventually they precipitate out, forming crystals that eventually become stones. This can be very painful, as the stones move down the urinary tract or out of the kidney via the ureters, and requires immediate medical attention.

Treatment with **varuna bark** makes the urine less likely to form stones, because it reduces calcium excretion and increases magnesium and sodium excretion. It can be used as a tincture, or made as a decoction. Bruise and boil 4 ounces of the bark in 1 ½ pints of water until it boils down to 1 pint. Strain and cool. Use 2 ounces two to three times per day.

Beggar-lice (jin qian cao or *Desmodium styracifolium)* gets its name from the small, loose fruits, which cling to clothing. Japanese researchers have discovered a compound in the plant that decreases the amount of calcium excreted in the urine and increases the amount of citrate excreted, substantially decreasing the likelihood of kidney stone formation.

Lemon juice is a very inexpensive form of citrate, and 4 ounces per day provides sufficient concentration to increase urinary citrate levels and lower urinary calcium excretion.

Also important if you have a tendency to form stones:

- Drink more water.

- Cut back on caffeine.

- Go easy on sugar.

- Avoid phosphoric acid in sodas.

- Avoid high-oxalate foods like chard, rhubarb, beets, parsley, coffee, spinach, cocoa, and black tea.

- Take extra magnesium (200–400 mg) and vitamin B_6 (100 mg) every day.

- Increase fiber in the diet.

Vaginal Yeast Infections (Candidiasis) / Vaginitis

Vaginal yeast infection results from overgrowth of *Candida albicans,* a type of yeast normally present in small amounts in the digestive tract, vagina, and mouth. Over the past 20 years, new, more toxic yeast strains have developed as a result of overuse of antibiotics, so these infections have become very common. Symptoms include burning, itching, irritation, and redness around the vaginal opening. Many patients also experience a thick cottage-cheese-like discharge. Frequent vaginal yeast infections often signal the existence of an intestinal yeast problem that feeds the vaginal infections. For information on treating intestinal yeast infections, refer to our discussion in Chapter 11.

Hormonal changes, birth control pills, antibiotics, steroids, blood sugar imbalances, excessive douching, and physical irritation during sex can all trigger new infections or exacerbate existing vaginal yeast infections. Good hygiene is extremely important for prevention and treatment. This should include daily washing of the vaginal area, including the folds in the vulva. Keep the area dry and avoiding excessive heat.

The **grapefruit seed extract solution** recommended earlier as a treatment for UTIs is also very useful for preventing yeast infections. To treat active infections, you can make a douche, adding 5–10 drops of the liquid **grapefruit seed extract** to a commercial douching solution. Alternatively, you can dip a tampon in the solution. A single treatment is often sufficient for clearing up minor infections, although more stubborn cases may require three or four applications. Nightly vaginal insertion of an acidophilus capsule for a few nights helps ensure the return of healthy flora. The same methods can be used to treat other forms of vaginitis.

TCM doctors treat vaginal yeast infections with a tea of **phellodendron bark, kochia fruit** (di fu zi or *Kochia scoparia),* and **cnidium seed** (she chuang zi or *Cnidium monnieri).* They soak cotton with the tea and insert it vaginally twice per day.

A note of caution: If any infection continues or worsens after a few days, promptly see a physician.

Sexually Related Disorders

Male Infertility

Male infertility is often associated with a low sperm count or weakened sperm motility. Average normal sperm counts range from 80 million to 100 million sperm per mL. Male infertility is usually quantified at a count of 20 million sperm per mL or less. There are some reports that male fertility in certain parts of the world has been falling in recent years at an alarming rate.

Under investigation is the possibility that pesticides and other forms of pollution are responsible, because many chemicals have been shown to impair fertility or lead to impaired prenatal and perinatal development in experimental studies. Such problems require a global improvement in environmental conditions to reverse. At the local level, your nutritional, vocational, and living-environment choices can hopefully minimize risk.

There are numerous tonic and aphrodisiac herbs that can affect general sex drive and desire and improve sperm counts. Since sex drive is part of one's general health, almost any general tonic herb can offer some help in this area. It is important to keep in mind that aphrodisiac herbs are usually only one part of a treatment program for infertility, and there are some differences to keep in mind. Some of these herbs are very warming and stimulating, while others are more nourishing and strengthening. Prescribe based upon signs and symptoms. Also, some of these are contraindicated during pregnancy.

- Warming, stimulating, aphrodisiac herbs include **epimedium herb, cistanche** (rou cong rong or *C. deserticola),* **deer antler, ginseng root, garlic bulb, morinda root** (ba ji tian root or *M. officinalis),* and **guduchi stem.** These herbs can sometimes be overstimulating and should not be used if there are signs of heat or inflammation.

- Nourishing aphrodisiac herbs include **wild asparagus root, ashwagandha root, muira puama tincture, saw palmetto berry, shilajatu, dang gui root, milky oat seed tincture, amla fruit, purified gunga seed** *(Abrus precatorius),* **cuscuta seed** (tu si zi seed or *C. chinensis),* and **purified cowhage seed** *(Mucuna prurita).* TCM doctors note that seeds in general tend to nourish hormonal energy, which explains why there are several types of seeds in this group.

- Lesser-known Ayurvedic herbs for semen production include the condensed extract of **kadamba bark** *(Anthocephalus),* **ikshubalika seed** *(Hydrophila spinosa),* and **hastanjali tuber** *(Orchid incarnata).*

Increased temperature in the genital region can sometimes cause a drop in sperm count. I saw a particularly interesting case of a diabetic patient who had a low sperm count. Physical examination revealed a fungal skin infection near the testicles, causing increased temperature. After we cleared up the infection with **tea tree oil,** genital temperature declined and his sperm count returned to normal. In a separate case, this time with low sperm motility, we made a formula using the herbs mentioned above, also adding some **astragalus root** because the young man showed the signs and symptoms of Qi deficiency. Within 2 weeks, a surprisingly short time, his sperm count returned to normal, offering support for earlier published in vitro experiments in which **astragalus root** increased sperm motility.

Research Highlights

- In one study, 28 men with low sperm counts received 7.5 grams daily of the standard TCM formula **rehmannia eight** for 2 to 6 months. According to examinations of semen, subjects experienced, on average, a 78% increase in number, and moderate increases in sperm motility (53%) and sperm volume (56%). They also showed improvement in blood hormone (estradiol-17 beta) levels (Usuki, 1986). Three of the ingredients in this **rehmannia eight** formula are **rehmannia root, astragalus root,** and **schisandra berries.**

Female Infertility

Female infertility can have many causes. In cases with mechanical blockages such as scarring of the fallopian tubes, herbal medicines are not effective. However, they can definitely help if the problems are hormonal, emotional, or nutritional.

Common gynecological problems such as fibroid tumors, endometriosis, and chronic vaginal infections—all of which can lead to or exist concomitantly with infertility—may improve with herbal medicine treatments. These conditions generally fall into the TCM category of heat and dampness in the pelvic area. Herbs that might be used include **poria mushroom, pinellia tuber, tangerine peel, white atractylodes rhizome,** and **phellodendron bark.** Dietary measures such as **the diet to reduce heat and dampness** can also be helpful (Chapter 10).

Problems in other endocrine glands, such as the thyroid or the pituitary, can cause a failure to ovulate. In these cases it is best to treat the causative factors in the gland where the problem originates before resorting to tonic herbs. If the thyroid is weak, follow the treatments discussed in Chapter 14. If there is a problem with pituitary gland regulation, use **chaste tree berry.**

TCM doctors use some very effective herbs for these female infertility cases, which I always refer to Nai-shing. Basically, any imbalance in the hormonal systems can lead to a failure to ovulate or inability to carry a pregnancy to term. Yin deficiency is the most common cause of these imbalances. We often use the following herbs: **ginseng root, wild asparagus root, white peony root, cooked rehmannia root, dang gui root, licorice root, cuscuta seed** (tu si zi or *C. chinensis),* **eucommia bark** (du zhong or *E. ulmoides),* **deer antler, lycium fruit** (gou qi zi or *L. chinense),* and **salvia root.** I recommend making a tea (3 to 4 cups per day) or administering the herbs as powders—6 to 9 grams per day of the 4:1 concentrated granules. Take for several months up to half a year or longer.

Liver Qi stagnation is another common cause, in which case we treat with **dang gui root, white peony root, bupleurum root, poria mushroom, moutan bark,** and **trichosanthes root.**

Once a woman becomes pregnant, it is important to continue to keep the system healthy and prevent miscarriage. A few Western herbs that offer benefit during pregnancy include:

- **Black haw** *(Viburnum prunifolium)* to relax, nourish, and tonify the female reproductive organs

- **Partridgeberry** *(Mitchella repens)* to nourish and strengthen during pregnancy

- **Cramp bark** *(Viburnum opulus)* to prevent miscarriages and prepare for birth

For an excellent discussion of all the many issues related to pregnancy and childbirth beyond the scope of this book, I highly recommend *The Natural Pregnancy Book* by herbalist and midwife Aviva Jill Romm, AHG.

Genital Herpes

Genital herpes simplex is a virus, spread by direct skin-to-skin contact. As with most chronic viral diseases, once you are infected you can experience recurring flare-ups. Symptoms include blisters on the genital area and anus, and occasionally the buttocks. After a few days, the blisters break open and leave painful, shallow ulcers that gradually crust over and fade. These attacks may be triggered by heat-producing factors like emotional stress, fatigue, sunburn, drugs (prescription or recreational), sexual activity, or dietary errors. In the period prior to an outbreak (called the prodrome), patients may experience itching, irritation, and tingling in the genital area.

The herpes virus is highly contagious during the prodrome phase, while blisters are present, and for a short period after the blisters have disappeared. Herpes is considered incurable, so prevention of recurrence is the best strategy. Essentially, if the frequency of outbreaks can be reduced to less than one every few years or so, it is functionally similar to a cure.

TAM doctors state that immediate treatment during the initial outbreak is the best way to prevent recurrence, followed by long-term detoxification treatment of both the fatty tissue and the blood. The first step is application of a topical paste made with **neem leaf.** Then the blood and fat are cleansed internally with a compound called **guduchiyoga,** the main ingredients of which are **amla fruit** and **guduchi stem.** Use the compound continuously for 3 to 6 months. It is also important to watch the diet carefully, especially avoiding excessive intake of fats and oils.

Western herbalists use **echinacea, wild indigo root** *(Baptisia tinctoria),* **cat's claw inner bark** (uña de gato or *Uncaria tomentosa),* and **St. John's wort** as internal treatments. A useful external preparation is a tea made from **lemon balm** *(Melissa officinalis).*

My personal favorite external treatment, however, is **Earl Grey tea bags** (see the review of **tea leaves** in Section Two). **Tea leaves** work better in the short term than the common allopathic internal treatment acyclovir, cost far less, and have fewer side effects. I have prescribed this regimen for many patients, and they all find that the lesions crust over more quickly, then disappear and do not recur for at least several months after treatment. Apparently the tannins in the tea inactivate the virus.

Chinese doctors treat herpes with heat-reducing antiviral herbs, such as **gentiana root** (long dan cao or *G. scabra),* **isatis root** and **leaves, kochia fruit** (di fu zi or *K. scoparia),* **phellodendron bark, scute root, moutan bark** (mu dan pi or *Paeonia suffruticosa),* **cnidium fruit** (she chuang zi or *C. monnieri),* and **dictamnus bark** (bai xian pi or *D. dasycarpus).*

Research Highlights

- One study examined traditional herbal medicines with activity against acute herpes simplex virus type 1 (HSV-1) in mice. The various herbal extracts arrested the progression of recurrent HSV-1 disease and shortened the period of severe recurrent lesions compared with controls. Prophylactic treatment limited the development of recurrent skin lesions (Kurokawa et al., 1997).

- **Teng li gen root** *(Actinidia chinensis)* is the basis of a new ophthalmic eyedrop used in China for recurrent herpes-caused keratitis (corneal inflammation). It is nontoxic to the corneal epithelium (Zhang JM et al., 1993). A clinical combined system trial of 22 "obstinate" eyes used herbal eyedrops along with internal TCM medicines and, when deemed necessary, irradiation. The combined treatment decreased or prevented recurrence, maintained visual acuity, and reduced the frequent relapses that often lead to blindness (Bao, 1992).

Menstrual Disorders

Premenstrual Syndrome (PMS)

Premenstrual syndrome is the constellation of symptoms that appear in the days prior to the onset of a menstrual period. Symptoms include anxiety, irritability, fatigue, depression, headache, breast pain, abdominal bloating, and fluid retention. Numerous hormonal changes have been implicated in PMS. Depending on the predominant symptoms, researchers have subdivided the condition into four general types: anxiety, food craving, depression, and fluid retention. This system of classification makes it much easier to prescribe herbs, as it divides the condition in a way similar to herbal energetics.

Most cases involve progesterone deficiency or estrogen excess. I usually start with a trial of **chaste tree berry tincture** *(Vitex agnus-castus),* which helps increase progesterone via an effect on the pituitary hormone prolactin. Often this is enough. Native American women would chew **evening primrose seeds** to relieve PMS. The benefit may result from gamma-linoleic acid (GLA), the fatty acid abundant in the seeds that helps the body make needed hormones.

Nai-shing uses a base combination of **bupleurum root, scute root, cyperus rhizome** (xiang fu or *C. rotundus),* **blue citrus peel** (qing pi or *C. reticulata),* and **white peony root.** Other herbs are added according to signs and symptoms. For example, with fluid retention, she adds small amounts of diuretic herbs such as **dandelion leaf, leonorus herb** (yi mu cao or *L. heterophyllus),* or **water plantain** (ze xie or *Alisma plantago-aquatica)* to her base formula. In cases with anxiety symptoms, you can use **skullcap herb tincture** or **kava root** to control those symptoms. Because **chaste tree berry** and the TCM combinations seem to work through different biochemical mechanisms, using one or the other, or sometimes both in combination, can usually solve even the most severe PMS problems.

Research Highlights

- A randomized controlled double-blind clinical trial of 100 women measured the effects of **chaste tree berry** (30 drops twice per day) on breast pain preceding menstruation. Intensity of breast pain diminished more quickly in the treated group (Halaska et al., 1998). An earlier study showed reduction in water retention (Amann, 1979).

In a series of animal experiments, a Japanese researcher showed that the six-herb combination called **dang gui and white peony powder** increased progesterone secretion. When the formula ingredients were analyzed in groups, **dang gui root, water plantain** (ze xie or *Alisma plantago-aquatica),* and **white peony root** increased progesterone accumulation in the blood, while the combination of **poria mushroom** and **white atractylodes** decreased these levels. The formula as a whole favored progesterone production and reduced one of the estrogens called estradiol (Usuki, 1988). This formula is traditionally used to reduce cramping pain and swelling in the abdomen and uterus and to prevent miscarriage.

Menorrhagia

Menorrhagia is the term for excessive blood loss due to heavy menstrual bleeding or an extended menstrual period. Decline in hormones, especially progesterone, as a woman nears menopause is the most common cause of menorrhagia. It is important to get a proper diagnosis before attempting to use natural medicine because you must determine whether the condition is caused by hormone changes, fibroids, polyps, endometriosis, or tumors. Another cause is von Willebrand's disease, a membrane bleeding disorder affecting an estimated 1% of the population worldwide. These all need to be treated separately, as in the case of another specific cause—low levels of vitamin A.

In a South African study, researchers found a statistically significant difference between the fasting serum vitamin A values of healthy controls and of patients with menorrhagia. Furthermore, vitamin A therapy alleviated menorrhagia in 92% of these patients.

After assessment and treatment of underlying pathology, you can control bleeding with astringent or hemostatic herbs chosen from all traditions, such as **tien chi root, asoka bark** *(Saraca indica),* **di yu root** *(Sanguisorba officinalis),* **cramp bark** *(Viburnum opulus),* **xian he cao herb** *(Agrimonia pilosa),* or **typha pollen** (pu huang or *T. angustifolia).* If the patient is weak or deficient, **astragalus root, lotus embryo** (lian zi or *Nelumbo nucifera),* or **cooked rehmannia root** may be helpful over the long run. If the weakness and blood loss have progressed to anemia, use iron supplements and herbs from the **blood-nourishing group.** To stop bleeding quickly, try the Eclectic formula called **erigeron-cinnamon compound,** available from Herb Pharm. Using these strategies at our clinic, we have been able to slow or stop many persistent cases of acute menorrhagia. Over a period of three to six cycles we have also stopped or reduced the tendency to bleed excessively.

Dysmenorrhea (Menstrual Cramps)

Dysmenorrhea is the medical term for pain and cramping associated with menstruation. The pain and cramping usually appear with the onset of menstruation. Biochemically speaking, excessive production of prostaglandins by the myometrium and endometrium are the cause of uterine contractions, pointing to nutritional problems. Cramping can spread throughout the entire abdomen and lumbosacral region and even cause pain in the vulva and anus. In some cases, pain can be sufficiently severe to cause fainting. There is often clotting, and the pain is usually relieved after the blood begins to flow smoothly. Herbal medicines can be very effective for this condition.

However, as with menorrhagia, unless the case is very mild, it is advisable to see your gynecologist to rule out more serious organic diseases. It is also important to correct nutritional deficiencies while using herbal treatments for a holistic treatment.

TAM doctors believe that chronic tension in the uterus or a small uterus is sometimes the cause, and they explain that this is why, in some women, the cramps cease after childbirth. TCM doctors see this condition as stagnation of blood and Qi. The primary treatment goals with Chinese herbs are to break up the blood stagnation (clotting) and relax the uterus.

Herbs that relax the uterus include **black cohosh root** *(Cimicifuga racemosa),* **cramp bark** *(Viburnum opulus),* **kava root,** and **black haw root** *(Viburnum prunifolium).* Among the many useful herbs to break up blood stagnation are **dang gui root, red peony root, red clover blossoms, carthamus flower,** and **raspberry leaf** (as a tea). From the TCM perspective, due to Qi stagnation it is important to also use **bupleurum root.** If pain is severe, you can use **Jamaican dogwood** *(Piscidia erythrina),* or **yan hu suo tuber** *(Corydalis yanhusuo).* All of these herbs can either be used alone or in balanced combinations.

Research Highlights

- In a controlled crossover study, 33 women followed a low-fat vegetarian diet to determine whether it would reduce dysmenorrhea and premenstrual symptoms. Pain intensity decreased significantly in comparison to baseline levels on the worst days, and water retention symptoms were also significantly reduced. Researchers attributed the benefits to dietary influences on estrogen activity (Barnard et al., 2000).

- A randomized, double-blind, controlled study involved 556 girls ages 12–21, all of whom suffered from moderate to very severe spasmodic dysmenorrhea. The subjects received vitamin B_1 (100 mg per day) for 90 days. Researchers reported that 87% were completely cured, 8% were relieved (pain ranged from reduced to almost none), and 5% showed no effect whatsoever. The results remained the same 2 months later. (Gokhale, 1996).

- A study on 181 healthy Danish women looked at the correlation between dietary habits, especially low intake of fish products and intakes of specific nutrients, and menstrual pain. Statistical analysis of results were highly significant, supporting the hypothesis that a higher intake of marine omega-3 fatty acids correlated with milder menstrual pain symptoms (Deutch, 1995).

Fibrocystic Breasts

The symptoms of fibrocystic breast disease (FBD) are swelling, pain, and tenderness of the breast and the presence of small or large cysts—abnormal sacs containing gas, blood, fluids, or semisolid (mucinous) waste material. The associated pain increases prior to menstruation, due to the rise in estrogen levels. The cystic areas are palpable, with a dense, irregular, and stonelike feel. A physician should examine any lump to ascertain the diagnosis, especially if there is any discharge from the nipples. This disease affects as many as 20–40% of premenopausal women, but the severity of the condition usually decreases or subsides after menopause.

Of interest is the recognition that cysts are "holding tanks" set up by the body to capture and cordon off toxic fluids and waste material. The correlation between these waste materials and disease processes closely resembles the Ayurvedic concept that, when not cleared quickly enough, toxic metabolic by-products mix with and alter normally healthy tissue components. When pancreas cysts are examined by needle aspiration and found to contain mucinous material, for example, they are more likely to become cancerous. Examination of breast cyst fluids from 148 patients with fibrocystic breast disease showed high levels of PSA (prostate-specific antigen), a well-established marker of prostate cancer now found associated with breast cancer. Blood levels were not elevated in the women with fibrocystic disease, just the fluid in the cyst.

In women with breast cancer, the PSA in the blood was on average five times that of women without cancer. This suggests both that breast cysts are related to abnormalities in hormone activity and that they are protective as long as they are able to prevent the abnormal hormonal metabolites from spilling over into the blood.

Based upon this analysis, treatment would be to restore balance to the hormonal systems and prevent factors that aggravate or enlarge the cysts. Many (but not all) authorities recommend removing all possible sources of caffeine from the diet, especially coffee, tea, chocolate, and soft drinks, as they seem to irritate the condition. It may also be helpful to reduce dietary intake of hormone-fed meats. The herbal PMS treatments discussed earlier can be used to balance hormones, along with treatments used to keep the liver healthy. TCM doctors note that this problem is often associated with liver congestion. The main herb they use is **immature green tangerine peel,** also called **blue citrus peel** (qing pi or *Citrus reticulata)*. A commercial formula for breast hyperplasia, called **blue citrus tablets,** is available from ITM.

I also often suggest **kelp tablets** to make sure patients are getting sufficient iodine, and I credit this insight to holistic physician Jonathan Wright, M.D. I began recommending iodine supplementation after I listened to one of his lectures, in which he discussed the softening of patients' fibrocystic breast lumps within hours of taking a physiologic dosage of iodine solution.

Research Highlights

- In various studies, FBD patients were found to have lower intake of cholesterol, niacin, and zinc, (Vobecky et al., 1993), lower levels of blood selenium (Schrauzer et al., 1985) and higher than normal intake of caffeine (Bullough et al., 1990).

- According to one epidemiological study, "The positive association of caffeine with estrone and its inverse association with bioavailable testosterone suggest that caffeine's reported association with several chronic conditions may be mediated by an effect on endogenous sex steroids" (Ferrini and Barrett-Connor, 1996).

- Another study instructed 147 women with FBD to abstain from methylxanthines (caffeine, theophylline, and theobromine). Of the 113 patients who complied, reducing their caffeine intake substantially, 61% reported a decrease or absence of breast pain (Russell, 1989).

Menopause

In keeping with the traditions of my practice, the first thing I tell patients is that menopause, the cessation of ovulation, is not a disease, and it should be welcomed rather than feared. It is a liberating life transition, a normal slowing of hormone production after passing the childbearing years.

By the way, don't think for a minute that men don't go through their own menopausal stage. They are usually just unaware of it. Menopause can last as long as 10 years for some people. Taking artificial hormones as a form of treatment, unless specifically needed, is a much less attractive choice than increasing foods and herbs to help move the process along. Healthy diet and exercise are the best medicine and, when understood, can usually accomplish all the things hormone replacement is supposed to do with much less risk.

When ovulation ceases there is a quick drop in the production of progesterone. As a result, the following problems may gradually develop in some women:

- Atrophy of vagina, cervix, uterus, and ovaries

- Weakening of muscle control in the bladder, rectum, and sphincter muscles

- Vaginal dryness

- Redistribution of body fat

- Loss of bone mass

- Hot flashes

- Fatigue and loss of sex drive

It is common knowledge that Oriental women experience fewer menopausal symptoms than their Western counterparts. The most popular current explanation is that Asian populations consume much more soy, which is high in phytoestrogens. While I do not necessarily disagree, I think this perspective is too narrow and not fully proven. I think it more likely that the difference is due to much larger cultural, dietary, and environmental issues.

During the long period of time during which women go through menopause, they experience changes in body fat distribution. Often seen as an entirely negative and undesirable occurrence, I believe this redistribution may have some functional value. Epidemiological studies show a clear correlation between increased body fat and mortality. However, recent scientific evidence has demonstrated that fat tissue is a very active tissue, almost like an endocrine gland, secreting a variety of peptides (such as leptin), cytokines (such as tumor necrosis factor), and complement factors. In addition, fat cells store and release several chemical substrates, such as glycerol and FFA.

Although I cannot currently prove it in a laboratory (unless someone gives me a few million dollars), it makes sense to me that a healthy diet throughout life, similar to the one followed by most residents of China, creates moderate fatty stores of healthy substrates, including phytoestrogens. At menopause, moderate increases in fat distribution allow for increased levels of substrates. Slight increases in weight are not problematic because they make up for the estrogen losses resulting from decreased production.

Hot flashes are the body's attempts to mobilize its fat stores to release stored estrogens, but if the stores are not there, the flashes will increase in intensity and frequency until estrogen is supplied externally or fatty stores are increased. If the fat stores remain insufficient, the body will actively seek out and store any available fat as it enters the body, eventually leading to obesity.

We have known for a long time that mortality rates are higher for obese people than for lean people. However, we have also learned more recently that unfit lean men have a higher risk of all-cause mortality than men who are fit and obese. Once again, science is telling us to get out there and exercise. Muscle mass is associated with longevity.

Exercise directly reduces the risk of cardiovascular disease and bone loss. Therefore, in our clinic we implement the following lifestyle measures in our treatment approach to menopause symptoms:

- A healthy diet, with an emphasis on soy foods, fruits, and vegetables to increase body levels and stores of both phytoestrogens and phytoprogesterones

- Regular exercise to sustain metabolic rate and reduce risks of cardiovascular disease and bone loss (for more detailed information about preventing and treating bone loss, refer to our discussion of osteoporosis in Chapter 15)

Lifestyle changes may not always be sufficient. In more difficult cases you might try one or more of the following herbal treatments for menopause symptoms. I have found that it often takes several months of herbal treatment to relieve symptoms. The herb choices depend on the situation, and although herbs with phytoestrogenic activity are important, they are not the only choices. The idea here is to keep a free-flowing cycle of intake and elimination of hormones and hormonelike plants, allowing your body to choose the necessary amount to keep in circulation and to store. A healthy liver also has the ability to get rid of xenoestrogens, artificial estrogenlike chemicals that are the by-products of environmental pollution.

- Nai-shing's basic formula for hot flashes is **lycium bark** (which is very effective in some cases), **phellodendron bark, ligustrum fruit** (nu zhen zi or *L. lucidum*), **shou wu root, raw rehmannia root, cornus fruit** (shan zhu yu or *C. officinalis*), and **moutan bark** (mu dan pi or *Paeonia suffruticosa*). TAM doctors use **white** and **red sandalwood.**

- Use herbs with phytoestrogenic activity to build up your available stores over several months. Many extracts made from **soybeans, red clover blossoms, black cohosh root,** and **alfalfa** are now commercially available. Do not use excessive doses, and alternate different types.

- Use **pomegranates** on a semiregular basis, because they contain small amounts of estrone, a weak but true estrogen. You can eat the ripe fruit, dried seed, or juice as desired.

- Use liver herbs such as **dandelion root, bupleurum root, burdock root,** and **white peony root** to improve liver conjugation of estrogen to enhance its elimination from the body. These are also useful for mood swings.

- Use **schisandra berries** for menopausal night sweats.

- Follow the recommendations in Chapter 15 for osteoporosis, and in Chapter 12 to keep the heart healthy.

Morning Sickness

Morning sickness is the characteristic nausea experienced by many pregnant women upon awakening in the morning. For minor cases either **ginger root** or **peppermint leaf,** taken in tea form, can offer sufficient relief. If the problem is more severe, I recommend making **ginger tea** using **fresh ginger** (use a garlic press) and honey, then adding powders of **pinellia tuber, tangerine peel, poria mushroom, agastache,** and **cardamom fruit** (Sha ren or *Amomum* species). For quick temporary relief, it also helps to chew on a piece of **lemon** or **orange peel.**

Endometriosis

Endometriosis is a condition that occurs most commonly in women of reproductive age, whereby endometrial tissue appears in abnormal locations. Because this is also a hormone-related condition, the dietary recommendations, hormone-balancing strategies, and lifestyle mentioned throughout this chapter should be combined with the following TCM formula. The main goal of Nai-shing's treatment strategy for endometriosis is to strongly move the blood to flush out stagnation.

Use a formula of **dang gui root, cyperus rhizome** (xiang fu or *C. rotundus),* **leonorus** (yi mu cao or *L. heterophyllus),* **fennel seed** (xiao hui xiang or *Foeniculum vulgare),* **cnidium** (chuan xiong or *Ligusticum wallichii),* **red peony root, carthamus flower,** and **persica seed** (tao ren or *Prunus persica).* If there is pain, add **corydalis tuber** (yan hu suo or *C. yanhusuo).* This condition is difficult to treat and requires professional support.

Interstitial Cystitis

Interstitial cystitis is a chronic bladder inflammation characterized by deterioration and tightening of the urinary bladder. The symptoms are painful, frequent, and burning urination, blood in the urine, reduced urinary capacity, and generalized lower abdominal pain over the bladder area. In gross appearance, there is hyperemia (blood congestion) in the mucosa, often with exudate. Eventually, it leads to a thickening and inelasticity of the bladder wall and a persistent fibrosis. Mast cells are often predominant, which means there may be an autoimmune component.

This disease is difficult to treat, due to the complex set of symptoms. The treatment strategy we use has several components:

- To quickly reduce tension and pain in the urinary bladder, use **kava root** (standardized to 250 mg kavalactones), at a dose of one pill four times per day.

- To remove common triggers of urinary inflammation, follow the directions for eliminating food allergies mentioned in Chapter 11.

- To help reduce immune-based inflammation and heal the bladder mucosa, use moderate doses of **flaxseed** or **evening primrose oils** or other EFA supplements for up to a year or more.

- To reduce congestion and restore elasticity to the bladder, use a tincture of **stoneroot, gotu kola, horse chestnut** *(Aesculus hippocastanum),* and **agrimony** *(A. pilosa),* about 45 drops three times per day.

- Construct a major formula to remove the fibrosis and blood stagnation, relax the bladder, reduce bleeding, and reduce inflammation. Choose among **madder root** (qian cao gen or *Rubia cordifolia),* **leonorus** (yi mu cao or *L. heterophyllus),* **astragalus root, pyrrosia leaf** (shi wei or *P. lingua),* **salvia root, cinnamon twig, red peony root, long pepper, gotu kola, reishi mushroom, gardenia fruit** (zhi zi or *G. jasminoides),* and **tien chi root.**

Progress with this disease is often slow and requires patience. Stress reduction and abdominal breathing exercises are essential.

CHAPTER 19

Longevity and the Immune System

I don't want to achieve immortality through my work; I want to achieve immortality through not dying.

—Woody Allen

Longevity has been a cherished goal of humankind since the beginning of time. Perhaps the oldest known comprehensive medical text is the *Charaka Samhita,* the Ayurvedic encyclopedia compiled by the physician Charaka based upon the original work of the sage Atreya, who lived about 2,500 years ago. The book begins, "Now I shall expound upon the subject of longevity. . . . When disease appears, it creates great impediments to penance, abstinence, study, religious observance, and life span. The holy sages, out of sympathy for all living creatures, assembled at the side of the Himalayas to seek a solution."

To these ancient sages, the ideal goal was for everyone to have a blessed life. By a "blessed life" they meant a long and healthy life, with time to develop skills, extraordinary memory, intellectual abilities, spiritual knowledge, clear perception, and a deeper understanding of reality. They found herbal medicines to be one of the greatest supports for achieving this end, and many spent their entire lives searching for rejuvenating herbal tonics. Tonification and nourishment are two of the most important keys to longevity, and herbal medicine excels in this arena. As I did in Chapter 1, I will start by asking the simplest question possible.

What Is Aging?

Fortunately, I don't have to give you my own answer. In their book *Biomarkers: The 10 Determinants of Aging You Can Control,* authors Evans and Rosenberg delineate many physical biomarkers associated with the aging process, including:

- Reduced flexibility and strength
- Decreased cardiovascular endurance

- Increased body fat

- Reduced resting energy expenditure

- Reduced kidney clearance

- Reduced cell-mediated immunity

- Increased hearing threshold

- Reduced close vision and dark accommodation

- Reduced taste and smell sensitivity

- Altered hormone levels

- Increased autoantibodies

To this we can add worsening memory and concentration, lowered sex drive, and just plain old feeling old. This gives us a starting point. The next question is, can anything be done about this? It is obvious that we can delay problems with strength, body fat, cardiovascular endurance, and flexibility by utilizing such measures as diet and exercise. Looking closely, we can see that most of the other markers are directly or indirectly related to our defensive and immune system function. Moreover, a review of the research studies highlighted throughout this book shows that each and every one of the markers listed above can be affected by herbal medicines.

As we proceed through this chapter, I will describe different ways of affecting our immune system and other defenses, and I will explain individual herbs and formulas known to benefit overall defensive function, as well as formulas and herbs for specific health problems. It is important to know that, as a rule, immune tonic herbs can be used both for prolonging life in the healthy and for overcoming disease in the sick. As well, many of the same mechanisms that are related to aging are also causative of serious illness such as cancer.

Strengthening Defensive Energy

We all have trillions of immune cells and other defensive mechanisms. These are generally divided into specific immunity and other nonspecific defenses, discussed in detail below. Our complex defensive system recognizes and destroys foreign substances that enter our body. If these defenses are strong, we can weather health challenges effortlessly and avoid tissue damage.

However, if defensive components are weakened or dysfunctional for any reason, external pathogenic or toxic influences can gain inroad, which results in cellular damage and the gradual or sudden appearance of physical symptoms. Many of the health problems often attributed to the aging process, such as senility and fatigue, are caused by simple nutrient deficiencies that weaken our immune system. The importance of immunity in preventing disease and damage makes it one of the keys to longevity.

Common indicators of potential immune system problems include:

- Allergies

- Chronic fatigue

- Frequent or persistent bacterial, viral, fungal, or parasitic infections

- Inflammatory disorders of all sorts

- Increased signs of aging

Three Magic Life Nutrients and One Essential

Although the focus of this book is herbal medicine, we should not lose sight of the bigger picture. The three magic life nutrients are *clean air, clean water,* and *sunlight.* The one essential is *pure love.* As simple as this may sound, these nutrients have a direct impact on your health and your immune system. Many if not most of my patients with chronic illness have a deficiency of one or more of these nutrients. It is my contention that in the long run, concentrating on these four elements can be an extremely effective means of preventing disease.

Unfortunately, our increasingly limited access to pure air and clean water will continue to wreak havoc on the health of all living creatures. If you are able to, I strongly suggest that you go to your local library and borrow a copy of the spring 2000 special edition of *Time* magazine, entitled "How to Save the Earth." I do not have the words to explain the importance of this issue. Suffice it to say that after a thorough analysis of global statistics, according to the journal *Epidemiology*, "Our estimate is that 25–33% of the global burden of disease can be attributed to environmental risk factors," and "Children under 5 years of age seem to bear the largest environmental burden."

Longevity Begins before Conception

Let's take a look at one of the many insights of ancient Ayurveda—the series of health practices used to prepare newly married women and men for child conception. The ancient Ayurvedics believed that various forms of meditation, fasting, and tonics would support the creation of healthy babies. They also employed specific health and nutritional practices to support the mother's health during pregnancy, including the simple admonition that pregnant women should shield themselves from stressful and emotionally disturbing conditions.

Modern scientists are reporting mounting evidence to support the early wisdom that conditions in the womb can strongly affect the risk of adult disease. Scientists are now referring to these links as "fetal programming." Following are several examples:

- Researchers have recently discovered a higher likelihood of obesity in children whose mothers are starved during pregnancy.

- Doctors have found low birth weight to be a strong predictor of adult heart disease.

- There is now evidence that links certain conditions in the womb to the eventual development of breast cancer.

- Researchers have long reported a reduction in the ratio of lung volume to body weight as a result of reduced prenatal caloric and nutrient intake.

Consequently, I recommend the following preparatory practices to ensure successful conception of a healthy baby with strong lungs, heart, and immune system.

Three Steps for Strengthening the Immune System

- Assess and correct lifestyle and dietary problems and ensure proper digestion, as defined in previous chapters. Sufficient intake of all major nutrients is especially important. I recommend taking a high-potency multivitamin and mineral combination.
- Devise a whole-system herbal tonification formula according to the principles of Western, TAM, or TCM medicine based on signs and symptoms.
- Choose specific immune system herbs or nutrients based upon individual patient needs.

- Husband and wife should both adopt healthy lifestyles and engage in periods of fasting and meditation.

- Eliminate all alcohol, tobacco, and drugs to avoid poisoning your child.

- Eat adequate levels of healthy high-quality fats, carbohydrates, and proteins to avoid toxemia during pregnancy and obesity later in your child's life.

- Take a good-quality prenatal vitamin.

- TCM doctors tell us that the mother needs healthy blood to create a healthy baby. Nai-shing uses a simple combination of **dang gui root, shou wu root, cooked rehmannia root,** and **American ginseng root.**

Strengthening Defensive Energy with Herbs and Nutrients

We now know, almost intuitively, that strengthening the immune system benefits general good health and may contribute to longevity. This idea has historical roots in TCM **Fu zheng** (support the vital force) therapy, as well as Ayurvedic **rasayana** therapy. Modern extensions of the ancient ideas can be found in practices so new that they have not yet been officially named. They involve the use of nutrients and herbs to strengthen, activate, or calm immune cells and potentiate or modify specific host defense mechanisms. We already know how to do this in a general way from our ancient herbal roots, and many herbalists would argue that they have known this from day one. However, it is also clear that holistic health care practitioners are gradually learning how to do this in a more specific way. Proposed names for this concept include "immunotherapy" and "biological response modification."

Modern testing methods now allow us to identify and monitor specific changes in the components of the immune system that occur with the use of herbs and nutrients. This enables us to constantly increase our knowledge and gain more insight into how specific nutrients and herbs affect different components of the immune system.

Here is an example of how immunotherapy can work. In the phenomenon called anergy, the immune system fails to recognize a threat so it does not mount a response. Anergy poses a major problem in diseases such as cancer and AIDS, as it allows tumors or viral particles to escape immune surveillance. To do this tumors utilize a variety of methods. They release inhibitory chemicals (such as interleukin-10), as well as chemicals that induce immune cell death (apoptosis via *fas signaling*—i.e., a protein whose activation leads to cell death), and disrupt normal immune cell-to-cell interactions. Below you will see how many different herbs have been shown to affect each of these areas of immune dysfunction, giving us potential tools to overcome these problems.

TCM Fu zheng Treatment of the Immune System

Western scientists are just beginning to understand how to strengthen nonspecific host resistance. However, TCM doctors have long had practical methods for strengthening the whole organism.

The group of tonics called **Fu zheng** are used by TCM doctors specifically for this purpose. Many of the herbs in these formulas are chosen primarily from the traditional category of Qi tonics. Qi tonics strengthen the digestion, restore energy, generate fluids, and build the blood. Some of the primary **Fu zheng** herbs include **astragalus root, ganoderma mushroom, codonopsis, white atractylodes, honey-fried licorice root,** and **ginseng root.** Formulations made from these herbs can be used to strengthen the immune system and are especially useful for immune deficiency problems such as HIV or cancer.

Physicians in the Department of Pharmacology, Toxicology, and Therapeutics at the University of Kansas Medical Center, Kansas City, performed extensive screenings of the major Fu zheng formulas. They selected the "Ten Significant Herb Great Tonic Decoction" (Shi quan da gu tang), which contains **astragalus** and nine other herbs, as the most effective potent biological response modifier. This formula is used traditionally against anemia, anorexia, extreme exhaustion, fatigue, Yin deficiency, digestive weakness, and general weakness, particularly after illness.

The Formula for the Ten Significant Herb Great Tonic

Ginseng root (ren shen): 6–9 grams

White atractylodes rhizome (bai zhu): 9–12 grams

Poria mushroom (fu ling): 12–15 grams

Honey-fried licorice root (zhi gan cao): 3–6 grams

Cooked rehmannia root (shu di huang): 15–18 grams

White peony root (bai shao): 12–15 grams

Dang gui root (*Angelica sinensis*): 12–15 grams

Chuan xiong rhizome (*Ligusticum chuanxiong*): 6–9 grams

Cinnamon bark (rou gui): 6–9 grams

Astragalus root (huang qi): 15–18 grams

According to numerous studies over 8 years, the Ten Significant Herb Great Tonic formula had extremely low toxicity while exhibiting very strong immunomodulatory and immunopotentiating effects (by stimulating blood immune factors and interleukin production in association with NK cells). It is usually given as a decoction in China with some **ginger root** and **jujube date.** It has also been shown to potentiate therapeutic activity in several chemotherapies (mitomycin, cisplatin, cyclophosphamide, and fluorouracil) and radiotherapy and to inhibit the recurrence of malignancies and prolong survival in cancer cases. The formula ameliorates or prevents the side effects, including GI disturbances such as anorexia, nausea, vomiting, hematotoxicity, immunosuppression, leukopenia, thrombocytopenia, anemia, and nephropathy, of many anticancer drugs.

Ayurvedic Rasayana Treatment

Ayurvedic medicine is divided into eight basic sections. The **Rasayana Tantra** is the section on rejuvenating medicines. Study in this section focused on two areas—the lives of sages and the uses and benefits of the rejuvenating or divine plants. Any herb or formula called **rasayana** is a strong tonic which is safe and can rejuvenate you and prolong your life. An examination of the story behind the early historical use of these plants offers us valuable lessons concerning the destructive effects of human attitudes and actions on precious plants.

According to Dr. Mana, among the 600 Ayurvedic herbs that have been thoroughly tested and analyzed, Ayurvedic physicians used about 50 plants specifically for "immortal life" (longevity), and the rest for medicinal purposes. Ancient scholars believed that, when used properly, these plants could extend survival for long periods of time. The Vedas (holy books), Puranas (mythological books), and Ayurvedic texts talk a lot about these plants, their extraordinary effects, and the proper ways to use them. The general term for these plants was *Soma,* meaning divine lunar cycle plants. Knowledge of their identity and locations in the forest was kept very secret, known only to a limited group of people. Historically, Sudras (persons of low caste) were never allowed access to these plants. Only learned priests, warriors, and rich businesspeople were permitted to use them, to increase their power and influence (like today).

The Sanskrit names of the most important Soma plants are Amshuman, Rajataprabha, Munjavan, Chandrama, Garudaharita, Swetaksha, Durvasoma, Kaniya, Kanakaprabha, Pratanavan, Talvrinta, Karavirya, Gayatrya, Traistubha, Panktya, Jagata, Tripadgayatrya, and Udupati. The plants in this group were said to have had 15 leaves, and the growing and falling of these leaves depended upon the cycles of the moon. To extend life and increase vitality, people drank the juice of the plant tubers.

Unfortunately, we can no longer locate these plants. Dr. Mana states that the ancient monopoly of use was the most likely cause. We do have written descriptions of a few of these plants that might possibly still be available, though they have not been seen for a long time. It is more likely that every last one of these powerful plants has been eradicated from the Himalayan areas where they used to flourish. This is yet another heartbreaking example of the disappearance of precious plants due to human greed.

Rasayana Plants Used Today

Fortunately, there are still some tonic rasayana plants that can help us today. The primary rasayana plants available include **pueraria tuber** *(Pueraria lobata),* **shilajatu, licorice root, long pepper, gotu kola, guggul gum, amla fruit, vibhitaki fruit, ashwagandha root, guduchi stem, bala, haritaki fruit, gokshura fruit, aguru wood, punarnava** *(Boerhavia diffusa),* and **hastikarnapalasa** *(Butea monosperma).*

There are many classical Ayurvedic tonic formulas in widespread use in India and Nepal. Some of the best-known tonics are **Chayavanaprash** (Chayavana rasyayna), **Amalaka rasayana, Nagabala rasayana, Shilajatu rasayana,** and **Guggul rasayana. Chayavanaprash** is now available in many health food stores and Indian grocery stores in America.

Over the years, researchers have studied the adaptogenic value and potential of rasayana plants from all over the world. Scientists at the Ayurveda Research Centre in Mumbai, India, evaluated the adaptogenic potential of six of the above Ayurvedic rasayana plants. They used the whole, aqueous, standardized extracts in animal experiments, testing the ability of these plants to exert a normalizing effect, irrespective of direction of pathological change. They discovered that the plants offered protection against a variety of biological, physical, and chemical stressors, as indicated by markers of stress responses and objective parameters for stress manifestations.

Shilajatu Rasayana Formula for Long Life/Anticancer

This is the classic formula for a well-known Ayurvedic rasayana tonic. Note that the rasayana tonic herbs **shilajatu** and **guggul gum** are the main ingredients, with small amounts of many other herbs, especially digestive aids.

Ingredients

- *One part each* **camphor leaves** *(Cinnamomum camphora)*, **vacha root** *(Acorus calamus)*, **mustaka rhizome** *(Cyperus rotundus)*, **kiratatiktam** *(Swertia chirata)*, **guduchi stem, devadaru wood** *(Cedrus deodara)*, **turmeric root, purified atis tuber** *(Aconitum heterophyllum)*, **daruharidra bark** *(Berberis nepalensis)*, **pipali root** *(Piper longum)*, **chitraka** *(Plumbago zeylanicum)*, **coriander seed** (dhanyakam or *C. sativum)*, **gajapippali** *(Piper chava)*, **vidanga seeds** *(Embelia ribes)*, **karipippuli** *(Scindaprus officinalis)*, **trikatu, gold ore oxide** (maksika bhasma), **barley plant alkali** (yavakshara), **yavasa alkali** *(Alhagi mourorum)*, **mineral salt** (saindhavam), **sea salt** (samudram), and salt made with **amla fruit.**
- *4 parts each* **trivrit root** *(Operculina turpenthum)*, **danti seeds** *(Baliospermum montanum)*, **patram leaves** *(Cinnamomum tamala)*, **cinnamon bark** (twak or *C. zeylanicum)*, **cardamom** (sukshmaila or *Elettaria cardamomum)*, and **bamboo manna** (vamsa or *Bambusa* species).
- *8 parts* **iron oxide** (lauha bhasma)
- *16 parts* **rock sugar**
- *64 parts* **shilajatu**
- *32 parts* **guggul gum**

Preparation: 1-gram pill

Dose: 2 or 3 pills two to three times per day with warm water

This formula is available from your Ayurvedic practitioner or from Chrysalis Natural Medicine Pharmacy (see Resource Guide).

Free Radical Theory

Life depends upon the proper combination of oxygen with food nutrients to create and release energy. It is through this process that we see the never-ending interplay between creative/nutritive forces and destructive/metabolic heat forces, echoing back to the eternal ideas of Yin and Yang, and Vata, Pitta, and Kapha.

Free radicals are highly reactive molecules that contain an odd number of electrons. These dangerous chemicals can damage cells, cell membrane surfaces, and even our genetic material (DNA). If you imagine your body as a house, you can think of free radicals as iron Ping-Pong balls bouncing around inside, knocking over lamps, denting the furniture, and chipping the paint on the walls.

However, free radicals are not always completely bad. Your body generates these molecules as by-products when your immune system destroys bacteria, viruses, and other foreign substances. Up to 5% of the oxygen we consume is transformed into free radicals.

The free radical called "superoxide" is the most reactive of all these chemicals. Your body uses a naturally occurring enzyme called SOD (superoxide dismutase) to destroy (quench) this reactive superoxide, thus protecting you from the millions of free radical "hits" each of your cells endures each second of your life. This quenching process leads to the production of hydrogen peroxide, which your body consequently eliminates with another antioxidant enzyme called catalase (CAT). These antioxidants are different from the well-known vitamin antioxidants (A, C, and E) in that they are synthesized by cells rather than supplied from without. Vitamins are cofactors (or coenzymes) which aid enzyme functioning. Other important cellular antioxidants are glutathione peroxidase and methionine reductase.

This sort of free radical damage is believed to be a primary cause of aging, especially when it affects nerve cells. Scientists can measure the levels of another chemical called malondialdehyde (MDA), a product of lipid peroxidation, to determine the extent of cell membrane damage.

The authors of the groundbreaking book *Antioxidant Adaptation: Its Role in Free Radical Pathology* propose a four-stage process of bodily self-defense. In stage one we are healthy but inundated by chemicals from our air, water, and food supplies. Eventually our defenses give out, and we begin to suffer ill health, indicating a decline into stage two. It becomes more difficult to stay healthy; we are more susceptible to infection, allergy, and stress; and our energy levels decrease. Then we get to stage three, where we are in the midst of a disease process and suffer from symptoms on a daily basis. In stage four tissue, destruction continues to the point where we become susceptible to increased aging processes and serious diseases like cancer.

We can reduce free radical damage by simply maintaining high antioxidant levels. This is accomplished easily by following a healthy diet high in fresh fruits and vegetables and avoiding unhealthy foods like low-quality fats and oils and stale food, which can contribute to the generation of free radicals, such as lipid peroxides (LPO).

To quickly build up your body's supply of the four major cellular antioxidants, I recommend **wheat sprouts** (see Chapter 2 for a detailed description), which are especially rich in SOD, glutathione peroxidase, catalase, and methionine reductase. One of the common misunderstandings I encounter daily in my clinic is thinking that individual antioxidants are panaceas. If you imagine a cell undergoing excessive free radical damage as a house on fire, then antioxidants are like giants who can dump water on the fire. Therefore, it would logically follow that a single giant with a big water bucket could handle the entire problem. This is why people sometimes prefer to take megadoses of individual vitamins. Unfortunately, the process of quenching free radicals works more like a bucket brigade. Many ordinary-sized people (equivalent to moderate amounts of numerous antioxidants) will quench the fire more effectively and more quickly than would a single "giant" (a megadose of one substance). This is very similar to what we get when we formulate herbs or simply eat diets high in fresh fruits and vegetables.

Research Highlights

- A controlled clinical trial treated elderly senile patients with a **cordyceps mushroom extract.** The subjects' levels of SOD were markedly lower than in younger patients, while levels of a free radical known as MDA were higher. The treatment significantly increased the SOD activity and significantly decreased MDA levels. Numerous symptoms declined, including dizziness, leg weakness, frequent urination, and coldness (Zhang ZJ et al., 1997).

- In a single-blind clinical trial of 45 elderly males who exhibited signs of aging (Kidney Yang deficiency), subjects were treated for 3 months with TCM tonics. Several immune parameters increased significantly, as did levels of plasma adrenocortical hormone (ACTH), testosterone (T), and cyclic adenosine monophosphate (cAMP). Blood levels of SOD also increased while LPO levels decreased. These results showed the herbs increased antioxidant levels and endocrine function (Yin GY, et al., 1995).

- In another single-blind clinical trial, 71 elderly patients were treated with two different forms of **American ginseng root** in an alcohol base. The blood cell SOD activity and SOD/LPO ratio increased remarkably, while blood levels of LPO decreased significantly in both groups. A calculation of functional physiological age showed that aging reversed by an average of about 8 months (Cui and Chen, 1991).

- In one study, researchers selected 80 men between the ages of 60 and 80 years with no overt disease who exhibited signs and symptoms of Kidney Yin deficiency. They administered a Yin tonic formula to 50 participants and a placebo to the remaining 30. Blood samples were taken before and after the treatment and were measured for levels of LPO, SOD, glutathione peroxidase (GP), and several hormones, including testosterone. For purposes of comparison, they performed the same tests on blood samples from 33 men in their 20s. Prior to treatment, subjects had elevated levels of LPO and female hormones and reduced levels of SOD, GP, and testosterone. After treatment for 5 weeks, there was a "remarkable" reduction of LPO and estrogen, and an increase in SOD and testosterone. Researchers concluded that the tonic retarded the aging process (Wang XM and Xie ZF, 1992).

The Immune System

The body's immune system is primarily responsible for protecting the body against foreign substances or organisms. To do this, it must distinguish between self and not-self. As currently understood, this complex system involves many, many organs, cells, systems, and chemicals that help protect the body against infection and disease. This is done through both specific **cellular immunity** and other nonspecific defense mechanisms. **Nonspecific immunity** (also called **natural immunity**) developed first in our evolution, which may account for its less specific action. Some natural immunity cells, like Kupffer cells, remain primarily in the liver where they neutralize toxins of all sorts. Our much more specific **cellular immunity** developed later and works like a well-trained detective squad which, after getting fingerprints and collecting crime scene evidence, identifies and arrests only specific, targeted criminals. In a strict scientific sense, only cellular immunity is called the immune system. However, for the purposes of this book, we will consider both specific and nonspecific defensive mechanisms to be coordinated arms of the body's overall immune system.

In this sense, the immune system as a whole consists of the lymph system organs, the white blood cells, and various specialized cells and chemicals such as antibodies. Think of it as a large army with many soldiers, tanks, guns, planes, bombs, computers, and various other resources. Many serious diseases, including HIV, Chronic Fatigue Immune Dysfunction Syndrome (CFIDS), candidiasis, multiple chemical sensitivities (MCS), chronic viral infections, and cancer are characterized by chronic immune system dysfunction.

Most of the studies listed in this chapter are pharmacological studies done in test tubes or studies done on animals. A few are high-quality double-blind clinical trials done on humans. As we stated before, scientific evidence from pharmacological and animal studies gives us clues about the expected actions of herbs but is not definitive by any stretch of the imagination. Human clinical trials are of much greater importance. For example, certain chemicals which inhibit histamine release from rat mast cells do not do the same thing in human cells, while others do. Also, because of the sparse investigation of many herbs to date, there will no doubt emerge many, many more herbs than those listed here as examples that have effects on all aspects of immunity. This information helps our evolving understanding, but always, always look to traditional understandings to know how to apply herbs in a clinical situation.

Since time immemorial, herbal medicines have excelled at improving weak immune function and toning down an overactive immune system. Our understanding of how and why this is true is advancing every day. The immune system is more than the cells and organs of which it consists. As always, it must be viewed in the context of the greater whole, and, like all other parts of the body, it depends on food choices, digestion, exercise, and mental attitude.

A Broad Understanding

In the simplest of simple understanding, the immune system can be overactive or underactive, in exact concordance with the ancient concepts of excess and deficiency. Immune deficiency states render us more susceptible to infections and tumors, and immune overactivity makes us vulnerable to unnecessary inflammation and tissue destruction.

Another aspect of immune dysfunction is now being recognized in diseases such as amyloidosis, in which abnormal deposits of proteins from fragments of immunoglobulins appear in tissues. Recalling that one of the purposes of the classic divisions of Ayurveda is to help us recognize universal patterns within the whole, we can divide immune problems into three large categories for ease of understanding:

- **Vata immune dysfunction:** immune deficiency where there is a failure to respond and regulate properly. Here it is often necessary to strengthen (nourish) or stimulate (wake up) immune and/or nervous system function, increasing immune cell numbers and activation.

- **Pitta immune dysfunction:** immune overactivity where there is a preponderance of destructive inflammation and heat. Here it is often necessary to calm (down-regulate) immune function and reduce inflammatory chemicals, mediators, and triggers.

- **Kapha immune dysfunction:** immune-related problems where abnormal secretions, growths, deposits, or plaques form quickly or over time. Here it is often necessary to reduce coagulation, break up stagnation, and improve circulation.

This is just one of many ways to think about the big picture. Having a global perspective such as this is important when trying to figure out treatments. Understanding the larger, more basic relationships allows one to see complex relationships that occur at different levels. For example, it is well known in Ayurvedic medicine that when Pitta increases, Vata and Kapha tend to decrease. Ayurvedic doctors noticed this when patients with inflammatory diseases developed digestive problems and/or nervous-related symptoms and vice versa. It is now known that at the cellular level, proinflammatory cytokine chemicals (discussed below) "reprogram" metabolism and are directly linked to altered nutrient uptake and utilization. In general, anabolic (Kapha) processes are interrupted or slowed and catabolic (Pitta) activities are amplified.

These observations have important clinical implications, and gave Ayurvedic practitioners philosophical "permission" to develop colon and digestive system treatments for seemingly unrelated inflammatory and nervous system problems eons ago. This cause is now being championed by researchers like Dr. Jeffrey Bland, author of the wonderful groundbreaking monthly tape series called *Functional Medicine Update* (see Resource Guide for more information).

Specific Understanding

Deficits or defects in specific immune cells favor specific types of infections. For example, a T-cell deficiency increases your chances of getting bacterial sepsis, CMV, Epstein-Barr, and yeast infections. A B-cell defect or deficiency increases your susceptibility to *Streptococci*, *Staphylococci,* enteroviral encephalitis, intestinal giardiasis, and chronic meningitis. Your general immunological characteristics, such as your ABO blood type, can affect your susceptibility to specific diseases. People with Type O blood get more peptic ulcers because the markers on the surface of their blood cells make it easier for *H. pylori* to attach to their stomach lining. Similarly, people with Type A blood get more gastric cancer. Because plant proteins called lectins bind to the surface of your cells and act like specific antibodies, there is no doubt that your blood type can also partially determine your individual response to specific herbs. In fact, the plants themselves use similar sensitive chemical recognition mechanisms to activate defense-related genes just as we do. This can certainly help explain why some people react differently to certain herbs and foods than do others, and is a fascinating area for future herbal research.

The Immune System and Herbs

Many people still believe that the effects of herbs either are very weak or can only stimulate or suppress immune function in a general way. We are now learning that individual herbs have powerful and often very specific effects on immune function—another exciting area of natural medicine. The ability to see these effects both in the clinic, with regard to blood tests and patient response, and in the laboratory is gradually changing our understanding toward greater respect for herbal medicines, awareness of potential dangers, and a desire to understand in greater detail what these medicines are capable of doing. However, it is still true that herbs, because they are complexes, tend to act in multifaceted ways.

Introducing the Immune System Team

The two arms of the immune system contain important blood cell players and important molecular weapons and signaling chemicals. The two most important white blood cell components are **lymphocytes** and **macrophages,** and the most important molecular chemical components are **antibodies** and **cytokines.** Lymphocyte blood cells work with antibody chemicals to destroy *specific* antigens (foreign particles) in **cellular immunity.** Macrophage blood cells work with cytokine chemicals for *general* destruction of invaders, damaged cells, and debris in **nonspecific immunity.** We will call the two branches of the immune system Team Cellular and Team Nonspecific.

Cellular Immune System Players

The White Blood Cells of Team Cellular

T-lymphocytes (T-cells) are formed in the thymus gland. T-cells comprise 60–70% of the lymphocytes in your blood. Each T-cell contains a genetically programmed receptor that allows it to recognize a specific "bad guy" antigen. Along with neutrophils (see below), T-cell proliferation acts as an aggressive first-strike process. T-lymphocytes and neutrophils are the body's primary specific defenses. There are three basic types of T-cells, which fit neatly into the Vata, Pitta, and Kapha overview:

- *Killer T-cells* (our aggressive Pitta T-cells) travel to the site of a problem, where their cell surface receptors allow them to target and release killing chemicals into our own cells that are damaged, infected, or cancerous. They release other chemicals that attract phagocytes to the area, as well as interferons, which prevent viral replication.

- Our Vata-like T-cells, or *helper T-cells,* work more as messengers, helping the killer T-cells to do their job. They secrete IL-2 (described below), which amplifies the immune response and "tells" the body to grow more killer T-cells. There are two forms of helper T-cells, called Th_1 and Th_2. Th_1 cells focus on response to bacteria, viruses, fungi, and parasites. Th_2 cells focus on allergic reactions.

- Kapha-like *suppressor T-cells* slowly arrive on the scene, sometimes days or weeks after an infection, where they suppress and turn off the killer T-cells. If suppressor T-cells are low, the inflammation continues and damages the body.

Garlic bulb, katuki rhizome *(Picrorhiza kurroa),* **ginseng root, scute root, astragalus root, shiitake mushroom** *(Lentinus edodes),* **cuscuta seed** (tu si zi or *C. chinensis),* **pycnogenol** (from *Pinus maritima),* and **licorice root** are among the many herbs and phytochemicals that have been shown to activate or modulate T-cells.

B-lymphocytes (B-cells) are produced in the bone marrow (of adults) and distributed to outlying lymph tissue (spleen, tonsils, gastrointestinal tract, etc.). They constitute 10–20% of the lymphocyte population in the blood. When some B-cells encounter and bind to foreign antigens, they are activated and transform into plasma cells, which produce a vast amount of antibodies (IgG, IgA, IgE, IgM, etc.) specific to that particular invader. Other B-cells transform into memory cells, which patrol the body for the next appearance of the bad guy antigen so they can signal a quick response.

Licorice root, ginseng root, ashwagandha root, Siberian ginseng root bark, astragalus root, oldenlandia (bai hua she she cao or *O. diffusa),* **pycnogenol, carthamus flower,** and several types of **seaweed** (particularly *Hizikia fusiformis,* a kind of algae, and *Meristotheca papulosa)* have been shown experimentally to modulate the activity of B-cells.

The Chemicals Used by Team Cellular

Antibodies are specific immunoglobulin proteins that act against the foreign substances called **antigens**. The antibody attaches to the invader, creating an antibody-antigen complex, after which it stimulates the immune system to recognize the invader. Think of the antibody as the "Neighborhood Watch 1" member who grabs a criminal in the street, holds on, and yells for the police. Antibody response can be either primary, occurring at the first exposure to an antigen, or secondary, after exposure to the same or similar antigen at a later date. This is called "sensitization." It is the reason that certain pollens, for example, affect only people who have become sensitized. The most common antibodies tested for by physicians are called "IgG," "IgA," and "IgE." High levels in the blood indicate you are fighting an invader.

A few of the many herbs shown experimentally to modulate antibody response include **rehmannia root, cuscuta seed, punarnava root** *(Boerhavia diffusa),* **echinacea root, goldenseal root, cordyceps mushroom, ginseng root, berberine** (from *Berberis* species plants), **bitter melon** *(Momordica charanta),* **ziziphus seed** (suan sao ren or *Z. spinosa),* **cowhage seeds** (kapikachu or *Mucuna pruriens),* and **guduchi stem** *(Tinospora cordifolia).*

In one dramatic (but unreplicated) study, a TCM formula containing **leonorus** (yi mu cao or *L. heterophyllus),* **white peony root, banksia rose** *(Rosa banksia),* **angelica root** (bai zhi or *A. archangelica),* and **Sichuan lovage root** *(Ligusticum chuanxiong)* was shown to prevent hemolytic disease caused by maternal-fetal blood group (Rh-type) incompatibility.

IgA (immunoglobulin type A) is an antibody found primarily in the secretions of mucosal surfaces, including those of the upper respiratory tract and the digestive tract, and in tears. There is IgA in mother's milk, which helps protect the delicate upper respiratory and gastrointestinal tracts of infants. Consequently, breastfeeding helps protect against allergies and infections. Think of IgA as your body's "Neighborhood Watch 2" member who signals the immune system at the first sign of an invader's arrival on the surface of your mucous membranes. His job: to prevent the degradation of the epithelial membrane surfaces in your mouth, lungs, and intestinal tract, which could reduce IgA levels and enable foreign proteins and microbes to settle in.

Scute root and **licorice root** increase IgA supply. Carotenes and vitamin A are essential for IgA. A TCM Yin-tonifying formula containing **cornus fruit** (shan zhu yu or *C. officinalis),* **dioscorea, moutan, poria mushroom, cooked rehmannia root, water plantain rhizome** (ze xie or *Alisma plantago-aquatica),* **schisandra berry,** and **honey-fried astragalus root** has been shown to significantly stimulate small intestine IgA secretion in an animal model.

IgG (immunoglobulin type G) is the most abundant antibody in the blood serum, composing about 60–70% of the total. In the early stages of infection, increasing IgG can improve the speed of the immune response. In many cases of chronic inflammation and allergy it is important to modulate IgG response downward to reduce the inflammation.

White atractylodes, licorice root, kochia fruit (Di fu zi or *Kochia scoparia),* and **guduchi stem** have been shown to modulate IgG response. Long-term oral administration of **ginseng root** extracts has also been shown in animal experiments to decrease certain subtypes of IgG, such as IgG1, IgG2a, IgG2b, and IgG3. Additionally, a clinical trial of the traditional treatment for the common cold, using **echinacea root** and **goldenseal root** *(Hydrastis canadensis),* increased production of IgG and IgM.

IgE (immunoglobulin type E) is found primarily in the linings of the respiratory and intestinal tract. It binds to mast cells and basophils and stimulates the release of inflammatory substances (such as histamine), making it the most common "neighborhood watch" member concerned with allergic reactions.

Echinacea, garlic bulb, ginkgo leaf, feverfew, goldenseal root, er bu shir tsao herb *(Centipeda minima),* **rehmannia root, salvia root,** and **turmeric root** are among the many herbs that may reduce or inhibit IgE-mediated allergic reactions. In one study, a water extract of an herbal formula prepared from the very cold TCM herbs **scute root, coptis rhizome** *(C. japonica),* **phellodendron bark,** and **gardenia fruit** (zhi zi or *G. jasminoides)* suppressed anaphylactic histamine release in a dose-dependent manner.

Nonspecific Immunity Players

The Blood Cells of Team Nonspecific

Phagocyte is a general term for the white blood cells that engulf and digest foreign bodies in a nonspecific manner (a process called phagocytosis). These cells either are chemically attracted to sites of inflammation by the release of histamine and other messengers into the blood, or lie in wait at specific locations. They are easiest to understand if you think of them as vacuum cleaners or vultures.

There are two types, based upon size—smaller microphages, which primarily ingest bacteria, and the larger macrophages, which gobble up and digest dead tissue and cellular debris. Phagocytes also release pyrogens, chemicals that induce fever in response to infection.

Monocytes, the precursors of **macrophages,** comprise about 3–7% of the circulating white blood cells. Macrophages are actually monocytes that have taken up residence in specific tissue areas such as the liver, spleen, connective tissue, or lymph nodes. In the liver, they are called "Kupffer cells"; in the skin, they are called "Langerhans cells"; in the spleen and lymph nodes they are called dendritic cells; in the lung they are called alveolar macrophages; in the connective tissue they are called histiocytes; in the brain they are called microglia.

Macrophages are capable of fusing together into huge **granulomas** to combat and engulf larger pathogens. All the above-mentioned phagocytic cells are collectively known as the reticuloendothelial system (RES).

Many, many herbs have been shown to increase the numbers and action of phagocytes, including **ginseng root, rehmannia root, isatis root, codonopsis root** (dang shen), **mistletoe** *(Viscum album),* **cordyceps mushroom, cat's claw inner bark** *(Uncaria tomentosa),* **licorice root, astragalus root, celosia seed, guduchi stem, ashwagandha root, olive leaf extract, garlic bulb, ganoderma mushroom, Siberian ginseng root bark, maitake mushroom, lycium fruit, white atractylodes,** and **echinacea.**

According to a systematic study of more than 200 TCM herbs and formulas used for Qi energy tonification, *all* had the ability to increase the phagocytic index of the RES from two to five times above normal.

Natural killer (NK) cells make up approximately 15% of all circulating white blood cells. They roam the body and are capable of acting spontaneously, rather than in response to orders from other immune components (such as antibodies). Individual NK cells can be compared to Dirty Harry: more deadly than even cytotoxic T-cells, NK cells are very important first-line fighters of cancer and AIDS. In fact, the level of NK activity is a good estimator of chances of survival in these types of deadly diseases. NK cells release interferons, chemicals that interfere with viral replication. A weakening or cessation of function in NK cells indicates that death is near.

Many herbs, especially medicinal mushrooms like **maitake mushroom, ganoderma mushroom, and shiitake mushroom,** are known to strongly increase NK cell activity. Other herbs that stimulate NK cell function include **celosia seeds, licorice root, garlic bulb, ziziphus fruit, ginseng root, gymnostemma, Western larch bark,** and **mistletoe.**

Neutrophils are short-lived cells stored in the bone marrow and called into action to prevent and treat bacterial infections. These aggressive cells engulf and destroy bacteria, fungi, parasites, foreign particulate matter, and cancerous cells, destroying themselves in the process. You can think of them as the body's kamikaze cells.

Garlic oil, ginseng root, guduchi stem, shiitake mushroom, black cumin seed (krisnajirakam or *Nigella sativa),* and **mistletoe** have been shown to increase neutrophil activity. Cooling herbs like **scrophularia root** (xuan shen or *S. ningpoensis)* reduce neutrophil activity, an important mechanism for controlling some inflammations.

Eosinophils and **basophils,** like other immune cells, secrete a wide variety of toxic chemicals that break down and destroy antigen-antibody complexes related to allergy. Basophils, for example, release heparin and histamine. Eosinophils release several major basic proteins, eosinophil cationic protein, eosinophil-derived neurotoxin, and eosinophil peroxidase. All of these chemicals can cause tissue injury in prolonged inflammation.

Boswellia gum, ephedra, feverfew, perilla leaves, and **turmeric root extract** all affect eosinophil function, as does the patent medicine **Pe Min Kan Wan** and several other TCM classical formulas. The TCM **Minor Blue-green Dragon Formula**—composed of **ephedra, cinnamon twig, ginger root, Chinese wild ginger** (xi xin or *Asarum sieboldii),* **schisandra berry, white peony root, pinellia tuber,** and **licorice root**—is traditionally used by TCM doctors for fever and chills, coughing, asthma, chronic bronchitis, wheezing, and flu. Its well-known effectiveness for these conditions may be due to the fact that it has been shown to significantly down-regulate eosinophils in animal studies.

In an article appearing in the journal *Carcinogenesis,* the combination of an antibiotic (ampicillin) and **Minor Bupleurum Decoction (bupleurum root, scute root, pinellia tuber, ginger root, ginseng root,** and **jujube fruit)** was tested for its effect on lung cancer formation in rats given a cancer-causing chemical. The combination was found to inhibit cancer formation completely. No tests have been done on humans so far.

Mast cells are tissue-based cells that have an affinity for blood vessels. They are activated when antigens bind to their surface IgE receptors, causing allergic reactions. Like basophils, they release histamine and other chemicals that increase vascular permeability and allow other immune cells to enter the tissues from the bloodstream. In chronic allergic situations, it is important to stabilize mast cell activity.

Among the many, many herbs that seem to help stabilize or inhibit the activity of mast cells are **shilajatu, aguru wood, licorice root, ganoderma mushroom, ginkgo leaf, cooked rehmannia root, er bu shir tsao herb** *(Centipeda minima),* **lavender oil, xi xian cao herb** *(Siegesbeckia pubescens),* **gunja seed** *(Abrus precatorius),* **katuki rhizome** *(Picrorhiza kurroa),* **salvia root, devadaru** *(Cedrus deodara),* **aged garlic extract, andrographis** (chuan xin lian or *A. paniculata),* **vasaca leaf** *(Adhatoda vasica),* and **milk thistle seed.**

In one study, the phytochemicals luteolin, baicalein, and quercetin were shown to inhibit the release of histamine, leukotrienes, and other immune chemicals from mast cells in a dose-dependent manner. Luteolin was the most potent. Dr. Duke's database reveals that luteolin is found in many anti-inflammatory plants, including **celery seed** *(Apium graveolens),* **water plantain, wild indigo, arjuna bark, buddleia flowers, echinacea, ginkgo leaf, devil's claw root, flaxseed, honeysuckle flower, peppermint leaf,** and **grapes.**

The Molecules Used by Team Nonspecific

Immune response involves multiple interactions between phagocytes, NK cells, basophils, neutrophils, and so on. Many of these responses happen from cell-to-cell contact. Nearby, however, interactions depend upon immune system messenger molecules called **cytokines.** The number of these chemicals is huge. Among the things they do are attack viruses, initiate nonspecific anti-inflammatory effects, up-regulate immune response, down-regulate immune response, activate immune cells, attract immune cells, stimulate blood cell formation, and interfere with viral replication. Cytokines secreted by monocytes are called monokines, and cytokines secreted by lymphocytes are called lymphokines.

As you might expect, many herbs affect cytokines in general and specific ways. Among the herbs that affect cytokines are several from the **immunity/longevity group—ginseng root, mistletoe, cooked rehmannia root, astragalus root, garlic bulb,** numerous **medicinal mushrooms, marine algae,** and **echinacea.**

Interferons are chemicals secreted by cells as a result of viral infection. These chemicals signal the killer T-cells to increase activity and, as their name implies, to interfere with viral replication and help noninfected cells resist viral penetration. There are three primary classes of interferons—"alpha," "beta," and "gamma"—as well as various subsets. Most cells can secrete interferon.

Herbs that have been shown to directly enhance interferon activity include **ginseng root, garlic bulb, mistletoe, ashwagandha root, noni fruit** *(Morinda citrifolia),* and numerous herbal formulas.

Interleukins are proteins that stimulate white blood cell activity. There are dozens of different kinds of interleukins. Think of them as immune system coffee. Interleukin-1 helps produce fever. Interleukin-2, also known as T-cell growth factor, is very important. This is because it not only stimulates T-cell production but also exerts potent effects related to nerve cell growth, survival, and bioelectric activities

Herbs or herbal extracts shown to modulate production of interleukins, by themselves or in formulas, include **ginseng root, astragalus root, bupleurum root, cordyceps mushroom, mistletoe, ashwagandha root, rehmannia root, garlic bulb, celosia seeds, sophora flower** (huai hua mi or *S. japonica*), **black cumin seed,** and **cat's claw inner bark.**

Complement is a group of blood proteins that helps to destroy invaders. Complement works like a tag team, releasing each protein sequentially. Complement proteins attach macrophages or neutrophils to antigen-antibody complexes. Think of the process as chaining a watchdog to a burglar who's broken into your home.

The complement cascade is also capable of burning holes into the invader.

Medicinal mushrooms that contain beta-glucan, such as **ganoderma** and **maitake,** enhance complement activity. Herbs containing rosmarinic acid, such as **prunella** (xie ku cao or *P. vulgaris)* and **bugleweed** *(Lycopus virginicus),* inhibit complement activation. The heartwood of **su mu** (*Caesalpinia sappan*), used traditionally in China to reduce swelling, pain, and numbness, also inhibits complement activation.

Tumor necrosis factor (TNF) is a chemical released by macrophages (TNF-alpha) and activated T-cells (TNF-beta). It causes fever and can kill some types of cancer cells by attacking their blood vessels. Other variegated systemic effects include increased sleep and decreased appetite. In some cases of cancer, overproduction of TNF-alpha leads to cachexia, a pathological state of appetite suppression and weight loss.

Dandelion root, ginseng root extracts, mistletoe, several types of **seaweed, garlic root** and **aged garlic extract, scute root, schizonepeta** (jing jie or *S. tenuifolia),* **carthamus flower,** and **ganoderma mushrooms** have been found to stimulate TNF. Conversely in animal and pharmacological models, **green tea, cooked rehmannia root, coptis root, milk thistle seed extract, ashwagandha root, turmeric root extract** (three different compounds) were all found either to inhibit TNF-alpha production and/or to block some of TNF's inflammatory actions.

The Lymphatic System

Lymphatic system is a collective name for the various lymph tissues and cells in the body. The central lymph tissues include the thymus gland, the bone marrow, the lymph nodes, the spleen and tonsils, and compartments found behind the epithelial layer of the gastrointestinal mucosa called gut-associated lymphoid tissue (GALT), described briefly in

Chapter 11. Our understanding of the importance of lymph tissue in immunological function throughout the body is gradually increasing, as researchers focus on the functions of LALT (larynx-associated lymphoid tissue), MALT (mucosa-associated lymphoid tissue), and VALT (vascular-associated lymphoid tissue).

I think of these lymph tissues as immune governments or police stations, where lymphocytes go to get their orders, identify criminals, coordinate activities, transmit information, and receive nutritional paychecks.

Lymph System Components

Lymph is a clear, colorless, alkaline fluid that circulates through the body along our lymph vessels. TAM doctors call lymph "sweet water." The liver produces about one-third of the lymph and the intestine another sixth. The rest is produced in tissue spaces throughout the body.

The lymph vessels contain filtration nodes where immune system cells gather to destroy foreign bodies, especially bacteria and cancer cells. They also drain the villi in the intestinal tract. Tiny lymph capillaries originate in distant parts of the body and form into lymph vessels as they flow, in one direction only. The vessels get larger as they move toward the center of the body, finally converging into the large thoracic lymph duct, which emptys into the largest vein in the body, the vena cava.

The thymus gland is a soft pinkish gray gland that sits above the heart and serves as the maturation host for T-cells. It helps in the production of T-lymphocytes, strong white blood cells that help the body resist infection by bacteria, fungi, and viruses. The thymus also secretes hormones that regulate immune function. The thymus gland requires a sufficient supply of zinc in order to function properly. Oysters are a rich source of this mineral, providing approximately 150 mg in a 3.5-oz serving.

Many herbs have been shown to enhance thymus activity, including **echinacea, ginseng root, neem leaf, Siberian ginseng root bark,** and **licorice root.** Herbs containing triterpenoid saponins also generally stimulate the thymus gland. These herbs include **ganoderma** and **poria mushrooms, ginseng root, bupleurum root,** and **licorice,** as well as herbs found in many Yin tonics for the lung, such as opiopogon and **anemarrhena rhizome** (zhi mu or *Anemarrhena asphodeloides).*

The most voluminous lymph-related (lymphoid) organ in the body is the **GALT** or **gut-associated lymphoid tissue.** This tissue is a separate mesoderm-derived compartment located directly behind your intestinal membranes, and its function is to maintain a diverse population of healthy lymphocytes capable of responding to the enormous numbers of antigens that enter your body every time you eat. Special M-cells efficiently envelop these macromolecules and microorganisms from the intestine and deliver them to the underlying GALT. This process produces a huge quantity of immunoglobulins, which are necessary for your immune system to properly tag each and decide whether to allow it safe passage (tolerance) or mark it for destruction. Think of the GALT as your body's own Immigration and Naturalization Service.

According to an article appearing in the *Journal of the American Medical Association,* problems in the GALT have been associated with inflammatory bowel disease, Whipple's disease, autoimmune gastritis, *Helicobacter pylori* infection, immunoproliferative small intestinal disease, hepatitis A, B, C, D, E, F, and G, autoimmune hepatitis, primary biliary cirrhosis, progressive sclerosing cholangitis, and vanishing bile duct syndrome.

GALT health is maintained with the same methods discussed in Chapter 11, especially with the use of **castor oil packs,** carotenoids, vitamin B complex, vitamin A, avoiding food you are allergic to, healthy diet, and paying attention to proper digestion and elimination.

The spleen is the "heart" of the lymph system. It is a filtration organ and participates in immune response to blood-borne pathogens. It is the site where the body traps and digests upwards of 50% of all dying red blood cells and platelets. The spleen also serves as a blood reservoir for both phagocytic cells and lymphoid cells, releasing blood cells in cases of sudden blood loss or infection. Spleen problems are almost always secondary to other systemic problems, and the main symptom is enlargement. This usually resolves as the causative problems are treated.

As a general rule for treating the spleen, 60–70% of your main formula should focus on the specific causative factor. Additionally, 30–40% can include herbs specifically for the secondary spleen enlargement.

Ayurvedic doctors use **shilajatu, eclipta, rohitaka stem** *(Rhododendron arboreum),* **hemaksiri** *(Argemone mexicana),* and **condensed aloe gum** for spleen enlargement. TCM doctors use **blood-moving herbs,** especially **tortoiseshell** (gui ban), **zedoaria root** (e zhu or *Curcuma zedoaria),* **salvia root,** and **prepared rhubarb root.** Western herbalists use **milk thistle seed, blue flag root** *(Iris versicolor),* **red root** *(Ceanothus americanus),* **barberry root bark** *(Berberis vulgaris),* **bear's foot leaf** or **root** *(Polymnia uvedalia),* and **dandelion root.**

The tonsils, a mass of lymphatic tissue, are located on the sides of the throat. Like all lymph components, the tonsils act as a filter, and aid in the formation of white blood cells. The close-by adenoids act in a similar way.

Echinacea, honeysuckle flower (jin yin hua or *Lonicera japonica),* **forsythia fruit** (lian qiao or *F. suspensa),* **isatis root** and **leaves, white sage** *(Salvia apiana),* and **elderberry** are effective treatments for infected tonsils. Drinking tea high in tannin concentration or gargling with diluted **grapefruit seed extract** (GSE) can be useful. Fresh or dried **honeysuckle flower tea** with honey is a pleasant and palatable tonsil treatment.

Diseases of Immunity

Age-Associated Deterioration of Learning and Memory

A weakened immune system can alter the function of the central nervous system. In fact, animal studies show that decreases in immune function can lead to decreases in learning ability.

In one study, researchers concluded that the improvement of immune function is closely related to the amelioration of age-associated deterioration of learning and memory. Through the simple use of **aged garlic extract,** scientists were able to restore learning ability. I would suggest using combinations containing several of the immune tonic herbs mentioned earlier.

Ayurvedic medicine has maintained for centuries that overstimulation of the brain (e.g., with too much noise or bright light) is bad for the nervous system, while understimulation leads to dullness and lethargy. Modern scientists have agreed with this theory ever since early studies showed the dependency of animal intelligence on stimulation. Recent studies confirm our early suspicions that the brain requires stimulation for proper function, while isolation leads to a loss of cognitive ability. Consequently, it is vital to remain mentally active, engaging regularly in activities that promote intellectual stimulation, such as reading.

Allergy

Chronic allergy is a hypersensitivity caused by exposure to an allergen resulting in a marked increase in immune system reactivity upon subsequent exposure. A patient once told me that after she arrived on U.S. soil, it seemed to her everyone in America had chronic allergy problems, while no one did in her home country of Korea. This simple observation is simply an acknowledgment of the massive increase of allergens we now are forced to cope with in our industrial society.

Allergy symptoms can range from a simple rash to life-threatening anaphylactic shock, requiring emergency treatment. In addition, allergy is often (very often) a contributing factor to numerous other disease processes.

We have already discussed single-cell immune response to foreign antigens. The whole process is that antigen-processing cells present the antigen to T-cells, which then help B-cells to change form into IgE-secreting cells (called plasma cells). The newly formed IgE attaches itself to mast cells, which are found in large quantities in the respiratory tract, GI tract, and skin. This is why allergy occurs mostly in these locations. When the antigen gets into your system again, it links to the mast cells, which then release histamine, leukotrienes, and other irritating cytokine chemicals, which cause the initial allergy symptoms to occur.

Later reactions occur because Th_2 cells are activated by the processed allergen, then release interleukins, which cause eosinophils, basophils, and neutrophils to release more allergy-causing cytokines.

Allergy Symptoms

The classic respiratory symptoms are sneezing, secretion of watery mucus, and membrane swelling that blocks the nasal passageways. In chronic cases, dark circles develop under the eyes, as well as fatigue and hacking due to an itching sensation in the roof of the mouth. Over time, respiratory allergy moves toward asthma, covered in Chapter 17.

- Gastrointestinal symptoms develop from allergens in foods. These can cause itching and burning in the mouth, nausea, vomiting, intestinal inflammation and increased permeability, gas and bloating, and diarrhea or constipation. In severe cases anaphylaxis can develop, with lowered blood pressure, tracheal edema, and cardiorespiratory distress. In infants and children, food allergies can cause projectile vomiting, eczema, or failure to thrive.

- Cutaneous symptoms can develop from external sources such as chemical or insect venom. If the allergen is strong, it can lead to anaphylaxis, or swelling of the lungs, which can lead to death. More often, there is a late-phase redness and swelling at the site of the injury or bite.

- When allergens or secondary by-products of intestinal allergy are absorbed into the blood, hives, fatigue, heat sensations, chronic inflammatory diseases, depression, emotional imbalance, itching skin, edema, headaches, joint pain and swelling, and smooth muscle contraction can result. These are more common as patients increase in age.

- Acute symptoms occur within minutes of exposure to an allergen and typically recede over the next 30–90 minutes. Symptoms can recur a few hours later and last for several hours. If exposure to the allergen is continuous, as with food allergies or pollutants in the home or work environment, late-phase reactions occur. Over time, tissue damage can occur.

Allergy is a difficult nut to crack. Originally it was enough to keep people away from triggering substances, such as chemicals, bacteria, parasites, dust, mold, foods, and pollen spores.

Consider what happened to the caveman Og. Og lives a few miles from a sulfur pit surrounded by a giant fungus. One day, as Og walked close to the pit, the sulfur/fungus fumes got into his eyes, which began to burn and itch. Of course, Og made tracks out of there. But, unbeknownst to him, his B-cells were releasing signals that created sulfur- and/or fungal-remembering mast cells that lay in wait for the next appearance of the chemicals. The next week, Og took his wife out for a walk. About a mile from the pit, Og began to sniffle, itch, and burn, rubbing his eyes. "Air bad. Go this way," he declared, turning and leaving the area.

Mrs. Og protested: "Air not bad. Og crazy." Mrs. Og did not react because she had not developed reactivity.

Og had it easy: all he had to do was stay away from the sulfur pit. Today, however, we face the problem of inundation from thousands of invisible chemicals, many undetectable until an allergy develops and we have symptoms. It is difficult if not impossible to completely turn off allergies without incapacitating the immune system.

This is what happens when immunosuppressant drugs are used. Antihistamines are a bit better because they have fewer side effects, but they tend to wear off. They do not extinguish the causes, and the immune system will simply find another way to do what it thinks it should to cope.

Our best approach is to know the following facts:

- Our reaction will depend upon exposure. We *can* modify our environment.

- The strength of our barrier defenses can limit entry even when we are exposed.

- Our immune responses can be modified with herbs and nutrients.

As an herbalist, I employ several approaches:

- Purify the home atmosphere to reduce exposure to allergen triggers. This is covered in Chapter 17. This works even though not all triggers can be avoided, because when the total allergy load is decreased, the response is often far less. This is especially true for food allergies.

- Test for and reduce exposure to food allergies. The method for doing this, as well as strengthening the intestinal membranes (to reduce allergen absorption), is covered in Chapter 11. Although many allergists limit identification to IgE antibodies, holistic physicians include IgG, IgM, and sometimes IgA. It may be important to have your health care provider test for elevated IgG antibodies if you are having trouble with identification.

- Prescribe specific herbs and nutrients to tone down the allergic response and make it less aggressive.

Treatment of allergies

Herbs choosen for allergies should be based upon signs and symptoms, using the following guidelines. Make sure to look for and correct underlying problems, such as exposures to allergy-causing foods or environment, intestinal health, and so on. Herbs for treating sinusitis are covered in Chapter 17.

- The severity of the general inflammatory response can be decreased by using healthful fats and oils and supplementing with **borage oil, fish oils,** and so on.

- TCM herbs with antiallergy effects include **scute root, chrysanthemum flower, schisandra berries, er bu shir taso herb** *(Centipeda minima),* **magnolia flower, honeysuckle flower,** and **forsythia fruit.** Most of these are contained in **Pe Min Kan Wan pills,** commercially available (see Chapter 4). If there are signs of mucus, add **pinellia tuber, tangerine peel,** and **ginger root.**

- Ayurvedic herbs with antiallergy effects include **neem leaves, turmeric root, eclipta, tulsi, boswellia gum, aguru wood, karchura root** *(Curcuma zedoaria),* **tamalaki** *(Phyllanthus nururi),* **karkatashingi gall** *(Pistacia intergerrima),* **katphalam bark** *(Myrica nagi),* **coleus** *(C. forskohlii),* **Malabar nut** (vasaka or *Adhatoda vasica),* and **anthrapachaka leaf** *(Tylophora indica).*

- Western herbs used for allergy include **lobelia, feverfew, echinacea, eyebright flowering herb** *(Euphrasia officinalis),* **stinging nettle, ginkgo leaf,** and **garlic bulb.** The combination of the flavonoid **quercetin** with **bromelain** is also useful.

- Some additional herbs that have specific antiallergy effects can be found in our earlier discussion of IgG, IgF, eosinophils, basophils, and mast cells.

Chronic Fatigue Syndrome

Chronic fatigue syndrome (CFS) is an immune system dysfunction characterized by severe unrelenting fatigue, low body temperature, sore throat, lymphadenopathy, arthralgia, fibromyalgia, and various neurological and mental symptoms. One day while browsing the shelves of the local university library, I was fortunate enough to happen upon perhaps the first book ever written about chronic fatigue. *Chronic Fatigue Intoxication: A Heretofore Inadequately Described Affection,* by Edward H. Ochsner, M.D., was published in 1923. The author pointed out that chronic fatigue occurred primarily in sensitive, overworked people, and he clearly outlined the existence of what are now called trigger points. Dr. Ochsner considered the trigger points to be toxic accumulations, and his primary treatment protocol involved bed rest, dietary modification, and massage.

As it happens, the good doctor was also a rancher, and in one fascinating set of experiments he tested his theories on plow horses. He made them plow long hours, week after week, without allowing for adequate rest. The more sensitive horses were always first to succumb to a chronic fatigue type of condition, exhibiting prominent symptoms of acidic breath and poor digestion. In each case, a good long rest proved to be an effective cure. Today we see what appears to be the same syndrome in CFS, also called myalgic encephalomyelitis (ME) in the United Kingdom. Results of a 1997 study in England suggested that as many as 11% of patients visiting primary care facilities had symptoms of chronic fatigue.

The medical community now recognizes several potential causes of CFS, though no one claims to fully understand the causes or the nature of the illness. It is interesting to note that many of Dr. Ochsner's early insights still apply.

Following are some of the more common possible causes of CFS:

- Severe emotional or physical stress

- Lack of physical tone, or poor metabolism due to lack of exercise

- Digestive problems and intestinal infections resulting from poor diet

- Metabolic or environmental disturbances that exhaust the glands or the cellular mitochondria that produce the body's energy

It is likely that viral illness, emotional stress, and exposure to environmental toxins act as triggers of CFS. Onset is typically sudden, presenting with symptoms that follow a variable course, often characterized by a pattern of alternation between relapse and remission. Symptoms include, but are not limited to, debilitating and persistent fatigue, low-grade fever, sore throat, fibromyalgia (muscle pain), sleep disorders, and mental fogginess.

Most cases of CFS involve a low-grade fever along with immune deficiency. Consequently, CFS patients experience numerous changes in immune parameters, often exhibiting lower levels of natural killer cells (NK), antibodies, and important cytokines. They may also present evidence of considerable neurological stress and symptomalogy. Symptoms are often made worse by exercise.

Pretreatment of CFS

A large percentage of CFS patients suffer from specific metabolic problems, and there are many signs of toxicity. I would estimate that more than 30% of the CFS patients I have seen require pretreatment for these conditions before I can begin to treat their fatigue. For example, excretion of certain urinary metabolites definitely increases in CFS cases, and there is a high incidence of chronic candidiasis. Thyroid imbalance is also a common problem, as is blood sugar imbalance. For these reasons, I have found it an important first step to treat these problems individually, especially in the GI tract, before treating CFS directly. (For a review, refer to our discussion of treatment of intestinal disorders in Chapter 11.) Such an approach can often provide very quick relief, offering a noticeable reduction of symptoms. Liver detoxification and elimination of food allergies is another useful starting strategy favored by holistic doctors and naturopaths, as is use of low-dose cortisone, about 5–10 mg per day.

Direct Herbal Treatment of CFS

One major prong of treatment is the use of a tonic formula or a combination of tonic herbs like **ginseng root, astragalus root,** and **white atractylodes.** Other tonics include **ashwagandha root, shilajatu, mica oxide bhasma, wild asparagus root, schisandra berries, codonopsis, Siberian ginseng root bark, maitake mushroom, ganoderma mushroom, licorice root, guduchi stem,** and **amla fruit.**

These herbs work directly against any hidden infection and tonify depressed immune cells, including NK cells. Choose based upon the patient's signs and symptoms, of course. For example, **ginseng** and **astragalus roots** are more heating and energizing, while **ashwagandha root** and **ganoderma mushroom** are more calming and neutral in energy.

A second prong of treatment is the use of herbs known to reduce low-grade fevers. Such herbs include **isatis root** and **leaves, raw rehmannia, qing hao herb** *(Artemisia annua),* **bupleurum root, dandelion root, tulsi, cat's claw** (uña de gato or *Uncaria tomentosa),* **elderberrry, pau d'arco inner bark** *(Tabebuia* species), and **wild indigo root tincture** *(Baptisia tinctoria).*

After choosing a group of perhaps three to six tonic herbs, composing about 60–70% of the formula, I would make some of the following modifications, either to fill out the formula or as separate concomitant formulas:

- If there are signs of dampness or mucus, such as a greasy tongue coating or nausea, add a small amount of drying herbs like **black atractylodes, poria mushroom, pinellia tuber,** and **dried tangerine peel** to your formula.

- If there are signs of coldness, you can add a few warming herbs like **dry ginger root, prickly ash bark,** or **cinnamon bark.** Always ask first if the patient can tolerate spicy foods.

- For nervous system agitation, be sure to use **wild milky oat seed tincture, skullcap tincture,** and/or **ashwagandha root.**

- Cases in which the sides of the tongue are red or the patient is irritable require additional herbs that remove toxins from the liver. Such herbs include **bupleurum root, dandelion root,** and **wheat sprouts.**

- In cases where the patient presents with a pale tongue and severe exhaustion, add nourishing herbs like **dang gui root** or **cooked rehmannia root.**

- It is imperative that CFS patients get plenty of daily rest and good sleep. Herbs like **valerian root, kava root,** or **skullcap tincture** can be useful if patients have difficulty sleeping.

- Studies indicate that short bursts of daily exercise (not for extended periods of time) can be of great benefit for CFS patients. Researchers recommend beginning slowly, with 10-minute rounds of activity, and slowly working up to longer periods of exercise.

Nai-shing recalls a young female CFS patient named Dina, who had been suffering from severe chronic fatigue for almost 10 years. She was also cold all the time, even though her thyroid function was normal. We counseled her on necessary dietary changes and identification of food allergies. Nai-shing then prepared for her a simple tonic of **astragalus root, ginseng root,** and **white atractylodes** to tonify the vital energy, some **dry ginger** and **purified aconite** to warm the body, and some **dang gui root** and **cooked rehmannia root** to nourish the blood. Within two weeks Dina's energy increased dramatically, and she continued to improve steadily during a 4-month course of herbs. She recovered completely within 6 months.

Fibromyalgia

Fibromyalgia, a condition characterized by chronic muscle pain, is a sister disease to CFS. I rarely see a CFS case without this chronic muscle and fibrous tissue pain.

In addition to the CFS protocols discussed above, I recommend the following treatments for fibromyalgia.

- Over the years I have had much success with the simple combination of malic acid (about 1,200 mg per day) and magnesium (about 300–400 mg) for pain relief. A placebo-controlled double-blind study confirmed the efficacy of this combination. Both malic acid and magnesium are available in many health food stores.

- To reduce inflammation, you can add **boswellia gum** or **turmeric root** to your herbal formula.

- Blood-moving herbs such as **dang gui root, salvia root,** and **red peony root** have also proven to be effective treatments for fibromyalgia.

HIV and AIDS

The acquired immune deficiency syndrome (AIDS) is caused by a retrovirus (HIV or human immunodeficiency virus) that has the rare and dangerous ability to reproduce itself inside immune cells. It is capable of rapid mutation, making it a formidable medical challenge. HIV selectively targets helper T-cells, removing their ability to activate other parts of the immune system. This allows for unimpeded viral growth and replication.

The infection presents initially with mild flulike symptoms and swollen glands. The symptoms usually appear for a few weeks and then disappear. Several months later the infected person will test positive for the presence of HIV antibodies, though it may take several years before opportunistic infections begin to appear, signaling the onset of full-blown AIDS.

There are no simple herbal answers for this plague. I always refer patients to local physicians who specialize in this field and inform them of the following additional resources and protocols.

- Dr. Mana has developed an herbal protocol for the treatment of HIV-positive patients. He has been prescribing the treatment for his Asian and European patients for the past 6 years and informs me that it restores CD_4 and CD_8 lymphocyte parameters (important immune markers) toward normal levels and delays the onset of AIDS. However, it is less effective once patients have developed full-blown AIDS (see Resource Guide).

- The Institute of Traditional Medicine (ITM) in Portland, Oregon, has emerged as a leader in using Chinese herbal therapies for treating cases of HIV. Doctors at the facility have developed several tonic formulas based upon Chinese research dating back as early as 1984. They use herbs like **astragalus root, codonopsis, white atractylodes, schisandra berries, licorice root, poria mushroom,** and **ophiogon root.** ITM has been expanding its work, and when patients contact the Institute they are referred to local practitioners trained in the use of their therapies (see Resource Guide).

- According to reports from ITM, eating three to five cloves of **garlic** per day is helpful in preventing opportunistic infections. Dr. Dharmananda, the director of the Institute, wrote a very informative paper entitled "Garlic as the Central Herb Therapy for AIDS."

- Herbal medications can be effective for controlling various HIV and AIDS symptoms such as nausea, weakened digestion, and alteration in fat metabolism. These should be individually prescribed according to the nature and severity of the symptom(s) in each patient.

- One of the most debilitating problems in AIDS cases is wasting due to chronic diarrhea. **Dragon's blood bark** (sangre de drago or *Croton lechleri)* contains a red latex used orally by indigenous and mestizo peoples in numerous South American countries to treat diarrhea, dysentery, gastritic, and stomach ulcers. Shaman Pharmaceuticals has developed an extract of this herb specifically for controlling the wasting diarrhea that typically occurs in AIDS patients. It works by pulling fluids out of the colon so the stool can form normally but, amazingly, does not seem to cause constipation. I have used it successfully for two patients with very serious chronic diarrhea.

- Twenty-eight patients with HIV were studied to see the effect of TCM tonic formulas for enhancing immunity and relieving clinical symptoms. The CD_4 and CD_8 lymphocytes and viral load numbers were tested before and after treatment. All 28 patients had weight gain after treatment. Seven cases with chronic fever and four with diarrhea had their symptoms disappear. After 5 months' treatment, lymphocytes increased in 50% of patients, and viral loads decreased in 80% of patients.

Some theorists make it clear that key elements of the HIV-AIDS hypothesis are unproven. I suggest you read the article, now on the Internet, "A critical analysis of the HIV–T$_4$-cell–AIDS hypothesis." One by one this paper critically reviews evidence that the HIV virus kills T$_4$ lymphocytes, that HIV causes the appearance of Kaposi's sarcoma, pneumocystis carinii pneumonia (PCP), and certain other "indicator" diseases, that HIV infection by itself can destroy T$_4$ lymphocytes, and that all AIDS patients are infected with HIV. The argument is scientifically elegant and needs to be independently read. One important result from the clinical perspective is that it gives evidence of the importance of avoidance of immunosuppressive behaviors (such as IV drug use) as critical to disease progression. I agree with this. It is not enough to take tonic herbs.

Refer to the Rethinking AIDS Homepage:
http://www.virusmyth.com/aids/data2/introduction.htm

Idiopathic Thrombocytopenic Purpura

Idiopathic thrombocytopenic purpura (ITP) is an autoimmune hemorrhagic disorder characterized by progressive platelet loss and bleeding. It is a systemic illness that produces purple patches caused by small hemorrhages from mucous membranes. Women are affected by this condition three times as often as men are. Platelet counts decline due to an immune attack triggered by antibodies that target specific antigens on the platelets. When the platelets enter the spleen, they are destroyed. Patients with this disease often have a history of nosebleeds, bruising, and hemorrhage, all of which increase as platelet levels decline. ITP becomes chronic in almost all adults and is generally acute and limited in children, although an estimated 10–30% of children will also become chronic. Mortality is high in patients with failed interventions.

Western Treatment Options

An expert panel established by the American Society of Hematology in 1994 extensively reviewed ITP-related research and published practice guidelines. It is clear that ITP management remains primarily empirical.

There are three basic treatment options. First, treatment with high-dose corticosteroids can be used to control the immune attack and put the disease in temporary remission. Most patients relapse after steroid doses are tapered. Second, intravenous immunoglobulin (IVIG) can be used to temporarily restore platelets. The presumed mechanism of action is thought to be by sparing of platelets via receptor site blockade. The beneficial effect of this treatment peaks at 2 weeks and lasts about 1 month on average. Because most platelet destruction occurs in the spleen, spleen removal is the third option, which results in a 50–60% remission rate. Spleen removal has been in use since 1913.

TCM Understanding and Treatment of ITP

TCM textbooks and journal articles universally report high levels of success in treating ITP in both children and adults. Several published Chinese studies have shown that the diagnoses given by TCM doctors closely correspond to measurable immune cell changes, including T-lymphocyte subsets, NK cells, and platelet-associated IgG. Furthermore, in a typical study of 66 patients, researchers reported improvement in platelet counts in four of five subgroups taking TCM prescriptions.

At the Shanghai Medical University Children's Hospital, the Institute of TCM-WM (combined Chinese and Western medicine) did a clinical study of 41 children. Of the 41 subjects, 36 had tiny hemorrhagic spots and larger purple skin patches, 28 had nasal hemorrhage, 5 had blood in the stool, and 1 had a subcutaneous hematoma. The basic herbal prescription contained **cooked rehmannia root, dang gui root** *(Angelica sinensis),* **red peony root** *(Paeonia rubra),* **qian cao gen root** *(Rubia cordifolia),* **psoralea seed** *(P. corylifolia),* **astragalus root** *(A. membranicus),* **cuscuta seed** *(C. chinensis),* and **da zao fruit** *(Ziziphus jujuba).* After average treatment duration of 5.02 months, researchers reported that 24 cases were cured, 6 recovered, 10 improved, and 1 failed to respond, with a total effective rate of 97.6%. Upon follow-up they discovered that 22 of the cured patients remained without recurrence for an average 10.4 months after withdrawal.

It is important to realize that all TCM doctors trained in the modern era are aware of modern immunological understanding, while herbs are empirically chosen and formulated based upon long-standing historical use for a variety of bleeding disorders. ITP in TCM is usually divided into two sets, traditionally called "Heat in the blood causing Yin deficiency" and "Spleen Qi deficiency failing to hold the blood in the vessels." These terms could be loosely translated as "inflammation-related hemorrhage" and "nutrient-deficiency-related hemorrhage." The basic herbal treatment formulations are similar for both groups, with a slightly increased emphasis on anti-inflammatory herbs for the former, and a slightly increased emphasis on herbs that improve digestion in the latter.

According to a very recent, thorough review of 15 Chinese clinical reports, the herbs used vary markedly from physician to physician in China. However, fewer than 30 herbs are generally used, and they fall within four clear groupings—anti-inflammatory, hemostatic, digestion-strengthening, and liver-nourishing. Administration of the various decoctions of herbs was reported to raise platelet levels to acceptable levels in many cases and to normal levels in a few cases. The number of patients who did not relapse was about equal to the number who did. Many who discontinued herbs did not relapse for periods of time up to several months or longer. IgG levels also decreased in several studies.

No independent verifications have ever been done in the West of these clinical reports. Possible mechanisms of action were shown in a series of in vitro pharmacological studies done in 1991 showing that platelet-producing cells in ITP patients were obviously underfunctioning. A 1% incubation of patient's serum with a TCM herbal extract was able to increase platelet numbers close to normal, suggesting that the herbs might inhibit the antiplatelet antibodies and/or facilitate reproduction, division, and maturity of the platelet-producing cells.

Combining Western and Eastern Methods to Treat ITP

Western practitioners have not yet considered either nutritional or TCM herbal protocols as viable treatment options. If we add TCM herbal treatment to the three known Western options, we end up with four main treatment methods:

- Corticosteroids (e.g., prednisone)

- IVIG/Anti-D (intravenous infusion of IgG)

- Splenectomy

- TCM herbs

Each of these treatment options presents a variety of clearly circumscribed problems. The side effects of prednisone treatment are serious and well known, and the effectiveness of the treatment declines over time. IVIG treatment is expensive and relatively free of side effects, although the FDA reported 15 cases of hemoglobinemia and/or hemoglobinuria between the March 1995 licensure and April 1999, giving an estimated 1.5% occurrence. The main problem besides expense is that the effectiveness of this treatment also declines over time.

The herbs commonly used for TCM herbal treatment of ITP have a very low side effect profile and are virtually devoid of serious side effects when acquired from a reputable TCM physician and properly administered. However, as mentioned, there is a deficiency of acceptable clinical proof of efficacy, and there have been no long-term studies to show whether the treatments will lose effectiveness over periods of time longer than 1 year. There is a strong history of simultaneous use of steroids with TCM herbs with no interactive problems, but the same is not true of IVIG therapy, so I advise a minimum withdrawal of TCM herbs 2 days prior and 3 days subsequent to IVIG therapy to avoid direct interaction. It might be equally advisable to discontinue TCM herbs for up to 3 weeks to completely ensure there is no negative interaction weakening the IVIG.

Splenectomy has a limited initial success rate of 50–60%, and fatal sepsis is always possible as time passes after the operation because opsonin—a "glue" that helps bind antigens—is manufactured only in the spleen. In children, the estimated success rate ranges from 70% to 90%. However, the long-term outcome of splenectomy in children has not been studied sufficiently. Most clinicians now believe the operation should be performed only when all other therapeutic options have been exhausted and the patient has a platelet count less than 25,000/microL and is hemorrhaging.

For these reasons, researchers at the Division of Hematology/Oncology and General

Internal Medicine at Northwestern University Medical School in Chicago hoped that maintenance therapy with IVIG treatment would "increase the rate of remission, allowing splenectomy to be avoided." Pediatric hematologists often postpone splenectomy, when there is a reasonable possibility of spontaneous recovery. This consideration is of great importance because after splenectomy, patients become ineligible for IVIG or prednisone treatment. However, there is no known reason why TCM therapy cannot still be used after the procedure, as long as you consider the sterility of the herbs.

Given this background, I propose that TCM treatment should be used for exactly the same reasons as IVIG or prednisone therapy. The evidence from China points to the possibility that herbs can improve platelet counts, though at a slower and less reliable rate than prednisone or IVIG therapy, while maintaining a low side effect profile.

If clinicians have a fourth option, the chances of successfully avoiding splenectomy increase, unless the TCM therapy is subsequently determined to be completely without merit.

Here is a case history of successful ITP treatment. It illustrates how combined treatment across several systems can be used to manage this life-threatening immune disease process.

Cindy (adult Caucasian female, age 44) came to us in February 2000, having been diagnosed with ITP in December 1999. She had been extremely fatigued 3 months prior to the diagnosis, and she was showing typical signs of easy bruising. Her blood pressure had been elevated (about 140/100) for the previous year. At that time her platelets were at 30,000/microL (30t) and she was given an injection of Winrho SDF (an IVIG), which increased her platelets to 167t. As expected, within a month her platelets declined to 47t.

Nai-shing performed a TCM diagnosis. Cindy's tongue was bright red and her pulse very rapid, and she had an unremitting headache. According to TCM understanding, all of these signs denote severe heat in the blood. Cindy had been placed on prednisone, 80 mg per day, 2 months before seeing us. She was experiencing side effects including puffy face and dizziness from the prednisone, and it was failing to control the drop in platelets. Her doctors had scheduled her for spleen removal.

Nutritional analysis revealed that the patient was taking none of the basic vitamins necessary for proper immune function, and her diet was deficient in fruits. To counter this we gave her a high-anthocyanadin syrup (made from berries) twice per day, a high-potency multivitamin, vitamin C 500 mg per day, alpha-lipoic acid 250 mg twice per day, and an omega-3 fish oil supplement.

Nai-shing prescribed the following herb formula, mostly hemostatic and cooling herbs, 3 grams three times per day of dried herbal decoction concentrates:

Ginseng root: 24 grams (to strengthen energy and stop bleeding)
Millettia stem: 18 grams (to generate platelets)
Mu dan pi bark *(Paeonia suffruticosa):* 18 grams (to reduce inflammation)
Qian cao gen root *(Rubia cordifolia):* 24 grams (to restrain hemorrhage)
Raw rehmannia root: 24 grams (to reduce inflammation)

Salvia root: 18 grams (to reduce inflammation)
Schisandra berries: 18 grams (for fatigue and wasting)
White atractylodes: 12 grams (to strengthen digestion)
Xian he cao herb *(Agrimonia pilosa):* 24 grams (to restrain hemorrhage)
Zi cao root *(Lithospermum erythrorhizon):* 24 grams (antiautoimmune action)

After 1 week on the formula, continuing prednisone at 80 mg, Cindy's platelets increased to 152t. She reported to us that she "still felt like a balloon being blown up." Prednisone was dropped to 40 mg, causing platelets to decrease to 88t within a few days. Nai-shing and I determined that inflammation was still severe, so we altered the formula by adding:

Tian qi root: 12 grams (hemostatic and anti-inflammatory)
Bai mao gen rhizome *(Imperata cylindrica):* 6 grams (hemostatic and anti-inflammatory)
Rose hips *(Rosa rugosa):* 6 grams (astringent)
Triphala (three-fruit compound): 6 grams (general tonic and anti-inflammatory)

On 3/1/00, platelets increased to 95t, and the prednisone was tapered to 30 mg per day.
On 3/6/00 platelets increased to 133t, and prednisone was dropped to 20 mg.
On 3/13/00 platelets at 138t, prednisone was reduced to 20 mg every other day.
On 3/21/00 platelets dropped to 118t, prednisone at 10 mg every other day.
On 4/3/00 platelets at 126t and prednisone discontinued.
On 4/10/00 platelets at 91t (after 1 week without prednisone).

Over the next month, her platelets stabilized at a count between 90t and 110t. At this stage, Cindy was in a good position. As we continue to monitor her blood counts weekly, she is currently almost symptom free, and the options of prednisone and Winrho are still available to her if there is any flare-up. I told her doctors that the TCM herbs should be discontinued for 1 week and up to 3 weeks if it becomes necessary to take Winrho again. The longer we can keep her blood counts above critical ranges, the greater her chances of avoiding splenectomy, and the greater her chances of entering into long-term remission.

Cancer

Cancer is not a single disease but rather a family of diseases characterized by abnormal cell growth. Cancer accounted for 23% of all deaths in the United States in 1998, and each year more than a million Americans find out they have cancer. In spite of victories in certain areas, there are continuing losses in others. For example, although numbers of deaths from female breast cancer are declining due to improvements in testing and treatment, the American Cancer Society calculates that lung cancer will rise to 25% of all female cancer deaths in the year 2000.

Rapidly growing cancerous cells are termed neoplasms, meaning "new growth." The vast majority of neoplasms are made of cells from a single germ layer. When examined under a microscope and compared to normal, healthy cells, cancer cells look damaged. When the rapidly dividing cells mass together with connective tissue and blood vessels they form tumors, which can be one of two types, benign or malignant. Benign tumors cannot invade neighboring tissues, they remain localized, and the cells are relatively normal in appearance. However, malignant tumors can spread through the system. The cells are often (but not always) primitive in appearance, irregular in shape and size, and sometimes have a large misshapen nucleus.

There are three basic forms of cancer in modern understanding:

- **Carcinomas** begin in epithelial tissue—the lining cells covering the surfaces and interior structures of our glands, vessels, and ducts.

- **Sarcomas** are much more rare and develop out of connective and fibrous tissue, or directly from blood vessels. They are usually fleshy.

- **Leukemias** and **lymphomas** are born in the blood-forming cells of our bone marrow and lymph nodes.

The most common cancers are those affecting, in descending order, the lungs, colon or rectum, breast, larynx, prostate, uterus, kidney, bladder, lymph tissue, mouth, stomach, blood cells (leukemias), and skin. All cancers go through several stages, called initiation, promotion, progression, invasion of neighboring tissue, and finally, metastasis to distant sites.

Initiating factors, known as carcinogens, cause the transformation of normal cells into cancer cells. Radiation and certain harmful chemicals and viruses are carcinogens. They damage the body's deoxyribonucleic acid (DNA), the carrier of genetic information which resides in every cell. The most common chemical carcinogens are chemical agents such as pesticides, herbicides and trihalomethanes, tobacco, and alcohol.

Fortunately, our body has DNA repair mechanisms, and this forms the basis of many herbal and preventative treatments. Rapid advances in genetics have identified two families of genes that control cancer in a Yin and Yang fashion. Oncogenes promote cancer, while tumor-suppressor genes inhibit tumor growth. Emerging evidence indicates that herbal medicines and nutrients can affect these genes. Quercetin, a flavone found in many herbs and vegetables including onions, **licorice root,** and **sophora flower,** and **chaga mushroom,** can inhibit defect formation in tumor suppressor gene p53, which is involved in cancer prevention.

Cancer Prevention

Once cancer develops it is very difficult to treat, as the cancer cells take on lives of their own. Currently, prevention is our best defense. Therefore, it is extremely important to follow the myriad preventive health practices known to foster prevention.

Following are some of the many reasons that cancer is such a difficult disease to treat and cure.

- By the time cancer is detected, it may have gone through millions of cell divisions or "doublings," growing from a microscopic state into a well-entrenched tumor. Doubling allows tumors to grow incredibly quickly.

- Individual tumors contain variants that can develop resistance to drugs.

- Tumors ignore the normal "stop" signals other cells usually obey. This ignorance mechanism enables cancer cells to invade adjacent tissue areas.

- Cancer cells can detach from a tumor and remain alive as they travel through the bloodstream, forming new tumors at distant sites. Normal cells cannot do this, as they must remain attached to the membranes that feed them.

- People who are born with less ability to repair their DNA are at a far greater risk of getting certain cancers.

- Cancer cells can send out chemical signals that cause the formation of new blood vessels so they can feed themselves.

- Tumors form a fibrous outer coat that protects them against immune system attack.

- Tumors have the ability to turn off the immune system—a process called anergy.

- Cancer cells defy the normal "programmed death" or apoptosis process that controls normal cells and causes them to die as they age or are damaged. Thus cancer cells are, in a sense, immortal.

Following are lists of many foods and nutritional supplements that are believed to help prevent or slow the progression of cancer. While not proven to be cures by themselves, all of them have shown the ability to influence the cancer process. It is very likely, almost certain, that compounding several of these nutrients can create superior effects, due to synergistic action.

I like to incorporate as many of the following nutrients as I can into my daily regimen. I favor the food agents and rotate the nutritional supplements. Considering that so many people do not eat adequate amounts of fruits and vegetables, I believe that reading this information is a graphic way to drive this prevention information into the consumer consciousness.

Foods. Foods that researchers believe can help prevent cancer include apples, beans (including soybeans), beets, broccoli, brussels sprouts, cabbage, cauliflower, celery, citrus fruits, cumin, flaxseed oil, garlic, grapes, green vegetables, kale, olive oil, onions, parsley, pineapple (a source of bromelain), raspberries, red pepper, soybean products, squash, tangerines, tomatoes (a source of lycopene), yogurt (a source of probiotics), strawberries, and wheat bran. Most of the research focuses on specific phytochemicals such as flavonoids and carotenoids.

Broad-spectrum Multivitamins and Multiminerals. Free radicals damage our DNA, so foods, vitamins, and herbs that neutralize free radicals are important preventive agents. There are numerous studies on the protective effects of antioxidants, so these nutrients are essential in any cancer prevention program, although there has been less research than one would imagine for many common nutrients. For the rest, however, the evidence is solid. For example, we know that selenium, at a dose of 200 mcg per day, reduces prostate cancer rates by two-thirds.

Cellular Antioxidants. Glutathione peroxidase, catalase, methionine reductase, and SOD help protect against cancer via antioxidant and cell growth regulatory effects and by helping in DNA repair. Glutathione is especially important and is found in **wheat sprouts.** Flavonoids found in fruits and plants (especially anthocyanins, anthocyanidins, proanthocyanins, and proanthocyanidins) help to recirculate and keep glutathione in circulation, as well as having many other anticancer effects.

Lipoic Acid. This unique water/fat soluble antioxidant has shown evidence of inhibiting NF kappa-B from activating cancer-causing oncogenes. Use 100–200 mg per day in divided doses.

Chinese Herbal Medicines. These have been shown in numerous studies to exhibit a wide variety of anticancer and chemotherapeutic protection effects, including increased remission rates, a slowing of progression, antioxidant effects, and immune system enhancement.

N-acetyl-cysteine (NAC). This nutrient is currently under investigation by the National Cancer Institute because it has the ability to significantly decrease the incidence of cancerous and precancerous lesions induced by several chemical carcinogens in rodents. Benefits were shown for lesions in the colon, lung, liver, bladder, skin, and breasts. It has also shown potential as an inhibitor of metastasis.

Medicinal Mushrooms. Many of the medicinal mushrooms, including **chaga mushroom, maitake mushroom, ganoderma mushroom,** and **cordyceps mushroom,** contain cancer-preventive and cancer-fighting actions. Research has focused on the polysaccharides with beta 1,3 glucan linkages.

Cruciferous Vegetables. Indole-3-carbinol is a nutrient found in large quantities in cruciferous vegetables. It is a potent antagonist of breast cancer, reducing formation of cancerous compounds from hormones and participating in blockage of cancer cell progression. A controlled clinical trial using 300 mg per day on 60 women confirmed it as a promising breast cancer prevention agent.

Turmeric Root. Studies show that curcumin (the active ingredient) inhibits cancer cell proliferation in a variety of ways and helps induce programmed cell death, or apoptosis.

Coenzyme Q$_{10}$. Numerous holistic physicians are reporting a benefit in preventing and treating breast cancer. The preventive dose is 50 mg per day, while for cancer treatment the dose is 200 mg three times per day. According to one report, "overt complete regression of the tumors in two cases of breast cancer . . . [and] numerous metastases in the liver of a 44-year-old patient 'disappeared,' and no signs of metastases were found elsewhere."

Milk Thistle Seed. The milk thistle extract **silymarin** has shown an anticarcinogenic effect in human breast cancer cells, arresting cell cycle progression. Use 140–250 mg standardized silymarin extract one to three times per day.

Soybean Extracts. Scientists have demonstrated the protective effects of soybean components, via a variety of mechanisms, on breast cancer, prostate cancer, and urinary tract cancer. The component called genistein has been shown not only to prevent cancer but also to impede proliferation and induce differentiation. Chinese women and men use soybean products about twice per week, so this appears to be a good level for protection. In response to concerns about promotion of cancer in women with estrogen-dependent tumors, the Clinical Nutrition and Risk Factor Modification Center at St. Michael's Hospital in Toronto, Ontario, Canada, did a controlled clinical study and concluded that soy consumption did not increase the risk for hormone-dependent cancers.

Tangerines. Dr. William Mitchell, N.D., reported evidence that bioflavonoids found in the peel of tangerine can strengthen epithelial cells in such a way as to inhibit metastasis of cancer. This bioflavonoid, called tangeritin, increases the functional integrity of E-cadherin, a cell-to-cell adhesive protein. Tangerines can therefore be used as a preventative. The recommended dose is one tangerine per day, making sure to eat the juice as well as the white parts behind the rind (scrape them off with your teeth). If the peel is organic, save it, dry it in the oven, and grind it up. You can add it to food, thus making use of the whole fruit. The recommended dose of dried peel is 1 to 2 teaspoons per day.

Ayurvedic Herbs and Herbal Formulas. Ayurvedic tonic herbs have a long history of use in cancer, and a few recent studies have shown extraordinary antioxidant effects.

Garlic Bulb. Numerous studies have shown immunological benefits, and a few studies indicate benefits for oral and prostate cancers.

Guggul Gum. This herb, used commonly for cholesterol reduction, has a long historical record of use by Ayurvedic doctors in treating cancer.

Green Tea. Numerous studies indicate preventive and anticancer effects via several mechanisms, including protection against chemical carcinogens, inhibition of tumor-promoting substances, inhibition of cell division, and the inducing of apoptosis. Drink 2 to 3 cups of tea per day.

PC-Spes. This herbal product drops PSA levels dramatically in prostate cancer patients. It is described in detail in the book *The Prostate Cancer Miracle* by Jesse Stoff, M.D. We use it for all our prostate cancer patients, along with other methods in this chapter. (See the resource guide for ordering information.)

Of course, prevention is far more involved than nutrients and herbs. Things such as cutting back on sugar intake, exercising regularly, avoiding excess sun and wearing sunglasses, using air filters, and other lifestyle choices all qualify as important preventive measures.

Research Highlights

The effects of preventive herbal medicine treatments are easier to measure when studies are done on precancerous lesions. If such lesions can be made to regress, it is a clear sign of the preventive power of the treatment.

- In one study, the Beijing Academy of TCM used the classic **rehmannia six formula** to treat patients with precancerous lesions of the esophagus. After 5 years, 8.4% of the treated group developed esophageal cancer, as compared to 25.5% of the untreated controls (Long and Mong, 1992).

- Scientists at the Hebei Cancer Institute did a similar study using **cang dou pills.** They followed 648 cases and after 2 years, 4.2% of the untreated controls developed esophageal cancer, in comparison to 1.5% of the treated group (Hou and Yan, 1992).

- In a multicenter, double-blind, controlled trial, beta-carotene was shown to produce regressions in patients with premalignant oral lesions. Subjects were given beta-carotene at a dose of 60 mg/day, or placebo for 6 months. Of the treated subjects, 52% responded with regressions (Garewal et al., 1999).

- In a controlled, blind clinical trial, a 400-IU dose of vitamin E was shown to regress small intestinal metaplasia (precancerous tissue changes). After 12 months, 10 of 14 patients (71%) showed no signs of metaplasia (Bukin et al., 1997).

Western Treatment of Cancer

The Western or allopathic treatment of cancer is based upon three major methods: surgery, radiation, and chemotherapy. As mentioned earlier, surgical removal of tumors has been recorded since the seventh century B.C. and remains very valuable to this day. It is difficult to shrink tumors. Surgical removal is sometimes called "debulking," a descriptive name that readily explains its value. Once a large bulk of cancerous tissue is removed, the job of removing the rest of the cancer cells is much easier, with one caveat. The cutting of tumors releases millions of cells into circulation, increasing the chance of spreading. For this reason, radiation and chemotherapy are considered necessary to remove these freed cells.

Chemotherapy kills damaged cancerous cells. Chemotherapeutic drugs are very toxic, so they also damage healthy cells and cause side effects. Radiation also kills cancer cells. It has an advantage because a beam of radiation can be localized to very specific sites, but side effects are also common with this form of treatment.

The Importance of Combined Treatment

The treatment of cancer is an excellent example of the need for combined and cooperative treatment. The history of medicine is replete with warring schools of thought. The Eclectic physicians of the last and early part of this century were almost wiped out by opposing forces, and today insurance and licensing issues hold a powerful grip on the practice of medicine. I predict this will change for three compelling reasons:

1. The history of freedom of choice and individual rights rooted in the American Constitution will eventually overcome restrictions, though this will no doubt require expensive court battles.

2. Scientific studies will continue to show the benefits of using natural medicines in combination with allopathic techniques and medicines.

3. Patients will continue to demand that they get the best medicines available, no matter what the source.

The book *Complementary Cancer Therapies* by Dan Labriola, N.D., gives an excellent simplified overview of the major chemotherapeutic chemicals and their side effects. These include bone marrow suppression, nausea and vomiting, kidney and liver toxicity, heart and lung toxicity, hair loss, mouth sores, nerve damage, and intestinal tract damage. Dr. Labriola is an expert on the integration of alternative and allopathic cancer treatments. He introduces the concept of the "protected zone," the time period when chemotherapy or radiation is attacking cancerous cells. He also theorizes that certain alternative treatments should be avoided at those times, pointing out that the avoidance of side effects with many nutritional treatments may interfere with the cancer-killing effects of the allopathic drugs in the protected zone.

On the other hand, a review of available evidence "demonstrates that exogenous antioxidants alone produce beneficial effects in various cancers, and, except for a few specific cases, animal and human studies demonstrate no reduction of efficacy of chemotherapy or radiation when given with antioxidants." The same holds true for many herbal combinations tested in China.

However, there are undoubtedly dangers, as shown by the negative study discussed below. My current clinical judgment is that until we know more, you should avoid strong antioxidant herbs or vitamins 2 days prior to and 4 days after a chemotherapy or radiation treatment, both as a precaution and to relieve anxiety in patients and oncologists. I still recommend use of herbal agents that have been shown to strengthen immune response, but only in strict accordance with signs and symptoms, and based upon a clear strategy.

Research Highlights

- In one study, herbal formulas with **ginseng root, astragalus root,** and other TCM herbs were used in combination with chemotherapy (vincristine, cyclophosphamide, methotrexate, and carmustine), radiotherapy, and immunotherapy to treat 54 cases of small-cell lung cancer. Survival rates increased dramatically, with some patients gaining an estimated 3–17 years of survival (Cha RJ et al., 1994).

- A Chinese study analyzed 285 cases of metastatic carcinoma in the supraclavicular lymph nodes. Patients were treated by five methods: Chinese medication, radiotherapy plus Chinese medication, chemotherapy plus Chinese medication, combined Chinese and Western medicine, and expectant (palliative) treatment. Researchers reported: "Analysis shows that radiotherapy plus Chinese medication has the best curative effect with an effective rate of 75.5%. The effective rates were 74.2% for the combined treatment, 55.5% for the chemotherapy plus medication, 12.5% for the Chinese medication, and none for expectant treatment" (Cui and Li, 1995).

- Injections of extracts of **ginseng root** and **astragalus root** were used with chemotherapy on 176 human cases of digestive tract tumors. Results showed that in comparison to controls, the injections reduced the toxic effects of the chemotherapy, significantly protected white blood cells, and reduced failure due to lowered WBC counts. In follow-up experiments on animals the injections also prolonged survival times (Li NQ, 1992).

- A placebo-controlled double-blind clinical study was done on primary liver cancer using TCM tonic herbs and radiation therapy. The 1-year, 3-year, and 5-year survival rates of the group that received herbs were higher than the control group survival by 20.0%, 23.4%, and 16.6% respectively (Han JQ et al., 1997).

- **Negative study.** A clinical trial of 60 cases of nasopharyngeal carcinoma used combined treatment of radiotherapy and TCM tonic herbs. A 5-year follow-up showed a metastatic rate 2.67 times higher for treated patients than for controls (Han JQ et al., 1995). The medicine used in the study (Fuchunpian) consists of very strongly warming tonic herbs rather than anti-inflammatory and nourishing herbs, demonstrating the importance of proper herbal choices.

The Ayurvedic Perspective on Cancer

In 1987, Dr. Mana completed a 5-year personal research project resulting in the publication of his book *The Ayurvedic Records of Cancer Treatment*. According to Dr. Mana, "It is not well known that much research work concerning the proper treatment of cancer has been recorded in different Ayurvedic texts, [and] I hope that the Ayurvedic knowledge of cancer treatment presented in this book will be a new alternative guideline for modern medical scholars who are really serious about research of cancer treatment."

Unfortunately, this book is available only in Nepal, so I have taken the liberty (with Dr. Mana's permission, of course) of editing and reprinting the following key paragraphs. I believe this is the first clear presentation in English of Ayurvedic cancer theory.

The English medical word *cancer* does not refer to a new disease. This word is used to indicate a malignant tumor, or any kind of abnormal growth. Abnormal growths, either malignant or not, are assigned particular names in English, dependent upon type and location. Some examples are *tumor, neoplasm, epithelioma, carcinoma, sarcoma, fibroma, myoma, lipoma, adenoma, angioma,* and *cyst.*

The Ayurvedic words for abnormal growths were also based on type and location and were assigned names in a similar fashion. *Granthi, Arbuda, Gulma, Asthila, Balmika,* and *Shaluka* are some of the words that were used. Thus, names assigned by both systems generally refer to neoplasms found within particular organs or body tissues.

In the West, neoplasms are divided into two pathogenic natures, benign and malignant. The Ayurvedic words *Tridosaja* abnormal growth and *Sannipataja* abnormal growth are used to indicate the malignant stage of the neoplasm; the word *Vataja* or *Pittaja* or *Kaphaja* or a combination of any two of them (e.g., *Vata-Pittaja* or *Vata-Kaphaja* or *Pitta-Kaphaja*) is used to signify a benign neoplasm.

Ayurveda explains that a malignant abnormal growth, or Tridosaja neoplasm, is one in which all the three major bodily control systems—Vata, Pitta, and Kapha—which should have mutual coordination for normal functioning of the body, are out of control.

A cystlike bluish abnormal growth with neuralgic pain is the main symptom indicating the presence of a Vataja neoplasm. A reddish or yellowish vascular growth with inflammation and burning pain characterizes the Pittaja neoplasm. A stonelike hard abnormal growth with a little pain and itching is descriptive of a Kaphaja neoplasm. The Sannipataja or Tridosaja neoplasm manifests all the characters of Vataja, Pittaja, and Kaphaja neoplasm. In the same way, a neoplasm with the name Vata-Pittaja, Vata-Kaphaja, or Pitta-Kaphaja will have a mixture of symptoms.

Following these definitions, Ayurveda has classified all kinds of neoplasm to delineate their malignant or nonmalignant nature for proper diagnosis and treatment. Readers who are interested in researching the field of Ayurveda should know these definitions. Otherwise, the Ayurvedic approach, which is not based on modern medical science, will not be clearly understood.

Ayurveda points out that the tissues of the inner layer of the dermis, or the same kind of tissues lining any part of the body, are regarded as the original birthplace of Granthi or Arbuda. The tissue of the inner layer of the skin is called "rohini." Literally, it means "tissue which has the nature of growth." Ayurvedic anatomy considers it to be a sixth layer of the skin. It seems clear that the word *rohini* is a synonym for the word *epithelium,* the group of cells found lining the skin, and surface layers of the mucous membranes, where many cancers start.

Pathogenic injuries to muscular tissues and blood can be caused by lifestyle errors, such as unhealthy foods, poor hygiene, or poor behavior. They can also result from physical trauma or imbalances of Vata, Pitta, and Kapha. Such injuries result in injury to the rohini tissue, and the formation of abnormal branches from the blood vessels. In this stage, early Granthis or Arbudas can develop, in the form of bubble-shaped glandular growths.

Because the injured rohini tissues have "the nature of growth," the process of healing often leaves behind tiny scars. That is, the rapidly growing cells have a tendency to form poorly vascularized tissue during repair. However, the injured rohini tissues cannot, in general, develop into harmful neutral cells. But it is well investigated that injured rohini tissues which exist within the milieu of muscular tissue, fats, and/or blood which are vitiated by pathogens (doshas) can and do develop into harmful neutral cells. Thus the epithelial cells become parasites.

At the time of Atreya and Dhanwantari (7th century B.C.), surgery was considered the best method of treatment. They found that the herbal medical treatments against cancer, in the form of either Granthi or Arbuda, were beneficial only in the beginning stage. Nonetheless, they recorded a group of successful treatments for use against Gulma and neoplasms of individual organs.

Vagbhata (8th century A.D.), a well-known Buddhist physician, composed two texts, *Astanga Hridaya* and *Astanga Sangraha*. These texts introduced some new understandings and a new medical approach to the treatment of cancer. For example, these texts have delineated some new types of Granthis and their treatments.

The Siddhas (7th to 13th century A.D.) are known as the founders of Buddhist and Hindu Tantrism. They made powerful contributions to the field of medicine. In particular, the science which became incorrectly known as "alchemy," but which was actually medicine making based upon their theories of the pharmacology of toxic materials, is the contribution which brought about a revolutionary change in the medical history of Ayurveda. As a consequence of their contributions, cancer was considered no longer incurable, if it was treated in the early stages. This was true for both the basic common neoplasms and neoplasms of the individual organs.

The *Chakradatta* composed by Dr. Chakrapani (10th century A.D.), the *Sarangadhara Samhita* by Dr. Sarangadhara (14th century A.D.), the *Bhavaprakasha Samhita* by Dr. Bhavamisra (15th century A.D.), the *Satmya Darpan Samhita* by Dr. Viswanath (16th century A.D.), the *Vaisajya Ratnabali* by Dr. Binoda Lala Sen Gupta (18th century A.D.), the

Rasatarangini by Dr. Sadananda Sharma (19th century A.D.), and so on are the Ayurvedic texts of internal medicine. These texts contain numerous well-tested remedies based on "alchemy" for internal and external cancers.

The fundamental theory of Ayurvedic treatment is based on the balance of Vata, Pitta, and Kapha. Within the body, these philosophical "regulatory energies" are represented by three major bodily systems: the nervous system, the venous system, and the arterial system. Observation shows that three regulatory systems are found connected to every internal organ; they regulate each organ, as well as the organism as a whole. This theory is called Tridosa Siddhanta.

As we mentioned earlier, the original Ayurvedic texts pointed out that the medical treatment against cancer based on the theory of Tridosha balance had no satisfactory results. Medicine based on the theory of balance has a mild or slow effect that cannot effectively counteract the rapid growth and the critical condition of most cancers. Therefore, the doctors of that time period emphasized surgery as the best application for the cure of cancer.

The effect of drugs based on the principle of "alchemy" is different and more powerful. Certain poisonous plants, heavy metals (such as mercury and arsenic), minerals, and animal products were found very useful in cancers when they were prepared by the process of alchemy, using various methods to alter the strong poisons and render them harmless. Their extensive research in this field focused on the idea of "rasayana," or rejuvenation, the term for the Ayurvedic school that focused on longevity (one of the eight original branches). With the intention of promoting long life and good health, the doctors studying rasayana therapies concentrated on the unique nature of certain plants and minerals which stimulated the body tissues to create extraordinary immunity against many forms of disease. Working in this field, ancient alchemists were proud to introduce some effective remedies for external and internal cancers.

The remainder of the book describes dozens of classic formulas and treatments used for various types of cancers (see the Resource Guide for instructions on how to obtain this information). Ayurvedic treatment for cancer requires a high level of skill in diagnosis and choice of medicines, so I will offer only a few sample formulas, in addition to the **shilajatu rasayana** formula presented earlier in this chapter:

This **"alchemical"** anticancer formula was presented by Dr. Vagbhata in the 13th century, in the 24th chapter of his book ***Rasaratna Samucchaya*. Purified mercury** is ground with **tanduliyam juice** *(Amaranthus polyganus),* **punarnava root** *(Boerhavia diffusa),* **naga** (a type of *Sida cordifolia),* **aloe gum** (kanya or *A. vera),* **bala,** and cow urine. **Note:** This medicine contains toxic ingredients and requires special preparation skills. Mercury preparations are not legal to import into the U.S. at the present time. Ayurvedic physicians, including Dr. Mana, have reported many successes using these formulas over the centuries.

Kaishora guggulu: 64 parts each of **haritaki fruit, vibhitaki fruit, amla fruit,** and **guduchi stem** are mixed together with 64 parts of **guggul gum** and boiled in an iron vessel. When the mixture becomes gummy, mix in:

3 parts each of **haritaki fruit, vibhitaki fruit, amla fruit**
4 parts of **guduchi stem**
6 parts of **trikatu**
2 parts of **vidanga seeds** *(Embelia ribes)*
1 part of **danti seeds** *(Baliospermum montanum)*
1 part of **trivrit root** *(Operculina turpenthum)*

Form into 1-gram pills. For cancer, this compound is given in doses of 2 to 4 pills with warm water two to three times per day. It is also used for boils, ulcers, gout, and other forms of inflammation (Pitta dosha).

General Ayurvedic Immune Treatment

Ayurvedic treatment is far more involved than just tonic formulas. In fact, there are not only specific treatment protocols for individual types of cancers, which are quite comprehensive, but also dietary, lifestyle, and hygiene protocols for prevention. Such suggestions include avoidance of excess amounts of greasy food and alcohol.

Regarding prevention of breast cancer, Dr. Mana told me in 1978 that herbalists have known for centuries that breastfeeding plays a very important role in preventing breast cancer. Blockage or distention of the vessels and lymphatic ducts in the breast is considered to be a precondition of dysplastic or cancerous changes. Dr. Mana gave three examples:

- At the time of menstruation, hormonal changes cause the breasts to expand with slight pain. The breasts should naturally return to their normal condition. If the breasts remain expanded with pain, or if the pain and swelling are excessive, this indicates that there are blockages in the blood vessels or ducts. For the health of the breasts, this condition must be corrected as soon as possible, using hot compress or hot fomentation to clean the duct system. Steam bathing or application of a hot fomentation (such as **castor oil** packs) is beneficial.

- Right after the birth of a child, whether male or female, the breasts of a healthy baby are naturally full of milky liquid. This liquid must be taken out daily for a period of 1 month. The best practice is to squeeze out gently the milky liquid once or twice a day. This prevents distention, resulting in healthier ducts throughout life. Later, when a female child reaches puberty, she will have fewer problems with blockage.

- If a woman avoids breastfeeding or has impurities in her breast milk, blockage in the ducts can occur. It is advised that right after childbirth the mother should make a simple test of the purity of her milk. Pure milk dropped in water will dissolve completely. If it does not dissolve, that indicates presence of an impurity in the milk that may create blockage and/or infection. In this condition, use of bitter herbs such as **turmeric root** is beneficial to purify the milk.

Epidemiological studies have now confirmed the Ayurvedic observation in the last statement, saying that there is "accumulating evidence that lactation may have a weak protective effect on breast cancer risk" and "Modest inverse associations appeared to persist even up to 50 years since first lactation . . . suggesting that lactation may have a slight and perhaps long-lasting protective effect on postmenopausal breast cancer risk."

In 1998 I asked Dr. Mana to provide me with some case histories for advanced cancers he had treated:

- Heidy (1985). This 32-year-old German woman was diagnosed with breast cancer and had both breasts removed in 1982. She came to Dr. Mana in Kathmandu in 1985 with a diagnosis of metastatic cancer of the lung, last stage. Her doctors had declared she had a maximum of 6 months to live, and she presented with extreme weakness, coughing, breathing difficulty, cachexia (weight loss), chest pain, and hemoptysis (spitting of blood). She was initially given three Ayurvedic medicines, **Lakshadiyoga, Kaishora guggulu,** and **Chandraprabha rasayana.** She felt better day by day after the treatment and went back to Germany with strong confidence. After 6 months she came back to the Kathmandu clinic reporting a recent medical checkup which was very, very satisfactory. The neoplasm of the lungs had almost disappeared. Treatment was given for 2 more years using various Ayurvedic tonics. By 1998 she was completely cured, and she still contacts Dr. Mana every year. Her doctors in Germany did not believe how she was cured. They thought it to be a result of her destiny.

- Sandra (1990). This 42-year-old American woman was diagnosed upon biopsy with malignant adenocarcinoma of the breast. She was advised to have immediate surgery, but she refused. She presented with both breasts enlarged with hard lumps, painful upon touch. She was given several Ayurvedic tonics, including **Kaishora rasayana** and **Shilajatu rasayana.** For 3 months there was only minor improvement, but the pain gradually decreased as the lumps became smaller. Her breasts gradually went down to normal size over the next 6 months, and she continued to take the medicine for 1 year without break. After the tumors were completely gone she was placed on supportive herbal therapy. She still calls Dr. Mana on the telephone from America and has had no relapse in 8 years.

- Champa Devi (1992). This 40-year-old Nepali woman came to Dr. Mana with acute jaundice, no appetite, nausea, extreme weakness, constipation, and enlarged liver. The local teaching hospital had done exploratory surgery and diagnosed her with obstructive jaundice with enlarged liver and liver neoplasm, but no treatment was deemed possible. She was given several Ayurvedic medicines for both cancer and jaundice, including **Kamalantaka** and **Manduravataka.** She improved day by day. After 1 month, the jaundice was gone, but the enlargement of her liver had not changed. After 3 months of treatment, her enlarged liver had decreased to half its previous size, after which she began to gain hope. She continued treatment for more than 1 year, until she was completely cured. She believes she was given a new life.

TCM and Cancer

Written records of the Chinese experience with cancer treatment date back to the time of the *Yellow Emperor's Inner Classic* (Huang di nei jing), second century B.C. This ancient book addresses symptoms similar to those of esophogeal, uterine, and bone cancer. Eighteen hundred years ago Dr. Zhang Zhong Jing described treatments for disease processes similar to cancers in his *Prescriptions from the Golden Cabinet* (Jin kui yao lue), as did Dr. Sun Si Miao in *One Thousand Golden Formulas* (Qian jin yao fang).

Causes of cancer in TCM are generally divided into internal and external causes. External causes were originally related to the general forces called wind, heat, damp, summer heat, dryness, and fire. In modern understanding diet, lifestyle, and chemical factors are included in the external causative group.

Internal causes can be divided into four groups:

1. Emotional imbalances, which arise from excessive or inappropriate joy, anger, worry (mental stress), anxiety (panic), grief, fear, and shock

2. Accumulation of toxins in the internal organs

3. Systemic imbalance of Yin and Yang

4. Deficiency of Qi

The basic idea is that the external causes cannot cause cancer unless or until the body has been weakened by internal causes. The various imbalances, called Qi stagnation, blood stasis, mucus accumulation, dampness stagnation, and heat toxins, gradually cause cancer to develop over time. Because the causative factors can be controlled and treated with lifestyle, diet, and herbal treatments, this becomes the primary TCM strategy for prevention. It differs from the aforementioned preventive measures only in that TCM-trained doctors are able to identify systemic imbalances within their paradigm and treat them in a more precise way.

Treatment of Chemotherapy and Radiation Side Effects with TCM Herbs

Combined treatment has been in continuous development and use in China for the past two decades. The following herbal strategies for combating side effects of radiation and chemotherapy are based upon the collection of data on common usage from physicians in the major hospitals in China, as reported in major journals, articles, and books.

These are general guidelines and can be modified by qualified doctors, of course. Western practitioners, if they understand the logic underlying the choices below, may substitute herbs with similar actions. For example, **milk thistle seed** could be used for liver toxicity. Ayurvedic practitioners might use herbs such as **guduchi stem** and **turmeric root.** Dosages and relative proportions of herbs should be determined based on signs and symptoms.

- **Nausea:** Use a combination of **pinellia tuber, white atractylodes, licorice root, agastache, tangerine peel,** and **poria mushroom.** May be used as a tea or dried decoction.

- **Reduction of white blood cells and platelets:** Use a formula with **astragalus root, polygonatum rhizome** (huang jing or *P. sibiricum),* **millettia stem, lycium fruit, tu si zi seed** *(Cuscuta chinensis),* **dang gui root, jujube fruit** (da zao or *Ziziphus jujuba),* **tortoiseshell** (gui ban), **ligustrum berry** (nu shen zi or *L. lucidum),* **poria mushroom,** and **deer antler.**

- **Liver toxicity:** Use a formula with **capillaris** (yin chen hao or *Artemisia capillaris),* **rhubarb root, gardenia fruit** (zhi zi or *G. jasminoides),* **salvia root, moutan bark** (mu dan pi or *Paeonia suffruticosa),* **dang gui root, curcuma tuber** (yu jin or *C. longa),* and **schisandra berry. Schisandra berry** can be used by itself in large quantity.

- **Depression, fatigue, diarrhea, dizziness, poor appetite, insomnia** (any two or three of these symptoms): Use the classic formulas **gui pi tang** or **rehmannia six.** Some of the major herbs in these formulas are **white atractylodes, ginseng root, astragalus root, poria mushroom, honey-fried licorice, dang gui root, cooked rehmannia root,** and **dioscorea root** (shan yao or *D. opposita).* I advise using relatively small amounts of **ginseng** or **astragalus roots** at first and put more emphasis on **honey-fried licorice** and **dioscorea root,** then adjust accordingly.

- **Cough, cough with blood, shortness of breath** (especially after lung, diaphragm, or esophogeal cancer): Use a formula of **glehnia root** (sha shen or *Adenophora tetraphylla),* **scrophularia root** (xuan shen or *S. ningpoensis),* **licorice root, apricot seed, ophiopogon root** (mai men dong), **rubia root** (qian cao gen or *R. cordifolia),* and **cordyceps mushroom.**

- **Local skin damage from radiation:** Externally, use **Golden Satisfaction Cream** (ru i huang jin san). In a cream base combine **rhubarb root, phellodendron bark, curcuma tuber** (yu jin or *C. longa)*, **angelica root** (bai zhi or *A. archangelica)*, **arisaema rhizome** (tian nan xing or *A. amurense)*, **tangerine peel, black atractylodes, magnolia bark, licorice root,** and **trichosanthes root.** Also effective is an ointment containing 4% **curcuma tuber** (e zhu). Internally, use a formula made of **forsythia fruit, honeysuckle flower, moutan bark, salvia root, red peony root, myrrh gum, mastic gum** (ru xiang or *Boswellia carterii)*, **astragalus root, millettia,** and **dried earthworm** (di long or *Pheretima aspergillum)*.

- **Bloating, gas, abdominal and stomach pain, and bleeding ulcer:** Use **white peony root, licorice root, dioscorea root, chih-ke, white atractylodes, poria mushroom, hawthorn fruit** (shan zha), **wheat sprouts** (fu xiao mai), and **germinated rice sprouts** (gu ya).

- **Kidney toxicity with urging and frequency:** Use **rehmannia six formula.** If there is blood in the urine and severe pain, add **poria mushroom, grifola mushroom** (zhu ling or *Polyporus umbellatus / Grifola umbellata)*, **plantago seed** (che quian zi), **imperata rhizome** (bai mao gen or *I. cylindrica)*, **rubia root, agrimony** (xian he cao or *A. pilosa)*, **di yu root** *(Sanguisorba officinalis)*, and **tien chi root.**

- **Intestinal inflammation and diarrhea or constipation, blood in the stool and pain:** Use **rubia root, tien chi root, di yu root, sophora flower** (huai hua mi or *S. japonica)*, **agrimony,** and **purslane** (ma chi xian or *Portulaca oleracea)*.

- **Neuropathy:** Use a formula made of **drynaria rhizome** (gu sui bu or *D. fortunei)*, **raw rehmannia root, epimedium, morinda root** (ba ji tian or *M. officinalis)*, **loranthes** (sang ji sheng), **salvia root, dang gui root, millettia stem, psoralea seed** (bu gu zhi or *P. corylifolia)*, **curculigo rhizome** (xian mao or *C. orchioides)*, and **cibotium rhizome** (gu ji or *C. barometz)*. Additional herbs are added depending on the location of the symptoms. For the face: add **angelica root** and **cnidium rhizome** (chuan xiong or *Ligusticum wallichii)*. For the upper limbs: add **mulberry twig** (sang zhi or *Morus alba)* and **curcuma tuber.** For the lower limbs: add **achyranthes root** (huan niu xi or *A. bidentata)* and **mu gua fruit** *(Chaenomelis lagenaria)*.

- **Heart damage with edema, breathing difficulty, heart pain, shortness of breath, palpitations, and angina:** Use **codonopsis root** (dang shen or *C. pilosula)*, **glehnia root, ginseng root, salvia root, sophora flower, schisandra berry, ophiopogon root, kudzu root,** and **cnidium rhizome.**

- **Hormone imbalances or endocrine disturbances, with reduced or absent menstruation or reduction in sperm count:** Use **ligustrum fruit** (nu shen zi or *L. lucidum)*, **eclipta, cinnamon bark, purified aconite** (fu zi or *Aconitum palmatum)*, epimedium, dang gui root, cnidium rhizome, salvia root, water plantain (ze xie or *Alisma plantago-aquatica),* leonorus (yi mu cao or *L. heterophyllus),* persica seed (tao ren or *Prunus persica),* and carthamus flower.

- **Hair loss:** Use a formula of **cooked** and **raw rehmannia root, ligustrum fruit, dang gui root, donkey skin gelatin** (e jiao), **deer antler, turtle shell, shou wu root, epimedium,** and **salvia root.**

- **Local skin discoloration from radiation:** Use a formula of **salvia root, dang gui root, cnidium rhizome, red peony root, carthamus flower, morinda root** (ba ji tian or *M. officinalis),* **cinnamon bark, deer antler, epimedium, tu si zi seed,** and **lycium fruit.**

- **Recovery from surgery:** Use **tien chi root** by itself, 2–4 grams twice a day, or make a formula with **astragalus root, ginseng root, red peony root, dang gui root, poria mushroom, American ginseng root, tien chi root,** and **wild asparagus root.**

Using Herbs to Strengthen the Effects of Chemotherapy

Many Chinese researchers have been focusing on simultaneously stopping the side effects and strengthening the anticancer effects of chemotherapy and radiation therapy. We can understand how this is possible if we correlate the general or systemic effects that herbs have (as understood in the traditional sense) with our previous discussion listing the very specific effects many herbs have on immune system parameters. There are at least four theoretical groupings:

1. With chemotherapy or radiation patients with signs of severe inflammation and toxins, use herbs with anticancer effects that also reduce heat. Examples are **subprostrata root** (shan dou gen or *Sophora subprostrata),* **scute root, oldenlandia herb** (bai hua she she cao or *O. diffusa),* and **prunella.**

2. With signs of Yin deficiency, use herbs with anticancer effects that also nourish the Yin. Examples are **raw rehmannia root** and **scrophularia root.**

3. With blood congestion or hyperviscosity, use herbs with anticancer effects that also move the blood. Examples are **salvia root, cnidium rhizome, tien chi root, millettia stem,** and **pinellia tuber.**

4. With signs of Qi deficiency and weakness, use herbs with anticancer effects that also tonify the Qi. Examples are **Siberian ginseng root bark, white atractylodes, ginseng root,** and **licorice root.**

It is important to understand that these individual herbs vary in their effects on specific types of cancers, so, although choices can be made based upon energetic considerations, it is wise to check Medline for the latest research findings.

Research Highlights

- Japanese researchers noted that enhancing production of tumor necrosis factor (TNF) can benefit cancer patients. In animal models, **subprostrata root** and **white atractylodes** were among the crude herbs able to do this without side effects (Xu QA et al., 1989).

- **Oldenlandia herb** inhibits Yoshida's sarcoma and Ehrlich's ascites sarcoma in vitro. It also inhibits sarcoma-180, ascitic lymphocarcoma, and uterine cancer in mice. **Scute root** strongly inhibits JTC-26 and inhibits sarcoma-37, Ehrlich's ascites sarcoma, and cerbroma-B22 in rats (reported in Dharmananda, 1997).

Traditional Western Herbal Formulas for Cancer

I first heard about the work of the late Dr. Eli Jones while listening to a lecture by David Winston, one of the few living herbalists who is fully trained in the Eclectic medicine traditions. Dr. Jones treated thousands of cancer patients at the end of the 19th century and was so respected in the field that members of opposing schools of medicine would go to him if they themselves developed cancer. In 1894, he began giving postgraduate instruction in cancer therapy to physicians from all parts of the country. In his out-of-print book *Cancer Treatment* (published in the late 1800s), now freely available on the Internet, he told us, "I have a record of cases of genuine cancer that have been cured for fifteen to twenty-five years, and there has not been a single symptom of the return of the disease." He also said, "No remedy or combination of remedies has ever been discovered, or ever will be discovered, that will cure all forms of cancer." He warned, "In the United States, in 1890 there were 18,536 deaths from cancer; in 1900 there were 29,222 deaths from this disease. At the present time the mortality cannot be less than 50,000 annually. In a paper before the Philadelphia Medical Society, Dr. John A. McGlinn says, 'One man out of every thirty-two and one woman out of every eleven die of cancer.'" (One wonders what he would think of today's statistics.)

Jones also states, "Good pure water, good pure air helps to make good healthy red blood. Unadulterated food, mostly vegetables, easily digested, leaving out tea and coffee, keep the nervous system strong and vigorous. Stop worrying." He tells us that we must "raise the nerve power, the vitality of the patient at or as near normal as possible. Many times I have noticed this fact that when the eye, the pulse, and the tongue showed the organs of the body secreting properly, good digestion, a strong, full, regular pulse, the disease itself would be at a standstill, but if the signs showed a weakened vitality, the disease would take on new life and activity."

Most of the first half of Dr. Jones's book is devoted to teaching the importance of treating the whole person, making sure the digestion and liver are functioning well, and properly dealing with stress and poor diet. He lists many specific remedies.

However, the jewel of the book for today's patient is his **Compound Scrophularia**

Syrup, which he describes as follows: "After many years of testing different remedies for the internal treatment of cancer to form a combination which could be dignified with the name 'Cancer Syrup'—a remedy that could be depended upon in the more advanced stages of cancer when the system has become saturated with the germs of cancer—I have devised the following formula. It has been the earnest study of my life to find such a combination that I could leave as a help to my brother physicians in their efforts to cure the more desperate forms of this disease. I have the utmost faith in the curative power of this combination. I have never mentioned this remedy to anyone and would not until I had thoroughly tested it in many difficult cases of genuine cancer so that I could conscientiously recommend it in my book on cancer."

The formula contains **scrophularia leaves/root** *(S. nodosa),* **poke root** *(Phytolacca americana),* **yellow dock root** *(Rumex crispus),* **false bittersweet root/bark** *(Celastrus scandens),* **turkey corn root** *(Corydalis formosa),* **mayapple root** *(Podophyllum peltatum),* **juniper berries** *(J. communis),* **prickly ash berries,** and **guiacum wood resin** *(G. officinalis).*

An analysis of this formula shows that it contains herbs that strongly reduce toxic heat and swelling, soften hardened tissue, nourish the blood, cleanse the liver, reduce pain, and reduce blood congestion. Because it contains many very strong herbs, it should be administered only under the direction of a qualified herbalist. This formula is made by Herbalist & Alchemist (see Resource Guide for information).

The Hoxey Formula

This classic formula was used by Harry Hoxey early in the 20th century to treat cancer. He developed quite a reputation and had many run-ins with the legal and medical systems of his day. He claimed the formula had been discovered by his grandfather, who used it to treat farm animals with cancers. In fact, the late Dr. John Christopher said in a lecture that similar or almost identical formulas existed in the Eclectic materia medica and were also in use by Native Americans. This formula is a classic "blood purifier," which can be used to cleanse the liver, blood, and lymphatics. It is particularly effective in treating swollen lymph nodes and swollen glands. I have used it successfully many times for chronic swollen glands unresponsive to antibiotics, usually combining it with **castor oil packs.**

Early in my career, a patient named Alice, the wife of a local professor, came to me with acute leukemia. At that time I had no experience in treating this disease, and she was under the care of an oncologist, so I simply gave her the Hoxey formula and some dietary changes. To my amazement, although she was taking no other medicine, the numbers of abnormal cells in her blood quickly began to decline, and she went into a complete remission. The remission lasted for 8 years. Tragically, after her best friend died suddenly, the leukemia returned within a month, and she died undergoing a bone marrow transplant.

This formula contains liquid extracts of **red clover blossoms, licorice root, buckthorn bark** *(Rhamnus frangula),* **burdock seed** *(Arctium lappa),* **stillingia root** *(Stillingia sylvatica),* **Oregon grape root** *(Berberis aquifolium),* **phytolacca root** *(P. americana),* **prickly ash bark, wild indigo root** *(Baptisia tinctoria),* and **potassium iodide.**

This compound should be administered only by a qualified herbalist or health professional. It is available from several herbal suppliers.

Putting It All Together

When Nai-shing and I work with cancer patients, we need to determine the type of cancer they have and the method of treatment being used by their oncologist. After that we examine them to determine their general condition, including digestive energy, nervous system condition, blood, emotions, vital force, and so on. Then we choose from the following essential strategies. These strategies can be used whether or not the patient is undergoing Western treatment.

- **Develop a personal and educational support network.** Cancer patients often feel helpless and, out of fear, go along with the treatments they are given at the outset. It is imperative to find a network of family, friends, therapists, and doctors who can work together and coordinate various treatments.

- **Make supportive dietary changes and supply basic nutrients.** Be sure to use a good variety of vitamins, minerals, and specific nutrients like coenzyme Q_{10}, lipoic acid, and so on. (See Chapter 10.)

- **Treat the whole person.** Contributing problems such as thyroid conditions, blood sugar problems, emotional problems, digestive power, and hormonal imbalances must all be taken into consideration and treated.

- **Timing is important.** Reduce strong antioxidants about 2 days before and 4 days after a chemotherapy or radiation treatment. Use herbs that strengthen the Western treatments instead.

- **Debulking is a viable option.** Surgical removal is the best method of debulking tumors whenever possible. After surgery, use herbs that stimulate wound healing for several weeks. Medicines that dissolve tumor masses are essential when the patient has solid tumors, even after surgery, as are immune tonics, to control metastasis. The standard Ayurvedic formula **Kanchanara guggulu** can be used, or one of the TCM "mass-resolving" formulas. I am hoping that more effective yet less toxic methods for breaking down tumors become available. One area of interest is the work of Dr. Nicholas Gonzalez in New York. Using porcine pancreatic enzymes combined with metabolic-based diets and detoxification, he has been very successful in stimulating tumor destruction. His work is based upon the theory that our pancreatic enzymes are a natural cancer fighter. More information is available at www.dr-gonzalez.com.

- **Use a generalized anticancer formula.** Choose from among standard formulas such as the **Hoxey formula, Kaisara guggulu, Compound Scrophularia Syrup, Gynostemma tablets,** or **Astragalus 10+** (both made by ITM). There are many TCM formulas of this sort as well, which combine various anticancer actions. These should be used throughout the therapy and may be rotated. Advanced practitioners may review the ingredients and choose those based upon patient needs.

- **External treatments can be useful.** If the tumor is on the surface, external herbal medicines (escharotic pastes) can be used. These are especially useful for skin cancers. Information on their use can be found on Michael Tierra's Planetary Herbs Web site. However, properly done surgery would be the first choice. **Castor oil packs** can be used over cancerous areas. Of great interest is the work of herbalist and certified nutritionist Donald Yance, AHG. His book (see below) contains information on the use of anticancer transdermal essential oils, which can be applied externally over solid tumors.

- **Regulate the blood.** There are many formula choices here. You can refer to information from Chapter 12. The treatment must be based upon individual signs and symptoms. Goals include improving blood circulation, removing toxins, improving liver function, nourishing the blood, removing fats and viscous matter. Toxin removal should be emphasized.

- **Treat side effects of chemotherapy and radiation as they occur.** This is described in detail on pages 498–500. These treatments are as needed.

- **Strengthen the immune system.** Throughout cancer treatment, and for months and years afterward, it is essential to use a formula of strong immune-system-strengthening herbs, emphasizing medicinal mushrooms, fu zheng, and rasayana herbs.

Note: For more information, I highly recommend that all cancer patients get a copy of these two books:

Herbal Medicine, Healing and Cancer, by Donald Yance, C.N., AHG. This book by an experienced practitioner outlines many successful treatments of cancer using herbs and nutrients.

Beating Cancer with Nutrition, by Patrick and Noreen Quillin. Dr. Quillin's book, in addition to its excellent content, has a comprehensive list of holistic doctors listed by ZIP code.

Parting Comments

At this point you are educated about the realities of global herbal medicine. You are in a far stronger position to select and choose for yourself among the vast array of therapies and modalities available today, with far less chance of making simple mistakes. Thank you for allowing me to participate in your health care. On a closing note, I wish you a lifetime of wellness. To determine if you're a good candidate, remember this Internet aphorism:

The 12 Warning Signs of Good Health

1. The persistent presence of a support network

2. Chronic positive expectations and a tendency to frame events in a constructive light

3. Episodic peak experiences

4. A sense of spiritual involvement

5. Increased sensitivity to the needs of the body

6. A tendency to easily adapt to changing conditions

7. An increased appetite for physical exercise, healthy foods, and herbs

8. A rapid response time to crisis and quick recovery

9. A tendency to identify and communicate feelings

10. Repeated episodes of gratitude, generosity, and related positive emotions

11. A compulsion to contribute to society

12. A persistent sense of humor

If five or more of these indicators are present, you may be at risk for full-blown good health.

APPENDIX:
HERBS LISTED BY
PHYSIOLOGICAL ACTION

Herbs That Affect Digestion

By Common Name

Aila *(Amomum* species)

Ardrakam *(Zingiber officinalis)*

Areca peel *(Areca catechu)*

Astragalus root *(Astragalus membranaceus)*

Badara *(Ziziphus jujuba)*

Bai dou kou *(Amomum kravana)*

Bai zhu *(Atractylodes macrocephala)*

Ban xia *(Pinellia ternata)*

Bitter orange fruit *(Citrus aurantium—immature)*

Black cumin seeds *(Nigella sativa)*

Black mustard seeds *(Sinapsis juncea)*

Black pepper *(Piper nigrum)*

Bromelain *(Ananas comusus)*

Bupleurum root *(Bupleurum chinensis)*

Capillaris *(Artemisia capillaris)*

Cardamom *(Amomum* species)

Cardamom *(Elettaria cardamomum)*

Cayenne pepper *(Capsicum frutescens)*

Chai hu *(Bupleurum chinensis)*

Chavyam *(Piper chava)*

Chebulic myrobalan *(Terminalia chebula)*

Chen pi *(Citrus reticulata)*

Chih-ke *(Citrus aurantium—mature)*

Chih-ko *(Citrus aurantium—mature)*

Chinese date *(Ziziphus jujuba)*

Cinnamon bark *(Cinnamomum* species)

Cloves *(Myrtus caryophyllus)*

Cluster *(Amomum kravana)*

Codonopsis *(Codonopsis pilosulae)*

Cumin seed *(Cuminum cynimum)*

Cyperus tuber *(Cyperus rotundus)*

Da fu pi *(Areca catechu)*

Da zao *(Ziziphus jujuba)*

Dang shen *(Codonopsis pilosulae)*

Dioscorea *(Dioscorea* species)

Gan cao *(Glycyrrhiza glabra)*

Gan jiang *(Zingiber officinalis*)

Ginger root *(Zingiber officinalis)*

Ginseng root *(Panax ginseng)*

Haritaki fruit *(Terminalia chebula)*

He zi *(Terminalia chebula)*

Hou po *(Magnolia officinalis)*

Hu jiao *(Piper nigrum)*

Huang jing *(Polygonatum sibiricum)*

Huang qi *(Astragalus membranicus)*

Indian plum *(Ziziphus jujuba)*

Jatiphalam *(Myristica fragrans)*

Jirakam *(Cuminum cynimum)*

Jujube date *(Ziziphus jujuba)*

Krisnajirakam seed *(Nigella sativa)*

Kushtha *(Saussurea* species / *Aucklandia lappa)*

Kut root *(Saussurea* species */ Aucklandia lappa)*
Lavangam *(Myrtus caryophyllus)*
Licorice root *(Glycyrrhiza glabra)*
Long pepper *(Piper longum)*
Madhukam *(Glycyrrhiza glabra)*
Magnolia bark *(Magnolia officinalis)*
Maricham *(Piper nigrum)*
Mu xiang *(Saussurea* species */ Aucklandia lappa)*
Mustaka *(Cyperus rotundus)*
Nutgrass *(Cyperus rotundus)*
Nutmeg seed *(Myristica fragrans)*
Omum seed *(Trachyspermum ammi)*
Oregano *(Origanum* species)
Papaya fruit *(Carica papaya)*
Peppers *(Piper* species)
Pineapple stem *(Ananas comusus)*
Pipali fruit *(Piper longum)*
Ren shen *(Panax ginseng)*
Rosemary leaf *(Rosmarinus officinalis)*
Rou dou kou *(Myristica fragrans)*
Rou gui *(Cinnamomum* species)
Sarsapi *(Sinapsis juncea)*
Saussurea *(Saussurea* species */ Aucklandia lappa)*
Sha ren *(Amomum* species)
Shan yao *(Dioscorea* species)
Sheng jiang *(Zingiber officinalis)*
Sneezewort *(Achillea ptarmica)*
Sunthi *(Zingiber officinalis)*
Tangerine peel *(Citrus reticulata)*
Thoroughwax root *(Bupleurum chinensis)*
Trikatu (three-pepper compound)
White atractylodes rhizome *(Atractylodes macrocephala)*
Wild yam *(Dioscorea* species)
Xiang fu *(Cyperus rotundus)*
Yavani *(Trachyspermum ammi)*
Yin chen hao *(Artemisia capillaris)*
Zhi gan cao *(Glycyrrhiza glabra)*
Zhi shi *(Citrus aurantium*—immature)

By Latin Name

Achillea ptarmica (Sneezewort)
Amomum kravana (Bai dou kou / Cluster)
Amomum species (Aila / Cardamom / Sha ren)
Ananas comusus (Bromelain / Pineapple stem)
Areca catechu (Areca Peel / Da fu pi)
Artemisia capillaris (Yin chen hao / Capillaris)
Astragalus membranaceus (Huang qi / Astragalus root)
Atractylodes macrocephala (Bai zhu / White atractylodes)
Bupleurum chinensis (Bupleurum / Chai hu / Thoroughwax root)
Capsicum frutescens (Cayenne pepper)
Carica papaya (Papita / Papaya)
Cinnamomum species (Twak / Cinnamon bark / Rou gui / Tvak)
Citrus species (Chih-ko / / Zhi shi / immature fruit of the bitter orange / Tangerine peel / Chen pi)
Codonopsis pilosulae (Codonopsis / Dang shen)
Cuminum cynimum (Jirakam / Cumin seed)
Cyperus rotundus (Mustaka / Cyperus tuber / Xiang fu / Korehijar / Nutgrass)
Dioscorea species (Shan yao / Dioscorea / Wild yam)
Elettaria cardamomum (Sukshmaila / Cardamom / Lesser cardamom)
Glycyrrhiza glabra (Madhukam / Licorice / Gan cao / Zhi gan cao)
Hordei germinatus (Hordeum gerinatis)
Magnolia officinalis (Hou po / Magnolia bark)
Myristica fragrans (Jatiphalam / Nutmeg seed / Rou dou kou)
Myrtus caryophyllus (Lavangam / Cloves)
Nigella sativa (Krisnajirakam seed / Black cumin)

Origanum species (Oregano)
Panax ginseng (Ren shen / Ginseng)
Pinellia ternata (Ban xia)
Piper chava (Chavyam)
Piper longum (Pipali fruit / Long pepper)
Piper nigrum (Maricham / Black pepper / Hu jiao)
Polygonatum sibiricum (Huang jing)
Rosmarinus officinalis (Rosemary leaf)
Saussurea species / *Aucklandia lappa* (Kushtha / Mu xiang / Saussurea / Kut root)

Sinapsis juncea (Sarsapi / Black mustard)
Terminalia chebula (Haritaki fruit / Chebulic myrobalan / He zi)
Trachyspermum ammi (Yavani / Omum seed)
Trikatu (Three-pepper compound)
Zingiber officinalis (Sheng jiang / Sunthi / Ginger root / Gan jiang)
Ziziphus jujuba (Badari / Da zao / Indian plum / Jujube / Chinese date)

Diuretic Herbs

By Common Name

Barley water (after cooking) *(Hordeum vulgare)*
Beggar-lice *(Desmodium styracifolium)*
Buchu leaves *(Barosma betulina)*
Cleavers herb *(Galium aparine)*
Desmodium *(Desmodium stryacipolium)*
Han fang ji root *(Stephania tetrandra)*
Indian kidney tea *(Orthosiphon aristata)*
Java tea leaves *(Orthosiphon aristata)*
Jin chien cao *(Desmodium styracifolium)*
Jin qian cao *(Desmodium styracifolium)*
Juniper berry *(Juniperus communis)*
Mu tong *(Akebia* species)
Open-ended wood *(Akebia* species)
Parsley piert *(Aphanes arvensis)*
Punarnava *(Boerhavia diffusa)*
Stephania root *(Stephania tetrandra*)
Uva ursi leaf *(Arctostaphylos uva-ursi)*
Water plantain *(Alisma plantago-aquatica)*
Ze xie *(Alisma plantago-aquatica)*

By Latin Name

Akebia species (Mu tong / Open-ended wood)
Alisma plantago-aquatica (Ze xie / Water plantain)
Aphanes arvensis (Parsley piert)
Arctostaphylos uva-ursi (Uva ursi leaf)
Barosma betulina (Buchu leaves)
Boerhavia diffusa (Punarnava plant and root)
Desmodium styracifolium (Desmodium / Jin qian cao / Jin chien cao / Beggar-lice)
Galium aparine (Cleavers herb)
Hordeum vulgare (Barley water—after cooking)
Juniperus communis (Juniper berry)
Orthosiphon aristata (Java tea leaves / Indian kidney tea)
Stephania tetrandra (Han fang ji / Stephania)

Laxative Herbs

By Common Name

Agar *(Gelidium* species)
Aloe gum *(Aloe* species)
Amlavetasa *(Rheum emodi, R. palmatum)*
Arka *(Calotropis gigantea)*
Belleric myrobolan *(Terminalia belerica)*
Buckthorn bark *(Rhamnus* species)
Cascara sagrada *(Rhamnus* species)
Castor oil *(Ricinus communis)*
Chebulic myrobalan *(Terminalia chebula)*
Da huang *(Rheum emodi / R. palmatum)*
Eranda *(Ricinus communis)*
Flaxseed oil *(Linum usitatissimum)*
Haritaki fruit *(Terminalia chebula)*
He zi *(Terminalia chebula)*
Hu huang lian *(Picrorhiza kurroa)*
Indian jalap *(Operculina turpenthum)*
Indian laburnum *(Cassia fistula)*
Kanya *(Aloe* species)
Katki *(Picrorhiza kurroa)*
Katuki rhizome *(Picrorhiza kurroa)*
Kumari *(Aloe* species)
Lu hui *(Aloe* species)
Mang xiao *(Depuratum mirabilitum)*
Milkweed plant *(Calotropis gigantea)*
Mirabilitum *(Depuratum mirabilitum)*
Nishotha resin *(Operculina turpenthum)*
Papaya fruit *(Carica papaya)*
Papita *(Carica papaya)*
Psyllium hulls *(Plantago* species)
Rajavriksa pod/fruit *(Cassia fistula)*
Rhubarb root *(Rheum emodi / R. palmatum)*
Senna *(Senna* species / *Cassia* species)
Triphala (three-fruits compound)
Trivrit root *(Operculina turpenthum)*
Vibhitaki fruit *(Terminalia belerica / belleric myrobalan)*

By Latin Name

Aloe species (Kumari / Aloe gum / Kanya / Lu hui)
Calotropis gigantea (Arka / Milkweed plant)
Carica papaya (Papita / Papaya fruit)
Cassia fistula (Rajavriksa pod/fruit / Indian laburnum)
Depuratum mirabilitum (Mang xiao / Mirabilitum)
Gelidium species (Agar)
Linum usitatissimum (Flaxseed oil)
Operculina turpenthum (Trivrit root / Nishotha resin / Indian jalap)
Picrorhiza kurroa (Katuki rhizome / Katki / Hu huang lian)
Plantago species (Psyllium hulls)
Rhamnus species (Cascara sagrada / Buckthorn bark)
Rheum emodi, R. palmatum (Amlavetasa / Da huang / Rhubarb root)
Ricinus communis (Eranda / Castor oil and root)
Senna species / *Cassia* species (Senna)
Terminalia belerica (Belleric myrobalan / Vibhitaki fruit)
Terminalia chebula (Haritaki fruit / Chebulic myrobalan / He zi)
Triphala (Three-fruits compound)

Blood-Thinning Herbs*

By Common Name

Anteater scales *(Manis pentadactyla / Manitis pentadactylae)*

Bromelain *(Ananas comusus)*

Carthamus flower *(Carthamus tinctorius)*

Chuan shan jia *(Manis pentadactyla / Manitis pentadactylae)*

Chuan xiong root *(Ligusticum chuanxiong)*

Dragon's blood *(Dracaena cambodiana / Draconis sanguis)*

E zhu *(Curcuma zedoaria)*

Ginkgo leaf *(Ginkgo biloba)*

Hong hua *(Carthamus tinctorius)*

Karchura *(Curcuma zedoaria)*

Khella *(Ammi visnaga / A. majus)*

Liquidambar fruit *(Liquidambar taiwaniana)*

Lu lu tong *(Liquidambar taiwaniana)*

Lycopus *(Lycopus lucidus)*

Mo yao *(Commiphora myrrha / C. molmol)*

Myrrh gum *(Commiphora myrrha / C. molmol)*

Peach kernel *(Prunus persica)*

Persica seed *(Prunus persica)*

Pineapple stem *(Ananas comusus)*

Prickly ash bark *(Xanthoxylum clavaherculis)*

Quinine *(Cinchona* species)

Red cinchona bark *(Cinchona* species)

Rue *(Ruta graveolens)*

Safflower flower *(Carthamus tinctorius)*

Salvia root *(Salvia miltiorrhiza)*

San leng *(Sparganium stoloniferum)*

Sappan *(Caesalpinia sappan)*

Sati *(Curcuma zedoaria)*

Sparganii *(Sparganium stoloniferum)*

Su mu *(Caesalpinia sappan)*

Sweet woodruff *(Melilotus officinalis)*

Tao ren *(Prunus persica)*

Xue jie *(Dracaena cambodiana / D. sanguis)*

Yellow Peruvian bark *(Cinchona* species)

Ze lan *(Lycopus lucidus)*

Zedoary *(Curcuma zedoaria)*

By Latin Name

Ammi majus (Khella)

Ammi visnaga (Khella)

Ananas comusus (Bromelain / Pineapple stem)

Caesalpinia sappan (Su mu / Sappan)

Carthamus tinctorius (Hong hua / Carthamus flower / Safflower flower)

Cinchona species (Yellow Peruvian bark / Red cinchona bark / Quinine)

Commiphora myrrha, C. molmol (Mo yao / Myrrh gum)

Curcuma zedoaria (Karchura / E zhu / Zedoary / Sati)

Dracaena cambodiana / Draconis sanguis (Xue jie / Dragon's blood)

Ginkgo biloba (Ginkgo leaf)

Ligusticum chuanxiong (Chuan xiong root)

Liquidambar taiwaniana (Lu lu tong / Liquidambar fruit)

Lycopus lucidus (Ze lan / Lycopus)

Manis pentadactyla / Manitis pentadactylae (Chuan shan jia / Anteater scales)

Melilotus officinalis (Sweet woodruff)

Prunus persica (Tao ren / Persica seed / Peach kernel)

Ruta graveolens (Rue)

Salvia miltiorrhiza (Salvia root / dan shen)

Sparganium stoloniferum (San leng / Sparganii)

Xanthoxylum clava-herculis (Prickly ash bark)

*These herbs have historically been reported to significantly thin the blood, which may increase the action of your medications. This list is not exhaustive.

Herbs That May Lower Blood Pressure

By Common Name

American hellebore rhizome/root *(Veratrum viride)*

Carolina jasmine root/rhizome *(Gelsemium sempervirens)*

Coleus rootstock *(Coleus forskohlii)*

Da suan *(Allium sativum)*

Devil's claw root *(Harpagophytum procumbens)*

False hellebore rhizome/root *(Veratrum viride)*

Gamberi vine stems and thorns *(Uncaria sinensis)*

Garlic bulb *(Allium sativum)*

Gastrodia rhizome *(Gastrodia elata)*

Gelsemium root/rhizome *(Gelsemium sempervirens)*

Gou teng vine stems and thorns *(Uncaria sinensis)*

Hawthorn leaf/berry *(Crataegus* species)

Jatamansi *(Nardostachys jatamansi / Valeriana wallichii / V. jatamansi)*

Linden flower *(Tilia cordata / T. platyphyllos)*

Mistletoe *(Viscum album)*

Muskroot *(Nardostachys jatamansi / Valeriana wallichii / V. jatamansi)*

Olive leaf *(Olea europaea)*

Rauwolfia root *(Rauwolfia serpentina)*

Ren shen / Ginseng root *(Panax ginseng)*

Sarpagandha root *(Rauwolfia serpentina)*

Tagara root *(Valeriana wallichii / V. jatamansi)*

Tian ma rhizome *(Gastrodia elata)*

Valerian root *(Valeriana* species)

Yellow jasmine root/rhizome *(Gelsemium sempervirens)*

By Latin Name

Allium sativum (Garlic bulb / Da suan)

Coleus forskohlii (Coleus rootstock)

Crataegus species (Hawthorn leaf/berry)

Gastrodia elata (Tian ma / Gastrodia rhizome)

Gelsemium sempervirens (Gelsemium root / Yellow jasmine / Carolina jasmine)

Harpagophytum procumbens (Devil's claw root)

Nardostachys jatamansi (Jatamansi / Muskroot)

Olea europaea (Olive leaf)

Panax ginseng (Ren shen / Ginseng root)

Rauwolfia serpentina (Sarpagandha root / Rauwolfia)

Tilia cordata / T. platyphyllos (Linden flower)

Uncaria sinensis (Gou teng vine stems and thorns / Gamberi)

Valeriana species (Valerian root / Tagara / Jatamansi)

Veratrum viride (American hellebore rhizome/root / False hellebore)

Viscum album (Mistletoe)

Herbs That May Stimulate the Heart Due to Cardiac Glycoside Content or Other Mechanisms

By Common Name

Aconite *(Aconitum* species)
Adonis *(Adonis vernalis)*
Arjuna bark *(Terminalia arjuna)*
Arnica *(Arnica montana)*
Astragalus root *(Astragalus membranaceus)*
Belladonna *(Atropa belladonna)*
Bishop's weed *(Ammi visnaga)*
Camphor *(Cinnamomum camphora)*
Cayenne *(Capsicum* species)
Coffee *(Coffea arabica)*
Digitalis *(Digitalis purpurea)*
Ephedra *(Ephedra* species / *Ma huang)*
Foxglove *(Digitalis purpurea / D. lanata)*
Fu zi *(Aconitum* species)
Ginseng *(Panax ginseng)*
Hawthorn berry *(Crataegous* species*)*
Huang qi *(Astragalus membranaceus)*
Indian hemp *(Apocynum cannabinum / A. androsaemifolium)*
Karavira *(Nerium indicum)*
Leonorus *(Leonorus* species)
Lily-of-the-valley *(Convallaria majalis)*
Ma huang *(Ephedra)*
Mate *(Ilex paraguariensis)*
Monkshood *(Aconitum* species)
Motherwort *(Leonorus* species)
Oleander leaves *(Nerium oleander)*
Pheasant's eye *(Adonis vernalis)*
Pleurisy root *(Asclepias tuberosa)*
Scotch broom *(Cytisus scoparius)*
Shan zha *(Crataegus* species)
Shepherd's purse *(Capsella bursa-pastoris)*
Spreading dogbane *(Apocynum cannabinum / A. androsaemifolium)*
Squill *(Drimia maritima)*
Squill *(Urginea maritima / Scilla maritima)*

Strophanthin *(Strophanthus* species)
Vatsanabha tuber *(Aconitum* species)
Yi mu cao *(Leonorus* species)

By Latin Name

Aconitum species (Vatsanabha tuber / Fu zi / Monkshood / Aconite)
Adonis vernalis (Adonis / Pheasant's eye)
Ammi visnaga (Bishop's weed)
Apocynum androsaemifolium (Spreading dogbane leaf / Indian hemp)
Apocynum cannabinum (Spreading dogbane leaf / Indian hemp)
Arnica montana (Arnica)
Asclepias tuberosa (Pleurisy root)
Astragalus membranaceus (Astragalus root / Huang qi)
Atropa belladonna (Belladonna)
Coffea arabica (Coffee)
Capsella bursa-pastoris (Shepherd's purse)
Capsicum species (Cayenne)
Cinnamomum camphora (Camphor)
Convallaria majalis (Lily-of-the-valley)
Crataegus species (Hawthorn berry / Shan zha)
Cytisus scoparius (Scotch broom)
Digitalis purpurea (Foxglove / Digitalis)
Drimia maritima (Squill)
Ephedra species (Ephedra / Ma huang)
Erysimum species (Unknown Russian name)
Ilex paraguariensis (Mate)
Leonorus species (Yi mu cao / Leonorus / Motherwort)
Nerium species (Oleander / Karavira)
Panax ginseng (Ginseng)
Scilla maritima (Squill)
Strophanthus species (Strophanthin)
Terminalia arjuna (Arjuna bark)
Urginea maritima (Squill)

Herbs That May Potentially Interact with MAO Inhibitors Due to Tyramine Content or Other Mechanisms

By Common Name

Calamus root *(Acorus calamus)*
California poppy *(Eschscholzia californica)*
Chaste tree berry *(Vitex agnus-castus)*
Ephedra *(Ephedra* species)
Gan cao root *(Glycyrrhiza glabra)*
Ginkgo leaf *(Ginkgo biloba)*
Jatiphalam *(Myristica fragrans)*
Licorice root *(Glycyrrhiza glabra)*
Ma huang herb *(Ephedra sinica)*
Madhukam root *(Glycyrrhiza glabra)*
Nutmeg *(Myristica fragrans)*
Rou dou kou *(Myristica fragrans)*
Scotch broom *(Cytisus scoparius)*
Shi chang pu root *(Acorus* species)
Sweet flag root *(Acorus* species)
Vacha root *(Acorus* species)
Yohimbe bark *(Corynanthe yohimbe / Pausinystalia yohimbe)*
Zhi gan cao root *(Glycyrrhiza glabra)*

By Latin Name

Acorus species (Acorus root / Vacha root / Calamus root / Shi chang pu root)
Corynanthe yohimbe (Yohimbe bark)
Cytisus scoparius (Scotch broom)
Ephedra sinica (Ma huang herb / Ephedra)
Eschscholzia californica (California poppy)
Ginkgo biloba (Ginkgo leaf)
Glycyrrhiza glabra (Madhukam / Licorice / Gan cao / Zhi gan cao)
Myristica fragrans (Rou dou kou / Nutmeg seed / Jatiphalam)
Pausinystalia yohimbe (Yohimbe bark)
Vitex agnus-castus (Chaste tree berry)

Herbs That May Lower Blood Sugar*

By Common Name

Agrimony *(Agrimonia eupatoria)*
Artichoke leaves *(Cynaria scolymus)*
Atirasa *(Taraxacum officinale)*
Bael fruit *(Aegle marmelos)*
Banaba leaves *(Lagerstroemia speciosa)*
Bean pod—without beans *(Phaseolus vulgaris)*
Bilberry *(Vaccinium myrtillus)*
Bilwa fruit *(Aegle marmelos)*
Bitter gourd *(Momordica charanta)*

Bitter melon *(Momordica charanta)*
Bitumenlike secretion (Shilajatu)
Black atractylodes rhizome *(Atractylodes lancea)*
Blueberry *(Vaccinium myrtilloides)*
Cang zhu rhizome *(Atractylodes lancea)*
Chaparral leaf *(Larrea tridentata)*
Cowhage seed *(Mucuna pruriens)*
Creosote bush *(Larrea tridentata)*
Damiana leaf and flower *(Turnera diffusa)*
Dandelion *(Taraxacum officinale)*

*These effects are generally minor.

Devil's club root bark *(Oplopanax horridum)*

Eucalyptus *(Eucalyptus globulus)*

Fenugreek leaf/seed *(Trigonella foenum-graecum)*

Fig leaf decoction *(Ficus carica)*

Ganoderma mushroom *(Ganoderma lucidum)*

Garlic *(Allium sativum)*

Ginseng root *(Panax ginseng)*

Goat's rue *(Galega officinalis)*

Green tea *(Camellia sinensis)*

Guayusa *(Ilex guayusa)*

Guduchi stem/leaf *(Tinospora cordifolia)*

Gurmar leaf *(Gymnema sylvestre)*

Gymnema leaf *(Gymnema sylvestre)*

Haldi rhizome *(Curcuma longa)*

Haridra root *(Curcuma longa)*

Heart-leaved moonseed *(Tinospora cordifolia)*

Hen-of-the-woods mushroom *(Grifola frondosa / Polyporus frondosus)*

Holy basil leaf *(Ocimum sanctum)*

Jambu seed *(Syzygium jambolanum / S. cumini)*

Jambul seed *(Syzygium jambolanum / S. cumini)*

Jiang huang root *(Curcuma longa)*

Juniper berry *(Juniperus communis)*

Karavella *(Momordica charanta)*

Kirata tikta *(Swertia chirata)*

Ku gua *(Momordica charanta)*

Ling zhi mushroom *(Ganoderma lucidum)*

Lotus plant tincture *(Nelumbo nucifera)*

Ma huang herb *(Ephedra sinica)*

Maitake mushroom *(Grifola frondosa / Polyporus frondosus)*

Malabar kino *(Pterocarpus marsupium)*

Mistletoe *(Viscum album)*

Neem leaf *(Azadirachta indica)*

Nimba leaf *(Azadirachta indica)*

Nopal stem *(Opuntia streptacantha)*

Onion *(Allium cepa)*

Opuntia *(Opuntia* species)

Oregano leaves *(Origanum* species)

Patha *(Stephania hernandifolia)*

Patola plant *(Tricosanthes dioica)*

Persian lilac leaves *(Azadirachta indica)*

Prickly pear cactus *(Opuntia* species)

Psyllium seed *(Plantago ovata)*

Pu gong ying *(Taraxacum officinale)*

Rajavriksa pods *(Cassia fistula)*

Reishi mushroom *(Ganoderma lucidum)*

Rosemary leaf extract *(Rosmarinus officinalis)*

Sang ye leaf *(Morus alba)*

Senega root *(Polygala senega)*

Shilajatu (Bitumenlike secretion)

Siberian ginseng root *(Eleutherococcus senticosus)*

Silajit (Bituminlike secretion)

Tulsi leaf *(Ocimum sanctum)*

Turmeric root *(Curcuma longa)*

Vilwa fruit *(Aegle marmelos)*

Yin chen hao *(Artemisia capillaris)*

Yu zhu *(Polygonatum officinale)*

By Latin Name

Aegle marmelos (Bael fruit / Vilwa / Bilwa)

Agrimonia eupatoria (Agrimony)

Allium cepa (Onion)

Allium sativum (Garlic)

Arocomia mexicana root

Artemisia capillaris (Yin chen hao)

Artocarpus heterophyllus leaves

Asteracanthus longifolia plant

Atractylodes lancea (Cang zhu / Black atractylodes rhizome)

Azadirachta indica (Neem leaf / Nimba / Persian lilac)

Bauhinia candicans

Biophytum sensitivum

Bryonia alba

Camellia sinensis (Green tea)
Cassia fistula (Rajavriksa pods)
Cecropia obtusifolia
Chromium picolinate
Cleome droserifolia
Curcurbita ficifolia
Curcuma longa (Haridra / Turmeric root / Jiang huang / Haldi)
Cynaria scolymus (Artichoke leaves)
Dioscorea dumetorum tubers
Eleutherococcus senticosus (Siberian ginseng root)
Ephedra sinica (Ma huang herb)
Eucalyptus globulus (Eucalyptus)
Euphorbia prostrata
Ficus carica (decoction of fig leaves)
Galega officinalis (Goat's rue)
Ganoderma lucidum (Ganoderma mushroom / Reishi / Ling Zhi)
Grifola frondosa / Polyporus frondosus (Maitake mushroom / Hen-of-the-Woods)
Guazuma ulmifolia
Gymnema sylvestre (Gurmar leaves)
Hedychium coronarium rhizome
Ichnocarpus frutescens flowers
Ilex guayusa (Guayusa)
Juniperus communis (Juniper berries)
Kalopanax pictus stem bark
Lagerstroemia speciosa (Banaba leaves)
Larrea tridentata (Creosote bush)
Lepechinia caulescens
Momordica charanta (Bitter gourd juice / Bitter melon / Karavella)
Morus alba (leaf)
Mucuna pruriens (Cowhage seeds)
Musa sapientum
Myrcia multiflora leaves
Nelumbo nucifera tincture
Ocimum sanctum leaf powder (Holy basil / Tulsi)

Oplopanax horridum (Devil's club root bark)
Opuntia species (Prickly pear / Opuntia cactus)
Opuntia streptacantha (Nopal stems)
Origanum species (Oregano leaves)
Panax ginseng (Ginseng root)
Pandanus odorus
Phaseolus vulgaris (pod without beans)
Phyllanthus amarus
Plantago ovata (Psyllium seed)
Polichia campestris
Polygala senega
Polygonatum officinale
Psacalium peltatum
Pterocarpus marsupium (Malabar kino)
Pycnanthus angolensis
Rhizophora mangle
Rosmarinus officinalis leaf extract
Rubus ulmifolius
Slanum verbascifolum
Stephania hernandifolia (Patha)
Swertia chirata (Kirata tikta)
Syzygium jambolanum / S. cumini (Jambu seeds / Jambul seeds)
Taraxacum officinale (Atirasa / Dandelion root and leaf / Pu gong ying)
Teucrium cubense
Tinospora cordifolia (Guduchi stem/leaves / Heart-leaved moonseed)
Tinospora crispa
Tournefortia hirsutissima
Tricosanthes dioica
Trigonella foenum-graceum (Fenugreek leaf/seed)
Turnera diffusa
Vaccinium species (blueberry / bilberry)
Vaccinium myrtillus (leaves)
Viscum album (mistletoe)
Zizyphus sativa leaves

Essential/Volatile Oils

By Common Name

Allspice *(Pimenta dioica)*
Anise *(Illicium verum)*
Basil *(Ocimum basilicum)*
Bay *(Pimenta racemosa)*
Bergamot *(Citrus bergamia)*
Bergamot mint *(Mentha citrata)*
Blue cypress *(Supressus sempervirens)*
Camphor *(Cinnamomum camphora)*
Cardamom *(Elettaria cardamomum)*
Cedarleaf *(Thuja occidentalis)*
Cedarwood *(Juniperus virginiana)*
Chamomile *(Matricaria recutita)*
Cinnamon *(Cinnamomum zeylanicum)*
Citronella *(Cymbopogon winterianus)*
Clary sage *(Salvia sclarea)*
Clove bud *(Syzygium aromaticum)*
Cubeb *(Piper cubeba)*
Eucalyptus *(Eucalyptus globulus)*
Fennel, sweet *(Foeniculum vulgare)*
Ginger *(Zingiber officinalis)*
Jasmine *(Jasminum grandiflorum)*
Juniper berry *(Juniper communis)*
Lavender *(Lavandula officinalis)*
Lemon *(Citrus limonum)*
Lemongrass *(Cymbopogon citratus)*
Lime *(Citrus aurantifolia)*
Marjoram, sweet *(Origanum marjorana)*
Mustard *(Brassica species)*
Naiouli *(Melaleuca quinquenervia)*
Neroli *(Citrus aurantium)*
Nutmeg *(Myristica fragrans)*
Orange *(Citrus sinensis)*
Oregano *(Origanum vulgare)*
Patchouli *(Pogostemon cablin)*
Peppermint *(Mentha piperita)*
Pine *(Pinus palustris)*
Rose *(Rosa species)*
Rosemary *(Rosmarinus officinalis)*

Sage *(Salvia officinalis)*
Sandalwood *(Santalum album)*
Spearmint *(Mentha spicata)*
Spruce *(Picea species)*
Tangerine *(Citrus reticulata)*
Tea tree *(Melaleuca alternifolia)*
Thyme *(Thymus vulgaris)*
Wintergreen *(Gaultheria procumbens)*
Witch hazel *(Hamamelis virginiana)*
Ylang ylang *(Cananga odorata)*

By Latin Name

Brassica species (Mustard)
Cananga odorata (Ylang ylang)
Cinnamomum camphora (Camphor)
Cinnamomum zeylanicum (Cinnamon)
Citrus aurantifolia (Lime)
Citrus aurantium (Neroli)
Citrus bergamia (Bergamot)
Citrus limonum (Lemon)
Citrus reticulata (Tangerine)
Citrus sinensis (Orange)
Cymbopogon citratus (Lemongrass)
Cymbopogon winterianus (Citronella)
Elettaria cardamomum (Cardamom)
Eucalyptus globulus (Eucalyptus)
Foeniculum vulgare (Fennel, sweet)
Gaultheria procumbens (Wintergreen)
Hamamelis virginiana (Witch hazel)
Illicium verum (Anise)
Jasminum grandiflorum (Jasmine)
Juniper communis (Juniper berry)
Juniperus virginiana (Cedarwood)
Lavandula officinalis (Lavender)
Matricaria recutica (Chamomile)
Melaleuca alternifolia (Tea tree)
Melaleuca quinquenervia (Naiouli)
Mentha citrata (Bergamot mint)
Mentha piperita (Peppermint)

Mentha spicata (Spearmint)
Myristica fragrans (Nutmeg)
Ocimum basilicum (Basil)
Origanum marjorana (Marjoram, sweet)
Origanum vulgare (Oregano)
Picea species (Spruce)
Pimenta dioica (Allspice)
Pimenta racemosa (Bay)
Pinus palustris (Pine)
Piper cubeba (Cubeb)
Pogostemon cablin (Patchouli)

Rosa species (Rose)
Rosmarinus officinalis (Rosemary)
Salvia officinalis (Sage)
Salvia sclarea (Clary sage)
Santalum album (Sandalwood)
Supressus sempervirens (Blue cypress)
Syzygium aromaticum (Clove bud)
Thuja occidentalis (Cedarleaf)
Thymus vulgaris (Thyme)
Zingiber officinalis (Ginger)

Herbs to Avoid During Pregnancy or Breast-Feeding

By Common Name

Achyranthes root *(Achyranthes bidentada)*
Aconite *(Aconitum* species)
Acorus root *(Acorus calamus)*
Adonis *(Adonis vernalis)*
Agave *(Agave americana)*
Ajamoda *(Carum copticum / C. roxburghi-anum / Apium graveolens)*
Alfalfa leaf *(Medicago sativa)*
Alkanet *(Alkanna tinctoria)*
Aloe gum *(Aloe* species—internal use only should be avoided)
American century *(Agave americana)*
American hellebore *(Veratrum viride)*
Amlavetasa *(Rheum emodi)*
Anemone *(Pulsatilla chinensis / Anemone pulsatilla)*
Angelica root *(Angelica archangelica)*
Anteater scales *(Manis pentadactyla / Manitis pentadactylae)*
Apamarga plant *(Achyranthes aspera)*
Apricot seed *(Prunus armeniaca)*
Areca peel *(Areca catechu)*
Arnica *(Arnica* species)
Asafoetida *(Ferula narthex)*

Asarabacca *(Asarum europaeum)*
Ashwagandha *(Withania somnifera)*
Ashwagandha root *(Convolvulus arbensis / Withania somnifera)*
Atis tuber *(Aconitum* species)
Ba dou *(Croton* species)
Babchi seeds *(Psoralea corylifolia)*
Bai tou weng *(Pulsatilla chinensis)*
Bai zhi root *(Angelica dahurica)*
Ban lan gen root *(Isatis tinctoria)*
Ban mao *(Mylabris phalerata)*
Ban xia rhizome *(Pinellia ternata)*
Barberry *(Berberis* species)
Bastard turnip *(Bryonia dioica / B. alba)*
Bedellium *(Commiphora mukul / Balsamodendron mukul)*
Beebalm *(Monarda* species)
Bei mu bulb *(Fritillaria* species)
Belladonna *(Atropa belladonna)*
Benefit mother herb *(Leonorus heterophyllus)*
Bermuda buttercup *(Oxalis pes-caprae)*
Betel leaf *(Piper betel)*
Beth root *(Trillium erectum)*
Bhallataka *(Semecarpus anacardium)*
Bishop's weed *(Ammi majus)*
Bitter apple *(Citrullus colocynthis)*

Bitter gourd *(Momordica charanta)*
Bitter melon *(Momordica charanta)*
Black cohosh root *(Cimicifuga racemosa)*
Black cumin seed *(Nigella sativa)*
Black horehound *(Ballota nigra)*
Black nightshade *(Solanum nigrum)*
Black pepper *(Piper nigrum)*
Black root *(Leptandra virginica)*
Bladderwrack *(Fucus vesiculosus)*
Blessed thistle *(Cnicus benedictus)*
Bloodroot *(Sanguinaria canadensis)*
Blue cohosh *(Caulophylum thalictroides)*
Blue flag *(Iris* species)
Blue vervain *(Verbena hastata)*
Borage *(Borago officinalis)*
Brahati vanavrinktaki *(Solanum indicum)*
Brahmi *(Centella asiatica / Hydrocotyle asiatica)*
Bryony *(Bryonia dioica / B. alba)*
Bu gu zhi fruit *(Cullen corylifolia)*
Bu gu zhi seed *(Psoralea corylifolia)*
Buchu leaves *(Barosma* species)
Buckthorn bark *(Rhamnus cathartica)*
Bugleweed herb *(Lycopus virginicus)*
Burdock root *(Arctium lappa)*
Butterbur root *(Petasites frigida)*
Cactus *(Euphorbia nerifolia)*
Calamus root *(Acorus calamus)*
California poppy *(Eschscholzia californica)*
Camphor tree leaves *(Cinnamomum camphora)*
Canada snakeroot *(Asarum canadense)*
Carolina jasmine *(Gelsemium sempervirens)*
Carthamus flower *(Carthamus tinctorius)*
Cascara sagrada bark *(Rhamnus purshiana)*
Castor oil plant *(Ricinus communis)*
Catnip herb *(Nepeta cataria)*
Cat's claw *(Uncaria tomentosa)*
Celandine *(Chelidonium majus)*
Chandanam *(Santalum album)*

Chandrasura *(Nasturtium officinale)*
Changeri *(Oxalis acetosella)*
Chaste tree berry *(Vitex agnus-castus)*
Chervil *(Anthriscus cerefolium)*
China tree root bark *(Melia azedarach)*
Chinese cork tree *(Phellodendron chinense)*
Chinese skullcap root *(Scutellaria baicalensis)*
Chinese wild ginger *(Asarum sieboldii)*
Chuan huang bai bark *(Phellodendron chinense)*
Chuan lian zi fruit *(Melia toosendan)*
Chuan niu xi root *(Cyathula officinalis)*
Chuan shan jia scales *(Manis pentadactyla / Manitis pentadactylae)*
Chuan xin lian *(Andrographis paniculata)*
Chuan xiong root *(Ligusticum chuanxiong)*
Cinchona bark *(Cinchona* species)
Cinnamon bark *(Cinnamomum verum)*
Cnidium *(Ligusticum chuanxiong)*
Cocaine *(Erythroxylon coca)*
Coffee *(Coffea arabica)*
Cola *(Cola nitida)*
Colocynth root *(Citrullus colocynthis)*
Coltsfoot flower *(Tussilago farfara)*
Comfrey leaf/root *(Symphytum officinalis)*
Coptis rhizome *(Coptis chinensis)*
Corydalis rhizome *(Corydalis yanhusuo)*
Cotton root bark *(Gossypium* species)
Cowhage seed *(Mucuna pruriens)*
Crab's eye *(Abrus precatorius)*
Culver's root *(Leptandra virginica)*
Cyathula root *(Cyathula officinalis)*
Da fu pi peel *(Areca catechu)*
Da huang *(Rheum palmatum)*
Da ji *(Euphorbia* species)
Da qing ye leaf *(Isatis tinctoria)*
Dadima rind *(Punica granatum)*
Dan shen *(Salvia miltiorrhiza)*
Dang gui root *(Angelica sinensis)*
Daruharidra bark *(Berberis* species)

Darvi *(Berberis asiatica)*

Datura *(Datura metal / D. stramonium)*

Deer musk *(Moschus moschiferus)*

Devil's claw root *(Harpagophytum procumbens)*

Devil's club *(Oplopanax horridum)*

Devil's dung *(Ferula* species)

Devil's turnip *(Bryonia dioica / B. alba)*

Di gu pi root bark *(Lycium chinense)*

Digitalis *(Digitalis purpurea)*

Dioscorea *(Dioscorea* species)

Dong quai root *(Angelica sinensis)*

Dragon's blood *(Croton* species)

Dragon's blood *(Dracaena cambodiana / Draconis sanguis)*

Dyer's broom *(Genista tinctoia)*

E zhu rhizome *(Curcuma zedoaria)*

Ekavira *(Lobelia pyramidalis)*

Elecampane *(Inula helenium)*

Ephedra *(Ephedra* species)

Epimedium *(Epimedium grandiflorum)*

Eranda plant *(Ricinus communis)*

False hellebore *(Veratrum viride)*

False unicorn rhizome *(Chamalirium luteum)*

Fan xie ye *(Cassia* species)

Fenugreek seed *(Trigonella foenum-graecum)*

Feverfew *(Chrysanthemum parthenium / Tanacetum parthenium)*

Forsythia flower *(Forsythia suspensa)*

Foxglove *(Digitalis purpurea)*

Fritillary bulb *(Fritillaria* species)

Fu zi tuber *(Aconitum* species)

Gan cao root *(Glycyrrhiza uralensis)*

Gelsemium root *(Gelsemium sempervirens)*

Giant fennel *(Ferula communis)*

Ginkgo leaf *(Ginkgo biloba)*

Goldenseal root *(Hydrastis canadensis)*

Gotu kola *(Centella asiatica / Hydrocotyle asiatica)*

Gou qi zi berry *(Lycium chinense)*

Gravel root *(Eupatorium purpureum)*

Gua lou fruit *(Trichosanthes kirilowii)*

Guan fang ji *(Aristolochia westlandii)*

Guan mu tong *(Aristolochia manshuriensis)*

Guggul gum *(Commiphora mukul / Balsamodendron mukul)*

Gunja *(Abrus precatorius)*

Haldi rhizome *(Curcuma longa)*

Haridra rhizome *(Curcuma longa)*

Hastikarnapalasa seed *(Butea monosperma)*

He huan pi *(Albizzia julibrissin)*

Helonius rhizome *(Chamalirium luteum)*

Henbane *(Hyoscyamus niger)*

Hercules' club bark *(Zanthoxylum* species)

Hibiscus flower *(Hibiscus rosa-sinensis)*

Hingu *(Ferula narthex)*

Ho po hua flower *(Magnolia officinalis)*

Holy basil *(Ocimum sanctum)*

Hong hua flower *(Carthamus tinctorius)*

Horehound / White horehound *(Marrubium vulgare)*

Horny goat weed *(Epimedium grandiflorum)*

Horsemint *(Monarda* species)

Horsetail *(Equisetum* species)

Hou po bark *(Magnolia officinalis)*

Hu jiao *(Piper nigrum)*

Hu lu ba seed *(Trigonella foenum-graecum)*

Huan niu xi root *(Achyranthes bidentata)*

Huang bai bark *(Phellodendron amurense)*

Huang lian rhizome *(Coptis chinensis)*

Huang qin root *(Scutellaria baicalensis)*

Hyssop *(Hyssopus officinalis)*

Indian jalap *(Operculina turpenthum)*

Indian licorice *(Abrus precatorius)*

Indian pennywort *(Centella asiatica / Hydrocotyle asiatica)*

Indian sorrel *(Oxalis acetosella)*

Indian tobacco *(Lobelia inflata)*

Indravaruni fruit *(Citrullus colocynthis)*

Ipecac *(Cephaelis ipecahuanha)*

Jaborandi *(Pilocarpus* species)

Japa flowers *(Hibiscus rosa-sinensis)*

Jatamansi *(Nardostachys jatamansi)*

Jatiphalam *(Myristica fragrans)*

Jequirity *(Abrus precatorius)*

Ji xue teng root *(Millettia reticulata / M. dielsiana / Spatholobus suberectus)*

Jiang huang rhizome *(Curcuma longa)*

Joe Pye weed *(Eupatorium purpureum)*

Jujube seeds *(Ziziphus spinosa)*

Juniper berry *(Juniperus* species)

Kakamachi *(Solanum nigrum)*

Kan jang *(Andrographis paniculata)*

Kantakari *(Solanum xanthocarpum / S. surattense)*

Kapi kacchu *(Mucuna pruriens)*

Kapikachu *(Mucuna pruriens)*

Karapura leaf *(Cinnamomum camphora)*

Karavella *(Momordica charanta)*

Karavira *(Nerium indicum / N. odorum)*

Karchura *(Curcuma zedoaria)*

Karpasa root bark *(Gossypium* species)

Kava root *(Piper methysticum)*

Kesaram stigmas *(Crocus sativus)*

Khella *(Ammi visnaga / Ammi majus)*

Kirta *(Andrographis paniculata)*

Kola nut *(Cola acuminata)*

Krisnadhattura *(Datura metal / D. stramonium)*

Krisnajirakam seed *(Nigella sativa)*

Ku gua *(Momordica charanta)*

Ku lian gen pi *(Melia azedarach)*

Kuan dong hua *(Tussilago farfara)*

Kumari *(Aloe* species—internal use only should be avoided)

Kumkumam stigmas *(Crocus sativus)*

Lavender *(Lavandula officinalis)*

Leech *(Hirudo nipponia)*

Lei gong teng *(Tripterygium wilfordii)*

Lemon balm *(Melissa officinalis)*

Lemongrass *(Cymbopogon citratus)*

Leonorus *(Leonorus heterophyllus)*

Lian qiao flower *(Forsythia suspensa)*

Licorice root *(Glycyrrhiza glabra)*

Life root *(Senecio aura)*

Lily-of-the-valley *(Convallaria majalis)*

Liquidambar fruit *(Liquidambar taiwaniana)*

Liverwort *(Hepatica* species)

Lobelia *(Lobelia inflata)*

Lomatium root *(Lomatium dissectum)*

Long pepper *(Piper longum)*

Lovage root *(Ligusticum levisticum)*

Lu hui *(Aloe* species—internal use only should be avoided)

Lu lu tong fruit *(Liquidambar taiwaniana)*

Lucerne *(Medicago sativa)*

Lycium fruit *(Lycium chinense)*

Lycopus *(Lycopus lucidus)*

Ma huang *(Ephedra sinica)*

Madagascar periwinkle *(Vinca rosea)*

Magnolia bark *(Magnolia officinalis)*

Mahanimba leaves *(Melia azedarach)*

Mai ya—germinated barley *(Hordeum vulgare)*

Maidenhead fern *(Adiantum pedatum)*

Major catkins *(Piper longum)*

Malabar nut *(Adhatoda vasica / Justicia vasica)*

Male fern *(Dryopteris filix-mas)*

Mandrake *(Podophyllum peltatum)*

Maricham *(Piper nigrum)*

Marijuana *(Cannabis* species)

Marking nut tree *(Semecarpus anacardium)*

Mastic gum *(Boswellia carterii)*

Mayapple *(Podophyllum peltatum)*

Meadow saffron *(Colchicum autumnale)*

Melia root bark *(Melia azedarach)*

Millettia root *(Millettia reticulata / M. dielsiana / Spatholobus suberectus)*

Mimosa tree bark *(Albizzia julibrissin)*

Ming dang shen root *(Changium smyrnoides)*

Mistletoe herb *(Viscum flavescens)*

Mo yao gum *(Commiphora myrrha / C. molmol)*

Monkshood *(Aconitum* species)

Motherwort *(Leonorus cardiaca)*

Moutan bark *(Paeonia suffruticosa)*

Mu dan pi bark *(Paeonia suffruticosa)*

Muskroot *(Nardostachys jatamansi)*

Mylabris *(Mylabris phalerata)*

Myrrh gum *(Commiphora myrrha / C. molmol)*

Neem leaf *(Azadirachta indica)*

Nettle *(Urtica dioica)*

Nilika plant *(Isatis tinctoria)*

Nishotha resin *(Operculina turpenthum)*

Niu bang zi root *(Arctium lappa)*

Northern prickly ash bark *(Zanthoxylum* species)

Nutmeg seed *(Myristica fragrans)*

Nux vomica *(Strychnos nux-vomica)*

Ocotillo stem *(Fouquieria splendens)*

Oregano leaf *(Origanum* species*)*

Oregon barberry root *(Mahonia* species)

Oregon grape root *(Berberis aquifolium)*

Oregon grape root *(Mahonia* species)

Osha root *(Ligusticum porteri)*

Oswego tea *(Monarda* species)

Palash *(Butea monosperma)*

Papaya fruit *(Carica papaya)*

Papita fruit *(Carica papaya)*

Parsley leaf and root *(Petroselinum crispum)*

Pasqueflower *(Pulsatilla chinensis / Anemone pulsatilla)*

Passionflower *(Passiflora incarnata)*

Peach kernel *(Prunus persica)*

Pennyroyal *(Mentha pulegium / Hedeoma pulegioides)*

Persica seed *(Prunus persica)*

Pheasant's eye *(Adonis vernalis)*

Phellodendron bark *(Phellodendron amurense / Phellodendron chinense)*

Pilocarpine *(Pilocarpus jaborandi)*

Pinellia rhizome *(Pinellia ternata)*

Pipali fruit *(Piper longum)*

Pleurisy root *(Asclepias tuberosa)*

Poke root *(Phytolacca americana)*

Pomegranate fruit *(Punica granatum)*

Prickly ash bark *(Xanthoxylum clava-herculis)*

Prickly ash bark *(Zanthoxylum* species)

Pulsatilla *(Anemone pulsatilla)*

Purslane *(Portulaca oleracea)*

Qian niu zi *(Pharbatis* species)

Qing hao *(Artemisia* species)

Quassia *(Picrasma excelsa / Quasia amara)*

Queen Anne's lace *(Daucus carota)*

Queen-of-the-meadow *(Eupatorium purpureum)*

Rauwolfia *(Rauwolfia serpentina)*

Red clover blossoms *(Trifolium pratense)*

Rhubarb root *(Rheum* species)

Rohitaka stem *(Rhododendron arboreum)*

Roman chamomile *(Chamaemelum nobile)*

Rosary pea *(Abrus precatorius)*

Rosemary leaf *(Rosmarinus officinalis)*

Rosy periwinkle *(Catharanthus roseus)*

Rou dou kou *(Myristica fragrans)*

Rou gui *(Cinnamomum zeylanicum / C. Cassia)*

Ru xiang gum *(Boswellia carterii)*

Rue *(Ruta graveolens)*

Safflower flower *(Carthamus tinctorius)*

Saffron stigmas *(Crocus sativus)*

Sage leaf *(Salvia officinalis)*

Salvia root *(Salvia miltiorrhiza)*

San leng rhizome *(Sparganium* species)

San qi root *(Panax notoginseng)*

Sappan bark *(Caesalpinia sappan)*

Sarpagandha root *(Rauwolfia serpentina)*

Sassafras root bark *(Sassafras officinale)*
Sati *(Curcuma zedoaria)*
She xiang *(Moschus moschiferus)*
Scirpus *(Sparganium* species)
Scotch broom *(Cytisus scoparius)*
Senega root *(Polygala senega)*
Senna *(Senna* species)
Senna leaf *(Cassia* species)
Sete sangrias *(Cuphea balsamona)*
Shan yao root *(Dioscorea opposita)*
Shang lu *(Phytolacca* species)
Shavegrass *(Equisetum* species*)*
Shepherd's purse *(Capsella bursa-pastoris)*
Shi chang pu root *(Acorus gramineus)*
Shui zhi *(Hirudo nipponia)*
Sichuan chinaberry fruit *(Melia toosendan)*
Sichuan lovage root *(Ligusticum chuanx-iong)*
Silk tree *(Albizzia julibrissin)*
Snuhi *(Euphorbia nerifolia)*
Southern prickly ash bark *(Zanthoxylum* species)
Sparganii rhizome *(Sparganium* species)
Spikenard, various types *(Aralia* species)
Spotted beebalm *(Monarda* species)
Squill *(Urginea maritima / Scilla maritima)*
St. John's wort *(Hypericum perforatum)*
Stillingia root *(Stillingia sylvatica)*
Stinging nettle *(Urtica dioica)*
Su mu bark *(Caesalpinia sappan)*
Suan zao ren seed *(Ziziphus spinosa)*
Swarnapatri *(Cassia* species)
Sweet flag *(Iris* species)
Sweet flag root *(Acorus calamus / A. gramineus)*
Sweet leaf *(Monarda fistulosa)*
Sweet-scented oleander *(Nerium indicum / N. odorum)*
Tambulam *(Piper betel)*
Tan xiang *(Santalum album)*
Tang kuai root *(Angelica sinensis)*

Tansy leaf *(Tanacetum vulgare / Chrysanthemum vulgare)*
Tao ren seed *(Prunus persica)*
Thornapple *(Datura metal / D. / stramonium)*
Thuja leaf *(Thuja occidentalis)*
Thunder god vine *(Tripterygium wilfordii)*
Thyme leaf *(Thymes vulgaris)*
Tian chi root *(Panax notoginseng)*
Tian nan xing rhizome *(Arisaema* species)
Tien-chi root *(Panax notoginseng)*
Tobacco leaf *(Nicotiana tabacum)*
Tree peony bark *(Paeonia suffruticosa)*
Tree turmeric *(Berberis* species)
Trichosanthes fruit *(Trichosanthes kirilowii)*
Trivrit root *(Operculina turpenthum)*
Tulasi *(Ocimum sanctum)*
Tulsi plant *(Ocimum sanctum)*
Turkey rhubarb *(Rheum* species)
Turmeric rhizome *(Curcuma longa)*
Tvak *(Cinnamomum zeylanicum / C. Cassia)*
Twak *(Cinnamomum zeylanicum / C. Cassia)*
Uña de gato *(Uncaria tomentosa)*
Uva ursi leaf *(Arctostaphylos uva-ursi)*
Vacha root *(Acorus calamus)*
Vakuchi seed *(Psoralea corylifolia)*
Vasaca leaf *(Adhatoda vasica / Justicia vasica)*
Vatsanabha tuber *(Aconitum* species)
Vetiver *(Vetiveria zizanoides)*
Visatinduka seed *(Strychnos nux-vomica)*
Water horehound *(Lycopus* species)
Watercress *(Nasturtium officinale)*
White sandalwood *(Santalum album)*
Wild bergamot *(Monarda* species)
Wild carrot seed *(Daucus carota)*
Wild celery *(Apium graveolens)*
Wild celery *(Carum copticum / C. roxburghianum)*
Wild cherry bark *(Prunus serotina)*

Wild indigo root *(Baptisia tinctoria)*
Wild yam *(Dioscorea* species)
Winter cherry *(Withania somnifera)*
Woad *(Isatis tinctoria)*
Wormwood *(Artemisia* species)
Xi xin herb *(Asarum sieboldii)*
Xing ren seed *(Prunus armeniaca)*
Xue jie *(Dracaena cambodiana / Draconis sanguis)*
Yan hu suo rhizome *(Corydalis yanhusuo)*
Yarrow flower *(Achillea millefolium)*
Yellow jasmine *(Gelsemium sempervirens)*
Yellow sandalwood *(Santalum album)*
Yi mu cao *(Leonorus heterophyllus)*
Yi yi ren / Coix *(Coix lachryma)*
Yin yang huo *(Epimedium grandiflorum)*
Yohimbe bark *(Corynanthe yohimbe)*
Ze lan *(Lycopus lucidus)*
Zedoary root *(Curcuma zedoaria)*
Zhang nai leaf *(Cinnamomum camphora)*
Zoapatle *(Montanoa tomentosa)*

By Latin Name

Abrus precatorius (Jequirity / Indian licorice / Rosary pea / Crab's eye / Gunja)
Achillea millefolium (Yarrow flower)
Achyranthes aspera (Apamarga plant)
Achyranthes bidentata (Achyranthes root / Huan niu xi root*)*
Aconitum species (Atis tuber / Aconite / Monkshood / Fu zi tuber / Vatsanabha tuber)
Acorus calamus (Acorus root / Vacha root / Calamus root)
Acorus calamus / A. gramineus (Sweet flag root)
Acorus gramineus (Shi chang pu root)
Adhatoda vasica / Justicia vasica (Vasaca leaves / Malabar nut)
Adiantum pedatum (Maidenhead fern)

Adonis vernalis (Pheasant's eye / Adonis)
Agave americana (American century / Agave)
Albizzia julibrissin (Mimosa tree bark / He huan pi / Silk tree)
Alkanna tinctoria (Alkanet)
Aloe species—internal use only should be avoided (Lu hui / Kumari)
Ammi majus (Bishop's weed)
Ammi visnaga / A. majus (Khella)
Andrographis paniculata (Kirta / Kan jang / Chuan xin lian)
Anemone pulsatilla (Pasqueflower / Anemone / Pulsatilla)
Angelica archangelica (Angelica root)
Angelica dahurica (Bai zhi root)
Angelica sinensis (Tang kuai root / Dong quai root / Dang gui root)
Anthriscus cerefolium (Chervil)
Apium graveolens (Wild celery / Ajamoda)
Aralia species (Spikenard, various types)
Arctium lappa (Burdock root / Niu bang zi root)
Arctostaphylos uva-ursi (Uva ursi leaf)
Areca catechu (Da fu pi peel / Areca peel)
Arisaema species (Tian nan xing rhizome)
Aristolochia manshuriensis (Guan mu tong)
Aristolochia westlandii (Guan fang ji)
Arnica species (Arnica*)*
Artemisia species (Wormwood / Qing hao)
Asarum canadense (Canada snakeroot)
Asarum europaeum (Asarabacca*)*
Asarum sieboldii (Chinese wild ginger / Xi xin herb)
Asclepias tuberosa (Pleurisy root)
Atropa belladonna (Belladonna*)*
Azadirachta indica (Neem leaves)
Ballota nigra (Black horehound)
Baptisia tinctoria (Wild indigo root)
Barosma species (Buchu leaves)
Berberis aquifolium (Oregon grape root)

Berberis asiatica (Darvi)

Berberis species (Barberry / Tree turmeric / Daruharidra bark)

Borago officinalis (Borage)

Boswellia carterii (Mastic gum / Ru xiang gum)

Bryonia dioica / B. alba (Devil's turnip / Bastard turnip / Bryony)

Butea monosperma (Palash / Hastikarnapalasa seeds)

Caesalpinia sappan (Sappan bark / Su mu bark)

Cannabis species (Marijuana)

Capsella bursa-pastoris (Shepherd's purse)

Carica papaya (Papaya fruit / Papita fruit)

Carthamus tinctorius (Safflower flower / Carthamus flower / Hong hua flower)

Carum copticum / C. roxburghianum (Ajamoda / Wild celery)

Cassia species (Fan xie ye / Swarnapatri / Senna leaf)

Catharanthus roseus (Rosy periwinkle)

Caulophylum thalictroides (Blue cohosh)

Centella asiatica / Hydrocotyle asiatica (Gotu kola / Brahmi / Indian pennywort)

Cephaelis ipecahuanha (Ipecac)

Chamaemelum nobile (Roman chamomile)

Chamalirium luteum (Helonius rhizome / False unicorn rhizome)

Changium smyrnoides (Ming dang shen root)

Chelidonium majus (Celandine)

Chrysanthemum parthenium / Tanacetum parthenium (Feverfew)

Chrysanthemum vulgare (Tansy leaves)

Cimicifuga racemosa (Black cohosh root)

Cinchona species (Cinchona bark)

Cinnamomum camphora (Zhang nai leaf / Camphor tree leaves / Karapura leaf)

Cinnamomum zeylanicum / C. Cassia (Tvak / Rou gui / Cinnamon bark / Twak)

Citrullus colocynthis (Bitter apple / Indravaruni fruit)

Citrullus colocynthis (Colocynth root)

Cnicus benedictus (Blessed thistle)

Coffea arabica (Coffee)

Coix lachryma (Yi yi ren / Coix)

Cola acuminata (Kola nut)

Cola nitida (Cola)

Colchicum autumnale (Meadow saffron)

Commiphora mukul / Balsamodendron mukul (Indian bedellium / Guggul gum)

Commiphora myrrha / C. molmol (Myrrh gum / Mo yao gum)

Convallaria majalis (Lily-of-the-valley)

Convolvulus arbensis / Withania somnifera (Ashwagandha root)

Coptis chinensis (Coptis rhizome / Huang lian rhizome)

Corydalis yanhusuo (Yan hu suo rhizome / Corydalis rhizome)

Corynanthe yohimbe (Yohimbe bark)

Crocus sativus (Kesaram stigmas / Saffron stigmas / Kumkumam stigmas)

Croton species (Dragon's blood)

Cullen corylifolia (Bu gu zhi fruit)

Cuphea balsamona (Sete sangrias)

Curcuma longa (Haldi rhizome Jiang huang rhizome / Turmeric rhizome / Haridra rhizome)

Curcuma zedoaria (E zhu rhizome / Zedoary root / Sati / Karchura)

Cyathula officinalis (Chuan niu xi root / Cyathula root)

Cymbopogon citratus (Lemongrass)

Cytisus scoparius (Scotch broom)

Datura metal / D. stramonium (Thornapple / Krisnadhattura / Datura)

Daucus carota (Queen Anne's lace / Wild carrot seed)

Digitalis purpurea (Digitalis / Foxglove)

Dioscorea opposita (Shan yao root)

Dioscorea species (Dioscorea / Wild yam)

Dracaena cambodiana / Draconis sanguis (Dragon's blood / Xue jie)

Dryopteris filix-mas (Male fern)

Ephedra sinica (Ma huang / Ephedra)

Epimedium grandiflorum (Horny goat weed / Epimedium / Yin yang huo)

Equisetum species (Shavegrass / Horsetail)

Erythroxylon coca (Cocaine)

Eschscholzia californica (California poppy)

Eupatorium purpureum (Qucen-of-the-meadow / Gravel root / Joe Pye weed)

Euphorbia nerifolia (Cactus / Snuhi / Da ji)

Ferula communis (Giant fennel)

Ferula narthex (Asafoetida / Hingu)

Ferula species (Devil's dung)

Forsythia suspensa (Forsythia flower / Lian qiao flower)

Fouquieria splendens (Ocotillo stem)

Fritillaria species (Bei mu bulb / Fritillary bulb)

Fucus vesiculosus (Bladderwrack)

Gelsemium sempervirens (Carolina jasmine / Yellow jasmine / Gelsemium root)

Genista tinctoria (Dyer's broom)

Ginkgo biloba (Ginkgo leaf)

Glycyrrhiza glabra (Licorice root)

Glycyrrhiza uralensis (Gan cao root)

Gossypium species (Karpasa root bark / Cotton root bark)

Harpagophytum procumbens (Devil's claw root)

Hedeoma pulegioides (Pennyroyal)

Hepatica species (Liverwort)

Hibiscus rosa-sinensis (Japa flowers / Hibiscus flowers)

Hirudo nipponia (Shui zhi / Leech)

Hordeum vulgare (Mai ya—germinated barley)

Hydrastis canadensis (Goldenseal root)

Hyoscyamus niger (Henbane)

Hypericum perforatum (St. John's wort)

Hyssopus officinalis (Hyssop)

Inula helenium (Elecampane)

Iris species (Sweet flag / Blue flag)

Isatis tinctoria (Woad / Nilika plant/ Da qing ye leaf / Ban lan gen root)

Juniperus species (Juniper berry)

Lavandula officinalis (Lavender)

Leonorus cardiaca (Motherwort)

Leonorus heterophyllus (Benefit mother herb / Leonorus / Yi mu cao)

Leptandra virginica (Black root / Culver's root)

Levisticum officinale (Lovage root)

Ligusticum chuanxiong (Cnidium / Sichuan lovage root / Chuan xiong root)

Ligusticum levisticum (Lovage root)

Ligusticum porteri (Osha root)

Liquidambar taiwaniana (Liquidambar fruit / Lu lu tong fruit)

Lobelia inflata (Lobelia / Indian tobacco/ Ekavira)

Lomatium dissectum (Lomatium root)

Lycium chinense (Di gu pi root bark / Gou qi zi berry / Lycium fruit)

Lycopus lucidus (Lycopus / Ze lan)

Lycopus species (Water horehound)

Lycopus virginicus (Bugleweed herb)

Magnolia officinalis (Ho po hua flower / Hou po bark / Magnolia bark)

Mahonia species (Oregon barberry root / Oregon grape root)

Manis pentadactylae / Manitis pentadactyla (Anteater scales / Chuan shan jia scales)

Marrubium vulgare (Horehound / White horehound)

Medicago sativa (Lucerne / Alfalfa leaf)

Melia azedarach (Mahanimba leaves/ Ku lian gen pi/ Melia root bark / China tree root bark)

Melia toosendan (Sichuan chinaberry fruit / Chuan lian zi fruit)

Melissa officinalis (Lemon balm)

Mentha pulegium / Hedeoma pulegioides (Pennyroyal)

Millettia reticulata / M. dielsiana / Spatholobus suberectus (Ji xue teng root / Millettia root)

Momordica charanta (Ku gua / Bitter melon / Bitter gourd / Karavella)

Monarda fistulosa (Sweet leaf)

Monarda species (Spotted beebalm / Horsemint / Wild bergamot / Oswego tea / Beebalm)

Montanoa tomentosa (Zoapatle)

Moschus moschiferus (Deer musk / She xiang)

Mucuna pruriens (Kapi kacchu / Kapikachu /Cowhage seeds)

Mylabris phalerata (Ban mao / Mylabris)

Myristica fragrans (Rou dou kou / Nutmeg seeds / Jatiphalam)

Nardostachys jatamansi (Muskroot / Jatamansi)

Nasturtium officinale (Watercress / Chandrasura)

Nepeta cataria (Catnip herb)

Nerium indicum / N. odorum (Sweet-scented oleander / Karavira)

Nicotiana tabacum (Tobacco leaf)

Nigella sativa (Black cumin seeds / Krisnajirakam seeds)

Ocimum sanctum (Tulasi / Holy basil / Tulsi plant)

Operculina turpenthum (Indian jalap / Nishotha resin / Trivrit root)

Oplopanax horridum (Devil's club)

Origanum species (Oregano leaf)

Oxalis acetosella (Indian sorrel / Changeri)

Oxalis pes-caprae (Bermuda buttercup)

Paeonia suffruticosa (Moutan bark / Mu dan pi bark / Tree peony bark)

Panax notoginseng (Tien-chi root / Tian chi root / San qi root)

Passiflora incarnata (Passionflower)

Petasites frigida (Butterbur root)

Petroselinum crispum (Parsley leaf and root)

Pharbatis species (Qian niu zi)

Phellodendron amurense (Huang bai bark / Phellodendron bark)

Phellodendron chinense (Chinese cork tree / Chuan huang bai bark / Phellodendron bark)

Phytolacca species (Poke root / Shang lu)

Picrasma excelsa (Quassia)

Pilocarpus jaborandi (Pilocarpine)

Pilocarpus species (Jaborandi)

Pinellia ternata (Ban xia rhizome / Pinellia rhizome)

Piper betel (Betel leaf / Tambulam)

Piper longum (Major catkins / Long pepper / Pipali fruit)

Piper methysticum (Kava root)

Piper nigrum (Hu jiao / Black pepper / Maricham)

Podophyllum peltatum (Mandrake / Mayapple)

Polygala senega (Senega root)

Portulaca oleracea (Purslane)

Prunus armeniaca (Xing ren sccd / Apricot seed)

Prunus persica (Peach kernel / Persica seed / Tao ren seed)

Prunus serotina (Wild cherry bark)

Psoralea corylifolia (Bu gu zhi seed / Vakuchi seed / Babchi seed)

Pulsatilla chinensis (Bai tou weng)

Punica granatum (Pomegranate fruit / Dadima rind)

Quasia amara (Quassia)

Rauwolfia serpentina (Rauwolfia / Sarpagandha root)

Rhamnus cathartica (Buckthorn bark)

Rhamnus purshiana (Cascara sagrada bark)

Rheum emodi (Amlavetasa)

Rheum palmatum (Da huang)

Rheum species (Rhubarb root / Turkey rhubarb)

Rhododendron arboreum (Rohitaka stem)

Ricinus communis (Castor oil plant / Eranda plant)

Rosmarinus officinalis (Rosemary leaf)

Ruta graveolens (Rue)

Salvia miltiorrhiza (Dan shen / Salvia root)

Salvia officinalis (Sage leaf)

Sanguinaria canadensis (Bloodroot)

Santalum album (Yellow Sandalwood / Tan xiang / White sandalwood / Chandanam)

Sassafras officinale (Sassafras root bark)

Scilla maritima (Squill)

Scutellaria baicalensis (Chinese skullcap root / Huang qin root)

Semecarpus anacardium (Marking nut tree / Bhallataka)

Senecio aura (Life root)

Senna species (Senna)

Solanum indicum (Brahati vanavrinktaki)

Solanum nigrum (Kakamachi / Black nightshade)

Solanum xanthocarpum (Kantakari)

Sparganium species (Sparganii rhizome / San leng rhizome / Scirpus)

Stillingia sylvatica (Stillingia root)

Strychnos nux-vomica (Nux vomica / Visatinduka seeds)

Symphytum officinalis (Comfrey leaf/root)

Tanacetum vulgare (Tansy leaf)

Thuja occidentalis (Thuja leaf)

Thymes vulgaris (Thyme leaf)

Trichosanthes kirilowii (Gua lou fruit / Trichosanthes fruit)

Trifolium pratense (Red clover blossoms)

Trigonella foenum-graecum (Hu lu ba seed / Fenugreek seed)

Trillium erectum (Beth root)

Tripterygium wilfordii (Lei gong teng / Thunder god vine)

Tussilago farfara (Coltsfoot flower / Kuan dong hua)

Uncaria tomentosa (Uña de gato / Cat's claw)

Urginea maritima (Squill)

Urtica dioica (Nettle / Stinging nettle)

Veratrum viride (False hellebore / American hellebore)

Verbena hastata (Blue vervain)

Vetiveria zizanoides (Vetiver)

Vinca rosea (Madagascar periwinkle)

Viscum flavescens (Mistletoe herb)

Vitex agnus-castus (Chaste tree berry)

Withania somnifera (Ashwagandha / Winter cherry)

Xanthoxylum clava-herculis (Prickly ash bark)

Zanthoxylum species (Hercules' club bark / Southern prickly ash bark/ Northern prickly ash bark / Prickly ash bark)

Ziziphus spinosa (Suan zao ren seed / Jujube seed)

Herbs to Avoid Unless Prescribed by a Doctor

By Common Name

Aconite *(Aconitum* species)

Adonis *(Adonis vernalis)*

American mistletoe *(Phoradendron leucarpum)*

Anemone *(Anemone pulsatilla)*

Apricot seed *(Prunus armeniaca)*

Arnica flower *(Arnica latifolia)*

Autumn crocus *(Colchicum autumnale)*

Bai tou weng *(Pulsatilla chinensis)*

Bastard turnip *(Bryonia* species)

Bitter almond *(Prunus dulcis)*

Belladonna *(Atropa belladonna)*

Blechnum *(Dryopteris filix-mas)*

Boxwood *(Buxus sempervirens)*

Bryony *(Bryonia* species)

Calamus *(Acorus calamus)*

Carolina jasmine *(Gelsemium* species)

Cedarwood *(Juniperus virginiana)*

Chuan liang zi *(Melia toosendan)*

Comfrey *(Symphytum* species—okay for external use)

Datura *(Datura* species)

Devil's turnip *(Bryonia* species)

Digitalis *(Digitalis purpurea)*

Eastern red cedar *(Juniperus virginiana)*

Ephedra *(Ephedra* species / *Ma huang)*

Fly agaric mushroom *(Amanita muscaria)*

Foxglove *(Digitalis purpurea)*

Fu zi *(Aconitum* species)

Gelsemium root *(Gelsemium* species)

Germander *(Teucrium* species)

Guan zhong *(Dryopteris filix-mas)*

Hellebore, various types *(Veratrum* species)

Henbane *(Hyoscyamus niger)*

Ipecac *(Cephaelis ipecahuanha)*

Ku lian pi *(Melia toosendan)*

Jaborandi *(Pilocarpus* species)

Jalap *(Ipomoea purga)*

Jimson weed *(Datura* species)

Lily-of-the-valley *(Convallaria majalis)*

Lobelia *(Lobelia* species)

Long birthroot *(Aristolochia* species)

Ma dou ling *(Aristolochia* species)

Ma huang *(Ephedra sinica)*

Madagascar periwinkle *(Catharanthus roseus)*

Mahanimba *(Melia azedarach)*

Male fern *(Dryopteris filix-mas)*

Mandrake *(Podophyllum peltatum / Mandragora officinarum)*

Mayapple *(Podophyllum peltatum)*

Meadow saffron *(Colchicum autumnale)*

Mistletoe *(Viscum flavescens)*

Monkshood *(Aconitum* species)

Nutmeg *(Myristica fragrans)*

Pasqueflower *(Anemone pulsatilla)*

Peach seed *(Prunus persica)*

Pennyroyal *(Mentha pulegium / Hedeoma pulegioides)*

Pheasant's eye *(Adonis vernalis)*

Pits of apricot, peach, or bitter almond *(Prunus* species)

Poke root *(Phytolacca americana)*

Pulsatilla *(Anemone pulsatilla)*

Qing mu xiang *(Aristolochia* species)

Rauwolfia *(Rauwolfia serpentina)*

Russian belladonna *(Scopolia carniolica)*

Sarpagandha root *(Rauwolfia serpentina)*

Scopolia *(Scopolia carniolica)*

Scotch broom *(Cytisus scoparius)*

Sichuan pagoda tree *(Melia toosendan)*

Squill *(Urginea maritima)*

Tansy *(Tanacetum vulgare / Chrysanthemum vulgare)*

Thornapple *(Datura* species)

Tian xian teng *(Aristolochia* species)

Tonka *(Dipteryx* species)

Virginia snakeroot *(Aristolochia* species)

Wahoo *(Euonymus atropurpureus)*
Xian mao *(Curculigo orchioides)*
Yellow jasmine *(Gelsemium* species)
Yohimbe bark *(Corynanthe yohimbe)*

By Latin Name

Aconitum species (Vatsanabha tuber / Fu zi / Monkshood / Aconite)

Acorus species (Calamus / Acorus)

Adonis vernalis (Adonis / Pheasant's eye)

Amanita muscaria (Fly agaric mushroom)

Aristolochia species (Long birthroot / Virginia snakeroot)

Arnica latifolia (Arnica flower)

Atropa belladonna (Belladonna)

Bryonia species (Bryony / Bastard turnip / Devil's turnip)

Buxus sempervirens (Boxwood)

Catharanthus roseus (Madagascar periwinkle)

Cephaelis ipecahuanha (Ipecac)

Colchicum autumnale (Meadow saffron / Autumn crocus)

Convallaria majalis (Lily-of-the-valley)

Corynanthe yohimbe (Yohimbe bark)

Curculigo orchioides (Xian mao)

Cytisus scoparius (Scotch broom)

Datura species (Jimson weed / Datura / Thornapple)

Digitalis purpurea (Foxglove / Digitalis)

Dipteryx species (Tonka)

Dryopteris filix-mas (Guan zhong / Blechnum / Male fern)

Ephedra sinica (Ma huang)

Euonymus atropurpureus (Wahoo)

Gelsemium species (Gelsemium root / Yellow jasmine / Carolina jasmine)

Hyoscyamus niger (Henbane)

Ipomoea purga (Jalap)

Juniperus virginiana (Cedarwood / Eastern red cedar)

Lobelia species (Lobelia)

Mandragora officinarum (Mandrake)

Melia azedarach (Mahanimba)

Melia toosendan (Chuan liang zi / Ku lian pi / Sichuan pagoda tree)

Mentha pulegium / Hedeoma pulegioides (Pennyroyal)

Myristica fragrans (Nutmeg)

Phoradendron leucarpum (American mistletoe)

Phytolacca americana (Poke root)

Pilocarpus species (Jaborandi)

Podophyllum species (Mayapple / Mandrake)

Prunus species (Pits of apricot, peach, or bitter almond)

Pulsatilla chinensis / Anemone pulsatilla (Anemone / Bai tou weng / Pulsatilla / Pasqueflower)

Rauwolfia serpentina (Sarpagandha root)

Scopolia carniolica (Russian belladonna)

Symphytum species (Comfrey—okay for external use)

Tanacetum vulgare / Chrysanthemum vulgare (Tansy)

Teucrium chamaedrys (Germander)

Urginea maritima (Squill)

Veratrum species (Hellebore, various types)

Viscum flavescens (Mistletoe)

Common Poisonous Indoor and Outdoor Plants and the Related Symptoms

Philodendron *(Philodendron* species)

Symptoms: Burning sensation in lips, mouth, throat; contact dermatitis; remote risk of edematous swelling in back of mouth and throat leading to closure of airways.

Mother-in-law plant *(Dieffenbachia* species / Diffenbachia / Dumbcane)
Symptoms: Same as philodendron, as well as speech impairment and superficial necrosis of tissue.

Poinsettia *(Euphorbia pulcherrima)*
Symptoms: Possibility of contact dermatitis, mild nausea, emesis.

Holly berries *(Ilex* species)
Symptoms: Nausea, persistent emesis, diarrhea.

Peppers *(Capsicum* species)
Symptoms: Painful but harmless burning sensation of lips, mouth, tongue.

Umbrella plant *(Brassaia* and *Schefflera* species / Schefflera)
Symptoms: Same as philodendron.

Poison ivy *(Toxicodendron radicans)*
Symptoms: Allergic contact dermatitis (similar reactions may occur with other *Toxicodendron* species including poison oak and poison sumac).

Devil's ivy *(Epipremnum aureum* / Pothos / Variegated philodendron)
Symptoms: Same as philodendron.

Yew *(Taxus* species)
Symptoms: Dizziness, dry mouth, nausea, emesis, rash, cyanotic lips, weakness, possible coma, bradycardia, arrhythmias, hypotension. Death has resulted.

Peace Lily *(Spathiphyllum* species / Spathe flower, White anthurium)
Symptoms: Same as philodendron.

Pokeweed *(Phytolacca americana* / Inkberry)
Symptoms: Nausea, gastroenteric cramps, sweating, vomiting, diarrhea.

Climbing Nightshade *(Solanum dulcamara* / **Bittersweet)**
Symptoms: Gastric irritation, fever and/or diarrhea after latent period of several hours, all of which may persist for days. Death has resulted in children.

Rhododendron *(Rhododendron* **species** / **Azalea)**
Symptoms: Burning in mouth, salivation, vomiting, diarrhea, prickly skin, headache, muscular weakness, dimness of vision, bradycardia, hypotension, coma, convulsions. Death has resulted.

Begonia *(Begonia* **species)**
Symptoms: Animal studies have shown this plant causes death in some mammals.

Chrysanthemum *(Chrysanthemum* **species** / **Mum)**
Symptoms: Allergic contact dermatitis, especially among floral trade workers.

Of these species, Chinese doctors use ilex and chrysanthemum flowers, and Western herbalists use peppers and pokeweed. Western doctors use yew to make taxol, a chemotherapeutic agent. All of these are pretty potent herbs and should be used only when prescribed by competent herbalists. Capsicum (pepper) is safe when used as directed for external use as long as you keep it away from your eyes and sensitive skin areas. It will burn your skin or your GI tract if you use too much.

For a more complete list of poisonous outdoor and indoor plants, see the Canadian Poisonous Plants Information System at http://res.agr.ca/brd/poisonpl/title.html.

Common Causes of Food Allergy

Alcohol
Apple
Banana
Beef
Benzoic acid
Carrot
Cheese
Chicken
Chocolate
Coffee
Corn
Cow's milk
Egg
Fish (particularly shellfish)
Grapes
Melon
Monosodium Glutamate (MSG)

Nuts (particularly almonds, cashews,
    peanuts, and walnuts)
Oats
Onion
Orange
Peach
Pork
Potato
Ricc
Rye
Soy
Strawberry
Sugar
Tea
Tomato
Wheat
Yeast

Note: All foods have the capacity to cause an allergic reaction. This list merely includes many of the most common food allergens.

RESOURCE GUIDE

General Help Guide

I know from experience as a patient that after reading about a medicine that can help me, I get very frustrated if I can't find it. On the other hand, I know as an herbalist that it takes skill to figure out exactly what is needed, and that what people want is not always what they need. In this section, I want to make it easier for you to find a good herbalist, good herbal medicines, good herbal companies, and good herbal information.

Contacting the Author

To contact the author's clinic/pharmacy, call **Chrysalis Natural Medicine** (in the United States), at (302) 994-0565, or fax to (302) 995-0653. You can also e-mail Alan at AlanT33@aol.com. If you can't find a local herbalist, feel free to call to set up a telephone conference with Alan or Nai-shing Tillotson. Virtually all medicines and formulas mentioned in this book can be purchased at the Chrysalis pharmacy.

Finding the Right Practitioner

At the current time, it is often difficult to find a well-trained herbalist, as there is a serious shortage. The herbalists who are in practice vary widely in training and expertise. Often, your best bet is to go to your local health food store and ask for a recommendation. Another method is to contact a holistic nurse (see information on holistic nurses on page 543). See whose name comes up frequently and at more than one location. You may also look in your Yellow Pages under "Holistic practitioner" or "Acupuncture." Call the local medical society and ask if there are any medical doctors with holistic credentials. You can use the Internet, but many lists contain just those people who happen to have seen the site and signed up. Many of the best practitioners are too busy to surf the net to sign up. The following lists do actual professional screening or require licensing checks.

To find a professsional herbalist, contact:

American Herbalists Guild
1931 Gaddis Rd.
Canton, GA 30115
Phone: (770) 751-6021
Fax: (770) 751-7472
E-mail: ahgoffice@earthlink.net
Web site: http://www.healthy.net/herbalists/index.html

The American Herbalists Guild was founded in 1989 as a nonprofit educational organization to represent the goals and voices of herbalists. It is the only peer-review organization in the United States for professional herbalists specializing in the medicinal use of plants. AHG membership consists of professionals, general members (including students), and benefactors. Professional members of this organization have been carefully screened and are all highly qualified. Call for a free information package, or visit the web site. They also provide a booklet with herbal medicine educational sources, if you want to further your training.

To find an Ayurvedic practitioner, contact:

American Ayurvedic Association
719 Old Hickory Rd., Suite F
Lancaster, PA 17601
Phone: (877) 598-8830
Fax: (717) 560-5614
E-mail: docdave@ptd.net

The AAA is a network of professionals committed to the practice of Ayurvedic principles for the prevention of disease as well as the promotion of health and longevity. Individuals approved for diplomate status must achieve proficiency in a variety of Ayurvedic topics, procedures, and ethical standards and must meet rigorous criteria of the diplomate programs.

To find a naturopathic physician, contact:

American Association of Naturopathic Physicians
601 Valley St., #105
Seattle, WA 98109
Phone: (206) 298-0125
Fax: (206) 298-0129
Web site: http://www.infinite.org/Naturopathic.Physicians/Welcome.html
Send $5 for list of practitioners, written requests only.

Naturopathic physicians listed by this group are all graduates of one of the naturopathic schools. Many practice in states that do not license, while others have state licenses. The training is the same. All naturopaths are qualified herbalists.

To find a practitioner skilled in TCM herbal medicine, contact one of these organizations:

American Association of Acupuncture and Oriental Medicine
433 Front St.
Catasauqua, PA 18032
Phone: (610) 266-1433
Fax: (610) 264-2768
E-mail: aaom1@aol.com
Web site: http://www.aaom.org

Send $5 for a list of members in any three states. Not all acupuncturists are fully trained in TCM herbal medicine. Acupuncturists who have been trained in Chinese medical universities are all fully qualified in herbal medicine.

Institute of Traditional Medicine
2017 SE Hawthorn
Portland, OR 97214
Phone: (503) 233-4907
Fax: (503) 233-1017
Web site: http://www.europa.com/~itm/

ITM has a practitioner list which screens for qualifications, and requires at least 3 years of professional practice, and ongoing education in herbal medicine.

To find a holistic M.D., contact:

American Holistic Medical Association
6728 Old McLean Village Dr.
McLean, VA 22101
Phone: (703) 556-9728
Fax: (703) 556-8729
Web site: http://www.holisticmedicine.org/

To contact Dr. Mana in Nepal:

Piyusavarsi Ausadhalaya Clinic
Mahaboudha, Kathmandu, Nepal
Phone (from the United States): 011 977 1 223-960
Fax: 011 977 1 428-743 (Be aware of time difference)

E-mail to Dr. Mana's son, Dr. Madhu Bajracharya: nccl@wlink.com.np
Web site: www.geocities.com/hotsprings/sauna/8859

To order medicines from Nepal, it is necessary to be aware of customs regulations and to have a method of monetary transfer. The best way is to use both e-mail and fax. Arrange your order and get the costs by sending an e-mail describing what your medical condition is and what you want. Instructions, costs, and/or follow-up questions will then be given to you on the return e-mail from Dr. Mana's son. Monies can then be sent by Western Union to the Western Union office in Kathmandu (there is only one), addressed to Dr. Madhu Bajracharya. To ensure passage through customs, you must at the same time fax a signed letter/order to Kathmandu affirming the following information:

1. The product was purchased for your personal use.

2. The product is not for commercial distribution, and the amount of product is not excessive (i.e., 3-month supply or less).

3. You must provide the name and address of a licensed physician in the United States responsible for monitoring your treatment with the product.

Your faxed letter will be received in Kathmandu and attached to the package, which will be sent by UPS to your address after receipt of your monies. You will be given a UPS tracking number by e-mail and can track the package in this manner until it arrives. If the order is stopped by customs in the United States, they will contact you to ensure you did request the Ayurvedic medicine. However, if you have sent the proper documentation, there should be no trouble, as it is in accordance with U.S. law.

Herbal Companies Mentioned Frequently

To locate specialty products mentioned in the text, it is best to have your herbalist or natural foods store contact these companies at the number listed, as they are wholesalers, not retailers. You can also contact the companies and ask for a store near you that distributes their products. You can also call the author's clinic/pharmacy at (302) 994-0565.

Frontier Herbs: (800) 669-3275
Frontier Herbs provides high-quality crude herbs and various herbal products.

Herbalist and Alchemist: (908) 689-9020
H & A was founded by herbalist David Winston, AHG, and provides some of the highest-quality herbal tinctures and herbal products available in the United States.

Herb Pharm: (800) 348-4372
Herb Pharm was founded by Ed Smith ("Herbal Ed"). They grow and wildcraft their own herbs and make a superb line of tinctures.

Heritage Store: (800) 862-2923
This company sells ipsab.

Institute of Traditional Medicine: (503) 233-4907
ITM makes a high-quality line of TCM herbal products available to practitioners only. Thus, if you contact them to locate a qualified TCM herbal practitioner, you are also being assured the practitioner is prescribing quality herbal medicines.

N.E.E.D.S. (800) 634-1380
P.O. Box 580
East Syracuse, NY 13057
http://www.needs.com
This company carries PC-SPES, used for prostate cancer.

Phyto-pharmica: (800) 553-2370
Phyto-pharmica makes several products mentioned in the text, including Hyporil, Osteoprime and Thyrosine Complex.

Planetary Formulas: (800) 606-6226
Planetary Formulas makes numerous products combining Western, Chinese, and Ayurvedic herbs, including Myelin Sheath Support, one of the formulas developed by Dr. Tillotson to help patients with multiple sclerosis and other neurological disorders.

Threshold Enterprises: (800) 777-5677

Threshold distributes many of the products mentioned in the text. They distribute periwinkle extract and Source Naturals products.

Vision Pharmaceuticals, Inc.: (800) 325-6789 or (605) 996-3356

Makers of Viva-drops.

Herbal Information on the Net:
Professional, Educational, Commercial, Internet Links, and More

I am going to list only some of my very favorite herbal places here. Once you go onto the Internet at any of these sites, they provide links to a huge number of other sites. Magazines and journals are listed separately.

NATIONAL LIBRARY OF MEDICINE: Your best bet for research:
http://www.ncbi.nlm.nih.gov/entrez/

This is the best place to go for retrieving scientific articles. Go to the web site and follow these directions. Just type in the name of the disease or subject you want in the white box. For example, if you type in the words "herbs, medicinal" or "TCM," you will retrieve articles about herbs or traditional Chinese medicine, respectively. For more complex searches, use (in capitals) the word AND or OR. If you type in "cancer AND herbs, medicinal," you will retrieve most of the articles on herbs that have some relationship to cancer. If you type in "cancer and TCM," you will retrieve articles on Chinese herbs used in cancer studies. You can use an asterisk (*) to wild card searches. For example, I usually use "Ayurved*," because it covers the words "Ayurveda" and "Ayurvedic." Use the clinical filters search box (click button in the blue area on the left) to find clinical double-blinded studies.

Jim Duke, Ph.D.
Father Nature's Farmacy: http://www.ars-grin.gov/duke/
Products: http://www.allherb.com

Formerly chief of the Medicinal Plant Resources Laboratory of the United States Department of Agriculture, Dr. Duke has spent more than 30 years traveling the world in search of medicinal plants, has published some 20 books, and has served as a consultant for the National Institutes of Health on using herbs to fight cancer and AIDS. He lectures extensively and teaches ethnobotany seminars in the Amazon rain forest. To get started, I suggest you purchase his book *The Green Pharmacy*. Father Nature's Farmacy web site is a fantastic way to train yourself on the Internet.

University of California, Santa Barbara Global Medicine Project
9550 Dos Pueblos Canyon Road
Goleta, CA 93117
Phone: (805) 685-0933
Fax: (805) 685-6576
http://www.globalmedicine.ucsb.edu/

The UCSB Global Medicine Project was begun with the intent to focus attention upon the great diversity of healing arts in the world community, and to stimulate opportunities for research and education in these medical traditions. The founders believed that it was time to create a dialogue among these various approaches to healing so that all people can benefit from both ancient and modern medical knowledge. The initial motivation behind the Global Medicine Project was to alleviate unnecessary suffering for people whose own culture's medicine is unable to help them when they are facing a serious illness. The project offers an annual international conference on global medicine, academic courses, library, collaborative research, translation and publication, and a medicinal plant project with a greenhouse, gardens, and a plant tissue culture lab. Dr. Dan Smith directs the educational programs, and Dr. Cynthia Husted directs the Center for the Study of Neurodegenerative Disorders. This project is outstanding in that they are working in a deeply respectful way to simultaneously integrate insights and knowledge from traditional herbal systems with the latest discoveries at the molecular biology level. The Global Medicine Project is designed to help people make more effective health choices by providing access to information about treatment and prevention, practitioners, and healing substances that are most relevant to their personal situation from a global perspective.

Contacts:

Dan K. Smith, Ph.D.
Associate Dean, International Students and Scholars
E-mail: smith-d@sa.ucsb.edu

Cynthia A. Husted, Ph.D.
Director, Center for the Study of Neurodegenerative Disorders
E-mail: husted@mambo.lscf.ucsb.edu

Alternative Health News Online
Frank Grazian, Editor and Publisher
http://www.altmedicine.com/

This is the most helpful alternative, complementary, and preventive health-news page on the Internet. It provides you with news and information that will keep you up to date on the latest happenings in this rapidly growing field.

Planetary Herbs web site of Dr. Michael Tierra, OMD, L.Ac.
http://www.planetherbs.com/

Dr. Tierra is one of the foremost authorities on herbal medicine in North America. He is a licensed acupuncturist in the state of California and has had a clinical practice for 30 years. He is trained in Chinese, Ayurvedic, and Western herbal medicine (as is his wife Lesley Tierra, L.Ac., AHG) and is a world-renowned author of several herb books, including *Way of Herbs, Way of Chinese Herbs, Planetary Herbology,* and *Chinese Traditional Herbal Medicine,* and the herbal education program "East-West Herbology Course." Dr. Tierra is the product formulator for Planetary Formulas and is an internationally recognized authority on the world's herbal traditions.

HealthWorld Online
http://www.healthworld.com/

HealthWorld Online is an Internet health network that integrates both alternative and conventional health information into a synergistic whole. The web site provides resources needed by individuals to make those choices, focusing on the idea of Self-Managed Care™. With access to comprehensive, integrated health and medical information, the *individual* can begin to take action for maintaining and restoring health—and can most appropriately and cost-effectively utilize our society's excellent natural and conventional health care systems. The founders see this as our society's natural transition from the managed care system's "disease management" approach—what one former United States Surgeon General called the "sick-care system"—to a well-care approach built around personal desires and actions. The "means" to achieve this transformation is information—clear, accurate, reliable information that covers the full spectrum of health care disciplines and options. This web site provides, generally at no charge, a full scope of empowering information, in an easily accessible format, to any individual who has a "need to know" and has access to an Internet-linked computer.

United Plant Savers
P. O. Box 98
East Barre, VT 05649
Phone: (802) 479-9825
Fax: (802) 476-3722
E-mail: info@plantsavers.org
http://www.plantsavers.org

United Plant Savers is a nonprofit, grassroots membership organization devoted to protecting and replanting at-risk native medicinal plant species and to raising public awareness of the plight of our medicinal plants. It is stewarded by board members who have been working for decades in the woods and fields to preserve our native medicinal species. UPS is staffed by people with dirt under their fingernails and firsthand knowledge of what it takes to replenish the land.

American Holistic Nurses Association
P. O. Box 2130
Flagstaff, AZ 86003-2130
Phone: (800) 278-AHNA
http://ahna.org/

The goal of the American Holistic Nurses Association is to bring concepts of holism to all areas of nursing practice. AHNA members often say that "Joining the AHNA is like coming home." Since 1981, AHNA members have worked to integrate holistic principles into their own lives, as well as into nursing, education, clinical practice, and nursing research.

Bastyr University
14500 Juanita Drive NE
Bothell, WA 98011
Phone: (206) 823-1300
http://www.njcommunity.org/hslanj/alternat.html

Located 12 miles north of Seattle, Washington, Bastyr University is a fully accredited, nonprofit institution that has been recognized internationally as a pioneer in the study of natural healing. Founded in 1978 by practicing naturopathic physicians, it is the only education and research center in the United States for alternative natural medicine. Bastyr University's curriculum integrates the knowledge of modern science with the wisdom of ancient healing methods and traditional cultures from around the world. Its mission is to serve as a leader in the improvement of the health and well-being of the human community through natural health education, research, and community health care.

Citizens for Health
P. O. Box 2260
Boulder, CO 80306
Phone: (800) 357-2211
http://www.citizens.org

Citizens for Health is a nonprofit, grassroots consumer advocacy group that champions public policies empowering individuals to make informed health choices. The group believes that good health is a right, not a benefit to be determined by government or based on economic and social status. Citizens for Health is a national and international network of thousands of individuals, young and old, at every level of society, who want to exercise their right to make informed choices regarding their health care.

Great Smokies Diagnostic Laboratory
63 Zillacoa Street
Asheville, NC 28801-1074
Phone: (800) 522-4762 or (828) 252-9303
http://www.gsdl.com/

Great Smokies Diagnostic Laboratory (GSDL) provides physicians worldwide with innovative, quality assessments of physiological function. From its first tests of digestive function (the Comprehensive Digestive Stool Analysis) to its more recent developments in the assessment of immune, nutritional, endocrine, and metabolic function, the lab consistently gets high marks for evaluations of physiological function. Have your physician order their extremely informative testing guide.

HealthComm / Dr. Jeffery Bland's Institute for Functional Medicine
P. O. Box 1729
Gig Harbor, WA 98335

Phone: (206) 851-3943
http://www.healthcomm.com/
http://www.fxmed.com/

HealthComm is a private nonprofit organization that promotes advanced research and education into a diverse range of topics related to Functional Medicine. It offers a unique array of educational services aimed at helping health care professionals better understand and treat chronic illness. Here you can find information on the work of Dr. Jeffery Bland, Ph.D. I highly recommend you or your health care providers subscribe to *Functional Medicine Update,* the monthly taped discussion of the latest research in the field.

SimpleCare
Medical Arts Center
4033 Talbot Road South, Suite 570
Renton, WA 98055
Phone: (888)-469-1112
Fax: (425)-254-1111
E-mail: membership@simplecare.com
http://www.simplecare.com

SimpleCare is a nonprofit program of the American Association of Patients and Providers. They provide an alternative to the sick insurance system in the United States, which basically makes patients beg for care, and doctors beg for money, usually unsuccessfully. I highly recommend you visit their web site or call them for information.

National College of Naturopathic Medicine
11231 SE Market Street
Portland, OR 97216
Phone: (503) 499-4343
E-mail: pro-services@ncnm.edu
http://www.ncnm.edu/

Founded in 1956, the National College of Naturopathic Medicine is the oldest accredited school of natural medicine in North America. As such, the college has been at the center of the profession, preserving and extending the legacy of naturopathic medicine. The profession has experienced a resurgence in the past two decades, as a health-conscious public has sought alternatives to conventional medicine.

The University of Bridgeport, College of Naturopathic Medicine
221 University Avenue
Bridgeport, CT 06601
Phone: (203) 576-4109
http://www.bridgeport.edu/

This is another recent addition to the growing number of colleges providing naturopathic education.

Wild Rose College of Natural Healing

1228 Kensington Road, NW, #400
Calgary, Alberta, Canada T2N 4P9
Phone: (403) 270-0936
Fax: (403) 283-0799
Toll-free: (888) WLD-ROSE (953-7673)
E-mail: coordinators@wrc.net
http://www.wrc.net/

Wild Rose College, established in 1975, offers diploma programs in Master Herbology and Wholistic Therapy, courses available year-round by correspondence, and evening and weekend classes September to June in Calgary.

National Center for Complementary and Alternative Medicine

P. O. Box 8218
Silver Spring, MD 20907-8218
Toll-free: (888) 644-6226
TTY/TDY (hearing impaired): (888) 644-6226 (same number)
http://nccam.nih.gov/

The NCCAM is located on the NIH campus in Bethesda, Maryland. It was established, by congressional mandate, to "facilitate the evaluation of alternative medical treatment modalities" to determine their effectiveness. The mandate also provides for a public information clearinghouse and a research training program. The NCCAM *does not* serve as a referral agency for various alternative medical treatments or individual practitioners. The primary activity of the NCCAM is to facilitate and conduct research. Written requests for routine information will be processed within 2 to 3 business days of receipt.

American Botanical Council (ABC)

P. O. Box 144345
Austin, TX 78714-4345
Phone: (512) 926-4900
For general information, E-mail: abc@herbalgram.org
http://www.herbalgram.org/

One of the nation's leading repositories of information on herbalism, the ABC is a nonprofit educational organization. The organization distributes scientific information and research findings on beneficial herbs and plants and encourages awareness of their potential in healing and medicine. The ABC is also the organization entrusted with the dissemination of the English translation of Germany's Commission E Monographs.

American Herbal Pharmacopoeia
Box 5159
Santa Cruz, CA 95063
Phone: (831) 461-6317
Fax: (831) 475-6219
E-mail: herbal@got.net
http://www.herbal-ahp.org/

It is the mission of the American Herbal Pharmacopoeia™ to disseminate authoritative and comprehensive information to the herbal industry, pharmacists, health care practitioners, educational institutions, regulatory agencies, retailers, and the general public through quality-control standards for the manufacture of herbal supplements and botanical medicines focused on a high degree of safety and effectiveness; to promote internal harmonization in the development of quality-control standards for herbal supplements and botanical medicines; and generally to encourage, investigate, direct, undertake, and perform all aspects and functions essential to the furtherance of the safe and effective use of herbal supplements and botanical medicines.

Institute for the Study of Human Knowledge (ISHK)
Box 176
Los Altos, CA 94023
Phone: (650) 948-9428
Fax: (650) 948-2687
E-mail: ishkbks@aol.com
http://www.ishkbooks.com/index.html

The Institute for the Study of Human Knowledge (ISHK) is an educational institution dedicated to publicizing useful research on the mind. ISHK Book Service publishes and distributes books, translations, and tapes on traditional psychology. With directors and associates who include educators, brain scientists, biologists, ecologists, physicians, sociologists, novelists, historians, and others, ISHK focuses on communicating new insights that come from a broad base of cutting-edge information, especially information overlooked by standard resources. For example, in 1975, research on the link between the mind and disease was conclusive, yet unrecognized in the medical profession and popular press. ISHK launched the Healing Brain Seminars, which were attended by over 10,000 doctors, nurses, and health professionals. The ISHK Book Service supported the publication and distribution of books such as *Healthy Pleasures* and *The Psychology of Consciousness*. Tapes on stress management and depression were commissioned from recognized experts. ISHK continues this work through *Mental Medicine Update*, Dr. David Sobel's newsletter. Today, in part due to ISHK, the link between the mind and health is widely acknowledged.

Other Web Sites of Interest

American Association of Naturopaths Homepage
www.naturopathic.org/welcome.html

IBIS (Integrative Medical Arts)
http://www.integrativemedicalarts.com/Interactions.html

Bastyr University Library
www.bastyr.edu/library

The Food Allergy Network
http://www.foodallergy.org/

CAM Courses Taught at Medical Schools Guide
http://cpmcnet.columbia.edu/dept/rosenthal

Enzymatic Therapy
www.enzy.com

Frontier Herbs
www.frontiercoop.com

Herbal Bookworm
www.teleport.com/~jonno

Herbal Hall
www.herb.com/herbal.html

HerbNet
www.herbnet.com

Herb Research Foundation
www.herbs.org

Henriette Kreiss Homepage
www.sunsite.unc.edu/herbmed

Howie Brounstein's Homepage
www.teleport.com/~howieb/howie.html

Lloyd Library and Museum
www.libraries.uc.edu/lloyd

National Nutritional Foods Association
www.nnfa.org

Rachel's Environment & Health Weekly
www.envirolink.org/pubs/rachel/contents.html

Publications

Robyn's Recommended Reading

Robyn Klein, AHG, herbal medicine instructor at the Sweetgrass School of Herbalism in Montana, publishes *Robyn's Recommended Reading,* a newsletter that reviews all sorts of publications related to herbal medicine. It is an excellent way to filter out the good from the bad and get access to rare and unusual resources. You can write or visit the web site.

Robyn's Recommended Reading
1627 W. Main
Suite 116
Bozeman, MT 59715
Web site: http://www.avicom.net/~rrr/journals.html

Subscription (4 issues): $15/year (U.S.)
         $20/year, Canada and overseas (U.S. funds only)
         ($5 for sample of current issue)

Note: Publications reviewed by Robyn will have her comments.

Alternatives Newsletter
Mountain Home Publishing
1201 Seven Locks Road
Rockville, ME 20854
Phone: (800) 219-8591

This newsletter offers very interesting and valuable information on natural medicine treatments from around the world.

American Herb Association Quarterly
P. O. Box 1673
Nevada City, CA 95959

Subscriptions (4 issues): $20/year, regular members (U.S.)
         $35/year, supporting members (U.S.)
         $24/year, Canadian members
         $28/year, foreign members
         (all fees are U.S. funds only)

The AHA is an association of medical herbalists. Membership is open to anyone interested in herbs. The goals of the AHA are to promote the understanding, acceptance, and ecological use of herbs. Research for the *AHA Quarterly* is done primarily at the University of California Medical Library in San Francisco. The AHA reviews over 60 medical journals, 40 international herb-related newsletters/magazines, and 28 major magazines and newspapers to bring its readers the latest herb information. Regular features include editorials, herbal views, herb reports, news and network, legal status, international news, book reviews, herbal clippings, calendar, classifieds, and advertisements. The average issue length is 20 pages in an 8x11-inch format.

Robyn says: There are dozens of herb newsletters, but this is the very best of them. The AHA has been publishing it since 1981, and it is still going strong. This is a great publication to start with if you are new to herbalism, and one which professional herbalists read eagerly.

Australian Journal of Medical Herbalism

National Herbalists Association of Australia
Office Manager
P. O. Box 61
Broadway, Australia 2007
E-mail: nhaa@nhaa.org.au

Subscription: $165/year, practitioners
$45/year, students
$75/year, companion

Note: These fees do not include additional required joining fee.

The *Australian Journal of Medical Herbalism* is a quarterly publication of the National Herbalists Association of Australia. This peer-reviewed journal publishes material concerning all aspects of medical herbalism, including the philosophy, phytochemistry, pharmacology, and clinical applications of medicinal plants. Regular features include Australian medicinal plant reviews, MEDPLANT abstracts, case studies, book reviews, calendar of events, and conference reports. The average issue length is 30–35 pages in a 7x10-inch format.

Robyn says: This journal contains lots of case histories, in-depth articles, and comments on recent research. Excellent for clinicians and professional herbalists.

The European Journal of Herbal Medicine (EJHM)

National Institute of Medical Herbalists
56 Longbrook Street
Exeter
Devon EX4 6AH, United Kingdom

Subscription (3 issues): £19.50/year (U.K.)
£29.50/year (Overseas)

The *EJHM* is the journal of the National Institute of Medical Herbalists (NIMH). The articles are written by NIMH members and other great herbalists. Regular features include editorials, letters, herbal world, interviews, materia medica, clinical notes, therapy, traditions, and book reviews. Average issue length is 50 pages in an 8x11-inch format.

Robyn says: An excellent professional journal.

HerbalGram
American Botanical Council
P. O. Box 201660
Austin, TX 78720
Phone: (512) 331-8868
Fax: (512) 331-1924
Web site: www.2.outer.net/herbalgram/abcmission.html
www.herbalgram.org

Subscription: $25/year (U.S.)
                $45/2 years (U.S.)
                $60/3 years (U.S.)
                (Foreign subscribers add $10 per year.)

HerbalGram is the journal of the American Botanical Council and the Herb Research Foundation. It is a full-color magazine offering an overview of herb research, herb market trends, herb news, and book reviews. The mail-order book department offers an excellent selection of books on topics such as pharmacognosy, herbs, herbal history, and natural products science. A watchdog of the media, the staff at *HerbalGram* is intimately involved in the politics of the use of herbs in the United States. It is a great resource for updates on the legislative world of herbs and the academic discipline of pharmacognosy. Regular features include editorials, news features, herb blurbs, media issues, herb monographs, research reviews, legal and regulatory news, conference reports, market reports, book reviews, letters, calendar, and classifieds. Average issue length is 80 pages in an 8x11-inch format.

Robyn says: A very informative publication for the general public and all professionals. Focus is on pharmacognosy and Western scientific views of herbalism.

Horizon Herbs Seed Catalog
P. O. Box 69
Williams, OR 97544
Phone: (541) 846-6704
Fax: (541) 846-6233
E-mail: herbseed@chatlink.com

Horizon Herbs is the place to get seeds for medicinal plants. Run by master medicine maker and herb grower Richo Cech, this company puts out a great catalog loaded with information on how to properly grow your herbs. Call or e-mail and get the catalog. You can also call and get Richo's new book *Making Plant Medicine*.

International Journal of Pharmacognosy (IJP)
Swets & Zeitlinger Publishers
P. O. Box 613
Royersford, PA 19468
Phone: (800) 447-9387
E-mail: pub@swets.nl

Subscription: $99/year for members of American Society of Pharmacognosy
$360/ycar for nonmembers

The purpose of *IJP* is to advance our knowledge and understanding of the efficacy and safety of natural product drugs.
For abstracts of articles, see: www.sun.swets.nl/sps/journals/ijp.html

Robyn says: An academic journal that publishes scientific research on natural products.

Journal of Ethnopharmacology
Elsevier Scicnce
Customer Support Department
P. O. Box 945
New York, NY 10159-0945
Web site: www.elsevier.nl/inca/publications/store/5/0/6/3/5

Subscription (12 issues): $1191

The *Journal of Ethnopharmacology* publishes original articles concerned with the observation and experimental investigation of the biological activities of plant and animal substances used in the traditional medicine of past and present cultures. An abstract section of about 50 abstracts per volume is published at the end of the journal on a regular basis, covering the most recent literature in the field. The journal's audience includes ethnopharmacologists, medical chemists, pharmacologists, toxicologists, anthropologists, and botanists.

Robyn says: For herbalists, this is one of the most valuable scientific journals relating to the medicinal use of plants. The table of contents for some back issues is available at their web site.

Medical Herbalism
P. O. Box 20512
Boulder, CO 80308
Phone: (303) 541-9552
Web site: www.medherb.com

Subscription: $36/year or $60/2 years (U.S.)
$39/year or $65/2 years (Canada)
$45/year or $80/2 years (Overseas)
$25/year, students (with photocopy of student I.D.)

Medical Herbalism is a newsletter for the clinical practitioner. Well-known herbal author and practitioner Paul Bergner researches and writes about herbs and their clinical use. He currently teaches (and directs the clinical education program) at the Rocky Mountain Center for Botanical Studies in Boulder, Colorado. He offers case studies from naturopathic physicians and licensed herbalists. Regular features include editorials, case histories, clinical comments, herb monographs, classifieds, and display ads. Average issue length is 24 pages in an 8x11-inch format.

Robyn says: A very informative quarterly offering case histories and lengthy herb articles for professional herbalists. The Medical Herbalism web site has very useful links.

The Modern Phytotherapist
Professional Health Products, Inc.
P. O. Box 80085
Portland, OR 97280
Phone: (800) 952-2219
OR
MediHerb Pty., Ltd.
P. O. Box 713
Warwick, Queensland, 4370

Subscription (3 issues): $40/year

Regular features include editorials, articles on herbal subjects, case histories, herbal monographs, and book reviews. Average issue length is 28 pages in an 8x11-inch format.

Robyn says: An excellent publication for clinicians and herbalists. Articles written mostly by Australian clinical herbalists. With Kerry Bone at the helm, this publication never ceases to impress me with its very useful information and attention to current issues in herbalism.

Nutrition Science News
New Hope Communications, Inc.
1301 Spruce Street
Boulder, CO 80302
Phone: (303) 939-8440
Web site: www.nutritionsciencenews.com

Subscription (12 issues): $36/year (U.S.)
$6 (+$3 s&h)/single copy (U.S.)
(Inquire about international rates.)

Nutrition Science News is a comprehensive and definitive information source for businesses interested in improving the quality of health and health care through the use of food and supplements. *Nutrition Science News* supports the growth of business with news, trends, product information, and scientifically validated nutrition research vital to successful industry development. Regular features include main articles, news, science briefs, industry analysis, new products, and display ads. Average issue length is 50 pages in an 8x11-inch format.

Robyn says: Though focused on the industry, I find many of the articles very informative and useful. Insights on the use of supplements, foods, and herbs. Sometimes the articles are written by seasoned freelance writers, and sometimes by really experienced clinicians and herbalists. A very good reference source. New Hope also publishes the Natural Foods Merchandiser, *which covers herbal politics as well as herbal products.*

The Review of Natural Products
Facts and Comparisons
111 West Port Plaza
Suite 300
St. Louis, MO 63146
Phone: (314) 878-2515

Subscription: $65/year

This publication is made up of short monographs on various medicinal plants and substances. These monographs compile the latest research on the subject.

Regular features include separate monographs on herbs and natural products including the following information: scientific names, common names, botany, history, chemistry, pharmacology, toxicology, summary, patient information, uses, side effects, and literature citations. Average issue length is 10–15 pages in an 8x11-inch format.

Robyn says: Informative monographs on herbs, dietary supplements, and natural products from the Western scientific viewpoint.

Townsend Letter for Doctors & Patients
The Examiner of Medical Alternatives
911 Tyler Street
Port Townsend, WA 98368
Phone: (360) 385-6021
Web site: www.tldp.com

Subscription (10 issues): $49/year
$88/2 years
$32/year, students (with copy of valid student I.D.)
(Inquire for international rates.)

Regular features include editorials, in the news, special features, letters to the editor, and book reviews. Average issue length is 150 pages in an 8x11-inch format.

Robyn says: This publication is chock-full of articles covering the whole range of alternative medicine subjects. Most authors are M.D.'s, N.D.'s, and Ph.D.'s. Some articles are written by seasoned freelance writers. I haven't found it to cover herbs very often, though there are a few really good articles on phytotherapy by N.D.'s now and then. A good place to learn about Western medicine treatment and its critics.

The Mind/Body Health Newsletter
Phone: (800) 222-4745

Breakthrough research and empowering techniques for the mental health care field. Edited by David Sobel, M.D., and Robert Ornstein, Ph.D.

Dr. Jonathan Wright's Nutrition & Healing
c/o Publishers Mgmt. Corp.
Box 84909
Phoenix, AZ 85071
Phone: (800) 528-0559 or (602) 252-4477
Fax: (602) 943-2362

This newsletter is the work of Drs. Jonathan Wright, M.D., and Alan Gaby, M.D., two leaders in the field of nutritional medicine. Each issue profiles specific health conditions and reports research findings. Each issue also contains a fabulous herbal article by herbalist and researcher Kerry Bone, director of Medi-Herb, an Australian leader in the field of herbal medicine.

Quality Manufacturers

Following is a list of herbal manufacturers who have gained a reputation in industry publications for following safe manufacturing practices. This list includes many of the market leaders but is far from complete. New companies are coming along every day. Absence from the list does not in any way imply lack of quality control in a particular company.

American Biologics
Arise & Shine Herbal Products
Arizona Natural Products
Arkopharma
Arrowhead Mills
Ayush Herbs
Barlean's Organic Oils
Barth's Nutra Products
Bayer Corporation
Bio-Botanica Inc.
Biodynamax
Bioforce of America Ltd.
Botanical Laboratories
Botanical Products Inc.
Botanicals International
Burroughs Wellcome
Celestial Seasonings, Inc.
Combe Inc.
Complementary Formulations
Country Life
Draco Natural Products
Dynapro International Inc.
East Earth Herb Inc.
Eclectic Institute Inc.
Eli Lilly and Company
Ellon USA Inc.
Energy Plus
Enrich International
Enzymatic Therapy
F & F Laboratories
Flag Fork Herb Farm
Flora Laboratories Inc.
Fmali Herb Company
Freeda Vitamins Inc.

Frontier Cooperative Herbs
Fujisawa USA
Futurebiotics
Gaia Herbs
General Nutrition Companies Inc.
Good 'N' Natural
Hall Laboratories
Health from the Sun
Herbalife International Inc.
Herbalist & Alchemist
Herb Pharm, Inc.
Herbs Etc.
Hobe Laboratories Inc.
Hsu's Ginseng Enterprises
IL Hwa American Corporation
Imperial Elixir
Irwin Naturals
Jarrow Formulas
J. R. Carlson Laboratories
Kroeger Herb Products
Kwai
Lederle Consumer Health Products
Leiner Health Products
Luyties Pharmacal
Madis Botanicals Inc.
Madys Co. Inc.
Maharishi Ayur-Ved
Martek
Matrix Health Products
MediHerb Pty. Ltd.
Michael's Health Products
Mon Tong
Modern Products Inc.
Montana Naturals International Inc.

Murdock Madaus Schwabe
Musashi North America
Natrol Inc.
Nat-Trop
Naturade Products Inc.
Naturally Vitamin Supplements Inc.
Nature Care Products Co.
Naturemost Laboratories Inc.
Nature's Answer
Nature's Apothecary
Nature Bounty Inc.
Nature's Herbs
Nature's Life
Nature's Plus Company
Nature's Pride
Nature's Secret
Nature's Sunshine Products Inc.
Nature's Way
New Vistas Inc.
NOW
Nutrition for Life
Old Mill Herb Company
Performance Labs Inc.
Peruvian Rainforest Botanicals
Philips Nutritionals
Phyto-Pharmica
Pines International
Planetary Formulas
Powerfood Inc.
Progenix Corporation
Pro-Liquitech
Pure-Gar/Quintessence

Quantum
Rainbow Light
Red Bull North America Inc.
Sabinsa
St. John's Herb Garden Inc.
San Francisco Herb & Natural Food Company
Schiff Products
Scientific Botanicals
Seven Forests
Silver Sage
Solaray Inc.
Solgar Vitamin and Herb Company Inc.
Spectrum Naturals
Spring Wind Herb Company
Standard Homeopathic Company
SuperNutrition Research Inc.
Thompson Nutritional Products
Threshold
Trace Minerals Research
Tree of Life
Twin Laboratories
Vale Enterprises Inc.
Vermont Ginseng Products Ltd.
Vincent Trading Company
Vitamin Specialties Company
Wakunaga of America Co. Ltd.
Whole Herb Company
World Organics Corporation
Yellow Emperor Inc.
Yogi Botanicals
Zand Herbal Formulas

American Association of Poison Control Centers

If you are having a serious adverse reaction to an herbal medication, contact your closest poison control center.

ALABAMA

Alabama Poison Center
Tuscaloosa, AL
(205) 345-0600

Regional Poison Control Center
The Children's Hospital of Alabama
Birmingham, AL
(205) 939-9201

ARIZONA

University of Arizona PCC
Arizona Poison and Drug Information
  Center
Tucson, AZ
(602) 626-6016

Samaritan Regional Poison Center
Good Samaritan Regional Medical Center
Phoenix, AZ
(602) 253-3334

CALIFORNIA

Central California Regional Poison Control
  Center
Valley Children's Hospital
Fresno, CA
(209) 445-1222

San Diego Regional Poison Center
UCSD Medical Center
San Diego, CA
(619) 543-6000

San Francisco Bay Area Regional Poison
  Control Center
San Francisco General Hospital
San Francisco, CA
(800) 523-2222

Santa Clara Valley Regional Poison Center
San Jose, CA
(408) 885-6000

University of California, Davis Medical
  Center
Regional Poison Control Center
Sacramento, CA
(916) 734-3692

COLORADO

Rocky Mountain Poison and Drug Center
Denver, CO
(303) 629-1123

DISTRICT OF COLUMBIA

National Capital Poison Center
Washington, DC
(202) 625-3333

FLORIDA

Florida Poison Information Center—
  Jacksonville
Jacksonville, FL
(904) 549-4480

The Florida Poison Information Center
   and Toxicology Resource Center
Tampa, FL
(813) 253-4444

GEORGIA

Georgia Poison Center
Atlanta, GA
(404) 616-9000

INDIANA

Indiana Poison Center
Indianapolis, IN
(317) 929-2323

KENTUCKY

Kentucky Regional Poison Center
   of Kosair Children's Hospital
Louisville, KY
(502) 629-7275

MARYLAND

University of Maryland Poison Center
Baltimore, MD
(410) 528-7701

MASSACHUSETTS

Massachusetts Poison Control System
Boston, MA
(617) 232-2120

MICHIGAN

Poison Control Center
Detroit, MI
(313) 745-5711

MINNESOTA

Hennepin Regional Poison Center
Minneapolis, MN
(612) 347-3141

Minnesota Regional Poison Center
St. Paul, MN
(612) 221-2113

MISSOURI

Cardinal Glennon Children's Hospital
   Regional Poison Center
St. Louis, MO
(314) 772-5200

NEBRASKA

The Poison Center
Omaha, NE
(402) 390-5555

NEW JERSEY

New Jersey Poison Information and
   Education System
Newark, NJ
(800) 962-1253

NEW MEXICO

New Mexico Poison and Drug Information
   Center
Albuquerque, NM
(505) 843-2551

NEW YORK

Hudson Valley Regional Poison Center
North Tarrytown, NY
(914) 366-3030

Long Island Regional Poison Control
  Center
Mineola, NY
(516) 542-2323

New York City Poison Control Center
New York, NY
(212) 340-4494

NORTH CAROLINA

Carolinas Poison Center
Charlotte, NC
(704) 355-4000

OHIO

Central Ohio Poison Center
Columbus, OH
(614) 228-1323

Cincinnati Drug & Poison Information
  Center and Regional Poison Control
  System
Cincinnati, OH
(513) 558-5111

OREGON

Oregon Poison Center
Portland, OR
(503) 494-8968

PENNSYLVANIA

Central Pennsylvania Poison Center
Hershey, PA
(800) 521-6110

The Poison Control Center serving the
  greater Philadelphia metropolitan area
Philadelphia, PA
(215) 386-2100

Pittsburgh Poison Center
Pittsburgh, PA
(412) 681-6669

RHODE ISLAND

Rhode Island Poison Center
Providence, RI
(401) 277-5727

TEXAS

North Texas Poison Center
Dallas, TX
(214) 590-5000

Southeast Texas Poison Center
Galveston, TX
(409) 765-1420
(713) 654-1701

UTAH

Utah Poison Control Center
Salt Lake City, UT
(801) 581-2151

VIRGINIA

Blue Ridge Poison Center
Charlottesville, VA
(804) 924-5543

WEST VIRGINIA

West Virginia Poison Center
Charleston, WV
(304) 348-4211

REFERENCE NOTE

More than 1,600 books, scientific abstracts, and articles were reviewed during the writing of this book. Selected references appear throughout the book under the heading "Research Highlights."

For all other references, please e-mail the author at: *AT33@aol. com*.

SPECIAL RESOURCE SECTION

HERBS

Botanical Herbs

LAREX, Inc.
(800) 386-5300
www.larex.com

ClearTrac™AG
This product is known as Larch Arabinogalactan (AG), a naturally occurring prebiotic fiber extracted from native larch trees that grow in abundance in the U.S. It uses a patented water-based, solvent-free manufacturing process. ClearTrac™AG has been used to stimulate the growth of beneficial gastrointestinal micro flora, specifically, Lactobacilli acidophilus and Bifidobacteria, in addition to being a great source of dietary fiber. ClearTrac™AG enhances a healthy colon by acting as a food source for the growth of friendly bacteria Bifidobactyeria and Lactobacilli and decrease potentially harmful colon bacteria such as *E.coli* and salmonella.

Andrographis Paniculata

Swedish Herbal Institute
1-800-744-9444
www.adaptogen.com

Kan Jang®
Scandinavia's best-selling cold and flu tablet. Each tablet contains 300mg of standardized andrographis paniculata (root) extract. Available in health food stores.

Swedish Flower Pollen

Graminex, L.L.C.
1-877-472-6469
www.graminex.com

Cernilton®
Long-term clinical research supports the benefits of Cernilton®, which contains Cernitin™ flower pollen extract, in promoting healthy prostate function. Studies show a reduction in prostate volume, residual urine volume, and the improvement of voiding difficulties. Other symptoms of BPH and prostatitis may be reduced. Cernitin™ flower pollen extract may improve the conditions of liver function, smooth muscle function and immune system function. The chemical analysis of Cernitin™ flower pollen extract shows that it contains most of the vitamins, minerals, amino acids and enzymes the body needs in micro nutrient quantities. It is a standardized, virtually allergen-free whole extract of selected pollen. Four tablets contain 250mg of pollen extract.

Herbal Combinations

Combining herbs can sometimes be extremely effective and even dramatic. A marvelous example is PC SPES.

PC SPES

In the late 1990s a group of doctors developed and began to test an herbal product called PC-SPES (meaning prostate cancer hope). It contains saw palmetto berry along with a group of Chinese herbs. This product is extraordinarily effective, and drops PSA levels close to zero in the majority of patients with minimal side effects. Slowing the disease in this manner buys lots of precious time.

An herbal combination that has been very effective in treating prostate cancer and dramatically reducing PSA levels, it also doesn't have as many side effects as with hormonal drugs. Available through the following company:

BotanicLab™
1-800-242-5555
www.botaniclab.com

BotanicLab™ is the primary distributor of PC SPES, which has had encouraging results in clinical trials involving prostate cancer patients at well-respected university research centers, including UCSF Medical Center, Columbia-Presbyterian Medical Center, the Cancer Institute of New Jersey, and the University of Kentucky. In addition, several *in vivo* and *in vitro* studies have been conducted at various well-known research laboratories and published in medical journals. For information about PC SPES, contact BotanicLab™ through their toll-free phone number or visit them on their web site.

Mail Order for Herbs

N.E.E.D.S.
1-(800) 634-1380
www.needs.com

If you can't find the herbal supplement you are looking for in your local health food store, try calling N.E.E.D.S. They carry virtually all of the top herbal lines and will supply a catalog upon request.

Living Tree Community Foods
1-800-260-5534
www.livingtreecommunity.com

Organically grown nuts and nut butters, including almonds (many varieties), macadamia nuts, pine nuts, pumpkin seeds, sunflower seeds, walnut quarters, raw almond butter, and raw cashew butter. They refrigerate their nuts, seeds and nut butters until the day they are shipped.

Raw Vermont Honey
Unfiltered and unheated. A taste of the wild, fruity and ebullient.

Poultry

Sheltons Poultry, Inc.
1-800-541-1844

Free-range chicken and turkey with no added antibiotics. Available in natural foods stores. Noted health expert, Andrew Weil, M.D., cautions people to avoid eating poultry and meat with added antibiotics, which the CDC has linked to drug-resistant strains of disease-causing bacteria.

Seafood

Available from the following companies:

Capilano Pacific
1-877-391-WILD (9453)
www.capilanopacific.com

Wildfish™

This company is a wonderful source for wild-caught salmon. Most of the salmon available in restaurants and stores are farm-raised. Usually this means medications such as antibiotics have been added to the feed, as well as synthetic coloring. Wild-caught salmon has none of these problems and a high level of omega-3 fatty acids and much less fat than farm-raised salmon. It tastes better as well. Also available: halibut, tuna and lox without any added chemicals.

Teas (Green)

Try switching from coffee to green tea and enjoy the benefits of antioxidants and less caffeine. Actually there is an amino acid in green tea (Camellia sinensis) that balances caffeine's effects and delivers a sense of relaxation.

Available from the following companies:

Great Eastern Sun
1-800-334-5809
www.great-eastern-sun.com

Haiku® Organic Japanese Teas

Organic Original Sencha Green Tea: the finest grade of green leaf tea available, made from the tender young leaves of selected tea bushes, cut at the peak of their flavor, rolled, steamed, and briefly dried. Contains 100% Nagata Japanese Organic Sencha Green Tea Leaves and Buds. Available in tea bags and bulk.

Organic Original Hojicha Roasted Green Tea: lower in caffeine than Sencha, Hojicha has a subtle smoky and rich flavor that is quite different from that of Sencha. Contains 100% Nagata Japanese Organic Hojicha Roasted Green Tea Leaves and Stems. Available in tea bags and bulk.

Great Eastern Sun carries a full line of delicious organic classic teas and flavored tea blends including:

Organic Ceylon Highland; Nothing but 100% famed mountain-grown Sri Lankan leaf from the Thotulagalla and Green Fields Organic Estates goes into this smooth, full flavored tea. Its rich yet delicate taste can be enjoyed any time of day (especially in the morning!) and is delicious hot or iced. Ingredients: Organic Ceylon Black Tea.

Organic Darjeeling Thunder Bolt: Grown exclusively for One World® on the Makaibari Organic Estate on the pristine slopes of the Himalayan Mountains of northern India, this refined tea has a flavor so unique it has been called "the champagne of teas." Fragrant aroma and rich taste make it the finest of India's unblended teas.

Organic Zanzibar Orange Spice: Meticulously formulated, One World®'s Organic Orange Spice is a superb combination of organic cut black teas flavored with organic Orange Peel, Organic Cloves, Organic Cinnamon and Organic Orange Oil.

Triple Leaf Tea, Inc.
1-800-552-7448
www.tripleleaf-tea.com
http://www.tripleleaf-tea.com
maryanne@tripleleaf-tea.com

Effective, authentic, traditional Chinese green, naturally decaffeinated green, medicinal and diet teas, made with authentic Chinese herbs and traditional herbal formulas, packaged in convenient tea bag form. All teas are GMO-free.

Triple Leaf Tea's Decaf Green Tea and decaf green tea blends use a natural solvent-free carbon dioxide decaffeination process that researchers have found maintains almost all of green tea's beneficial antioxidants, including EGCG, while leaving no chemical residue. Two other decaffeination methods use either a chemical solvent, ethyl acetate, which researchers have found to remove much of the antioxidants, or water, which also is likely to lose the antioxidants, since they are extremely water-soluble.

If you drink a lot of green tea and don't want the caffeine this is the ideal tea to use.

Jasmine Green Tea
Made from jasmine flowers combined with green tea, creating a delicious aromatic tea. Jasmine was traditionally used for its calming, relaxing and warming properties, for brightening the mood and as a soothing digestive tea.

100% Ginger Root Tea is a delicious and spicy tea bag that is a terrific boost during the day. Also available: 100% American Ginseng Root Tea, to support balance, health and well-being.

NATURAL DETOXIFICATION AND CLEANSING

When taking charge of your health, it is very important to avoid toxins in the food you eat, the water you drink, the air you breathe, and in virtually every product you use, from shampoos and toothpaste to cleansers and cosmetics. The companies listed here are of the highest quality. If you cannot find their products at your local health food store, please contact these companies directly for the store nearest you.

Dental Products

Woodstock Natural Products, Inc.
The Natural Dentist™
1-800-615-6895

Toothpaste: mint, cinnamon and fluoride-free mint
Mouth rinse: mint, cinnamon, cherry-flavored

There is a holistic connection between the health of your teeth and gums and your whole body. This is especially true for diabetics, who need to be vigilant about their teeth and gums because they have a tendency to develop periodontal disease. Woodstock Natural Products are formulated by a holistic dentist and contain soothing and healing herbs, with no alcohol, sugar, or harsh chemicals. These products have been clinically proven to kill germs that cause gum disease. In a study published in the *Journal of Clinical Dentistry* in 1998, researchers at the New York University College of Dentistry in New York City, found that The Natural Dentist toothpaste removed plaque more effectively than the leading commercial brand. The same group also found that The Natural Dentist mouth rinse killed more germs than the leading commercial brand.

Desert Essence®
1-888-476-8647
www.desertessence.com

Oral Care Collection
A complete line of antiseptic and cleansing oral care products using tea tree oil for deep cleaning and disinfecting of teeth and gums. All products are animal and eco-friendly and made without artificial colors, sweeteners or harsh abrasives.

Tea Tree Oil Dental Floss: creates a germ-free mouth and cleans between teeth
Tea Tree Oil Dental Tape: provides same benefits as floss with a wider ribbon
Tea Tree Oil Dental Pics: cleans between teeth with antiseptic power
Tea Tree Oil Breath Freshener: contains natural and organic essential oils

Mail Order for Environmental Products

N.E.E.D.S
1-800-634-1380
www.needs.com

An excellent mail order company for top-of-the-line environmental products. They also carry a full line of supplements.

Aireox Air Purifier (Model 45)
Removes mold spores, pollen dust, formaldehyde, and more.

Aireox Car Air Purifier (Model 22)
A very effective purifier for your car that will eliminate toxins while you're driving.

Allens Naturally
A full line of toxin-free household cleansers, including dishwashing and laundry detergents and all-purpose cleaners.

Water Filters
N.E.E.D.S. carries a variety of high-quality water filters

Elite Shower Filter and Massager
For removing chlorine, heavy metals and bacteria.

Far Infrared Therapy Sauna for Detoxification

High Tech Health
1-800-794-5355
www.hightechhealth.com

Thermal Life® Far Infrared Therapy Sauna
This highly effective low-temperature sauna (100F to 130F) employs heaters that emit rays at a special wavelength designed to push heavy metal toxins, including mercury and other toxins, out of the body through the sweat glands. There have been reports of high mercury levels coming down substantially—some cases have become mercury-free in 90 days. More than 300 doctors in the U.S. are now providing this therapy for their patients. The best part of this sauna is its ease of use. It requires no pre-heating, doesn't need any water, and it can be moved anywhere in the home or apartment. Unit sizes available for 1-5 persons.

Environmental Physician

Dr. Sherry Rogers is a pre-eminent authority in environmental medicine and specializes in finding the environmental causative factors of disease. She is available for personal phone consultations, (315) 488-2856. Her most recent book, *No More Heartburn,* is a must read for all patients with colon problems. Get this and her other dozen books and referenced monthly subscription newsletter (free sample available) from 1-800-846-6687.

Index